Intrinsically Motivated Learning in Natural and Artificial Systems

Gianluca Baldassarre • Marco Mirolli
Editors

Intrinsically Motivated Learning in Natural and Artificial Systems

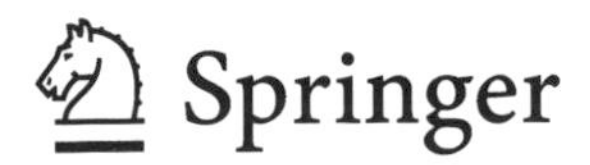

Editors
Gianluca Baldassarre
Marco Mirolli
Istituto di Scienze e Tecnologie
della Cognizione
Consiglio Nazionale delle
Ricerche
Rome, Italy

ISBN 978-3-642-32374-4 ISBN 978-3-642-32375-1 (eBook)
DOI 10.1007/978-3-642-32375-1
Springer Heidelberg New York Dordrecht London

Library of Congress Control Number: 2013930554

ACM Computing Classification (1998): I.2, J.4, J.5

Printed on acid-free paper

Springer is part of Springer Science+Business Media (www.springer.com)

Contents

Part III Novelty-Based Intrinsic Motivation Mechanisms

Part IV Competence-Based Intrinsic Motivation Mechanisms

Part V Mechanisms Complementary to Intrinsic Motivations

Part VI Tools for Research on Intrinsic Motivations

Intrinsically Motivated Learning Systems: An Overview

Gianluca Baldassarre and Marco Mirolli

Abstract This chapter introduces the field of intrinsically motivated learning systems and illustrates the content, objectives, and organisation of the book. The chapter first expands the concept of intrinsic motivations, then introduces a taxonomy of three classes of intrinsic-motivation mechanisms (based on predictors, on novelty detection, and on competence), and finally introduces and reviews the various contributions of the book. The contributions are organised into six parts. The contributions of the first part provide general overviews on the concept of intrinsic motivations, the possible mechanisms that may implement them, and the functions that they can play. The contributions of the second, third, and fourth parts focus on the three classes of the aforementioned intrinsic-motivation mechanisms. The contributions of the fifth part discuss mechanisms that are complementary to intrinsic motivations. The contributions of the sixth part introduce tools and experimental paradigms that can be used to investigate intrinsic motivations.

1 Intrinsically Motivated Learning

The capacity to learn autonomously and in a cumulative fashion is one of the hallmarks of intelligence. Higher mammals, especially when young, engage in a number of exploratory activities with the environment (e.g. think about children at play; von Hofsten 2007). These activities are not directed to pursue goals that are directly relevant for the survival and reproduction of the organism, but are driven by *intrinsic motivations*, that is, motivations such as curiosity, interest in novel stimuli or surprising events, and interest in learning new behaviours. The adaptive value of intrinsically motivated activities is that they allow the cumulative acquisition

G. Baldassarre (✉) · M. Mirolli
Institute of Cognitive Sciences and Technologies, CNR, Roma, Italy
e-mail: gianluca.baldassarre@istc.cnr.it; marco.mirolli@istc.cnr.it

G. Baldassarre and M. Mirolli (eds.), *Intrinsically Motivated Learning in Natural and Artificial Systems*, DOI 10.1007/978-3-642-32375-1_1,

of knowledge and skills that can be later used (e.g. in adulthood) to accomplish fitness enhancing goals (Baldassarre 2011; Singh et al. 2010). Intrinsic motivations continue to operate also during adulthood, and indeed in humans they underlie lifelong learning and other typically human activities such as art and scientific discovery (Schmidhuber 2010). Interestingly, intrinsic motivations are also the basis of processes that strongly affect human well-being, such as the sense of competence, self-determination, and self-esteem (Ryan and Deci 2000).

The concept of intrinsic motivation was introduced in the 1950s in animal psychology (Harlow 1950) and was further elaborated in human psychology (Deci 1975; Deci and Ryan 1985), where it is now widely applied, especially in the fields of educational psychology (e.g. Kohn 1993), developmental psychology (e.g. Harter 1981), and organisational psychology (Houkes et al. 2001).

Furthermore, recent neuroscientific research on the learning signals used by real brains, in particular with respect to the learning of novel actions (e.g. Redgrave and Gurney 2006) and the memorisation of novel information (e.g. Lisman and Grace 2005), is starting to uncover the basic brain mechanisms underlying intrinsic motivations.

Recently, the concept of intrinsic motivation was introduced in machine learning and developmental robotics (Barto et al. 2004; Oudeyer et al. 2007; Schembri et al. 2007c) as a means for developing artificial systems that can autonomously learn several different skills. The idea is that intelligent machines and robots could autonomously acquire skills and knowledge under the guidance of intrinsic motivations, and later exploit such knowledge and skills so to accomplish the tasks that are useful for the user in a more efficient and faster way than if they had to acquire them from scratch. This possibility would clearly enhance the utility and autonomy of intelligent artificial systems. For this reason, the investigation of intrinsically motivated learning systems is becoming a central research topic in machine learning and autonomous robotics.

Notwithstanding the importance of this emerging field, up to now there has not been any attempt to draw a unifying picture. The present book provides a general and highly interdisciplinary overview of recent research on intrinsic motivations. While the principal target of this book is the community that tries to synthesise autonomous learning artificial systems, either for applicative purposes or as a means to understand real organisms, this book contains also a number of contributions from researchers in the empirical sciences, because we think that a close dialog between the natural and the artificial sciences is the most fruitful way to address the problems related to intrinsically motivated learning. As a result, this book contains contributions from several different fields of researchers, including robotics (Hart and Grupen 2012; Natale et al. 2012; Nehmzow et al. 2012; Oudeyer et al. 2012), machine learning (Barto 2012; Schmidhuber 2012), computational modelling (Baldassarre and Mirolli 2012; Dayan 2012; Gurney et al. 2012; Merrick 2012; Mirolli and Baldassarre 2012), psychology (Schlesinger 2012; Stafford et al. 2012; Taffoni et al. 2012), and neuroscience (Otmakova et al. 2012; Redgrave et al. 2012).

The research on intrinsic motivations is indeed very new, and as such it is still not fully structured. For example, within conferences and projects concerning intrinsic motivations, it is not rare to see researchers animatedly debating the very notion of intrinsic motivations, their functions, and the possible mechanisms that can be used to implement them. In this respect, much effort was spent to improve the clarity of the presentation and the use of a common language to facilitate comparison. As a result, this book is also a means to foster the emergence of common views at the broad theoretical and taxonomical level.

Overall, this book has two fundamental goals. The first aim is to present the state of the art of the research on intrinsically motivated learning. To this purpose, it collects the contributions of most of the important researchers of the field, who have achieved the most important milestones within it. The authors were asked to review their major contributions and to frame them within the broader relevant literature. These criteria ensured that this book covers the important research in the field. The second aim of this book is to identify the scientific and technological open challenges related to intrinsically motivated learning and the most promising research directions to tackle these challenges. In this respect, all contributors were asked not only to present a review of the work done within their topic of interest but also to leverage on this to present the most important challenges raised by such investigations and, when possible, to envisage possible solutions for them.

2 Structure of the Book

Beyond this introductory chapter, this book is structured in six parts. Part I contains contributions that introduce the reader to the general issues of intrinsic motivations. This allows the reader to familiarise himself with the notion of intrinsic motivation, with the literature on it, with the different functions it can play within organisms and intelligent artificial systems, and with the different classes of mechanisms that can be used to implement it.

Parts II–IV constitute the "central" parts of this book. Each of these parts is dedicated to a different major class of intrinsic-motivation mechanisms. While according to us the fundamental function of intrinsic motivations is that of guiding the learning system in the acquisition of novel skills, different mechanisms can be envisaged to subserve this function (see Mirolli and Baldassarre 2012). In particular, the first two classes of mechanisms (prediction based and novelty based, discussed in Parts II and III, respectively) are based on some form of knowledge that the learning system is acquiring, while the third class (discussed in Part IV) is directly based on the acquisition of competence. We now briefly expand on the relation of the three parts with these classes of mechanisms.

Part II focuses on intrinsic-motivation mechanisms relying on "diachronic knowledge", that is, on the *prediction* of future states based on current states and (possibly) planned actions: in this respect, experiences that are less predictable are potentially more interesting than those more predictable, that is, well known.

For example, these types of intrinsic motivations may allow a child to focus her attention on a bottle that unexpectedly fell on the ground after she hit it by mistake. This focusing may allow her to learn a new potential effect of her actions, and the knowledge so acquired might be useful in a later stage to perform various tasks as an adult. This is a key capability at the core of human intelligence: flexibility, and creativity, maximally apparent in children at play. To date, prediction-based mechanisms are surely the most developed and studied kind of intrinsic-motivation mechanisms.

Part III focuses on intrinsic-motivation mechanisms relying on "synchronic knowledge", that is, on the sensory appearance and inner structure of world states in a given instant: in particular, these mechanisms classify new experiences on a continuous scale from novel, hence interesting, to familiar, hence less/not interesting. These mechanisms are, for example, related to the fact that you see a picture for the first time (e.g. an original painting), and this attracts your attention so that your brain can store information about it, or to the fact that you see two familiar objects together for the first time (e.g. a pigeon on your desktop when you get to your office in the morning). This novelty detection is fundamental to focus learning resources on novel objects. This kind of knowledge-based mechanism has been less studied in robotics than those based on prediction but might nonetheless play an important role for intrinsically motivated learning both in natural and artificial systems.

Part IV focuses on competence-based intrinsic-motivation mechanisms that measure the acquisition of competence, that is, of the skills (*sensorimotor mappings* or *action policies*) that allow the agent to act on, and change, the world as desired. For example, succeeding in inserting a toy-cube in the appropriate hole of a toy-box can motivate a child to keep on playing with the toys (Ornkloo and Hofsten 2006). Competence-based intrinsic motivations, whose existence and importance has been recently highlighted, are an emergent new important subtopic within the field of intrinsic motivations. Their importance is due to the fact that they directly measure the acquisition of skills that allow us to best act in the world. For this reason, they represent fundamental mechanisms for driving the maximisation of skill acquisition.

Part V is dedicated to mechanisms complementary to intrinsic motivations, namely, to mechanisms that, working in synergy with intrinsic motivations, may enhance their functioning. Indeed, learning processes supporting cumulative learning in organisms, in particular in children, do not work in isolation but rely upon other mechanisms that can implement other important sub-functions that in turn can support learning. Examples of these are mechanisms for bottom-up attention guidance that support intrinsic motivations in finding novel patterns and information and developmental constraints like the use of appropriate sensorimotor primitives and space representations, maturation processes, and social guidance.

Finally, Part VI is dedicated to research "tools" that can be used for investigating intrinsic motivations. Different kinds of tools are covered by the different contributions: the first contribution is on a behavioural experimental paradigm usable with rats, humans, and robots; the second contribution is on a mechatronic board usable for running behavioural experiments with monkeys, children, and robots; and the third contribution involves a robotic hardware platform (the iCub robot) that can be used to build and test developmental models on intrinsic motivations. The significance of this part of this book lies in the "infancy" of the field of intrinsic motivations: the development of new tools of research is of great value, and their spreading among the community is of great importance for the further development of the field.

3 Contents

3.1 Part I: General Overviews on Intrinsic Motivations

The first part of the book contains three contributions that introduce the reader to the general issues related to intrinsic motivations.

Intrinsic Motivation and Reinforcement Learning. The first contribution is by *Andrew Barto*, who introduced the notion of intrinsic motivations in the fields of machine learning and robotics (e.g. Barto et al. 2004; Singh et al. 2005). As you will see from the various contributions of this book, a fair amount of computational work on intrinsic motivations is based on the computational reinforcement learning framework. After introducing both reinforcement learning and the psychological literature on intrinsic motivation, Barto's contribution explains why the reinforcement learning framework is particularly well suited for incorporating intrinsic motivations. Moreover, it discusses an evolutionary perspective according to which there is a continuum between extrinsic and intrinsic motivations as the two kinds of motivations differ only in how directly they are related to the evolutionary success of the behaviours they prompt: while extrinsic motivations drive the agent to pursue activities more directly related to survival and reproduction, intrinsic motivations lead the agent to develop behaviours less directly related to basic needs, such as play [see Baldassarre (2011) for a proposal of a stronger distinction between the two types of motivations done on this basis].

Functions and Mechanisms of Intrinsic Motivations: The Knowledge Vs. Competence Distinction. The second contribution of this part, by *Marco Mirolli* and *Gianluca Baldassarre*, clarifies the distinction between knowledge and competence with respect to both the functions and the mechanisms of intrinsic motivations. The contribution starts by reviewing both the psychological and the computational literature on intrinsic motivations on the basis of this distinction. Then, it proposes that the *general function* of all kinds of intrinsic motivations is allowing intelligent systems to acquire skills rather than knowledge. However, especially in hierarchical and modular learning systems, different sub-function can be identified, which can be implemented by different mechanisms. In particular, the paper suggests that knowledge-based intrinsic-motivation mechanisms can be used for discovering which skills can be acquired, whereas competence-based mechanisms can be used for deciding which skills to train and when.

Exploration from Generalization Mediated by Multiple Controllers. The last contribution of this part is from *Peter Dayan*, one of the most active computational theoreticians on brain and behaviour. In his contribution, he gives a general perspective on intrinsic motivations from the point of view of recent computationally oriented research on brain and behaviour, in particular based on reinforcement learning. In particular, the contribution relates intrinsic motivations to the reinforcement learning notions of exploration bonuses (Kakade and Dayan 2002) and generalisation. Bonuses can arise from the generalisation of knowledge from known worlds to successively experienced environments. Different controllers endowed with different architectures and implementing different functions can realise different bonuses. This normative grounding contributes to define the structure of the field and to establish links between various concepts in reinforcement learning, psychology, and neuroscience.

3.2 Part II: Prediction-Based Intrinsic-Motivation Mechanisms

This part is formed by three contributions focused on intrinsic-motivation mechanisms based on measures of knowledge intended as prediction capability.

Maximising Fun by Creating Data with Easily Reducible Subjective Complexity. This contribution is by *Jürgen Schmidhuber*, who proposed seminal systems on intrinsic motivations in the 1990s (Schmidhuber 1991a,b) and has later been developing a coherent theory on intrinsic motivations from the machine learning point of view (Schmidhuber 2010). The core idea of his work is that an agent can use the improvement of prediction capability or, at a more abstract level, the improvement in the compression of the internal representation of information, as an intrinsic reinforcement. In this way, the agent will learn to act so as to maximise the agent's information intake. In his chapter, he presents an extensive review of all the works that generated such theory during the last 20 years, gives a clear and direct presentation of the key principles of such theory, reviews the major experimental results, and proposes interesting theoretical implications of the theory (e.g. to explain a number of different phenomena, from scientific discovery to creativity in art).

The Role of the Basal Ganglia in Discovering Novel Actions. The second contribution of this part is from *Peter Redgrave* (a neuroscientist) and colleagues, and presents an important neuroscientific theory on action discovery and learning (Redgrave and Gurney 2006; Redgrave et al. 2011) that is clearly related to the notion of intrinsic-motivation mechanisms related to prediction. The theory challenges the major tenets of the standard theory related to the neuromodulator dopamine and reinforcement learning processes in the brain. By taking into account empirical data that are difficult to explain with the received view, the proposed theory provides a coherent picture that explains how action discovery might be realised in real brains on the basis of intrinsic-motivation signals. These signals are produced by events (e.g. the sudden onset of a light detected by the superior colliculus, a brain area closely connected with the retina) that are unpredicted by the agent and are capable of guiding the learning processes that lead the agent to acquire the actions that cause the unexpected events to happen.

Action Discovery and Intrinsic Motivation: A Biologically Constrained Formalisation. The last contribution of this part is by *Kevin Gurney* and colleagues, who develop and formalise the theoretical framework proposed in the previous contribution. The main idea of this contribution is that intrinsic-motivation learning signals, in particular those caused by unexpected salient events, drive the acquisition of different types of information in the brain, in particular the acquisition of "forward models" (i.e. the capacity to predict future states on the basis of current states and planned actions), and "inverse models" (i.e. the capacity to associate the correct actions to desired outcomes and perceived world states). While forward models contribute to establish the unpredictability of salient events, and hence to generate the related (intrinsic) learning signals, inverse models implement the capacity to act so to realise desired states, which can be acquired on the basis of intrinsic motivations. In general, this contribution represents a biologically motivated formal framework for modelling intrinsically motivated action discovery and acquisition.

3.3 Part III: Novelty-Based Intrinsic-Motivation Mechanisms

This part is formed by three contributions that are focused on intrinsic-motivation mechanisms based on measures of knowledge intended as novelty/familiarity of percepts.

Novelty Detection as an Intrinsic Motivation for Cumulative Learning Robots. The first contribution of this part is from *Ulrich Nehmzow*'s research team. Nehmzow, who recently passed away, did pioneering work with autonomous robots and *habituable neural networks* (Neto and Nehmzow 2007; Vieiraneto and Nehmzow 2007). These are systems that allow a robot to learn new perceptual patterns, get progressively familiar with them, and then exploit this knowledge for accomplishing various tasks (e.g. a patrolling robot might understand if a certain infrastructure has been damaged from the last check). This chapter first clarifies the relationship existing between intrinsic motivations and novelty detection, for example, as studied in machine learning and statistical research. Then it presents a critical review of the methods of novelty detection previously developed by the authors. Finally, it illustrates the key open challenges that need to be considered in the design of novelty detection systems and the types of solutions that might be investigated to face them.

Novelty and Beyond: Towards Combined Motivation Models and Integrated Learning Architectures. The second contribution of this part is by *Kathryn Merrick*, who has pioneered the application of novelty-based intrinsic motivations based on habituable neural networks in both robotics and interactive software and video games (Merrick and Maher 2009). This contribution presents a critical review of the author's work in the field, including attempts to model competence-seeking motivations. In particular, it discusses four architectures that combine components related to intrinsic-motivation mechanisms in different ways. Moreover, the contribution frames the reviewed applications within the broader perspective of "motivated agents", proposing research road maps to build agents that integrate various types of intrinsic and extrinsic motivations.

The Hippocampal-VTA Loop: The Role of Novelty and Motivation in Controlling the Entry of Information into Long-Term Memory. The last contribution of the chapter is by *John Lisman* (a theoretical neuroscientist) and co-workers, who have carried out fundamental work on the brain circuits and mechanisms underlying the acquisition of novel information (Lisman and Grace 2005). The main idea proposed here is that the complex cerebral loop that involves the hippocampus (fundamental for the acquisition and recognition of novel patterns) and the dopaminergic neurons (providing motivational and learning signals) allows the brain to understand whether a certain perceptual pattern is new so to enhance its memorisation. The contribution also discusses the most advanced open problems in the biological investigation of these issues and possible ways to face them. Interestingly, the mechanisms presented in this work may represent the brain basis of novelty-based intrinsic motivations, which complement the mechanisms discussed in the contributions by Redgrave and co-workers related to prediction-based intrinsic motivations.

3.4 Part IV: Competence-Based Intrinsic-Motivation Mechanisms

This part is formed by two contributions that focus on intrinsic-motivation mechanisms based on measures of the system's ability to reach a certain goal.

Deciding Which Skill to Learn When: Temporal-Difference Competence-Based Intrinsic Motivation (TD-CB-IM). The first contribution of this part, by *Gianluca Baldassarre* and *Marco Mirolli*, reviews one of the first models on competence-based intrinsic motivations (Schembri et al. 2007a,b,c). This is also the first model casting intrinsic motivations in an evolutionary perspective, where intrinsic motivations play the key adaptive function of guiding learning of skills in the absence or paucity of extrinsic motivations (e.g. as happens in the childhood of humans); the skills so acquired can be readily exploited in later phases of life (e.g. in adulthood). This contribution first discusses the importance of competence-based intrinsic motivations for autonomous skill acquisition by focusing, in particular, on the problem of deciding which skill to train in each moment. Then the contribution reviews the work of the authors on a competence-based intrinsic-motivation mechanism that is based on the idea of using the TD-error signal of standard reinforcement learning models as an intrinsic reinforcement for a selector that has to decide which skill to train when. Finally, the contribution discusses a number of open issues related to competence-based intrinsic motivations.

Intrinsically Motivated Affordance Discovery and Modelling. The last contribution of this part is by *Stephen Hart* and *Roderic Grupen*, two roboticists who have proposed some of the most advanced robotic applications based on intrinsic motivations (Hart and Grupen 2011). Their system is based on a two-level hierarchical system where the lower level is formed by dynamic motor primitives and the higher level is a reinforcement learning system that learns to suitably assemble the primitives of the lower level represented in an abstract format. The system includes a model that learns to predict in which states the motor primitives can be executed with success. The enlargement of the set of states where this happens is used to generate learning signals that so mark the improvement of the primitives and the recognition of their enhanced applicability (called here "affordance"). The authors review various experiments showing that the system can guide a robot to autonomously acquire a rich repertoire of primitives (e.g. for object reaching, grasping, and displacement) and discuss possible improvement of the systems in future work.

3.5 Part V: Mechanisms Complementary to Intrinsic Motivations

This part is formed by two contributions that present some mechanisms that can work in synergy with intrinsic-motivation systems to foster the learning processes guided by them.

Intrinsically Motivated Learning of Real-World Sensorimotor Skills with Developmental Constraints. The first contribution of this part is from *Pierre-Yves Oudeyer, Adrien Baranes*, and *Frédéric Kaplan*, who have had a fundamental role in promoting the study of intrinsic motivations in the robotic community (e.g. Oudeyer and Kaplan 2007; Oudeyer et al. 2007). The contribution reviews the principles and main outcomes of recent research by the authors on how intrinsic motivations can be complemented by other factors so as to improve the capacity of robots to undergo a truly open-ended development. In particular, the authors present several developmental constraints that can be useful for overcoming the difficulties given by the high dimensionality and unboundedness of the sensorimotor space of robots, including sensorimotor primitives, task space representations, maturation processes, and social guidance. The nature and operation of these constraints is illustrated on the basis of robot experiments, which are also used to highlight the open challenges of this research.

Investigating the Origins of Intrinsic Motivation in Human Infants. The second contribution of this part is by *Matthew Schlesinger* (a developmental psychologist), who proposes a new perspective on novelty-based intrinsic motivations by investigating the mechanisms that guide attention itself. Consider, for example, the eyes of a child who does not have a particular goal in mind and is engaged in exploring the environment. With high probability, the child will direct his gaze to areas where the surface of objects has a high contrast, a high luminosity, or a high motion: all these areas have a high saliency as they are informative with respect to the surrounding portions of the environment (e.g. a high contrast on a homogeneous surface or movement in a static background). Goal-directed, top-down attentional skills are gradually acquired by building on these basic capabilities and under the guidance of more sophisticated forms of novelty detection as those reviewed in previous parts. Three theoretical developmental perspectives that try to explain the development of visual exploration are compared. Furthermore, the contribution reviews a model on the development of perceptual completion which offers a case study on the development of visual exploration and the role of oculomotor skills. Finally, a number of open challenges that are suggested by this work are discussed.

3.6 Part VI: Tools for Research on Intrinsic Motivations

The final part of this book presents three contributions that illustrate new important research tools for investigating intrinsic motivations.

A Novel Behavioural Task for Researching Intrinsic Motivations. The first contribution is from *Tom Stafford* and co-workers (a team of experimental psychologists) and illustrates a new experimental paradigm, called the "joystick task". In contrast to standard reinforcement learning paradigms, which have been developed to study how the deployment of already acquired actions is affected by extrinsic rewards, the joystick task has been explicitly designed to investigate intrinsically motivated action discovery and acquisition. Flexibility is one of the important features of the novel experimental paradigm: the paradigm allows us to generate a multitude of experimental conditions with the desired level of difficulty. Moreover, different versions of the paradigm are proposed for studying action learning with different types of participants and species including rats, monkeys, humans, human patients, and robots. Beyond discussing the rationale of the task, its potential for future research on intrinsically motivated action learning, its main features, and its range of applicability, the contribution reviews also some preliminary results that have been obtained with different kinds of subjects (rats and humans), thus showing the potential of the task for comparative research.

The "Mechatronic Board": A Tool to Study Intrinsic Motivations in Humans, Monkeys, and Humanoid Robots. The second contribution of this part is by *Fabrizio Taffoni* and colleagues, which include researchers from four different groups: a group of bioengineers led by *Eugenio Guglielmelli*, a group of developmental neuroscientists and psychologists led by *Flavio Keller*, a group of primatologists led by *Elisabetta Visalberghi*, and a group of computational modelists led by *Gianluca Baldassarre* and *Marco Mirolli*. The contribution illustrates a new experimental tool (called the mechatronic board) that has been explicitly designed to investigate the acquisition of actions on the basis of free exploration and intrinsic motivations. The tool has been designed (in terms of materials, size, modularity, complexity, etc.) to be used with different types of participants and species: monkeys, children, human adults, and even robots. In the mechatronic board, different types of manipulators can be inserted (the number and kind of objects that might be used to elicit interest and exploration is open), and a feedback panel provides different kinds of effects (sounds, lights, opening of boxes) depending on the actions of the participants. All aspects of the board are programmable, and all events can be automatically recorded. For these reasons, the mechatronic board represents an important research tool for the investigation of intrinsic motivations. This is also shown by illustrating some preliminary results obtained in pilot experiments involving children, monkeys and robots.

The iCub Platform: A Tool for Studying Intrinsically Motivated Learning. The last contribution is from *Lorenzo Natale* and co-workers, a group of roboticists led by *Giorgio Metta* and *Giulio Sandini*. The contribution presents the humanoid robot iCub, a recently developed robotic platform designed to model developmental phenomena in children. The robot's size, physical structure, level of sophistication of the sensors, and motor plant have all been designed for this purpose. The design of the robot hardware, its drivers, and the library of control programs that have been developed for it are all open source, as the robot has been developed with the aim of becoming an open research tool for developmental robotic research. Indeed, the robot is already in use in several robotic labs and is becoming the standard tool for research on bio-inspired autonomous robotics in Europe. For all these reasons, the iCub represents a valuable tool for robotic research on intrinsic motivations.

4 Conclusion

In summary, this book aims at becoming a reference point in the field of intrinsically motivated learning by (a) establishing the theoretical foundations of the field, (b) describing the most significant achievements accomplished so far and the most important open challenges, (c) illustrating the scientific and technological potentials of the field, and (d) presenting new methods and tools for carrying out investigations in the field.

Given the importance of intrinsic motivations for humans and for autonomous intelligent robots and machines, we hope this book will recruit new researchers and foster further investigations in this emergent and fascinating research field.

Acknowledgements This chapter and a large part of the research reported in this book were supported by the project "IM-CLeVeR: Intrinsically Motivated Cumulative Learning Versatile

Robots" funded by the European Commission under the 7th Framework Programme (FP7/2007-2013) and "Challenge 2: Cognitive Systems, Interaction, Robotics", Grant Agreement No. ICT-IP-231722. Support or co-support from other institutions, where present, is described in the "Acknowledgment" section of each chapter. The editors of this book thank the EU reviewers (Benjamin Kuipers, Luc Berthouze, and Yasuo Kuniyoshi) and the EU project officer (Cécile Huet) for their valuable advice and their encouragement. For more information on the IM-CLeVeR project and for additional multimedia material, see the project website: http://www.im-clever.eu/. We also thank Simona Bosco for her editorial help with some contributions.

References

Baldassarre, G.: What are intrinsic motivations? A biological perspective. In: Cangelosi, A., Triesch, J., Fasel, I., Rohlfing, K., Nori, F., Oudeyer, P.-Y., Schlesinger, M., Nagai, Y. (eds.) Proceedings of the International Conference on Development and Learning and Epigenetic Robotics (ICDL-EpiRob-2011), pp. E1–E8. Frankfurt Germany, 24–27 August, 2011

Baldassarre, G., Mirolli, M.: Deciding which skill to learn when: Temporal-difference competence-based intrinsic motivation (TD-CB-IM). In: Baldassarre, G., Mirolli, M. (eds.) Intrinsically Motivated Learning in Natural and Artificial Systems. Springer, Berlin (2012, this volume)

Barto, A., Singh, S., Chentanez, N.: Intrinsically motivated learning of hierarchical collections of skills. In: International Conference on Developmental Learning (ICDL), La Jolla, CA, 20–22 October, 2004

Barto, A.G.: Intrinsic motivation and reinforcement learning. In: Baldassarre, G., Mirolli, M. (eds.) Intrinsically Motivated Learning in Natural and Artificial Systems. Springer, Berlin (2012, this volume)

Dayan, P.: Exploration from generalisation mediated by multiple controllers. In: Baldassarre, G., Mirolli, M. (eds.) Intrinsically Motivated Learning in Natural and Artificial Systems. Springer, Berlin (2012, this volume)

Deci, E.: Intrinsic Motivation. Plenum, New York (1975)

Deci, E.L., Ryan, R.M.: Intrinsic motivation and self-determination in human behavior. Plenum, New York (1985)

Gurney, K., Lepora, N., Shah, A., Koene, A., Redgrave, P.: Action discovery and intrinsic motivation: A biologically constrained formalisation. In: Baldassarre, G., Mirolli, M. (eds.) Intrinsically Motivated Learning in Natural and Artificial Systems. Springer, Berlin (2012, this volume)

Harlow, H.F.: Learning and satiation of response in intrinsically motivated complex puzzle performance by monkeys. J. Comp. Physiol. Psychol. **43**, 289–294 (1950)

Hart, S., Grupen, R.: Learning generalizable control programs. IEEE Trans. Auton. Mental Dev. **3**(1) (2011)

Hart, S., Grupen, R.: Intrinsically motivated affordance discovery and modeling. In: Baldassarre, G., Mirolli, M. (eds.) Intrinsically Motivated Learning in Natural and Artificial Systems. Springer, Berlin (2012, this volume)

Harter, S.: A new self-report scale of intrinsic versus extrinsic orientation in the classroom: Motivational and informational components. Dev. Psychol. **17**, 100–112 (1981)

Houkes, I., Janssen, P., de Jong, J., Nijhuis, F.: Specific relationships between work characteristics and intrinsic work motivation, burnout and turnover intention: A multi-sample analysis. Eur. J. Work Org. Psychol. **10**, 1–23 (2001)

Kakade, S., Dayan, P.: Dopamine: Generalization and bonuses. Neural Netw. **15**(4–6), 549–559 (2002)

Kohn, A.: Punished by Rewards. Houghton Mifflin Boston, MA (1993)

Lisman, J.E., Grace, A.A.: The hippocampal-VTA loop: Controlling the entry of information into long-term memory. Neuron **46**(5), 703–713 (2005)

Merrick, K., Maher, M.: Motivated Reinforcement Learning: Curious Characters for Multiuser Games. Springer, Berlin (2009)

Merrick, K.E.: Novelty and beyond: Towards combined motivation models and integrated learning architectures. In: Baldassarre, G., Mirolli, M. (eds.) Intrinsically Motivated Learning in Natural and Artificial Systems. Springer, Berlin (2012, this volume)

Mirolli, M., Baldassarre, G.: Functions and mechanisms of intrinsic motivations: The knowledge versus competence distinction. In: Baldassarre, G., Mirolli, M. (eds.) Intrinsically Motivated Learning in Natural and Artificial Systems. Springer, Berlin (2012, this volume)

Natale, L., Nori, F., Metta, G., Fumagalli, M., Ivaldi, S., Pattacini, U., Randazzo, M., Schmitz, A., Sandini, G.: The iCub platform: A tool for studying intrinsically motivated learning. In: Baldassarre, G., Mirolli, M. (eds.) Intrinsically Motivated Learning in Natural and Artificial Systems. Springer, Berlin (2012, this volume)

Nehmzow, U., Gatsoulis, Y., Kerr, E., Condell, J., Siddique, N.H., McGinnity, M.T.: Novelty detection as an intrinsic motivation for cumulative learning robots. In: Baldassarre, G., Mirolli, M. (eds.) Intrinsically Motivated Learning in Natural and Artificial Systems. Springer, Berlin (2012, this volume)

Neto, H.V., Nehmzow, U.: Visual novelty detection with automatic scale selection. Robot. Auton. Syst. **55**(9), 693–701 (2007)

Ornkloo, H., Hofsten, C.v.: Fitting objects into holes: On the development of spatial cognition skills. Dev. Psychol. **43**(2), 404–416 (2006)

Otmakova, N., Duzel, E., Deutch, A.Y., Lisman, J.E.: The hippocampal-VTA loop: The role of novelty and motivation in controlling the entry of information into long-term memory. In: Baldassarre, G., Mirolli, M. (eds.) Intrinsically Motivated Learning in Natural and Artificial Systems. Springer, Berlin (2012, this volume)

Oudeyer, P.-Y., Banares, A., Frédéric, K.: Intrinsically motivated learning of real world sensorimotor skills with developmental constraints. In: Baldassarre, G., Mirolli, M. (eds.) Intrinsically Motivated Learning in Natural and Artificial Systems. Springer, Berlin (2012, this volume)

Oudeyer, P.-Y., Kaplan, F.: What is intrinsic motivation? A typology of computational approaches. Front. Neurorobot. **1**, 6 (2007)

Oudeyer, P.-Y., Kaplan, F., Hafner, V.V.: Intrinsic motivation systems for autonomous mental development. IEEE Trans. Evol. Comput. **11**(2), 265–286 (2007)

Redgrave, P., Gurney, K.: The short-latency dopamine signal: A role in discovering novel actions? Nat. Rev. Neurosci. **7**(12), 967–975 (2006)

Redgrave, P., Gurney, K., Stafford, T., Thirkettle, M., Lewis, J.: The role of the basal ganglia in discovering novel actions. In: Baldassarre, G., Mirolli, M. (eds.) Intrinsically Motivated Learning in Natural and Artificial Systems. Springer, Berlin (2012, this volume)

Redgrave, P., Vautrelle, N., Reynolds, J.N.J.: Functional properties of the basal ganglia's re-entrant loop architecture: Selection and reinforcement. Neuroscience vol. 198 pp. 138–151 (2011)

Ryan, R.M., Deci, E.L.: Self-determination theory and the facilitation of intrinsic motivation, social development, and well-being. Am. Psychol. **55**(1), 68–78 (2000)

Schembri, M., Mirolli, M., Baldassarre, G.: Evolution and learning in an intrinsically motivated reinforcement learning robot. In: Almeida e Costa, Fernando, Rocha, L.M., Costa, E., Harvey, I., Coutinho, A. (eds.) Advances in Artificial Life. Proceedings of the 9th European Conference on Artificial Life (ECAL 2007), Lisbon, Portugal, 10–14 September 2007. Lecture Notes in Artificial Intelligence, vol. 4648, pp. 294–333. Springer, Berlin (2007a)

Schembri, M., Mirolli, M., Baldassarre, G.: Evolving childhood's length and learning parameters in an intrinsically motivated reinforcement learning robot. In: Berthouze, L., Dhristiopher, P.G., Littman, M., Kozima, H., Balkenius, C. (eds.) Proceedings of the Seventh International Conference on Epigenetic Robotics, vol. 134, pp. 141–148 Lund, Sweden. Lund University Cognitive Studies vol. 149 (2007b)

Schembri, M., Mirolli, M., Baldassarre, G.: Evolving internal reinforcers for an intrinsically motivated reinforcement-learning robot. In: Demiris, Y., Mareschal, D., Scassellati, B., Weng, J. (eds.) Proceedings of the 6th International Conference on Development and Learning, pp. E1–E6. Imperial College, London, UK, 11–13 July (2007c)

Schlesinger, M.: Investigating the origins of intrinsic motivations in human infants. In: Baldassarre, G., Mirolli, M. (eds.) Intrinsically Motivated Learning in Natural and Artificial Systems. Springer, Berlin (2012, this volume)

Schmidhuber, J.: Curious model-building control systems. In: Proceedings of the International Joint Conference on Neural Networks, vol. 2, pp. 1458–1463. Singapore 18–21 November (1991a)

Schmidhuber, J.: A possibility for implementing curiosity and boredom in model-building neural controllers. In: Meyer, J.-A., Wilson, S. (eds.) From Animals to Animats: Proceedings of the First International Conference on Simulation of Adaptive Behavior, pp. 222–227. Paris, France, December, 1990. The MIT Press, Cambridge (1991b)

Schmidhuber, J.: Formal theory of creativity, fun, and intrinsic motivation (1990–2010): IEEE Trans. Auton. Mental Dev. **2**(3), 230–247 (2010)

Schmidhuber, J.: Maximizing fun by creating data with easily reducible subjective complexity. In: Baldassarre, G., Mirolli, M. (eds.) Intrinsically Motivated Learning in Natural and Artificial Systems. Springer, Berlin (2012, this volume)

Singh, S., Barto, A., Chentanez, N.: Intrinsically motivated reinforcement learning. In: Saul, L.K., Weiss, Y., Bottou, L. (eds.) Advances in Neural Information Processing Systems 17: Proceedings of the 2004 Conference, Vancouver, British Columbia, Canada, 13–18 December 2004. MIT, Cambridge (2005)

Singh, S., Lewis, R., Barto, A., Sorg, J.: Intrinsically motivated reinforcement learning: An evolutionary perspective. IEEE Trans. Auton. Mental Dev. **2**(2), 70–82 (2010)

Stafford, T., Walton, T., Hetherington, L., Thirkettle, M., Gurney, K., Redgrave, P.: A novel behavioural task for researching intrinsic motivation. In: Baldassarre, G., Mirolli, M. (eds.) Intrinsically Motivated Learning in Natural and Artificial Systems. Springer, Berlin (2012, this volume)

Taffoni, F., Formica, D., Schiavone, G., Scorcia, M., Tomassetti, A., Polizzi di Sorrentino, E., Sabbatini, G., Truppa, V., Mirolli, M., Baldassarre, G., Visalberghi, E., Keller, F., Guglielmelli, E.: The "mechatronic board": A tool to study intrinsic motivation in humans, animals and robots. In: Baldassarre, G., Mirolli, M. (eds.) Intrinsically Motivated Learning in Natural and Artificial Systems. Springer, Berlin (2012, this volume)

Vieiraneto, H., Nehmzow, U.: Visual novelty detection with automatic scale selection. Robot. Auton. Syst. **55**, 693–701 (2007)

von Hofsten, C.: Action in development. Dev. Sci. **10**(1), 54–60 (2007)

Part I
General Overviews on Intrinsic Motivations

Intrinsic Motivation and Reinforcement Learning

Andrew G. Barto

Abstract Psychologists distinguish between extrinsically motivated behavior, which is behavior undertaken to achieve some externally supplied reward, such as a prize, a high grade, or a high-paying job, and intrinsically motivated behavior, which is behavior done for its own sake. Is an analogous distinction meaningful for machine learning systems? Can we say of a machine learning system that it is motivated to learn, and if so, is it possible to provide it with an analog of intrinsic motivation? Despite the fact that a formal distinction between extrinsic and intrinsic motivation is elusive, this chapter argues that the answer to both questions is assuredly "yes" and that the machine learning framework of reinforcement learning is particularly appropriate for bringing learning together with what in animals one would call motivation. Despite the common perception that a reinforcement learning agent's reward has to be extrinsic because the agent has a distinct input channel for reward signals, reinforcement learning provides a natural framework for incorporating principles of intrinsic motivation.

1 Introduction

Motivation refers to processes that influence the arousal, strength, and direction of behavior. "To be motivated means *to be moved* to do something" (Ryan and Deci 2000). Psychologists distinguish between *extrinsic motivation*, which means doing something because of some externally supplied reward, and *intrinsic motivation*, which refers to "doing something because it is inherently interesting or enjoyable" (Ryan and Deci 2000). Intrinsic motivation leads organisms to engage in

A.G. Barto (✉)
University of Massachussetts, Amherst, MA, USA

Institute of Cognitive Sciences and Technologies, CNR, Roma, Italy
e-mail: barto@cs.umass.edu

G. Baldassarre and M. Mirolli (eds.), *Intrinsically Motivated Learning in Natural and Artificial Systems*, DOI 10.1007/978-3-642-32375-1_2,

exploration, play, and other behavior driven by curiosity in the absence of externally supplied rewards.

This chapter focuses on how to frame concepts related to intrinsic motivation using the computational theory of reinforcement learning (RL) as it is studied by machine learning researchers (Sutton and Barto 1998). It is a common perception that the computational RL framework[1] can only deal with extrinsic motivation because an RL agent has a distinct input channel that delivers reward signals from its external environment. In contrast to this view, this chapter argues that this perception is a result of not fully appreciating the abstract nature of the RL framework, which is, in fact, particularly well suited for incorporating principles of intrinsic motivation. It further argues that incorporating computational analogs of intrinsic motivation into RL systems opens the door to a very fruitful avenue for the further development of machine learning systems.

RL is a very active area of machine learning, with considerable attention also being received from decision theory, operations research, and control engineering, where it has been called "heuristic dynamic programming" (Werbos 1987) and "neurodynamic programming" (Bertsekas and Tsitsiklis 1996). There is also growing interest in neuroscience because the behavior of some of the basic RL algorithms closely correspond to the activity of dopamine-producing neurons in the brain (Schultz 1998). RL algorithms address the problem of how a behaving agent can learn to approximate an optimal behavioral strategy, usually called a *policy*, while interacting directly with its environment. Viewed in the terms of control engineering, RL consists of methods for approximating closed-loop solutions to optimal control problems while the controller is interacting with the system being controlled. This engineering problem's optimality criterion, or objective function, is analogous to the machinery that delivers primary reward signals to an animal's nervous system. The approximate solution to the optimal control problem corresponds to an animal's skill in performing the control task. A brief introduction to RL is provided in Sect. 2.

Providing artificial learning systems with analogs of intrinsic motivation is not new. Lenat's (1976) AM system, for example, included an analog of intrinsic motivation that directed search using heuristic definitions of "interestingness." Scott and Markovitch (1989) presented a curiosity-driven search method by which an agent's attention was continually directed to the area of highest uncertainty in the current representation, thus steadily reducing its uncertainty about the whole of the experience space. Schmidhuber (1991a,b, 1997, 1999) introduced methods for implementing curiosity by rewarding an RL agent for improving its prediction ability. Sutton's (1991) "exploration bonus" rewards an agent for visiting states in proportion to how much time has passed since they were previously visited, thus encouraging wide coverage of the state space. The author's efforts on this

[1]The phrase *computational RL* is used here because this framework is not a theory of biological RL despite what it borrows from, and suggests about, biological RL. Throughout this chapter, RL refers to computational RL.

topic began when he and colleagues realized that some new developments in RL could be used to make intrinsically motivated behavior a key factor in producing more capable learning systems. This approach, introduced by Barto et al. (2004) and Singh et al. (2005), combines intrinsic motivation with methods for temporal abstraction introduced by Sutton et al. (1999). The reader should consult Barto et al. (2004) and Singh et al. (2005) for more details on this approach.

Not all aspects of motivation involve learning—an animal can be motivated by innate mechanisms that trigger fixed behavior patterns, as the ethologists have emphasized—but what many researchers mean by motivated behavior is behavior that involves the assessment of the consequences of behavior through learned expectations (e.g., Epstein 1982; McFarland and Bösser 1993; Savage 2000). Motivational theories therefore tend to be intimately linked to theories of learning and decision making. Because RL addresses how predictive values can be learned and used to direct behavior, RL is naturally relevant to the study of motivation.[2]

The starting point for addressing intrinsic motivation using the RL framework is the idea that learning and behavior generation processes "don't care" if the reward signals are intrinsic or extrinsic (whatever that distinction may actually mean!); the same processes can be used for both. Schmidhuber (1991b) put this succinctly for the case of curiosity and boredom: "The important point is: the same complex mechanism which is used for "normal" goal-directed learning is used for implementing curiosity and boredom. There is no need for devising a separate system ...." As we shall see in what follows, this idea needs clarification, but it underlies all of the approaches to using RL to obtain analogs of intrinsic motivation: it becomes simply a matter of defining specific mechanisms for generating reward signals.

Although this approach is attractive in its simplicity and accords well with prevalent—though controversial—views about the pervasive influence of brain reward systems on behavior (e.g., Linden 2011), other theoretical principles—not discussed here—have been proposed that can account for aspects of intrinsic motivation (e.g., Andry et al. 2004; Baranes and Oudeyer 2010; Friston et al. 2010; Hesse et al. 2009). Further, contemporary psychology and neuroscience indicate that the nature of reward signals is only one component of the complex processes involved in motivation (Daw and Shohamy 2008). Despite these qualifications, restricting attention to the nature of reward signals within the RL framework illuminates significant issues for the development of computational analogs of motivational processes.

Several important topics relevant to motivation and intrinsic motivation are beyond this chapter's scope. There has been a great increase in interest in affect and emotion in constructing intelligent systems (e.g., Picard 1997; Trappl et al. 1997). Motivation and emotion are intimately linked, but this chapter does not address computational theories of emotion because it would take us too far

[2]RL certainly does not exclude analogs of innate behavioral patterns in artificial agents. The success of many systems using RL methods depends on the careful definition of innate behaviors, as in Hart and Grupen (2012).

from the main focus. Also not discussed are social aspects of motivation, which involve imitation, adult scaffolding, and collective intentionality, all of which play important roles in development (e.g., Breazeal et al. 2004; Thomaz and Breazeal 2006; Thomaz et al. 2006).

This chapter also does not attempt to review the full range of research on motivational systems for artificial agents, to which the reader is referred to the extensive review by Savage (2000). Even research that explicitly aims to combine intrinsic motivation with RL has grown so large that a thorough review is beyond the scope of this chapter. The reader is referred to Oudeyer and Kaplan (2007) and Oudeyer et al. (2007) for a review and perspective on this research.

The concept of motivation in experimental and psychoanalytic psychology as well as in ethology has a very long and complex history that is discussed in many books, for example, those by Arkes-Garske (1982), Beck (1983), Cofer and Appley (1964), Deci and Ryan (1985), Klein (1982), Petri (1981), and Toates (1986). This chapter only touches the surface of this extensive topic, with the goal of giving a minimal account of issues that seem most relevant to computational interpretations of intrinsic motivation. Another goal is to describe some of the old theories to which the recent computational approaches seem most closely related.

This chapter begins with a brief introduction to the conventional view of RL, which is followed by two sections that provide some historical background on studies of motivation and intrinsic motivation. These are followed by two sections that respectively relate RL to motivation in general and intrinsic motivation in particular. Discussion of what an evolutionary perspective suggests about intrinsic motivation is next, followed by a brief summary, discussion of prospects, and finally some concluding comments.

2 Reinforcement Learning

RL is the process of improving performance through trial-and-error experience. The term reinforcement comes from studies of animal learning in experimental psychology, where it refers to the occurrence of an event, in the proper relation to a response, that tends to increase the probability that the response will occur again in the same situation (Kimble 1961). Although the specific term "reinforcement learning" is not used by psychologists, it has been widely adopted by theorists in artificial intelligence and engineering to refer to a class of learning tasks and algorithms. Early uses of this term were by Minsky (1961), Waltz and Fu (1965), and Mendel and McLaren (1970) in describing approaches to learning motivated in part by animal learning studies. The simplest RL algorithms are based on the commonsense idea that if an action is followed by a satisfactory state of affairs, or an improvement in the state of affairs, then the tendency to produce that action is strengthened, that is, reinforced, following Thorndike's (1911) "law of effect."

The usual view of an RL agent interacting with its environment is shown in Fig. 1. The agent generates actions in the context of sensed states of this environment, and

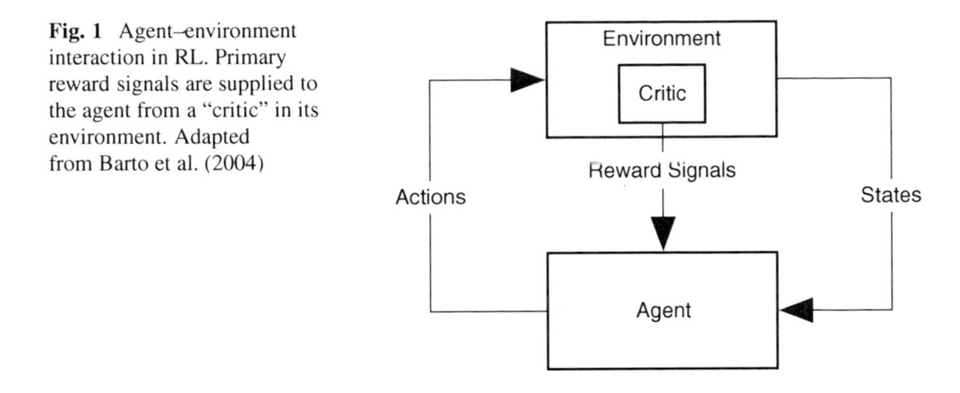

Fig. 1 Agent–environment interaction in RL. Primary reward signals are supplied to the agent from a "critic" in its environment. Adapted from Barto et al. (2004)

its actions influence how the environment's states change over time. This interaction is typically viewed as happening in discrete time steps, $t = 1, 2, 3, \ldots$, that do not represent the passage of any specific amount of real time. The environment contains a "critic" that provides the agent at each time step with an evaluation (a numerical score) of its ongoing behavior.[3] The critic maps environment states (or possibly state-action pairs or even state-action-next-state triples) to numerical reward signals. The agent learns to improve its skill in controlling the environment in the sense of learning how to cause larger magnitude reward signals to be delivered from its environment over time. The signal the critic conveys to the agent corresponds to what psychologists call *primary reward*, generally meaning reward that encourages behavior directly related to survival and reproductive success, such as eating, drinking, and escaping. The mapping from states to reward signals implemented by the critic is called a *reward function*. In RL the reward function is an essential component in specifying the problem the agent must learn to solve.

The agent's objective is to act at each moment of time so as to maximize a measure of the total quantity of reward it expects to receive over the future. This measure can be a simple sum of the reward signals it expects to receive over the future or more frequently, a discounted sum in which later reward signals are weighted less than earlier ones. The value of this measure at any time is the agent's *expected return*. Because the agent's actions influence how the environment's state changes over time, maximizing expected return requires the agent to exert control over the evolution of its environment's states. This can be very challenging. For example, the agent might have to sacrifice short-term reward in order to achieve more reward over the long term. The simplest RL agent's attempt to achieve this objective by adjusting a *policy*, which is a rule that associates actions to observed environment states. A policy corresponds to a stimulus–response (S–R) rule of animal learning theory. But RL is not restricted to simple S–R agents: more

[3]The term critic is used, and not "teacher", because in machine learning a teacher provides more informative instructional information, such as directly telling the agent what its actions *should have been* instead of merely scoring them.

complicated RL agents learn models of their environments that they can use to make plans about how to act appropriately.

Note that since return is a summation, a reward signal equal to zero does not contribute to it. Thus, despite the fact that the critic provides a signal at every moment of time, a signal of zero means "no reward." Many problems are characterized by reward signals for which nonzero values are relatively rare, occurring, for example, only after the completion of a long sequence of actions. This creates what is called the *problem of delayed rewards*, and much of RL is devoted to making learning efficient under these conditions.

The approach that has received the most attention focuses on RL agents that learn to predict return and then use these predictions to evaluate actions and to update their policies instead of using the primary reward signal itself. For example, in one class of methods, called *adaptive critic* methods (Barto et al. 1983), the agent contains a prediction component—an adaptive critic—that learns to predict return. An action that improves the likelihood of obtaining high return, as predicted by the adaptive critic, is reinforced. An increase in the prediction of return, then, acts as a reward itself. With these methods learning does not have to wait until a final goal is achieved.[4] This predictive ability of an adaptive critic mimics the phenomenon of *secondary*, or *conditioned*, reinforcement observed in animal learning (Mackintosh 1983). A secondary reinforcer is a stimulus that has become a reinforcer by virtue of being repeatedly paired in an appropriate temporal relationship with either a primary reinforcer or with another secondary reinforcer. In other words, a secondary reinforcer is a stimulus that has acquired, through a learning process, the ability to act as reinforcer itself.

Before going further, it is critical to comment on how this abstract RL formulation relates our view of an animal or a robot. An RL agent should not be thought of as an entire animal or robot. It should instead be thought of as the component *within* an animal or robot that handles reward-based learning. Thus, the box labeled "Environment" in Fig. 1 represents not only what is in the animal or robot's external world but also what is external to the reward-based learning component *while still being inside the animal or robot*. In particular, the critic in Fig. 1 should be thought of as part of an animal's nervous system and not as something in the animal's external world. Similarly, an RL agent's "actions" are not necessarily like an animal or robot's overt motor actions; they can also be actions that affect the agent's internal environment, such as the secretion of a hormone or the adjustment of a processing parameter.

It is also important to note that although the critic's signal at any time step is usually called a "reward" in the RL literature, it is better to call it a "reward signal" as it is labeled in Fig. 1. The reason for this is that psychologists and neuroscientists distinguish between rewards and reward signals. Schultz (2007a,b), for example,

[4]It is important to note that the adaptive critic of these methods is *inside* the RL agent, while the different critic shown in Fig. 1—that provides the primary reward signal—is in the RL agent's environment.

writes: "Rewards are objects or events that make us come back for more," whereas reward signals are produced by reward neurons in the brain. It is much more appropriate to think of the critic's signal as analogous to the output of a brain reward system than as an object or event in the animal's external world. These observations are important for understanding how the RL framework accommodates intrinsic reward signals. We return to these observations in Sect. 6.

Despite the fact that its roots are in theories of animal learning, RL is—with some exceptions—a collection of computational tools for use in artificial systems rather than a collection of animal behavior models. A wide range of facts about animal motivation are not usefully captured by the current RL framework. Dayan (2001), for example, correctly comments as follows:

> Reinforcement learning (RL) bears a tortuous relationship with historical and contemporary ideas in classical and instrumental conditioning. Although RL sheds important light in some murky areas, it has paid less attention to research concerning *motivation* of stimulus–response (SR) links.

A major reason for this neglect is that the mathematical framework of RL, as it is conventionally formulated (Sutton and Barto 1998), takes the existence of a reward signal as a given: the theory is not concerned with processes that generate reward signals. All that a well-posed RL problem requires is the specification of some (bounded) real-valued function from states to reward signals (or, in some cases, from state-action pairs or from state-action-next-state triples to reward signals). This not only sidesteps the entire subject of utility theory, which relates scalar measures to agent preferences, it also sidesteps many of the issues relevant to what (for an animal) would be called motivation.

Instead of being a shortcoming of the conventional RL framework, however, this level of abstraction has been a distinct advantage. It has allowed the theory of RL to progress in the absence of specific assumptions about how reward signals are generated in special cases. As a result, RL has been useful for a great many different types of problems, and it readily lends itself to being incorporated into a wide variety of comprehensive architectures for autonomous agents, in each of which different assumptions are made about how reward signals are generated. The abstract nature of RL is perhaps a major reason that it has been able to shed important light, as Dayan remarked, on some murky areas of biological data. Luckily, an account of intrinsic motivation in RL terms can be produced with only minor reduction in the framework's level of abstraction by introducing some assumptions about the nature of an RL agent's environment and reward signals. This is taken up in Sect. 6.

3 Motivation

Describing what the "hypothetical man on the street" means when asking why someone has behaved in a particular way, Cofer and Appley (1964) list three categories of factors: (1) irresistible external influences; (2) an internal urge, want, need, drive, plan, etc.; or (3) an external object or situation acting as a goal or incentive. The first of these exert their influence largely independently of the internal state of the organism as, for example, a reflexive withdrawal from a painful stimulus. The second two, in contrast, involve hypothesized internal states regarded as being necessary to explain the behavior. Incentive objects are external but are endowed with their behavior-controlling ability through the assignment to them of a state-dependent value by the organism. Motivational explanations of the strength and direction of behavior invoke an organism's internal state.

A clear example of the influence of internal motivational state on behavior is an experiment by Mollenauer (1971) as described by Dickinson and Balleine (2002). Rats were trained to run along an alleyway to obtain food. Rats in one group were trained while hungry, being food deprived before each training session, while rats in another group were nondeprived. The hungry rats consistently ran faster than did the sated rats. It might simply be that when rats are trained while they are hungry, they tend to run faster when the results of learning are tested. But the second part of Mollenauer's experiment showed that a shift in deprivation state had an immediate effect on the rat's performance. Rats in a third group were trained while hungry but tested when nondeprived. These rats immediately ran slower after this motivational shift. Instead of having to experience reduced reward for eating in the nondeprived state, their nondeprived state somehow exerted a direct and immediate influence on behavior. The kind of rapid behavioral change illustrated in this experiment and many others required theorists to postulate the existence of multiple internal motivational states. This experiment also illustrates the view taken by psychologists studying animal learning about how motivation and learning are intimately linked. Motivational factors can influence learning through their control over the effectiveness of reward and their control over how the results of learning are expressed in behavior.

The starting point for including motivational factors in the RL framework is to be clear about what we mean by an "internal state." In an extensive review of motivation for artificial agents, Savage (2000) focused on an "interactive view of motivation," attributed to Bindra (1978) and Toates (1986), that explains motivation in terms of a *central motive state* that depends on the interaction of an internal state and an external incentive factor:

$$\text{central motive state} = (\text{internal state}) \times (\text{incentive factor})$$

In Bindra's (1978) account, a central motive state arises through the interaction of an internal "organismic state" (such as arousal level, blood-sugar level, cellular dehydration, estrus-related hormonal levels) and features of an incentive object (such as features indicating the palatability of a food object).

The elaboration of the RL framework in Sect. 6 roughly follows this interactive view by factoring the RL problem's state into two components: a component internal to the animal or robot, and a component external to the animal or robot. This means that the RL problem's state at any time t is represented as a vector $s_t = (s_t^{\mathrm{i}}, s_t^{\mathrm{e}})$, where s_t^{i} and s_t^{e} are respectively the internal (cf. "organismic") and external state components (each of which can itself be a vector of many descriptive feature values). The nature of the dependency of reward signals on the internal dimensions is of particular importance for including intrinsic motivational factors in the RL framework.

There are many grounds for disputing this view of motivation, but at a commonsense level, it should be clear what is intended. If an organism is active in the sense of not being driven totally by environmental stimuli—a view that by now must be universal—then the organism must not implement a memoryless mapping from stimuli to responses, that is, there must be more than one internal state. Going further, McFarland and Bösser (1993) argue that for motivational descriptions of behavior to be meaningful, the agent has to have some degree of autonomy, that is, it must be capable of self-control, by which they mean that changes in behavior are the result of explicit decision processes that weigh behavioral alternatives. Thus, it would not be useful to talk about the behavior of a clockwork automaton in motivational terms even though it may have many internal states.

Among the influential theories of motivation in psychology are the drive theories of Hull (1943, 1951, 1952). According to Hull, all behavior is motivated either by an organism's survival and reproductive needs giving rise to primary drives (such as hunger, thirst, sex, and the avoidance of pain) or by derivative drives that have acquired their motivational significance through learning. Primary drives are the result of physiological deficits—"tissue needs"—and they energize behavior whose result is to reduce the deficit. A key additional feature of Hull's theories is that a need reduction, and hence a drive reduction, acts as a primary reward for learning: behavior that reduces a primary drive is reinforced. Additionally, through the process of secondary reinforcement in which a neutral stimulus is paired with a primary reward, the formerly neutral stimulus acquires the reinforcing power of the primary reward. In this way, stimuli that predict primary reward, that is, a reduction in a primary drive, become rewarding themselves. Thus, according to Hull, all behavior is energized and directed by its relevance to primal drives, either directly or as the result of learning through secondary reinforcement.

Hull's theories follow principles adapted from the concept of physiological homeostasis, the term introduced by Cannon (1932) to describe the condition in which bodily conditions are maintained in approximate equilibrium despite external perturbations. Homeostasis is maintained by processes that trigger compensatory reactions when the value of a critical physiological variable departs from the range required to keep the animal alive. This negative feedback mechanism maintains these values within required bounds. Many other theories of motivation also incorporate, in one form or another, the idea of behavior being generated to counteract disturbances to an equilibrium condition.

Although many of their elements have not been supported by experimental data, this and related theories continue to influence current thinking about motivation. They have been especially influential in the design of motivational systems for artificial agents, as discussed in Savage's review of artificial motivational systems (Savage 2000). Hull's idea that reward is generated by drive reduction is commonly used to connect RL to a motivational system. Often this mechanism consists of monitoring a collection of important variables, such as power or fuel level, temperature, etc., and triggering appropriate behavior when certain thresholds are reached. Drive reduction is directly translated into a reward signal for some type of RL algorithm.

Among other motivational theories are those based on the everyday experience that we engage in activities because we enjoy doing them: we seek pleasurable experiences and avoid unpleasant ones. These hedonic theories of motivation hold that it is necessary to refer to affective mental states to explain behavior, such as a "feeling" of pleasantness or unpleasantness. Hedonic theories are supported by many observations about food preferences which suggest that "palatability" might offer a more parsimonious account of food preferences than tissue needs (Young 1966). Animals will enthusiastically eat food that has no apparent positive influence on tissue needs; characteristics of food such as temperature and texture influence how much is eaten; animals that are not hungry still have preferences for different foods; animals have taste preferences from early infancy (Cofer and Appley 1964). In addition, nondeprived animals will work enthusiastically for electrical brain stimulation (Olds and Milner 1954).

Although it is clear that biologically primal needs have motivational significance, facts such as these showed that factors other than primary biological needs exert strong motivational effects.

4 Intrinsic Motivation

In addition to observations about animal food preferences and responses to electrical brain stimulation, other observations showed that something important was missing from drive-reduction theories of motivation. Under certain conditions, for example, hungry rats would rather explore unfamiliar spaces than eat; they will endure the pain of crossing electrified grids to explore novel spaces; monkeys will bar-press for a chance to look out of a window. Moreover, the opportunity to explore can be used to reinforce other behavior. Deci and Ryan (1985) chronicle these and a collection of similar findings under the heading of *intrinsic motivation*.[5]

The role of intrinsically motivated behavior in both children and adults is commonly noted as, for example, in this quotation from Deci and Ryan (1985):

> The human organism is inherently active, and there is perhaps no place where this is more evident than in little children. They pick things up, shake them, smell them, taste them, throw them across the room, and keep asking, "What is this?" They are unendingly curious, and they want to see the effects of their actions. Children are intrinsically motivated to learn, to undertake challenges, and to solve problems. Adults are also intrinsically motivated to do a variety of things. They spend large amounts of time painting pictures, building furniture, playing sports, whittling wood, climbing mountains, and doing countless other things for

[5] Deci and Ryan (1985) mention that the term intrinsic motivation was first used by Harlow (1950) in a study showing that rhesus monkeys will spontaneously manipulate objects and work for hours to solve complicated mechanical puzzles without any explicit rewards.

which there are not obvious or appreciable external rewards. The rewards are inherent in the activity, and even though there may be secondary gains, the primary motivators are the spontaneous, internal experiences that accompany the behavior. (Deci and Ryan 1985, p. 11)

Most psychologists now reject the view that exploration, manipulation, and other curiosity-related behaviors derive their motivational potency only through secondary reinforcement, as would be required by a theory like Hull's. There are clear experimental results showing that such behavior is motivationally energizing and rewarding on its own and not because it predicts the satisfaction of a primary biological need. Influential papers by White (1959) and Berlyne (1966) marshaled abundant experimental evidence to argue that the intrinsic reward produced by a variety of behaviors involving curiosity and play are as primary as that produced by the conventional biologically relevant behaviors. Children spontaneously explore very soon after birth, so there is little opportunity for them to experience the extensive pairing of this behavior with the reduction of a biologically primary drive that would be required to account for their eagerness to explore. In addition, experimental results show that the opportunity to explore retains its energizing effect without needing to be re-paired with a primary reward, whereas a secondary reward will extinguish, that is, will lose its reinforcing quality, unless often re-paired with the primary reward it predicts.

Berlyne summarized the situation as follows:

As knowledge accumulated about the conditions that govern exploratory behavior and about how quickly it appears after birth, it seemed less and less likely that this behavior could be a derivative of hunger, thirst, sexual appetite, pain, fear of pain, and the like, or that stimuli sought through exploration are welcomed because they have previously accompanied satisfaction of these drives. (Berlyne 1966, p. 26)

Note that the issue was not whether exploration, manipulation, and other curiosity-related behavior are important for an animal's survival and reproductive success. Clearly they are if deployed in the right way. Appropriately cautious exploration, for example, contributes to survival and reproductive success because it can enable efficient foraging, successful escape, and increased opportunities for mating. The issue was whether these behaviors have motivational valence because previously *in the animal's lifetime*, they predicted decreases in biologically primary drives or whether this valence is built in by the evolutionary process. Section 7 looks more closely at the utility of intrinsic motivation from an evolutionary perspective.

Researchers took a variety of approaches in revising homeostatic drive-reduction theories in light of findings like those described above. The simplest approach was to expand the list of primary drives by adding drives such as a curiosity drive, exploration drive, or manipulation drive, to the standard list of drives. Postulating primary "needs" for these behaviors, on par with needs for food, drink, and sex, marked a break from the standard view while retaining the orthodox drive-reduction principle. For example, an experiment by Harlow et al. (1950) showed that rhesus monkeys would learn how to unerringly unlatch a complex mechanical puzzle through many hours of manipulation without any contingent rewards such as food or water. They postulated a "strong and persistent manipulation drive" to explain how this was possible in the absence of extrinsic reward. Other experiments showed that giving an animal the opportunity to run in an activity wheel could act as reward for learning, suggesting that there is an "activity drive."

Postulating drives like these was in the tradition of earlier theorists who advanced broader hypotheses. For example, in a treatise on play, Groos (1901) proposed a motivational principle that we recognize as a major component of Piaget's (1952) theory of child development:

> The primitive impulse to extend the sphere of their power as far as possible leads men to the conquest and control of objects lying around them... We demand a knowledge of effects, and to be ourselves the producers of effects. (Groos 1901, p. 95)

Similarly, Hendrick (1942) proposed an "instinct to master" by which an animal has "an inborn drive to do and to learn how to do."

In a 1959 paper that has been called "one of the most influential papers on motivation ever published" (Arkes and Garske 1982), Robert White (1959) argued that lengthening the list of primary drives in this way would require such fundamental changes to the drive concept as to leave it unrecognizable. Drives for exploration, manipulation, and activity do not involve "tissue needs"; they are not terminated by an explicit consummatory climax but rather tend to decrease gradually; and reinforcement can result from the increase in such a drive rather than a decrease: for example, when an exploring animal seeks out novelty rather than avoids it. If decreasing exploratory drive corresponds to boredom, one does not normally think of boredom as a reinforcer for exploration.

White proposed that instead of extending the list of the standard drives, it would be better to emphasize the similarity of urges toward exploration, manipulation, and activity, and how they differ from the homeostatic drives. He proposed bringing them together under the general heading of *competence*, by which he meant *effective interaction with the environment*, and to speak of a general *effectance motivation* to refer to "an intrinsic need to deal with the environment." Like other critics of homeostatic theories, White did not argue that such theories are completely wrong, only that they are incomplete. With respect to effectance motivation, for example, he wrote that

> ...the effectance urge represents what the neuromuscular system wants to do when it is otherwise unoccupied or is gently stimulated by the environment. ... [it] is persistent in the sense that it regularly occupies the spare waking time between episodes of homeostatic crisis. (White 1959, p. 321)

The psychology literature is less helpful in specifying the concrete properties of experience that incite intrinsically motivated behavior, although there have been many suggestions. White (1959) suggested that Hebb (1949) may have been right in concluding that "difference in sameness" is the key to interest, meaning that along with many familiar features, a situation that is interesting also has novel ones, indicating that there is still more learning to be done. Berlyne (1954, 1960, 1971) probably had the most to say on these issues, suggesting that the factors underlying intrinsic motivational effects involve novelty (with a distinction between relative and absolute novelty, and between short-term and long-term novelty), surprise and incongruity (when expectations or hypotheses are not vindicated by experience), or complexity (depending on the number and similarity of elements in a situation).

Uniting these cases, Berlyne hypothesized a notion of conflict created when a situation incites multiple processes that do not agree with one another. He also hypothesized that moderate levels of novelty (or more generally, arousal potential) have the highest hedonic value because the rewarding effect of novelty is overtaken by an aversive effect as novelty increases (as expressed by the "Wundt Curve," p. 89, of Berlyne 1971). This is consistent with many other views holding that situations intermediate between complete familiarity (boredom) and complete unfamiliarity (confusion) have the most hedonic value: the maximal effect of novelty being elicited by "... a stimulus that is rather like something well known but just distinct enough to be 'interesting' " (Berlyne 1960). Many of these hypotheses fall under the heading of optimal level theories, which we describe in more detail below.

The role of surprise in intrinsic motivation that Berlyne and others have suggested requires some discussion in order to prevent a common misunderstanding. Learning from surprise in the form of mismatch between expectations and actuality is built into many learning theories and machine learning algorithms. The Rescorla-Wagner (1972) model of classical conditioning and the many error-correction learning rules studied under the heading of *supervised learning* by machine learning researchers, such as perceptrons (Rosenblatt 1962) and error back-propagation neural networks (Rumelhart et al. 1986), adjust parameters on the basis of discrepancies between expected and experienced input. Tolman's (1932) theory of latent learning, for example, postulated that animals are essentially *always learning* cognitive maps that incorporate confirmed expectancies about their environments. But according to Tolman, this learning is unmotivated: it does not depend on reinforcing stimuli or motivational state. This is different from Berlyne's view that surprise engages an animal's motivational systems. Therefore, it is necessary to distinguish between learning from surprise as it appears in supervised learning algorithms and the idea that surprise engages motivational systems.

4.1 Optimal Level Theories

To provide alternatives to homeostatic drive-reduction theories, and to avoid postulating additional drives for exploration, manipulation, etc., motivational theorists proposed a number of influential theories characterized as optimal level theories. This section describes one of these at some length because it suggests useful principles anticipating several recent computational theories. This account is drawn largely from Arkes and Garske (1982).

Dember et al. (1957) conducted an experiment involving an animal's preferences for stimuli of differing levels of complexity. They placed rats in a figure-eight runway having walls with vertical black and white stripes on one loop and horizontal black and white stripes on the other. To the moving rat, the horizontal stripes provided a roughly constant visual stimulus, whereas the vertical stripes provided a more complex time-varying stimulus pattern. With one rat in the runway at a time, they recorded the amount of time each rat spent in each loop. They found that a rat that initially preferred the loop with the horizontal stripes would later spend the preponderance of its time in the loop with the vertical stripes. Rats that initially preferred the vertical-striped loop rarely shifted preference to the horizontal-striped loop. In another experiment, the horizontal stripes provided the more complex stimulus (compared to plain white or plain black walls), and the rats shifted preference to the horizontal stripes, thus ruling out the possibility that the behavior was due to some peculiarity of horizontal and vertical stripes.

Dember et al. (1957) proposed an explanation for this behavior, elaborated by Dember and Earl (1957) as "the pacer principle." It is based on two key ideas. The first is that animals get used to a certain level of environmental complexity, and if they continue too long with stimuli of that complexity, they will become bored since they had already learned about stimuli of that complexity. A slightly more complex stimulus, on the other hand, will be interesting to them and will arouse curiosity, while an extremely more complex stimulus will be confusing or even frightening. So an animal will maximally prefer stimuli that are moderately more complex than what they are used to. Dember and Earl used the term *pacer*, presumably from horse racing, to refer to the level of stimulus complexity that is maximally preferred. The second idea, which is common to other optimal level theories, is that as a result of experience with a stimulus, the stimulus becomes simpler to the animal. As Dember and Earl (1957) state, this is due to "the ability of stimuli to increase the psychological complexity of the individual who perceives them." Consequently, an animal's experience with a preferred stimulus situation causes their preferences to shift toward situations of moderately increased complexity: experience with a pacer causes the pacer to shift toward increased complexity. This generates a motivational force causing the animal to constantly seek stimuli of increasing complexity.

Berlyne's (1954, 1960, 1971) ideas, mentioned above, also fall under the heading of optimal level theory, and much of his work focused on trying to determine the stimulus properties that underlie an animal's preferences. He considered properties such as novelty, incongruity, and surprisingness as contributing to the arousal potential of a stimulus and that an animal will prefer some intermediate level of arousal potential.

Optimal level theories have been very influential, with applications in child development, where both excessive and deficient amounts of stimulation may be detrimental to cognitive growth, in architecture, city planning, esthetics, economics, and music (Arkes and Garske 1982). The recent computational theory of Schmidhuber (2009) that places information-theoretic compression at the base of intrinsic motivation might be regarded as a modern descendant of optimal level theories.

4.2 Intrinsic Motivation and Competence

In his classic paper, White (1959) argued that intrinsically motivated behavior is essential for an organism to gain the *competence* necessary for autonomy, where by autonomy he meant the extent to which an organism is able to bring its environment under its control, to achieve mastery over its environment. Through intrinsically motivated activity, an organism is able to learn much of what is possible in an environment and how to realize these possibilities. A system that is competent in this sense has *broad set of reusable skills* for controlling its environment; it is able to interact effectively with its environment toward a wide variety of ends. The activity through which these broad skills are learned is motivated by an intrinsic reward system that favors the development of broad competence rather than being directed to more specific externally directed goals.

White's view of competence greatly influenced this author's thinking and that of his colleagues and students about the utility of analogs of intrinsic motivation for RL systems. Being competent in an environment by having a broad set of reusable skills enables an agent to efficiently learn how to solve a wide range of specific problems as they arise while it engages with that environment. Although the acquisition of competence is not driven by specific problems, this competence is routinely enlisted to solve many different specific problems over the agent's lifetime. The skills making up general competence act as the "building blocks" out of which an agent can form solutions to specific problems. Instead of facing each new challenge by trying to create a solution out of low-level primitives, it can focus on combining and adjusting its higher-level skills. This greatly increases the efficiency of learning to solve new problems, and it is a major reason that the relatively long developmental period of humans serves us so well.

By combining this view of competence with the theory and algorithms of hierarchical RL (Barto and Mahadevan 2003), the author and colleagues have taken some small steps toward developing artificial agents with this kind of competence, calling the approach *intrinsically motivated RL* (Barto et al. 2004; Singh et al. 2005). Evaluating the performance of these agents requires taking into account performance over ensembles of tasks instead of just single tasks. Intrinsically motivated RL therefore addresses the well-known shortcoming of many current machine learning systems—including RL systems—that they typically apply to single, isolated problems and do not yet allow systems to cope flexibly with new problems as they arise over extended periods of time. This brings the study of intrinsically motivated RL together with what cognitive scientists, roboticists, and machine learning researchers call "autonomous mental development" (Weng et al. 2001), "epigenetic robotics" (Prince et al. 2001), or "developmental robotics" (Lungarella et al. 2003), approaches aiming to develop analogs of the developmental processes that prepare animals over long time periods for a wide range of later challenges.

This competence-based view of intrinsically motivated RL contrasts with the view most prominently put forward in the work of Schmidhuber (2009) that intrinsic motivation's sole purpose is to facilitate learning a world model in order to make accurate predictions. The competence view, in contrast, emphasizes the utility of learning skills that allow effective environmental control. Of course, learning such skills can benefit from the learning of models, and machinery for doing so is built into hierarchical RL algorithms (Barto and Mahadevan 2003; Sutton et al. 1999), but such models need only be limited, local models that focus on environmental regularities relevant to particular skills. On a deeper level, this view arises from the conviction that control rather than prediction must have played the dominant role in the evolution of cognition. The utility of prediction arises solely through its role in facilitating control. Although we cannot control the weather, we use weather predictions to control its impact on us: we cancel the picnic, carry an umbrella, etc. Of course, because prediction is so useful for control, we would expect intrinsic motivational mechanisms to exist that encourage accurate prediction, but according to the competence view, this is not the sole underlying purpose of intrinsic motivation.[6]

5 Motivation and Reinforcement Learning

Although many computational models of RL contributed to how it is now studied in machine learning (e.g., Clark and Farley 1955; Mendel and Fu 1970; Mendel and McLaren 1970; Michie and Chambers 1968; Minsky 1954; Narendra and Thathachar 1989; Widrow et al. 1973), a most influential collection of ideas are those of A.H. Klopf—especially as it concerns the author and his students and our influence on RL. Klopf (1972, 1982) argued that homeostasis should not be considered the primary goal of behavior and learning and that it is not a suitable organizing principle for developing artificial intelligence. Instead, he argued that organisms strive for a maximal condition:

> It will be proposed here that homeostasis is not the primary goal of more phylogenetically advanced living systems; rather, that it is a secondary or subgoal. It is suggested that the primary goal is a condition which . . . will be termed heterostasis. An organism is said to be in a condition of heterostasis with respect to a specific internal variable when that variable has been maximized. (Klopf 1982, p. 10)

This proposal is built into all RL systems, where maximization—or, more generally, optimization—is the guiding principle instead of equilibrium seeking. This basis of RL commonly generates several questions that deserve comment. First, what is the difference between maximization and equilibrium seeking? There is clearly no logical difference between maximizing and minimizing (one simply changes a sign: both are optimization) and is not an equilibrium-seeking

[6]Schmidhuber (2009) would argue that it is the other way around—that control is a result of behavior directed to improve predictive models, which in this author's opinion is at odds with what we know about evolution.

system engaged in minimizing, specifically, minimizing the discrepancy between the current and the desired state? It is correct that equilibrium seeking involves minimizing, but it is a restricted variety of minimization based on assumptions that are not true in general. Consider the difference between searching for something that you will recognize when you find it, such as a specific web site, and searching for the "best" of something, such as (what you consider to be) the best-tasting wine. In the former case, when the desired item is found, the search stops, whereas in the latter, the search must go on—at least in principle—until you have sampled every variety (and year) of wine. The former case is like equilibrium seeking: the search is looking for zero discrepancy between the current and desired state, whereas the latter is like RL, where incessant exploration is called for.

A second question that comes up with regard to RL's focus on optimization is this one: does this not conflict with the commonly made observation that nature does not seem to optimize, at either ontogenetic or phylogenetic scales? Since biological adaptation does not produce optimal solutions, any view of nature based on optimization must be incorrect. The answer to this is that adopting an optimization framework does not imply that the results are always optimal. Indeed, in many large-scale optimization problems, globally optimal results are hardly ever achieved, and even if they were, one would never know it. The focus is on the *process*, which involves incessant exploration, and not the desired outcomes—which are almost never achieved.

Its emphasis on optimization instead of equilibrium seeking makes RL closer to hedonic views of motivation than to Hullian views. However, whereas a hedonic view of motivation is usually associated with affective mental states, RL—at least as described by Sutton and Barto (1998)—does not venture in to this territory. There is no mention of a "feeling" of pleasantness or unpleasantness associated with reward or penalty. This may be excluding an important dimension but that dimension is not an essential component of a framework based on optimization. What is essential is RL's attitude toward the following questions put forward by Cofer and Appley (1964):

> Is organismic functioning conservative or growth oriented? ... Does the organism's behavior serve primarily to maintain a steady state or equilibrium, that is, is it homeostatically organized and conservative? Or, alternatively, does the organism's behavior serve to take it to new levels of development, unfolding potentialities that a conservative principle could not encompass? (Cofer and Appley 1964, p. 15)

This nonconservative view of motivation, as contrasted with one based on maintaining equilibrium, is a good summary of what makes RL and other frameworks based on optimization attractive approaches to designing intelligent agents.

The importance of this for learning, especially machine learning, is that the learning algorithms most commonly studied are suitable only for supervised learning problems. As discussed above, these algorithms work by making adjustments directed toward eliminating mismatches between expectations and what actually occurs. They are therefore essentially equilibrium-seeking mechanisms in the sense of attempting to zero out an error measure. Indeed, learning algorithms such as

Rosenblatt's (1962) perceptron and Widrow and Hoff's Adaline (Widrow and Hoff 1960), and their many descendants, explicitly employ the negative feedback principle of an equilibrium-seeking servo mechanism. An RL algorithm, in contrast, is attempting to extremize a quantity, specifically a measure of reward. Although supervised learning clearly has its place, the RL framework's emphasis on incessant activity over equilibrium seeking makes it essential—in the author's opinion—for producing growth-oriented systems with open-ended capacities.[7]

6 Intrinsically Motivated RL

In the RL framework, an agent works to maximize a quantity based on an abstract reward signal that can be derived in many different ways. As emphasized in Sects. 1 and 2, the RL framework "does not care" where the reward signal comes from. The framework can therefore encompass both homeostatic theories of motivation in which reward signals are defined in terms of drive reduction, as has been done in many motivational systems for artificial agents (Savage 2000), and non-homeostatic theories that can account, for example, for the behavioral effects of electrical brain stimulation and addictive drugs. It can also include intrinsic reward signals.

In presenting the basic RL framework in Sect. 2, we emphasized that an RL agent should not be thought of as an entire animal or robot, and that the box labeled "Environment" in Fig. 1 represents not only an animal's or robot's external world but also components within the animal or robot itself. Figure 2 is a refinement of Fig. 1 that makes this explicit by dividing the environment into an *external environment* and an *internal environment*. The external environment represents what is outside of the animal or robot (which we will refer to as an "organism", as labeled in the figure), whereas the internal environment consists of components that are inside the organism.[8] Both components together comprise the environment of the RL agent.[9]

This refinement of the usual RL framework makes it clear that *all reward signals are generated within the organism*. Some reward signals may be triggered by sensations produced by objects or events in the external environment, such as a pat on the head or a word of praise; others may be triggered by a combination of external stimulation and conditions of the internal environment, such as drinking water in a state of thirst. Still other reward signals may be triggered solely by activity of the

---

[7] These comments apply to the "passive" form of supervised learning and not necessarily to the extension known as "active learning" (Settles 2009), in which the learning agent itself chooses training examples. Although beyond this chapter's scope, active supervised learning is indeed relevant to the subject of intrinsic motivation.

[8] We are relying on a commonsense notion of an organism's boundary with its external environment, recognizing that this may be not be easy to define.

[9] Figure 2 shows the organism containing a single RL agent, but an organism might contain many, each possibly having its own reward signal. Although not considered here, the multi-agent RL case (Busoniu et al. 2008) poses many challenges and opportunities.

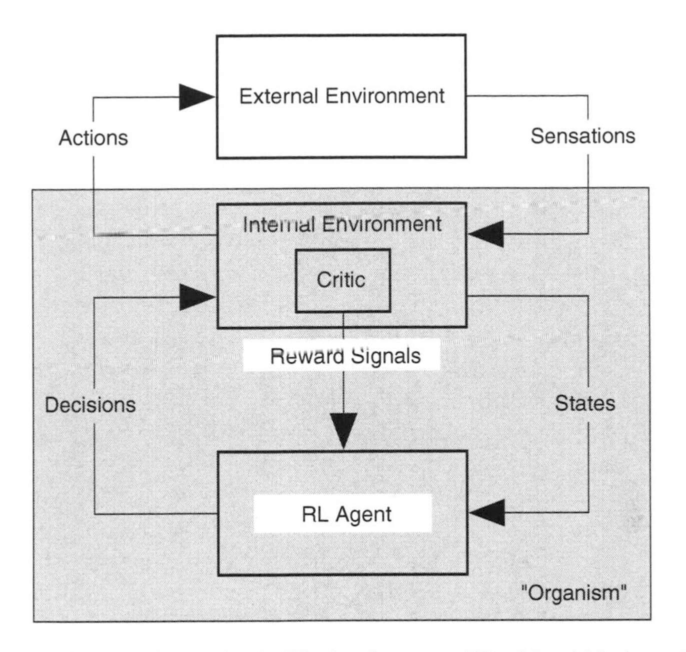

Fig. 2 Agent–environment interaction in RL. A refinement of Fig. 1 in which the environment is divided into an internal and external environment, with all reward signals coming from the former. The *shaded box* corresponds to what we would think of as the "organism." Adapted from Barto et al. (2004)

internal environment, such as entertaining a thought or recalling a memory. All of these possibilities can be accommodated by the RL framework as long as one does not identify an RL agent with a complete organism.

It is tempting to directly connect the distinction between the external and internal environments with the distinction between extrinsic and intrinsic reward signals: extrinsic reward signals are triggered by objects or events in the external environment, whereas intrinsic reward signals are triggered solely by activity of the internal environment. Unfortunately, this view does not do justice to the complexity and variability of either extrinsically or intrinsically rewarding behavior.

According to Bindra's (1978) account mentioned in Sect. 3, for example, an organism's internal state, such as arousal level, blood-sugar level, and hormone levels, interacts with features of an object or event signaled by external stimulation to generate a central motive state. Assuming this central motive state influences the generation of reward signals, this account clearly involves both the organism's internal and external environments. Even putting aside Bindra's account, it is clear that the state of an organism's internal environment modulates how external stimulation is transduced into reward signals. Moreover, for many instances of what we would consider intrinsically motivated activity, for example, when behavior is the result of pure curiosity, an organism's external environment is often a key player: objects and events in the external environment trigger curiosity, surprise, and other constituents of intrinsically motivated behavior.

Despite the difficulty of aligning extrinsic and intrinsic reward signals with an organism's external and internal environments, the internal environment may play a larger—or at least, a different—role in generating reward signals associated with intrinsic motivation. For example, a salient external stimulus might generate a reward signal to the degree that it is unexpected, where the expectancy is evaluated by processes in the internal environment and information stored there. Novelty, surprise, incongruity, and other features that have been hypothesized to underlie intrinsic motivation all depend on what the agent has already learned and experienced, that is, on its memories, beliefs, and internal knowledge state, all of which are components of the state of the organism's internal environment. One can think of these as the "informational," as opposed to the vegetative, aspects of the internal environment.

The approach to intrinsically motivated RL taken by the author and colleagues is to include these kinds of rewards as components of the RL agent's primary reward function. This is consistent with the large body of data alluded to above showing that intrinsically motivated behavior is not dependent on secondary reinforcement, that is, behavior is not intrinsically motivated because it had previously been paired with the satisfaction of a primary biological need in the animal's own experience (Deci and Ryan 1985). It is also in accord with Schmidhuber's (1991b, 2009) approach to curious RL systems where both normal and curious behavior use the same mechanism. *Some* behavior that we might call intrinsically motivated could be motivated through learned secondary reward signals, but this is not a necessary feature.

If the internal/external environment dichotomy does not provide a way to cleanly distinguish between extrinsic and intrinsic reward signals, what does? The author's current view is that there is no clean distinction between these types of reward signals; instead, there is a continuum ranging from clearly extrinsic to clearly intrinsic. This view is the result of considering the issue from an evolutionary perspective, which is taken up next.

7 Evolutionary Perspective

Intrinsically motivated behavior is not anomalous from an evolutionary perspective. Intrinsically motivated behavior and what animals learn from it clearly contribute to reproductive success. The evolutionary success of humans (up to the present at least) owes a lot to our intrinsic urge to control our environments. It is not surprising, then, that machinery has evolved for ensuring that animals gain the kinds of experiences from which they can acquire knowledge and skills useful for survival and reproduction. Building in reward mechanisms to motivate knowledge-acquiring and skill-acquiring behavior is a parsimonious way of achieving this—enlisting motivational processes to appropriately direct behavior. From an evolutionary perspective, then, there is nothing particularly mysterious about intrinsically motivated behavior. But can an evolutionary perspective help us understand the relationship between intrinsic and extrinsic motivation and reward signals?

Inspired in part by economists Samuelson and Swinkels (2006), who asked the following question:

> ... given that successful descendants are the currency of evolutionary success, why do people have utility for anything else? (Samuelson and Swinkels 2006, p. 120),

Singh et al. (2009, 2010) placed reward processes in an evolutionary context, formulating a notion of an *optimal reward function* given an evolutionary fitness function and a distribution of environments. Results of computational experiments suggest how both extrinsically and intrinsically motivated behaviors may emerge from such optimal reward functions. The approach taken in these studies was to evaluate entire primary reward functions in terms of how well simulated RL agents' learning according to these reward functions performed as evaluated by a separate "evolutionary fitness function." An automated search in a space of primary reward functions could then be conducted to see which reward function would confer the most evolutionary advantage to the learning agent. Key to this approach is that each agent's behavior was evaluated across multiple environments, where some features remained constant across all the environments and others varied from environment to environment.

Readers should consult Singh et al. (2009, 2010) for details, but a main lesson from these studies is that the difference between intrinsic and extrinsic reward may be one of degree rather than one that can be rigorously defined by specific features. When coupled with learning, a primary reward function that rewards behavior that is *ubiquitously useful across many different environments* can produce greater evolutionary fitness than a function exclusively rewarding behavior directly related to the most basic requisites of survival and reproduction. For example, since eating is necessary for evolutionary success in all environments, we see primary reward signals generated by eating-related behavior. But reward functions that in addition reward behavior less directly related to basic needs, such as exploration and play, can confer greater evolutionary fitness to an agent. This is because what is learned during exploration and play contributes, within the lifetime of an animal, to that animal's ability to reproduce. It is therefore not surprising that evolution would give exploration, play, etc. positive hedonic valence, that is, would make them rewarding.

A possible conclusion from this evolutionary perspective is that what we call extrinsically rewarding stimuli or events are those that have a relatively immediate and direct relationship to evolutionary success. What we call intrinsically rewarding activities, on the other hand, bear a much more distal relationship to evolutionary success. The causal chain from these behaviors to evolutionary success is longer, more complex, and less certain than the chain from what we typically call extrinsically motivated behavior. This makes it difficult to recognize evolutionarily beneficial consequences of intrinsically motivated behavior. Berlyne (1960) used the term "ludic behavior" (from the Latin *ludare*, to play) which "... can best be defined as any behavior that does not have a biological function that we can clearly recognize." It is not clear that this property adequately characterizes all intrinsically motivated behavior, but it does capture something essential about it.

The relationship between intrinsic reward and evolutionary success is analogous to the relationship between learned, or secondary, reward and primary reward. In the latter case, a stimulus or activity comes to a generate reward signals to the extent that it predicts future primary reward. This is the basic mechanism built into RL algorithms that estimate value functions. Behavior is selected on the basis of predictions of the total amount of primary reward expected to accrue over the future, as represented by the learned value function (see Sect. 2). Through this process, good actions can be selected even when their influence on future primary reward is only very indirect. Imagine, for example, an early move in a game of backgammon that helps to set the stage for a much later advance, which ultimately results in winning the game. An RL algorithm such as the one used in the program TD-Gammon (Tesauro 1994) uses the value function it learns to effectively reward this move immediately when it is taken.

A similar situation occurs in the case of intrinsic reward, except that in this case a stimulus or activity comes to elicit a *primary* reward signal to the extent that it predicts eventual *evolutionary* success. In this case, the evolutionary process confers a rewarding quality to the stimulus or activity. Although this is clearly different from what happens with secondary reward, where a stimulus becomes rewarding through learning that takes place within the lifetime of an individual animal, in both cases the rewarding quality arises due to a predictive relationship to a "higher-level" measure of success: reproductive success in the case of evolution and primary reward in the case of secondary reinforcement.

This evolutionary context provides insight into the kinds of behavior we might expect an evolved reward function to encourage. We might expect a reward function to evolve that "taps into" features that were constant across many ancestral generations, but we would not expect one to evolve that exploits features that change from generation to generation. For example, if food tends to be found in places characterized by certain fixed features, we might expect a primary reward signal to be elicited by these features to encourage approach behavior. However, we would not expect approach to specific spatial locations to be rewarding unless these locations were the loci of sustenance for generation after generation. Learning can exploit features that maintain relatively fixed relationships to reward within a single agent's lifetime, whereas the evolutionary process is able to exploit larger-scale constancies that transcend individual agents and environments.

As a consequence, an animal's reward systems will promote behavior that is *ubiquitously useful across many different environments*. In some cases, this behavior's utility is easily recognizable and appears to be directed toward a proximal goal with obvious biological significance. In other cases, the behavior's utility is difficult to recognize because it contributes more indirectly and with less certainty to evolutionary success: its purpose or goal may be so far removed from the behavior itself that it may appear to have no clear purpose at all.

A somewhat similar relationship exists between basic and applied, or programmatic, research. In arguing for the importance of basic research in his famous report to the United States president, Vannevar Bush (1945) wrote

> Basic research is performed without thought of practical ends. It results in general knowledge and an understanding of nature and its laws. This general knowledge provides the means of answering a large number of important practical problems, though it may not give a complete specific answer to any one of them. The function of applied research is to provide such complete answers. The scientist doing basic research may not be at all interested in the practical applications of his work, yet the further progress of industrial development would eventually stagnate if basic scientific research were long neglected ... Basic research leads to new knowledge. It provides scientific capital. It creates the fund from which the practical applications of knowledge must be drawn. (Bush 1945)

It is not misleading to think of basic research as intrinsically motivated, whereas applied research is extrinsically motivated, being directed toward a specific identifiable end. Bush was asserting that basic research has enormous practical utility, but it is not an immediate or certain consequence of the activity.

Although the distinction between basic and applied research seems clear enough, one may be hard pressed to point to features of specific research activities that would mark them, out of a broader context, as being conducted as part of a basic or an applied research project. The same seems true of intrinsically and extrinsically motivated behavior. The evolutionary perspective suggests that there are no hard and fast features distinguishing intrinsic and extrinsic reward signals. There is rather a continuum along which the directness of the relationship varies between sources of reward signals and evolutionary success. The claim here is that what we call intrinsically rewarding behavior is behavior that occupies the range of this continuum in which the relationship is relatively indirect. Whether it is direct or indirect, moreover, this relationship to evolutionary success is based on environmental characteristics that have remained relatively constant, though of varying reliability, over many generations.

This leads to a final observation that reconciles this view of intrinsic reward signals with others that have been put forward, for example, by Oudeyer and Kaplan (2007). Prominent among environmental features that maintain a relatively constant relationship to evolutionary success are features of the internal portion of an organism's environment, as depicted in Fig. 2. What is labeled there the internal environment is carried along in relatively unchanging form from generation to generation. The internal environment is clearly being altered as a result of evolution, but these changes are very slow compared to the changes in the external environment that occur from generation to generation. Therefore, we would expect an animal's primary reward function to encourage a variety of behaviors that involve features of this part of the learning system's environment. This would include behaviors that we think of as involving curiosity, novelty, surprise, and other internally mediated features usually associated with intrinsic reward. Thus, in addition to suggesting why it seems so difficult to place the distinction between intrinsic and extrinsic reward on a rigorous footing, the evolutionary perspective suggests an explanation for why the prototypical examples of activities that we think of as intrinsically rewarding tend to heavily depend on variables that describe aspects of an animal's internal environment.

There is clearly much more to understand about the relationship between evolution and learning, and there is a large literature on the subject. Less has been written about the evolution of reward structures, though a number of computational studies have been published (Ackley and Littman 1991; Damoulas et al. 2005; Elfwing et al. 2008; Littman and Ackley 1991; Schembri et al. 2007; Snel and Hayes 2008; Uchibe and Doya 2008). In addition to Singh et al. (2009, 2010), the most relevant computational study of which the author is aware is that of Ackley and Littman (1991). Sorg et al. (2010) provide computational results to support the view that a key role played by reward functions is to attenuate the negative consequences of various types of agent limitations, such as lack of information, lack of adequate time to learn, or lack of efficient learning mechanisms. This view is critical to reaching a better understanding of intrinsic motivation, and it is consistent with observations from economists who study the *evolution of preferences* in the context of game theory (Samuelson 2001).

8 Summary and Prospects

This chapter focuses on review and perspective while saying little about architectures and algorithms for intrinsically motivated artificial agents. However, some general conclusions are supported by the views presented here that can help guide the development of competently autonomous artificial agents:

1. *RL is particularly suited for incorporating principles of motivation into artificial agents, including intrinsic motivation.* This chapter argues that an approach to building intelligent agents based on principles of optimization, instead of solely equilibrium seeking, gives agents the kind of incessant activity that is essential for growth-oriented systems with open-ended capacities. A base in optimization does not mean that optimal solutions need ever be found: it is the process that is important.
2. *The distinction between an RL agent and its environment at the base of the RL formulation has to be looked at in the right way.* An RL agent is not the same as an entire animal or robot. Motivational processes involve state components that are internal to the animal or robot while at the same time being external to the RL agent. The sources of reward signals are, as is usual in the RL framework, external to the RL agent (so it cannot exert complete control over them) while still being within the animal or robot.
3. *State components that influence an RL agent's reward signals can include features of a robot's memories and beliefs in addition to "vegetative" features.* This follows from item (2) directly above since this information is part of the RL agent's environment. In fact, a robot's current policy, value function, and environment model are all possible influences on reward signals since they are

components of the state of the RL agent's environment. This opens the possibility for defining many interesting reward functions.

4. *The view that motivation can be equated with the nature of an RL reward function is only part of the story.* In a reward-maximizing framework, there is a natural correspondence between the reward function and the forces that direct agent activity. However, this does not imply that the nature of a reward function accounts for all aspects of an agent's motivations. In both modeling biological agents and building artificial agents, other components are important as well. For example, there are prominent roles for complex structures of built-in behaviors, and there may be multiple optimizing components with different objectives, requiring arbitration mechanisms to coordinate among competing goals. Further, interesting theories relevant to intrinsic motivation but not based on RL should not be overlooked (e.g., Andry et al. 2004; Baranes and Oudeyer 2010; Friston et al. 2010; Hesse et al. 2009).
5. *There is no hard and fast distinction between extrinsic and intrinsic reward signals.* There is rather a continuum along which reward signals fall, ranging from signals clearly related to proximal goals with obvious biological utility to signals with less direct and less reliable biological utility. These latter signals underlie what we think of as intrinsically motivated behavior. This view is suggested by recent computational studies by Singh and colleagues (Singh et al. 2009, 2010), which explore the concept of evolutionarily optimal reward functions as discussed in Sect. 7.
6. *Despite the difficulty in giving the extrinsic/extrinsic distinction a completely satisfactory formal definition, the distinction is still useful.* In particular, the psychologist's definition, where extrinsic motivation means doing something because of some specific rewarding outcome and intrinsic motivation means "doing something because it is inherently interesting or enjoyable" (Ryan and Deci 2000), is adequate for most purposes. It alerts us to the possible benefits of defining reward functions that depend on a wider range of factors than those usually considered in RL. Specifically, reward functions can depend on the state of a robot's internal environment, which includes remembered and learned information.
7. *It is not likely that there is a single unitary principle underlying intrinsic motivation.* Although the evolutionary perspective presented here does not give detailed information about what architectures and algorithms we should develop to produce intrinsically motivated artificial agents, it does suggest that the best reward functions will depend on the distribution of tasks at which we wish the agent to excel. Therefore, although some principles are undoubtedly widely applicable—such as some of those already receiving attention in the literature—skepticism is justified about the proposition that one principle suffices to account for all aspects of intrinsic motivation.
8. *Analogs of intrinsic motivation are destined to play important roles in future machine learning systems.* In the same way that intrinsic motivation plays a crucial role in directing human behavior for both children and adults, we can expect computational analogs to be important for directing the behavior of

machine learning systems that are able to exert some control over their input by being embedded in physical or virtual worlds. Moreover, the progress occurring in making computational power a ubiquitous resource means that learning systems can be constantly active, even when they are not engaged in solving particular problems. Intrinsic motivation is the means for making the most of such idle times in preparation for problems to come. In the introduction to his 1960 treatise on curiosity, Berlyne wrote the following:

> Until recently, rather little has been done to find out how animals behave, whether in the wild or in captivity, when they have nothing particular to do. (Berlyne 1960, p. 1)

Although we may know—or at least hope we know!—what our computers are doing when they have nothing particular to do, it is clear that, like animals, they could be working to build the competencies needed for when they are called to action.

9 Conclusion

Building intrinsic motivation into artificial agents may bring to mind all the warnings from science fiction about the dangers of truly autonomous robots. But there are good reasons for wanting artificial agents to have the kind of broad competence that intrinsically motivated learning can enable. Autonomy is becoming a more common property of automated systems since it allows them to successfully operate for extended periods of time in dynamic, complex, and dangerous environments about which little a priori knowledge is available. As automated systems inevitably assume more "unpluggable" roles in our lives, *competent autonomy* is becoming increasingly essential to prevent the kind of catastrophic breakdowns that threaten our society. In a real sense, we already depend on systems, such as the power grid, that are essentially autonomous but seriously lacking in competence. Providing them with intrinsic motivations carefully crafted to embody desirable standards may be a path toward making artificial agents competent enough to fulfill their promise of improving human lives.

Acknowledgements The author thanks Satinder Singh, Rich Lewis, and Jonathan Sorg for developing the evolutionary perspective on this subject and for their important insights, and colleagues Sridhar Mahadevan and Rod Grupen, along with current and former members of the Autonomous Learning Laboratory who have participated in discussing intrinsically motivated reinforcement learning: Bruno Castro da Silva, Will Dabney, Jody Fanto, George Konidaris, Scott Kuindersma, Scott Niekum, Özgür Şimşek, Andrew Stout, Phil Thomas, Chris Vigorito, and Pippin Wolfe. The author thanks Pierre-Yves Oudeyer for his many helpful suggestions, especially regarding non-RL approaches to intrinsic motivation. Special thanks are due to Prof. John W. Moore, whose expert guidance through the psychology literature was essential to writing this chapter, though any misrepresentation of psychological thought is strictly due to the author. This research has benefitted immensely from the author's association with the European Community 7th Framework Programme (FP7/2007-2013), "Challenge 2: Cognitive Systems, Interaction, Robotics", Grant Agreement No. ICT-IP-231722, project "IM-CLeVeR: Intrinsically Motivated

Cumulative Learning Versatile Robots." Some of the research described here was supported by the National Science Foundation under Grant No. IIS-0733581 and by the Air Force Office of Scientific Research under grant FA9550-08-1-0418. Any opinions, findings, conclusions, or recommendations expressed here are those of the author and do not necessarily reflect the views of the sponsors.

References

Ackley, D.H., Littman, M.: Interactions between learning and evolution. In: Langton, C., Taylor, C., Farmer, C., Rasmussen, S. (eds.) Artificial Life II (Proceedings Volume X in the Santa Fe Institute Studies in the Sciences of Complexity, pp. 487–509. Addison-Wesley, Reading (1991)

Andry, P., Gaussier, P., Nadel, J., Hirsbrunner, B.: Learning invariant sensorimotor behaviors: A developmental approach to imitation mechanisms. Adap. Behav. **12**, 117–140 (2004)

Arkes, H.R., Garske, J.P.: Psychological Theories of Motivation. Brooks/Cole, Monterey (1982)

Baranes, A., Oudeyer, P.-Y.: Intrinsically motivated goal exploration for active motor learning in robots: A case study. In: Proceedings of the IEEE/RSJ International Conference on Intelligent Robots and Systems (IROS 2010), Taipei, Taiwan 2010

Barto, A.G., Mahadevan, S.: Recent advances in hierarchical reinforcement learning. Discr. Event Dynam. Syst. Theory Appl. **13**, 341–379 (2003)

Barto, A.G., Singh, S., Chentanez, N.: Intrinsically motivated learning of hierarchical collections of skills. In: Proceedings of the International Conference on Developmental Learning (ICDL), La Jolla, CA 2004

Barto, A.G., Sutton, R.S., Anderson, C.W.: Neuronlike elements that can solve difficult learn-ingcontrol problems. **13**, 835–846 (1983). IEEE Trans. Sys. Man, Cybern. Reprinted in J.A. Anderson and E. Rosenfeld (eds.), Neurocomputing: Foundations of Research, pp. 535–549, MIT, Cambridge (1988)

Beck, R.C.: Motivation. Theories and Principles, 2nd edn. Prentice-Hall, Englewood Cliffs (1983)

Berlyne, D.E.: A theory of human curiosity. Br. J. Psychol. **45**, 180–191 (1954)

Berlyne, D.E.: Conflict, Arousal., Curiosity. McGraw-Hill, New York (1960)

Berlyne, D.E.: Curiosity and exploration. Science **143**, 25–33 (1966)

Berlyne, D.E.: Aesthetics and Psychobiology. Appleton-Century-Crofts, New York (1971)

Bertsekas, D.P., Tsitsiklis, J.N.: Neuro-Dynamic Programming. Athena Scientific, Belmont (1996)

Bindra, D.: How adaptive behavior is produced: A perceptual-motivational alternative to response reinforcement. Behav. Brain Sci. **1**, 41–91 (1978)

Breazeal, C., Brooks, A., Gray, J., Hoffman, G., Lieberman, J., Lee, H., Lockerd, A., Mulanda, D.: Tutelage and collaboration for humanoid robots. Int. J. Human. Robot. **1** (2004)

Bush, V.: Science the endless frontier: Areport to the president. Technical report (1945)

Busoniu, L., Babuska, R., Schutter, B.D.: A comprehensive survey of multi-agent reinforcement learning. IEEE Trans. Syst. Man Cybern. C Appl. Rev. **38**(2), 156–172 (2008)

Cannon, W.B.: The Wisdom of the Body. W.W. Norton, New York (1932)

Clark, W.A., Farley, B.G.: Generalization of pattern recognition in a self-organizing system. In: AFIPS' 55 (Western) Proceedings of the March 1–3, 1955, Western Joint Computer Conference, Los Angeles, CA, pp. 86–91, ACM, New York (1955)

Cofer, C.N., Appley, M.H.: Motivation: Theory and Research. Wiley, New York (1964)

Damoulas, T., Cos-Aguilera, I., Hayes, G.M., Taylor, T.: Valency for adaptive homeostatic agents: Relating evolution and learning. In: Capcarrere, M.S., Freitas, A.A., Bentley, P.J., Johnson, C.G., Timmis, J. (eds.) Advances in Artificial Life: 8th European Conference, ECAL 2005. Canterbury, UK LNAI vol. 3630, pp. 936–945. Springer, Berlin (2005)

Daw, N.D., Shohamy, D.: The cognitive neuroscience of motivation and learning. Soc. Cogn. **26**(5), 593–620 (2008)

Dayan, P.: Motivated reinforcement learning. In: Dietterich, T.G., Becker, S., Ghahramani, Z. (eds.) Advances in Neural Information Processing Systems 14: Proceedings of the 2001 Conference, pp. 11–18. MIT, Cambridge (2001)
Deci, E.L., Ryan, R.M.: Intrinsic Motivation and Self-Determination in Human Behavior. Plenum, New York (1985)
Dember, W.N., Earl, R.W.: Analysis of exploratory, manipulatory, and curiosity behaviors. Psychol. Rev. **64**, 91–96 (1957)
Dember, W.N., Earl, R.W., Paradise, N.: Response by rats to differential stimulus complexity. J. Comp. Physiol. Psychol. **50**, 514–518 (1957)
Dickinson, A., Balleine, B.: The role of leaning in the operation of motivational systems. In: Gallistel, R. (ed.) Handbook of Experimental Psychology, 3rd edn. Learning, Motivation, and Emotion, pp. 497–533. Wiley, New York (2002)
Elfwing, S., Uchibe, E., Doya, K., Christensen, H.I.: Co-evolution of shaping rewards and meta-parameters in reinforcement learning. Adap. Behav. **16**, 400–412 (2008)
Epstein, A.: Instinct and motivation as explanations of complex behavior. In: Pfaff, D.W. (ed.) The Physiological Mechanisms of Motivation. Springer, New York (1982)
Friston, K.J., Daunizeau, J., Kilner, J., Kiebel, S.J.: Action and behavior: A free-energy formulation. Biol. Cybern. (2010). Pubished online February 11, 2020
Groos, K.: The Play of Man. D. Appleton, New York (1901)
Harlow, H.F.: Learning and satiation of response in intrinsically motivated complex puzzle performance by monkeys. J. Comp. Physiol. Psychol. **43**, 289–294 (1950)
Harlow, H.F., Harlow, M.K., Meyer, D.R.: Learning motivated by a manipulation drive. J. Exp. Psychol. **40**, 228–234 (1950)
Hart, S., Grupen, R.: Intrinsically motivated affordance discovery and modeling. In: Baldassarre, G., Mirolli, M. (eds.) Intrinsically Motivated Learning in Natural and Artificial Systems. Springer, Berlin (2012, this volume)
Hebb, D.O.: The Organization of Behavior. Wiley, New York (1949)
Hendrick, I.: Instinct and ego during infancy. Psychoanal. Quart. **11**, 33–58 (1942)
Hesse, F., Der, R., Herrmann, M., Michael, J.: Modulated exploratory dynamics can shape self-organized behavior. Adv. Complex Syst. **12**(2), 273–292 (2009)
Hull, C.L.: Principles of Behavior. D. Appleton-Century, New York (1943)
Hull, C.L.: Essentials of Behavior. Yale University Press, New Haven (1951)
Hull, C.L.: A Behavior System: An Introduction to Behavior Theory Concerning the Individual Organism. Yale University Press, New Haven (1952)
Kimble, G.A.: Hilgard and Marquis' Conditioning and Learning. Appleton-Century-Crofts, Inc., New York (1961)
Klein, S.B.: Motivation. Biosocial Approaches. McGraw-Hill, New York (1982)
Klopf, A.H.: Brain function and adaptive systems—A heterostatic theory. Technical report AFCRL-72-0164, Air Force Cambridge Research Laboratories, Bedford. A summary appears in Proceedings of the International Conference on Systems, Man, and Cybernetics, 1974, IEEE Systems, Man, and Cybernetics Society, Dallas (1972)
Klopf, A.H.: The Hedonistic Neuron: A Theory of Memory, Learning, and Intelligence. Hemisphere, Washington (1982)
Lenat, D.B.: AM: An artificial intelligence approach to discovery in mathematics. Ph.D. Thesis, Stanford University (1976)
Linden, D.J.: The Compass of Pleasure: How Our Brains Make Fatty Foods, Orgasm, Exercise, Marijuana, Generosity, Vodka, Learning, and Gambling Feel So Good. Viking, New York (2011)
Littman, M.L., Ackley, D.H.: Adaptation in constant utility nonstationary environments. In: Proceedings of the Fourth International Conference on Genetic Algorithms, San Diego, CA pp. 136–142 (1991)
Lungarella, M., Metta, G., Pfeiffer, R., Sandini, G.: Developmental robotics: A survey. Connect. Sci. **15**, 151–190 (2003)

Mackintosh, N.J.: Conditioning and Associative Learning. Oxford University Press, New York (1983)

McFarland, D., Bösser, T.: Intelligent Behavior in Animals and Robots. MIT, Cambridge (1993)

Mendel, J.M., Fu, K.S. (eds.): Adaptive, Learning, and Pattern Recognition Systems: Theory and Applications. Academic, New York (1970)

Mendel, J.M., McLaren, R.W.: Reinforcement learning control and pattern recognition systems. In: Mendel, J.M., Fu, K.S. (eds.) Adaptive, Learning and Pattern Recognition Systems:Theory and Applications, pp. 287–318. Academic, New York (1970)

Michie, D., Chambers, R.A.: BOXES: An experiment in adaptive control. In: Dale, E., Michie, D. (eds.) Machine Intelligence 2, pp. 137–152. Oliver and Boyd, Edinburgh (1968)

Minsky, M.L.: Theory of neural analog reinforcement systems and its application to the brain-model problem. Ph.D. Thesis, Princeton University (1954)

Minsky, M.L.: Steps toward artificial intelligence. Proc. Inst. Radio Eng. **49**, 8–30 (1961). Reprinted in E.A. Feigenbaum and J. Feldman (eds.) Computers and Thought, pp. 406–450. McGraw-Hill, New York (1963)

Mollenauer, S.O.: Shifts in deprivations level: Different effects depending on the amount of preshift training. Learn. Motiv. **2**, 58–66 (1971)

Narendra, K., Thathachar, M.A.L.: Learning Automata: An Introduction. Prentice Hall, Englewood Cliffs (1989)

Olds, J., Milner, P.: Positive reinforcement produced by electrical stimulation of septal areas and other regions of rat brain. J. Comp. Physiol. Psychol. **47**, 419–427 (1954)

Oudeyer, P.-Y., Kaplan, F.: What is intrinsic motivation? A typology of computational approaches. Front. Neurorobot. 1:6, doi: 10.3389/neuro.12.006.2007 (2007)

Oudeyer, P.-Y., Kaplan, F., Hafner, V.: Intrinsic motivation systems for autonomous mental development. IEEE Trans. Evol. Comput. **11**, 265–286 (2007)

Petri, H.L.: Motivation: Theory and Research. Wadsworth Publishing Company, Belmont (1981)

Piaget, J.: The Origins of Intelligence in Children. Norton, New York (1952)

Picard, R.W.: Affective Computing. MIT, Cambridge (1997)

Prince, C.G., Demiris, Y., Marom, Y., Kozima, H., Balkenius, C. (eds.): Proceedings of the Second International Workshop on Epigenetic Robotics: Modeling Cognitive Development in Robotic Systems. Lund University Cognitive Studies, vol. 94. Lund University, Lund (2001)

Rescorla, R.A., Wagner, A.R.: A theory of Pavlovian conditioning: Variationsin the effectiveness of reinforcement and nonreinforcement. In: Black, A.H., Prokasy, W.F. (eds.) Classical Conditioning, vol. II, pp. 64–99. Appleton-Century-Crofts, New York (1972)

Rosenblatt, F.: Principles of Neurodynamics: Perceptrons and the Theory of Brain Mechanisms. Spartan Books, Washington (1962)

Rumelhart, D., Hintont, G., Williams, R.: Learning representations by back-propagating errors. Nature **323**(6088), 533–536 (1986)

Ryan, R.M., Deci, E.L.: Intrinsic and extrinsic motivations: Classic definitions and new directions. Contemp. Educ. Psychol. **25**, 54–67 (2000)

Samuelson, L.: Introduction to the evolution of preferences. J. Econ. Theory **97**, 225–230 (2001)

Samuelson, L., Swinkels, J.: Information, evolution, and utility. Theor. Econ. **1**, 119–142 (2006)

Savage, T.: Artificial motives: A review of motivation in artificial creatures. Connect. Sci. **12**, 211–277 (2000)

Schembri, M., Mirolli, M., Baldassarre, G.: Evolving internal reinforcers for an intrinsically motivated reinforcement-learning robot. In: Proceedings of the 6th International Conference on Development and Learning (ICDL2007), Imperial College, London 2007

Schmidhuber, J.: Adaptive confidence and adaptive curiosity. Technical report FKI-149-91, Institut für Informatik, Technische Universität München (1991a)

Schmidhuber, J.: A possibility for implementing curiosity and boredom in model-building neural controllers. In: From Animals to Animats: Proceedings of the First International Conference on Simulation of Adaptive Behavior, pp. 222–227. MIT, Cambridge (1991b)

Schmidhuber, J.: What's interesting? Technical report TR-35-97. IDSIA, Lugano (1997)

Schmidhuber, J.: Artificial curiosity based on discovering novel algorithmic predictability through coevolution. In: Proceedings of the Congress on Evolutionary Computation, vol. 3, pp. 1612–1618. IEEE (1999)

Schmidhuber, J.: Driven by compression progress: A simple principle explains essential aspects of subjective beauty, novelty, surprise, interestingness, attention, curiosity, creativity, art, science, music, jokes. In: Pezzulo, G., Butz, M.V., Sigaud, O., Baldassarre, G. (eds.) Anticipatory Behavior in Adaptive Learning Systems. From Psychological Theories to Artificial Cognitive Systems, pp. 48–76. Springer, Berlin (2009)

Schultz, W.: Predictive reward signal of dopamine neurons. J. Neurophysiol. **80**(1), 1–27 (1998)

Schultz, W.: Reward. Scholarpedia **2**(3), 1652 (2007a)

Schultz, W.: Reward signals. Scholarpedia **2**(6), 2184 (2007b)

Scott, P.D., Markovitch, S.: Learning novel domains through curiosity and conjecture. In: Sridharan, N.S. (ed.) Proceedings of the 11th International Joint Conference on Artificial Intelligence, Detroit, MI pp. 669–674. Morgan Kaufmann, San Francisco (1989)

Settles, B.: Active learning literature survey. Technical Report 1648, Computer Sciences, University of Wisconsin-Madison, Madison (2009)

Singh, S., Barto, A.G., Chentanez, N.: Intrinsically motivated reinforcement learning. In: Advances in Neural Information Processing Systems 17: Proceedings of the 2004 Conference. MIT, Cambridge (2005)

Singh, S., Lewis, R.L., Barto, A.G.: Where do rewards come from? In: Taatgen, N., van Rijn, H. (eds.) Proceedings of the 31st Annual Conference of the Cognitive Science Society, Amsterdam pp. 2601–2606. Cognitive Science Society (2009)

Singh, S., Lewis, R.L., Barto, A.G., Sorg, J.: Intrinsically motivated reinforcement learning: An evolutionary perspective. IEEE Trans. Auton. Mental Dev. **2**(2), 70–82 (2010). Special issue on Active Learning and Intrinsically Motivated Exploration in Robots: Advances and Challenges

Snel, M., Hayes, G.M.: Evolution of valence systems in an unstable environment. In: Proceedings of the 10th International Conference on Simulation of Adaptive Behavior: From Animals to Animats, Osaka, M. Asada, J.C. Hallam, J.-A. Meyer (Eds.) pp. 12–21 (2008)

Sorg, J., Singh, S., Lewis, R.L.: Internal rewards mitigate agent boundedness. In: Fürnkranz, J., Joachims, T. (eds.) Proceedings of the 27th International Conference on Machine Learning, Haifa, Israel, Omnipress pp. 1007–1014 (2010)

Sutton, R.S.: Reinforcement learning architectures for animats. In: From Animals to Animats: Proceedings of the First International Conference on Simulation of Adaptive Behavior, J.-A. Meyer, S.W.Wilson (Eds.) pp. 288–296. MIT, Cambridge (1991)

Sutton, R.S., Barto, A.G.: Reinforcement Learning: An Introduction. MIT, Cambridge (1998)

Sutton, R.S., Precup, D., Singh, S.: Between mdps and semi-mdps: A framework for temporal abstraction inreinforcement learning. Artif. Intell. **112**, 181–211 (1999)

Tesauro, G.J.: TD—gammon, a self-teaching backgammon program, achieves master-level play. Neural Comput. **6**(2), 215–219 (1994)

Thomaz, A.L., Breazeal, C.: Transparency and socially guided machine learning. In: Proceedings of the 5th International Conference on Developmental Learning (ICDL) Bloomington, IN (2006)

Thomaz, A.L., Hoffman, G., Breazeal, C.: Experiments in socially guided machine learning: Understanding how humans teach. In: Proceedings of the 1st Annual conference on Human-Robot Interaction (HRI) Salt Lake City, UT (2006)

Thorndike, E.L.: Animal Intelligence. Hafner, Darien (1911)

Toates, F.M. (1911): Motivational Systems. Cambridge University Press, Cambridge (1911)

Tolman, E.C.: Purposive Behavior in Animals and Men. Naiburg, New York (1932)

Trappl, R., Petta, P., Payr, S. (eds.): Emotions in Humans and Artifacts. MIT, Cambridge (1997)

Uchibe, E., Doya, K.: Finding intrinsic rewards by embodied evolution and constrained reinforcement learning. Neural Netw. **21**(10), 1447–1455 (2008)

Waltz, M.D., Fu, K.S.: A heuristic approach to reinforcement learning control systems. IEEE Transactions on Automatic Control **10**, 390–398 (1965)

Weng, J., McClelland, J., Pentland, A., Sporns, O., Stockman, I., Sur, M., Thelen, E.: Autonomous mental development by robots and animals. Science **291**, 599–600 (2001)

Werbos, P.J.: Building and understanding adaptive systems: A statistical/numerical approach to factory automation and brain research. IEEE Trans. Sys. Man Cybern. **17**, 7–20 (1987)

White, R.W.: Motivation reconsidered: The concept of competence. Psychol. Rev. **66**, 297–333 (1959)

Widrow, B., Gupta, N.K., Maitra, S.. Punish/reward: Learning with a critic in adaptive thresholdsystems. IEEE Trans. Sys. Man Cybern. **3**, 455–465 (1973)

Widrow, B., Hoff, M.E.: Adaptive switching circuits. In: 1960 WESCON Convention Record Part IV, pp. 96–104. Institute of Radio Engineers, New York (1960). Reprinted in J.A. Anderson and E. Rosenfeld, Neurocomputing: Foundations of Research, pp 126 134. MIT, Cambridge (1988)

Young, P.T.: Hedonic organization and regulation of behavior. Psychol. Rev. **73**, 59–86 (1966)

Functions and Mechanisms of Intrinsic Motivations

The Knowledge Versus Competence Distinction

Marco Mirolli and Gianluca Baldassarre

Abstract Mammals, and humans in particular, are endowed with an exceptional capacity for cumulative learning. This capacity crucially depends on the presence of intrinsic motivations, that is, motivations that are directly related not to an organism's survival and reproduction but rather to its ability to learn. Recently, there have been a number of attempts to model and reproduce intrinsic motivations in artificial systems. Different kinds of intrinsic motivations have been proposed both in psychology and in machine learning and robotics: some are based on the knowledge of the learning system, while others are based on its competence. In this contribution, we discuss the distinction between knowledge-based and competence-based intrinsic motivations with respect to both the functional roles that motivations play in learning and the mechanisms by which those functions are implemented. In particular, after arguing that the principal function of intrinsic motivations consists in allowing the development of a repertoire of skills (rather than of knowledge), we suggest that at least two different sub-functions can be identified: (a) discovering which skills might be acquired and (b) deciding which skill to train when. We propose that in biological organisms, knowledge-based intrinsic motivation mechanisms might implement the former function, whereas competence-based mechanisms might underlie the latter one.

M. Mirolli (✉) · G. Baldassarre
Istituto di Scienze e Tecnologie della Cognizione, Consiglio Nazionale delle Ricerche, Rome, Italy
e-mail: marco.mirolli@istc.cnr.it; gianluca.baldassarre@istc.cnr.it

G. Baldassarre and M. Mirolli (eds.), *Intrinsically Motivated Learning in Natural and Artificial Systems*, DOI 10.1007/978-3-642-32375-1_3,

1 Introduction

The capacity of autonomous cumulative learning demonstrated by complex organisms like mammals, and humans in particular, is astonishing. This capacity is likely to have its roots in *intrinsic motivations*, that is, motivations not directly related to extrinsic rewards such as food or sex, but rather to what the animal knows (curiosity, novelty, surprise) or can do (competence). Both animal and human psychologists have found evidence indicating that intrinsic motivations play an important role in animals' behavior and learning (Berlyne 1960; Deci 1975; Deci and Ryan 1985; White 1959).

Recently, the study of intrinsic motivations has been gaining increasing attention also in machine learning and robotics, as researchers in these fields have recognized that truly intelligent artificial systems need to develop their own abilities while autonomously interacting with their environment (Weng et al. 2001). The potentially open-ended complexification of a system's skills might require the use of learning signals that are non-task specific and hence intrinsic. As a result, several computational models of intrinsically motivated learning have been proposed so far, but the study of artificial intrinsically motivated cumulative learning systems is still in its infancy.

The aim of the present chapter is to aid the development of this field by clarifying issues related to different kinds of intrinsic motivations, both with respect to the possible mechanisms that might implement intrinsic motivations and to the possible functions that they might play in cumulative learning. In particular, the paper focuses on the distinction between knowledge-based and competence-based intrinsic motivations, that is, intrinsic motivations that are based on what the system *knows* versus on what the system *can do*. Note that what the system knows can include also knowledge (e.g., predictions) about the results of the system's actions. And, vice versa, competence-based intrinsic motivations might involve the use of predictions for obtaining measures related to competence. What really distinguish knowledge-based from competence-based systems is that the former use measures that are related to the capacity of the system to model its environment (including the system's body and the interactions between the system and the environment), whereas the latter use measures that are related to the system's ability to have specific effects on the environment.

We start (Sect. 2) by reviewing the psychological literature on intrinsic motivations, highlighting the distinction between intrinsic motivations driven by what a system knows (knowledge-based) and those driven by what it can do (competence-based). Then we review the computational modeling literature from the perspective of an analogous distinction between knowledge-based and competence-based intrinsic motivation systems (Sect. 3). In Sect. 4, we suggest that the distinction between knowledge-based and competence-based systems can and should be made not only with respect to the *mechanisms* of intrinsic motivations but also with respect to their *functions*, that is, with respect to what kind of learning they support, and we argue that the ultimate function of intrinsic motivation is to support the cumulative learning of skills rather than knowledge. Unfortunately, this is not the case for many of the computational models proposed in the literature so far (Sect. 5), in particular for those employing knowledge-based mechanisms. Indeed, we suggest that purely knowledge-based systems might not be particularly well suited for driving the cumulative acquisition of skills (Sect. 6). Finally, we consider the problem of intrinsic motivations from the point of view of a hierarchical learning system (Sect. 7): here, we argue that different kinds of intrinsic motivations might play different functional roles at different levels of the hierarchy, and we refer to the possible neural bases of both knowledge-based and competence-based intrinsic motivations in real brains. Section 8 concludes the paper by summarizing our contributions and discussing promising directions for future research.

2 Intrinsic Motivations in Psychology

Interest in intrinsic motivations first arose in the 1950s in the field of animal psychology, as several researchers discovered a number of phenomena that were in apparent contrast to the seminal theory of motivation proposed by Hull (1943). According to Hull's theory, animal behavior was motivated by drives, conceived as temporary physiological deficits that the organism is led to reduce in order to achieve homeostatic equilibrium. Typical examples of drives are hunger and thirst, which make the animal work for achieving respectively food and water so as to satisfy its needs for energy and liquid. According to Hull, all motivations are either physiological primary drives or secondary drives derived from primary ones through learning (as it happens in classical conditioning experiments).

Notwithstanding the popularity of Hull's theory, soon animal psychologists reported phenomena that were difficult to reconcile with the drive concept. For example, Harlow and coworkers (Harlow 1950; Harlow et al. 1950) reported that rhesus monkeys might spend long periods of time in trying to solve mechanical puzzles without any reward. Kish and colleagues reported that operant conditioning phenomena (i.e., phenomena related to the fact that the rate of responding to a manipulandum can be influenced by the consequences of these responses) could be elicited in mice not only by primary rewards but also by apparently neutral stimuli that had never been associated with rewards, such as "microswitch clicks, relay noises, and stimuli produced by a moving platform" (Kish 1955; Kish and Antonitis 1956). Similarly, Butler showed that rhesus monkeys could learn a discrimination task by using as a reinforcement just the possibility to look at other conspecifics from a window (Butler 1953).

Some authors, such as Montgomery (1954), tried to reconcile these findings with Hull's theory by postulating the existence of other drives, like drives to manipulate, to play, or to explore. But this move was hard to accept because exploratory drives do not seem to possess any of the two fundamental characteristics of primary drives: they are not related to any internal deficit and they do not seem to have any homeostatic function.

2.1 Knowledge-Based Views

The considerations reported above led several psychologists to develop explanations of intrinsic motivations that were not based on the drive concept. Among them, probably the most influential proposal was the one of Berlyne (1960). According to him, animal exploration and intrinsically motivated activities in general depend on the fact that animals are attracted by optimal levels of novelty of stimuli, of their complexity, and of surprise, conceived as a falsification of the animal's expectations. As it can be noted, all the intrinsic motivations proposed by Berlyne are knowledge-based in that they are related to the properties of the stimuli that the animal perceives and on their relation to the animal's knowledge (note that Berlyne never made the distinction between knowledge and competence that we are discussing here: this is our interpretation of his work). Several similar knowledge-based proposals have been made in the psychological literature. These postulated either that animals are motivated to receive an optimal level of stimulation (or of novelty of stimuli) (e.g., Hebb 1955; Hunt 1965) or that they are motivated to reduce the discrepancy (or incongruity or dissonance) between their knowledge and their current perception of the environment (e.g., Dember and Earl 1957; Festinger 1957; Kagan 1972).

2.2 Competence-Based Views

On the other hand, in his seminal review on motivations, White (1959) strongly advocated a competence-based view of intrinsic motivations, proposing that animals have a fundamental motivation for *effectance*, that is, for the capacity to have effective interactions with their environment. White's paper had a great influence on subsequent research on motivation. In particular, in the fields of educational and human psychology, the link between intrinsic motivations and the concept of competence has remained quite strong since then (Deci 1975). For example, according to *self-determination theory* (Deci and Ryan 1985), there is a continuum between extrinsically and intrinsically motivated activities. Among the most important factors that make an activity intrinsically motivated are the sense of *autonomy*, that is, the perception that the activity is self-determined, and the sense of *competence*, that is, the perception that we have (or are getting) mastery of the activity (Ryan and Deci 2000). Similarly, De Charms proposed that personal causation, that is, the sense of having control over one's environment, was a fundamental driving force of human behavior (De Charms 1968). Likewise, the *theory of flow* of Csikszentmihalyi postulates that humans are motivated to engage in activities that represent an appropriate level of learning challenge, that is, that are neither too easy nor too difficult to master given the individual's current level of competence (Csikszentmihalyi 1991).

3 Computational Models of Intrinsic Motivations

The distinction between knowledge-based and competence-based intrinsic motivations can also be appropriately applied within the context of the computational literature on intrinsic motivations. In this field, a useful and typical way of framing the problem of intrinsic motivations consists in considering it within the computational framework of reinforcement learning (e.g., Barto et al. 2004; Oudeyer and Kaplan 2007; Schembri et al. 2007c; Schmidhuber 1991b, see also Barto 2012). Reinforcement learning algorithms are developed so as to maximize the sum of future rewards, where a reward is defined as a numerical value that is continuously received by the learning agent (Sutton and Barto 1998). In this context, intrinsic motivations can be conceived as components of the rewards that are not directly related to the task that the agent must solve but are rather task independent.

3.1 Knowledge-Based Models

Most of the proposed models of intrinsic motivations are knowledge-based as they depend on the *stimuli* perceived by the learning system (and on their relations with the system's expectations, including those related to the results of the system's actions) rather than on the system's *skills*. For example, the first model of intrinsic motivations for an artificial reinforcement learning agent was proposed by Schmidhuber (1991b). It consisted in adding to a reinforcement learning agent an adaptive world model that learned to predict the next perception given the current perception and the planned action, and in using the errors in these predictions as an intrinsic reward for the system. The intrinsic reward complemented the extrinsic reward related to the task at hand. The rationale of this proposal was that in this way, the "curious" reinforcement learning agent would be pushed not only to maximize external rewards but also to improve its own world model, thus exploring poorly known parts of the environment.

This kind of system would get stuck in parts of the environment that are unpredictable or if the predictor has not enough computational power: in both cases, the prediction error would never decrease, and the system would keep on being reinforced to stay where it is. The recognition of this problem led Schmidhuber to propose the use of a measure of the learning progress of the world model (namely, the decrease in prediction error) as the intrinsic reward signal (Schmidhuber 1991a). An analogous idea has been recently explored in the context of developmental robotics by Oudeyer and colleagues under the name of *intelligent adaptive curiosity*, together with a mechanism for automatically dividing the whole sensorimotor space into subregions within which to compute the learning progress and on which to focus learning (Oudeyer et al. 2007). Several other models have been presented in which the intrinsic motivation consists of some form of perceived novelty, prediction error, or learning progress of a world model (Huang and Weng 2002; Lee et al. 2009; Marshall et al. 2004; Merrick and Maher 2009; Saunders and Gero 2002; Storck et al. 1995, see also Merrick 2012; Schmidhuber 2012).

3.2 Competence-Based Models

Contrary to what has been stated by Oudeyer and Kaplan in their useful review (Oudeyer and Kaplan 2007), there are also a few computational models of artificial systems whose learning is driven by some form of competence-based intrinsic motivations. The first of such systems is the *intrinsically motivated reinforcement learning* (IMRL) system proposed by Barto and colleagues (Barto et al. 2004; Stout et al. 2005), which is based on the reinforcement learning framework of *options* (Sutton et al. 1999). In short, an option is a temporally extended action defined by an initiation set (the set of states in which the option can be initiated), a policy (the states-actions mapping followed during the execution of the option), and a termination set (the set of states in which the option terminates). In practice, an option defines a skill that can be recalled each time the agent needs to achieve one of the option termination states. These states can be considered as the option goals. In IMRL options are created for reaching different *salient events*, where salient events are specified by the experimenter and are constituted, for example, by the opening of a door, the ringing of a bell, or the switching on of a light. Intrinsic rewards, perceived when the salient events are reached, are defined as $1 - p$, where p is the (estimated) probability of reaching the salient event with the executed option. In other words, the intrinsic reinforcement is given on the basis of the unpredicted occurrence of salient events. As the authors themselves explicitly state, this is a form of prediction error, and so, in this respect, it is analogous to the knowledge-based intrinsic motivations discussed above. However, the prediction error in this case is not calculated at every state, but only with respect to the goal states of the options (whenever these are reached). Hence, the intrinsic reward is given on the basis of the (lack of) ability of the system to reach one of its goal states. Hence, in this case the intrinsic reward should be considered as competence-based rather than knowledge-based.

The use of competence-based intrinsic rewards is more explicit in a model we have proposed (Schembri et al. 2007a,b,c). This was directly inspired by the IMRL framework, but instead of using options, it implements skills on the basis of *experts*, each of which is an instance of the actor-critic reinforcement learning architecture (Barto et al. 1983) trained with the temporal differences (TD) learning algorithm (Sutton 1988). The model is hierarchical and so it is also formed by a *selector* which assigns the control of action (and the possibility of learning) to experts. Each expert is assigned a reward function, and when given the control, it improves the policy of its actor (states-actions mapping) on the basis of its *TD error*, that is, the error of its critic related to the prediction of future discounted rewards. The selector learns to assign the control to experts on the basis of an intrinsic reward signal represented by the TD error of the expert selected at each step. The rationale of this is that the TD error of an expert can be considered as a good estimate of the improvement of its policy. Indeed, a positive average TD error of an expert means that it is behaving better than expected by its own critic, which means that it is improving its ability to maximize rewards. Vice versa, a zero average TD error indicates that it is behaving as expected, meaning that it is not improving. By receiving the TD error of the selected expert as its reward, the selector will learn to give the control to the expert that, in a given context, is expected to improve its skill the most.

Here it is clear, even more than in Barto's IMRL, that even though the intrinsic motivation signal for the selector (the TD error of the selected expert) is a form of prediction error, it is a competence-based signal, since the prediction error is relative to the rewards obtained by the experts, and hence it is a measure of skill improvement rather than of the agent's ability (or inability) in modeling its environment. This is clear if one considers that what is given as a reward to the selector is the TD error as such, and not its absolute value. If the signal regarded the *knowledge* of the system, then the absolute value of the error would be used because to measure knowledge one needs the amount of prediction error, irrespective of its sign. But here we are dealing with the TD error *as a measure of improvement in skill acquisition*, for which the sign is paramount because skills are improving only if the TD error is positive.

The fact that the TD error is a signal that is related to performance has important consequences for the possible problem of unlearnability. As discussed above, an intrinsically motivated knowledge-based system that uses the prediction error as a reward will get stuck in parts of the environment that are not predictable. In contrast, a system that uses the TD error as its intrinsic reward will not get stuck in parts of the environment where the reward is unpredictable because in that case the evaluations (predictions of future discounted rewards) will become equal to the average received reward and the TD error will be sometimes positive (when the reward is received) and sometimes negative (when the reward is not received). Hence, the reinforcement learning system will learn to predict that the average reward is zero and will pass to explore other parts of the environment where some skill learning progress can be made. In fact, in contrast to the method proposed by Barto and colleagues, this kind of competence-based intrinsic motivation is able to solve not only the problem of unpredictability of rewards but also the problem of unlearnability of a skill, and for the same reason. If, for whatever reason, a skill cannot be learned, the evaluations of the expert will equal the average received reward, the TD error signal will average to zero, and the selector will learn that the skill cannot be trained and will prefer experts that can improve their performance.

Two more recent models of competence-based intrinsic motivations are Stout and Barto (2010), which is quite similar to our own, and Baranes and Oudeyer (2010), which is not based on reinforcement learning but on control theory.

4 Functions Versus Mechanisms and the Primacy of Competence Over Knowledge

Up to now we have reviewed the psychological and computational modeling literature on intrinsic motivations from the point of view of the distinction between knowledge-based and competence-based hypotheses. Following Oudeyer and Kaplan (2007), we have so far related this distinction to the *mechanisms* that drive intrinsically motivated behavior and/or learning processes. An analogous but even more important distinction can be done with respect to the *function* that intrinsic motivations are considered to play within the overall system. Whereas there is a general agreement on the fact that intrinsic motivations serve the role of driving the learning of a system, it is much less clear (but it is important to clarify) which kind of learning they are supposed to support: is it learning of *knowledge* or learning of *competence*? In other words, do intrinsic motivations help the system in building *increasingly accurate models* or do they allow the discovery of *more effective ways of acting on* the environment?

The answer will probably reflect a more general and fundamental (we might call it *philosophical*) attitude that one takes in considering human beings and other animals as well as in building artificial intelligent systems. What is more important, knowledge or action? No doubt, the western culture has been giving prominence to knowledge over action: from Plato's *World of Ideas* to Descartes' *cogito ergo sum*, to Kant's primacy of the Critics of *Pure Reason* over the Critics of Practical Reason, and so on. This strong cultural legacy is evident also in modern *cognitive* science, which poses at the very center of the study of psychology the study of how human beings process information inside their heads rather than of how they behave and interact with their environment. Since their birth in the 1950s, the same general attitude has also informed the *sciences of the artificial* (Simon 1996), that is, disciplines such as artificial intelligence and machine learning. For decades the focus of research in these disciplines has been on reasoning, problem solving, knowledge representation on one hand (Russell and Norvig 2003), and perception and categorization on the other (Mitchell 1997), whereas the study of behavior has been almost neglected. This state of affairs has started to change, at least from the point of view of artificial systems, in the 1990s, when classical artificial intelligence was criticized and "invaded" by new robotics (Brooks 1991), artificial life (Langton 1989), adaptive behavior research (Meyer and Wilson 1990), and reinforcement learning (Sutton and Barto 1998), which started to gain increasing attention within machine learning. Indeed, what is common to all these new approaches and clearly distinguishes them from the old ones is their attitude with respect to the knowledge versus competence issue: all of them emphasize the primacy of behavior over representation, of action over cognition, and of competence over knowledge (Clark 1997; Pfeifer and Scheier 1999).

The rationale behind this fundamental shift lies in evolutionary considerations: animals evolved on the basis of their capacity to survive and reproduce, and survival and reproduction depend primarily on what organisms *do*, not on what they *know*. What is selected for is the capacity to adaptively interact with one's own environment in ever increasingly complex and efficient ways, not the capacity to accurately represent the environment in one's head (on this point, see also Barto 2010). This does not mean that the capacity to represent the world is useless and should not be investigated. Rather, it means that knowledge is ancillary to behavior, rather than the other way round. Hence, in general, the capacity to model the environment should be considered as one possible (but not necessary) tool for improving an agent's capacity of interacting with the environment, and not as the ultimate goal of an organism or of an artificial system. In other words, *some* form of knowledge might be useful in *some* circumstances for *some* purposes. But it should be kept in mind that perfect knowledge is not the ultimate goal of any living organism, and it should not be the goal of any useful artificial system. Indeed, understanding which kind and level of knowledge can be useful for which kind of behaving system in which circumstances is a fundamental challenge for both the empirical and the synthetic behavioral and brain sciences.

5 Functional Roles of Intrinsic Motivations in Computational Models

Coming back to the question about the ultimate function of intrinsic motivation which we introduced in the previous section, it should now be clear what our stance is, and why: whatever the *mechanisms* which implement intrinsic motivations, their primary and fundamental *function* is to allow a system to develop a cumulative repertoire of useful skills (rather than an increasingly accurate knowledge of the environment). We think not only that this is true for real organisms but that this should be the standpoint from which to consider the endeavor of building intrinsically motivated artificial systems. We feel the need to underscore this point because it is not clear to what extent this position is shared among computational modelers.

Surprisingly as it might seem, the majority of computational models of intrinsic motivations not only use knowledge-based *mechanisms* but have the acquisition of knowledge as their only *function*. For example, Schmidhuber's (1991a) curious agent is a "model builder," whose goal is the improvement of its predictions. The same is true for the robots used to test the intelligent adaptive curiosity algorithm of Oudeyer and colleagues (2007) and for almost all other systems whose intrinsic motivations are based on knowledge (e.g., Huang and Weng 2002; Lee et al. 2009; Marshall et al. 2004; Merrick and Maher 2009). On the contrary, competence-based intrinsic motivation mechanisms have been always used for improving skills (Baranes and Oudeyer 2010; Barto et al. 2004; Schembri et al. 2007a; Stout and Barto 2010).

It is important to note that this need not necessarily be the case. Indeed, the distinction between the functions of knowledge-based and competence-based intrinsic motivations is different from the one related to the mechanisms underlying them. It is possible of for knowledge-based intrinsic motivation mechanisms to help improve the learning agent's skills (as it happens, e.g., in Schmidhuber 2002), as it is possible for competence-based mechanisms to serve the acquisition of knowledge. But these possibilities in principle must be demonstrated in practice, and in doing so there might be some difficulties. As the focus here is in the use of intrinsic motivations for the acquisition of skills, the next section discusses only the possible problems related to the use of knowledge-based mechanisms for accumulating competence, while it does not consider the less relevant possibility of using competence-based intrinsic motivations for acquiring knowledge.

6 Knowledge-Based Mechanisms and Competence

As a representative example of a purely knowledge-based system (i.e., a system which uses only knowledge-based mechanisms), let us consider the work of Oudeyer et al. (2007). In the presented experiments, the authors show how the proposed system demonstrates an interesting developmental trajectory: it starts by focusing its learning on those parts of the sensorimotor space where predictions are easier, and when knowledge in those parts has been acquired, the system shifts its attention to the parts where predictions are more difficult. But while it is clear that through this developmental history the system accumulates increasingly complex *knowledge* about the sensorimotor contingencies of its world (and of the robot's body-world interactions), the authors never show that any *competence* (i.e., ability to *do* something) has been acquired. All you can observe is that the actions that are chosen at the beginning of learning are different from those that are chosen at the end, but *no accumulation of skills is demonstrated*. The same happens in most other works on knowledge-based intrinsic motivation systems (e.g., Huang and Weng 2002; Lee et al. 2009; Marshall et al. 2004; Schmidhuber 1991b; Storck et al. 1995, but see Baranes and Oudeyer 2009 for a case in which the use of the knowledge acquired through intrinsic motivations for control, i.e., competence, *is* demonstrated).

What are then the relationships between such knowledge-based systems and the acquisition of competence? There might be different answers to this question, the first of which simply stating that the ultimate goal of learning is not to acquire skills, but rather knowledge. For the reasons discussed above, however, we are not satisfied by this position. Indeed, if one is interested in understanding the mechanisms underlying the intelligent *behavior* of organisms, or in building robots which can *act* intelligently, one has to solve the problem of how knowledge can support the acquisition of skills.

One possibility is that once an accurate model of the sensory consequences of actions has been acquired, this model can directly guide behavior through its *inversion*, as it is done in some forms of model-based control (Hof et al. 2009): given the current goal of the system and the current context, the agent might internally simulate the consequences of all its actions and choose to perform the one whose predicted consequence are more similar to the goal (this is the approach taken, e.g., by Baranes and Oudeyer 2009; see also Baldassarre 2002b). This approach has the problem that it may be computationally very expensive, and it might become just unfeasible in realistic conditions, where the spaces of states and actions are high-dimensional and/or continuous. In these conditions, as primitive actions cannot usually directly lead to desired states, sequences of actions must be used, and so the complexity of the search grows exponentially.

Another possibility might be to suggest that the acquired model can be used for training the behavioral controller (as it happens, e.g., in the *distal teacher* framework: see Jordan and Rumelhart 1992). Notwithstanding the attractiveness of this idea, this seems to represent a very indirect route to skill learning. Indeed, consider that this solution would involve (a) the training of a behavioral system (on the basis of knowledge-based intrinsic motivations) so that (b) its behavior favors the training of a predictor (c) which then is used for training a second behavioral system (or for retraining the first one) to pursue its goals. Why not following a more straightforward route and directly train the skills? We do not want to deny that building models of the effects of the agent's own actions is useful for learning kills. In fact, we do think that prediction plays fundamental roles for action execution and learning. What we are questioning here is the idea that models are learnt *before* and *independently from* the skills that they are supposed to support. Hence, in our view, modeling abilities should *complement* and *aid* acquisition of skills, not *replace* them.

Yet another possibility is to claim that using knowledge-based intrinsic rewards can directly help the system not only in improving its knowledge but also in improving its skills (this is the position taken by Schmidhuber 2012). The idea is that by being rewarded by some form of prediction error (or improvement in prediction), a behaving system will tend to reproduce the actions that lead to unexpected consequences. Once the capacity to systematically reproduce those consequences has been acquired, a good model can be developed, the prediction error (improvements) will decrease together with the intrinsic rewards, and the system will move on and try to learn something else. Though we think that this idea is on the right track, it might still suffer of some important limitations.

The fundamental problem is that in order for a purely knowledge-based mechanism to optimally support the acquisition of a cumulative collection of skills, one should assume a very strict and direct link between knowledge and competence that seems difficult to justify. For example, what can assure that the predictions related to the system's own actions are in general more interesting than those that depend only on the environment? If this cannot be guaranteed, what would prevent a purely knowledge-based intrinsic motivation system to stop moving and spend its time in passively observing and modeling interesting parts of the environment *instead of* focusing on learning useful skills?

Furthermore, there are certainly a lot of situations that are challenging to predict but for which the actions are relatively trivial or even irrelevant. For example, imagine a humanoid robot that has the goal of clearing a table full of different objects by pushing them on the floor. Predicting the effects of own actions is surely possible but very complex. Instead, the action of pushing all objects on the floor is rather easy to be learned and accomplished. If the system is intrinsically motivated only to increase its knowledge, what would prevent the system in spending its time moving all the objects in all possible positions instead of focusing on the simple actions that would satisfy the goal? Of course, here the level of detail of the prediction is of the most importance, as for example, predictions regarding the presence or absence of objects on the table (rather than their exact location) would be easier to learn and suitable to drive the acquisition of the skill of clearing the table. But the problem is that *which is the right level of detail for the prediction depends on the competence you want to acquire*; how can a purely knowledge-based system decide which is the level of abstraction that is appropriate for improving competence?

And for many difficult skills, there might even be no level of detail in predictions that would be appropriate for the learning system. If the problem is too difficult, the desired consequences might be just too unlikely to manifest for the skill to be learned through knowledge-based intrinsic motivations alone. For example, think about the ability to juggle three balls: how could one acquire this ability through purely knowledge-based intrinsic motivations? If predictions are done at the level of the positions of the balls in space, the system would go on forever in learning the irrelevant predictions about all possible results of its actions of throwing the balls in all directions. But even if the predictions regard a more appropriate representation of the state space, for example, regarding whether or not a ball has been caught, the task is so difficult that after some unsuccessful attempts, the predictor will learn that the behaving system is not able to catch the ball on the fly, the prediction error (and prediction improvements) will go to zero, and the system will lose interest in the activity and pass to something else. The general point is that when I want to learn juggling, my behavior seems to be driven by a motivation that is directly related to the acquisition of that particular skill, and not just to the general predictions of the consequences of my movements.

Finally, another key problem of the knowledge-based intrinsic motivation models proposed so far is related to the cumulativity of learning. When the behaving system has learnt to systematically reproduce a certain consequence and the rewarding prediction improvements decrease to zero, the reinforcement learning system will begin to receive less rewards than expected and start to *unlearn* the just acquired behavior. This is exactly what happens, for example, in the system of Schmidhuber (1991b): once predictions within a given part of the sensorimotor space are learnt, the system gets bored and learns to *avoid* the actions just acquired. Hence, after training the system has cumulated knowledge but no competence. For an intrinsically motivated system to be cumulative in the acquisition of skills, it is necessary not only to temporarily focus its training on different sensorimotor activities but also to have a means for storing skills after they have been successfully discovered so that the system's repertoire can increase and old skills can be reused and combined to learn new ones. Hence, it seems impossible to study intrinsic motivations for cumulative learning without considering the architectural issue of how skills can be cumulated.

7 Intrinsic Motivations and Skills Accumulation

7.1 *Hierarchy and Modularity of Skill Organization*

A multitask cumulative learning system seems to need two key ingredients: (a) some form of structural modularity, where different skills are at least partially stored in different parts of the system and (b) some form of hierarchical organization, where a higher-level system is responsible for selecting which low-level module (expert) to use and train in each context. The need for a structurally modular and hierarchical organization of action has sometimes been questioned, most notably by the work of Botvinick and Plaut (2004) and of Tani and colleagues (e.g., Tani et al. 2008; Yamashita and Tani 2008). But the two basic features of structural modularity and hierarchy are common to the vast majority of computational models that deal with the acquisition of several skills, even though they are instantiated in different ways within different systems (Baldassarre 2002a; Barto et al. 2004; Caligiore et al. 2010; Dayan and Hinton 1993; Dietterich 2000; Doya et al. 2002; Haruno et al. 2001; Parr and Russell 1997; Schembri et al. 2007a; Singh 1992; Tani and Nolfi 1999; Wiering and Schmidhuber 1997, see Barto and Mahadevan 2003 for a review).

Furthermore, action selection and learning in real brains seem in fact to display a considerable level of modular and hierarchical organization (Fuster 2001; Grafton and Hamilton 2007; Meunier et al. 2010; Miller and Cohen 2001; Redgrave et al. 1999). Action selection is supposed to be implemented in the basal ganglia (Mink 1996; Redgrave 2007), a group of subcortical structures that is also thought to be responsible for the processes underlying reinforcement learning phenomena (Barto 1995; Doya 2000; Houk et al. 1995; Joel et al. 2002). Interestingly, the basal ganglia form a number of parallel loops with most of the cortex and in particular with those parts that are most directly related to action, that is, the whole frontal cortex and associative parietal and temporal areas (Alexander et al. 1986; Joel and Weiner 1994). These parallel loops can be observed at different levels of abstractions. First, loops are present at the level of macro-areas, thus forming different networks supposed to implement different functions: for example, a limbic network (with orbitofrontal cortex), an associative network (with dorsal prefrontal cortex, parietal cortex, and temporal cortex), and a sensorimotor network (with motor and premotor cortex) (Yin and Knowlton 2006). Second, parallel loops are present *within* each macro-area, for example, distinguishing parts of the motor cortex related to the control of different actuators, for example, an arm (Romanelli et al. 2005). Finally, *within* each subarea dedicated to a specific actuator, different loops might be responsible for implementing different actions (Gurney et al. 2001).

If one assumes that the accumulation of skills requires a learning architecture that is at least partially modular and hierarchical, the problem of identifying good intrinsic learning signals splits in two subproblems, as different levels of the hierarchy are likely to require different signals. In a system composed of several experts implementing different skills and a selector that arbitrates between them, the problem for each expert consists in identifying which skill to acquire and how, whereas the problem for the selector consists in deciding what to learn and when, that is, which skill to train in each context (Baldassarre and Mirolli 2012). What kind of learning signals can help to solve these problems? We argue that knowledge-based rewards might be used for training the experts, while competence-based learning signals might be used for training the selector.

7.2 *Knowledge-Based Signals for Skill Acquisition*

In line with most machine learning research, here we consider a skill as the ability to reach a certain final state (goal) in some conditions. This is also in line with how behavior seems to be organized in real brains, where actions are defined, at least at the cortical level, by their end states, that is, their outcomes, rather than by the specific movements that are performed by the subject (Graziano 2006; Rizzolatti and Luppino 2001). In this respect, probably the most important problem that an autonomous learning system should solve is the identification of the skills that it is worth acquiring. In other words, an autonomous cumulative learning agent must learn not only how to reach certain states but also which states of the world can be achieved in certain contexts given the appropriate behavior. We think that knowledge-based intrinsic motivation mechanisms might represent appropriate solutions to both these problems. In particular, both the discovery of which are the possible skills to be acquired, and the training of these skills might be driven by the same reinforcement signals provided by the detection of *unpredicted* events.

A possible way in which this might happen in real brains has recently been proposed in the neuroscientific literature by Redgrave and Gurney (2006, see also Gurney et al. 2012; Redgrave et al. 2012) as the repetition bias hypothesis. If the detection of an unpredicted change in the environment is immediately followed by a learning signal that biases the agent to reproduce the actions performed before the change, this might lead the system to focus learning on the change and to identify which are the specific aspects of the behavior that caused the event. This result will be achieved on the basis of the statistics of the agent–environment interactions: those aspects of the behavior that cause the environmental change will be reinforced more than those that do not, thus further increasing the probability of being deployed. As the behavior of the system is sculpted and starts to reliably produce the same environmental change, the change becomes predictable on the basis of the performed actions and so stops producing intrinsic rewards (Mirolli et al. 2012; Santucci et al. 2010).

This hypothesis can explain otherwise puzzling findings related to the neural basis of reinforcement learning, in particular, regarding the phasic activation of the neuromodulator dopamine. Phasic dopamine is released in the basal ganglia when rewards like food are received, and this enhances the plasticity of striatal synapses (Reynolds and Wickens 2002). Furthermore, after learning has taken place, phasic dopamine is no more released in conjunction with reward delivery but is rather anticipated at the time of the presentation of the stimulus that allowed predicting the reward (conditioning). If after learning the reward is omitted, a dip in baseline dopamine release is observed at the time of the predicted reward (Schultz 1998). All these data have led to propose that phasic dopamine constitutes the biological analog of the TD error signal of reinforcement learning models and represents the reward prediction error that drives biological reinforcement learning (Houk et al 1995; Schultz et al. 1997; Schultz and Dickinson 2000).

But there are several known phenomena that do not fit the reward prediction error hypothesis of phasic dopamine, which are not discussed here as they are reviewed at length in Redgrave et al. (2012). The most important point for the present discussion is the fact that phasic dopamine is triggered not only in the presence of rewards (or reward predicting stimuli, see above) but also in response to all kinds of unpredicted salient events, including sudden luminance changes and sounds (Dommett et al. 2005; Horvitz 2000), likely based on the processes taking place in a subcortical brain structure named *superior colliculus*. This supports the hypothesis discussed above that unpredicted events can generate intrinsic reinforcement signals that support the acquisition of novel actions.

Interestingly, dopamine release is triggered not only by the superior colliculus in response to unexpected simple environmental changes but also by the *hippocampus* in response to the detection of novel situations (Lisman and Grace 2005, see also Otmakova et al. 2012). Indeed, the novelty signals of the hippocampus seem to depend on the detection of associative novelty, that is, novelty in the contextual, spatial, and temporal association between perceived stimuli. For these reasons, we speculate that the release of dopamine in the presence of novel situations might underlie the intrinsically motivated learning of skills of increasing complexity, where the outcomes of the actions to be acquired are defined not only by simple instantaneous events but also by spatial and temporal relationships between objects in the environment.

It is important to note that these dopamine signals that are supposed to drive the intrinsically motivated acquisition of skills are simple signals related to unpredicted (or novel) events and states, *not to prediction learning progress*, as predicted by sophisticated knowledge-based intrinsic motivation models (Oudeyer et al. 2007; Schmidhuber 1991a, see also Schmidhuber 2012). How then can biological intrinsic motivation systems avoid getting stuck in trying to learn and reproduce events that are not predictable? The solution can be in the presence of competence-based intrinsic motivation mechanisms at the higher level of the hierarchy.

7.3 Competence-Based Signals for Deciding Which Skill to Train

If, as discussed above, cumulative learning depends on a hierarchical system where different modules learn different skills and a higher-level system selects which module must control behavior in each moment, then the unpredictability problem need not be addressed at the level of the single skills, but can be solved at the level of the selector. Indeed, as the selector is in charge of making strategic decisions about the system activities, it is the selector that has to avoid wasting time in situations where there is nothing to be learned. And this can be done in case the selector is trained with some form of competence-based intrinsic reward signal.

A working example is the use of the TD error of the experts as the reinforcement for the selector in the modular hierarchical reinforcement learning system presented in Sect. 3 (Schembri et al. 2007a,b,c). As mentioned there, such an intrinsically motivated system does not risk getting stuck in unlearnable situations as the TD learning of experts used to train the selector is a measure of the *learning progress* of the experts themselves, so the selector will learn to use, in each context, the expert that is learning the most. This works equally well whatever the reason why an expert cannot learn: an ability too difficult to be acquired or intrinsic stochasticity of action effects and rewards. In any case, the selector will use an expert only as long as it can learn something; when no competence learning progress is made, the TD error will average to zero, and the selector will prefer to move to something else.

Importantly, in order for such a solution to work, the competence-based intrinsic reward to the selector must measure the *learning progress of a skill* (as it is the case for Schembri et al. 2007a,b,c and for the more recent model of Stout and Barto 2010). If the reward reflects the inability of an expert to reach its goal state, as in the original proposal of intrinsically motivated reinforcement learning of Barto et al. (2004), the overall system is subject to the problem of unlearnability just as a purely knowledge-based system trained by prediction errors. In this case, the system could easily get stuck trying to pursue states (or changes of states) that do not depend on its own actions or that are just completely random.

While the biological knowledge-based signal that is supposed to drive the learning of the single skills can be identified with the release of phasic dopamine on the basis of unexpected events (and possibly with the information about associative novelty originating in the hippocampus), the identification of the possible biological implementation of a competence-progress intrinsic motivation signal is a completely open issue. As the signal should be related to the improvements in the acquisition of the agent's ability to systematically produce some environmental change, then it should originate in parts of the brain that may monitor the outcomes of the agent's actions (and, as we are talking about intrinsically motivated learning, the possible action outcomes should not be innately provided with value). Finally, since these signals should drive the reinforcement learning of the high-level selector, it might be related to dopamine, as the lower-level learning signal.

Interestingly, the prelimbic cortex, a part of the prefrontal cortex of the rat, might have the prerequisites to be involved in such a competence-progress evaluation. First, it is a brain region that is known to be involved in goal-directed action-outcome learning (Dalley et al. 2004; Heidbreder and Groenewegen 2003). Second, it receives a direct input from the hippocampus, where signals regarding the novelty of situations are generated. Third, it represents one of the major excitatory inputs of the ventral tegmental area dopaminergic neurons (Geisler et al. 2007), and the activation of these connections are known to produce dopaminergic release

(Taber et al. 1995). As we are not aware of any hypothesis about the functional role of the connections from the prelimbic cortex to the dopaminergic neurons, it would be interesting to investigate the possibility that they underlie competence-based intrinsic motivation signals.

8 Summary and Open Challenges

In this contribution we have discussed the different functions that intrinsic motivations might play in cumulative learning and the different mechanisms that may support these functions in both natural and artificial learning systems. With respect to the *function*, we have argued that the ultimate role of intrinsic motivations is supporting the cumulative acquisition of increasingly complex skills and that computational research on this issue would significantly benefit from making this point more explicit in the proposed models: in our view, models of intrinsic motivations should aim at letting artificial agents increase their *skills*, with the eventual accumulation of *knowledge* playing only a supporting role.

With respect to the *mechanisms*, we have argued that both knowledge-based and competence-based mechanisms might play important roles. The cumulative acquisition of skills might require some sort of modular and hierarchical architecture, in which different experts acquire different skills and a selector decides which expert to use in each situation. In such a hierarchical learning system, intrinsic motivations might play two sub-functions: (1) driving the learning of the experts by setting which are the skills that are to be acquired and (2) driving the decisions of the selector regarding which expert to train in each context. On the basis of biological evidence, we have suggested that knowledge-based mechanisms like the detection of unpredicted events might support the former function, while we have speculated that competence-based mechanisms measuring the progress in skill acquisition might support the latter. Several important challenges need to be tackled in future research, in particular with respect to the goal of modeling the intrinsically motivated cumulative learning of real organisms.

A first interesting research direction has to do with knowledge-based intrinsic motivations. In particular, with the intrinsic reinforcements that are supposed to support the acquisition of single skills through the discovery of which are the environmental changes that depend on the behavior of the learning agent and that thus can become target outcomes for the actions to be learned. As discussed above, such knowledge-based intrinsic motivations might be represented by *unexpected changes*, as seems to be the case for the signals that are triggered by the superior colliculus, or by the *novelty signals* that seem to be produced by the hippocampus. There are a very few models targeting real experimental data of these kinds of mechanisms (e.g., Fiore et al. 2008; Sirois and Mareschal 2004). In the most recent of them, we have shown how intrinsic reinforcements due to unexpected events might be particularly appropriate for driving the accumulation of skills that can be then deployed for maximizing extrinsic rewards (Mirolli et al. 2012; Santucci et al. 2010). However, reinforcement signals that are so simple can only represent the very basic ingredients of intrinsically motivated learning. Complex actions can be acquired only on the basis of more complex learning signals, which we have argued might be represented by the dopaminergic signals triggered by the hippocampus on the basis of the perception of novel stimuli or of novel associations between stimuli. Modeling these more complex forms of intrinsically motivated learning is a completely open challenge.

A second fundamental issue for future research is checking whether our hypothesis about competence-based intrinsic motivations in real animals can be supported by animal research and, in case it is, trying to understand which are the brain mechanisms that implement competence-based motivation signals. In fact, while the study of competence-based intrinsic motivations is a fundamental research topic in the psychological literature on motivations in humans (Csikszentmihalyi 1991; De Charms 1968; Ryan and Deci 2000), the topic of intrinsic motivations is now far less investigated within the field of animal psychology, and this literature has been generally focusing more on demonstrating the existence of knowledge-based intrinsic motivations like novelty, surprise, and curiosity (Butler 1953; Kish 1955; Reed et al. 1996). Analogously, while we have identified the putative neural bases of knowledge-based intrinsic motivations (as the activation of the dopaminergic system by the detection of unexpected changes from the superior colliculus and, possibly, by the detection of novelty from the hippocampus), the identification of the possible neural mechanisms of competence-based intrinsic motivation signals (if any) is much harder at the moment and hence constitutes a very important challenge for future research.

A further open issue is the identification and development of *hierarchical/modular* architectures that can support the kind of intrinsically motivated cumulative acquisition of skills that we have discussed so far (Baldassarre and Mirolli 2010). Two key requirements for such architectures are that they must (a) work with *continuous* state and action spaces and (b) be capable of *learning autonomously*, in particular on the basis of (intrinsic) reinforcement learning signals. In particular, the capacity of these architectures to learn autonomously and with continuous state and action spaces would make them relevant both for controlling robots and for modeling real organisms (in particular if based on neural-network components). Various hierarchical architectures have been proposed in the literature, but the majority of them are either dependent on abstract/symbolic representations of space and/or actions (Dayan and Hinton 1993; Dietterich 2000; Parr and Russell 1997; Singh 1992; Wiering and Schmidhuber 1997; see Barto and Mahadevan 2003 for a review), or is trained in a supervised fashion (e.g., Haruno et al. 2001). Although there are exceptions (Caligiore et al. 2010; Doya et al. 2002; Konidaris and Barto 2009; Provost et al. 2006; Schembri et al. 2007c), much more work is needed in this area, given its importance for implementing intrinsically motivated cumulative learning.

A last important open issue is related to what we might call *goal-driven learning*. With this expression, we refer to the possibility that intrinsic motivations might let a system form *goals* and that it is these goals that drive the subsequent acquisition of skills. The computational literature on hierarchical reinforcement learning has proposed several ways of creating goals but mostly as subgoals derived from the final goal related to the task at hand (but for exceptions see Jonsson and Barto 2006; Vigorito and Barto 2010). Here we refer instead to a situation in which there is no task to accomplish, but the system is endowed with intrinsic motivations that allow it to autonomously form goals with respect to which to acquire a competence, that is, the capacity to pursue them in an efficient way. This capacity might be important for at least two reasons. First, the representation of the goal could allow the system to generate an intrinsic reward when the system succeeds in producing the action or the combination of actions that allow it to achieve the goal. This might be crucial for allowing the system to learn the action or the action combination, that is, to acquire the competence which reliably leads to the achievement of the goal itself. Second, it might make the system activate a number of perceptual and motor processes focused on the acquisition of a specific competence while temporarily ignoring other stimuli which might generate other interfering intrinsic signals. For example, the system might focus attention on the portion of space and objects relevant for achieving the goal under focus or might produce only those actions which are related to achieving goals similar to the pursued one. Even this focusing mechanism might be crucial for learning complex skills. The importance of goals is evident, for example, in the IMRL systems proposed by Barto et al. (2004), where options are created for leading the system to salient events (goals), but in that case, goals are decided by the experimenter and hand-coded. Developing models in which goals are autonomously formed by the agent on the basis of intrinsic motivations and drive skill acquisition is another fundamental challenge for future research.

Acknowledgements Thanks to Pierre-Yves Oudeyer, Andrew Barto, Kevin Gurney, and Jochen Triesh for their useful comments that substantially helped to improve the paper. Any remaining omission or mistake is our own blame. This research has received funds from the European Commission 7th Framework Programme (FP7/2007-2013), "Challenge 2: Cognitive Systems, Interaction, Robotics," Grant Agreement No. ICT-IP-231722, Project "IM-CLeVeR: Intrinsically Motivated Cumulative Learning Versatile Robots."

References

Alexander, G., DeLong, M., Strick, P.: Parallel organization of functionally segregated circuits linking basal ganglia and cortex. Annu. Rev. Neurosci. **9**, 357–381 (1986)

Baldassarre, G.: A modular neural-network model of the basal ganglia's role in learning and selecting motor behaviours. J. Cogn. Syst. Res. **3**, 5–13 (2002a)

Baldassarre, G.: Planning with neural networks and reinforcement learning. Ph.D. Thesis, Computer Science Department, University of Essex (2002b)

Baldassarre, G., Mirolli, M.: What are the key open challenges for understanding autonomous cumulative learning of skills? AMD Newslett. **7**(2), 2–3 (2010)

Baldassarre, G., Mirolli, M.: Deciding which skill to learn when: Temporal-difference competence-based intrinsic motivation (td-cb-im). In: Baldassarre, G., Mirolli, M. (eds.) Intrinsically Motivated Learning in Natural and Artificial Systems. Springer, Berlin (2012, this volume)

Baranes, A., Oudeyer, P.-Y.: R-iac: Robust intrinsically motivated exploration and active learning. IEEE Trans. Auton. Mental Dev. **1**(3), 155–169 (2009)

Baranes, A., Oudeyer, P.-Y.: Intrinsically motivated goal exploration for active motor learning in robots: A case study. In: Proceedings of the International Conference on Intelligent Robots and Systems (IROS 2010). Taipel, Taiwan (2010)
Barto, A.: Adaptive critics and the basal ganglia. In: Houk, J.C., Davis, J., Beiser, D. (eds.) Models of Information Processing in the Basal Ganglia, pp. 215–232. MIT, Cambridge (1995)
Barto, A., Singh, S., Chentanez, N.: Intrinsically motivated learning of hierarchical collections of skills. In: International Conference on Developmental Learning (ICDL), La Jolla (2004)
Barto, A., Sutton, R., Anderson, C.: Neuron-like adaptive elements that can solve difficult learning control problems. IEEE Trans. Syst. Man Cybern. **13**, 834–846 (1983)
Barto, A.G.: What are intrinsic reward signals? AMD Newslett. **7**(2), 3 (2010)
Barto, A.G.: Intrinsic motivation and reinforcement learning. In: Baldassarre, G., Mirolli, M. (eds.) Intrinsically Motivated Learning in Natural and Artificial Systems. Springer, Berlin (2012, this volume)
Barto, A.G., Mahadevan, S.: Recent advances in hierarchical reinforcement learning. Discr. Event Dyn. Syst. **13**(4), 341–379 (2003)
Berlyne, D.E.: Conflict, Arousal., Curiosity. McGraw-Hill, New York (1960)
Botvinick, M., Plaut, D.: Doing without schema hierarchies: A recurrent connectionist approach to routine sequential action and its pathologies. Psychol. Rev. **111**, 395–429 (2004)
Brooks, R.A.: Intelligence without representation. Artif. Intell. J. **47**, 139–159 (1991)
Butler, R.A.: Discrimination learning by rhesus monkeys to visual-exploration motivation. J. Comp. Physiol. Psychol. **46**(2), 95–98 (1953)
Caligiore, D., Mirolli, M., Parisi, D., Baldassarre, G.: A bioinspired hierarchical reinforcement learning architecture for modeling learning of multiple skills with continuous states and actions. In: Proceedings of the Tenth International Conference on Epigenetic Robotics, vol. 149. Lund University Cognitive Studies, Lund (2010)
Clark, A.: Being There: Putting Brain, Body and World Together Again. Oxford University Press, Oxford (1997)
Csikszentmihalyi, M.: Flow: The Psychology of Optimal Experience. Harper Perennial, New York (1991)
Dalley, J.W., Cardinal, R.N., Robbins, T.W.: Prefrontal executive and cognitive functions in rodents: Neural and neurochemical substrates. Neurosci. Biobehav. Rev. **28**(7), 771–784 (2004)
Dayan, P., Hinton, G.E.: Feudal reinforcement learning. In: Advances in Neural Information Processing Systems 5, pp. 271–278. Morgan Kaufmann, San Francisco (1993)
De Charms, R.: Personal Causation: The Internal Affective Determinants of Behavior. Academic, New York (1968)
Deci, E.: Intrinsic Motivation. Plenum, New York (1975)
Deci, E.L., Ryan, R.M.: Intrinsic Motivation and Self-determination in Human Behavior. Plenum, New York (1985)
Dember, W., Earl, R.: Analysis of exploratory, manipulatory and curiosity behaviors. Psychol. Rev. **64**, 91–96 (1957)
Dietterich, T.: Hierarchical reinforcement learning with the maxq value function decomposition. J. Artif. Intell. Res. **13**, 227–303 (2000)
Dommett, E., Coizet, V., Blaha, C.D., Martindale, J., Lefebvre, V., Walton, N., Mayhew, J.E.W., Overton, P.G., Redgrave, P.: How visual stimuli activate dopaminergic neurons at short latency. Science **307**(5714), 1476–1479 (2005)
Doya, K.: Complementary roles of basal ganglia and cerebellum in learning and motor control. Curr. Opin. Neurobiol. **10**(6), 732–739 (2000)
Doya, K., Samejima, K., Katagiri, K.-i., Kawato, M.: Multiple model-based reinforcement learning. Neural Comput. **14**(6), 1347–1369 (2002)
Festinger, L.: A Theory of Cognitive Dissonance. Stanford University Press, Stanford (1957)
Fiore, V., Mannella, F., Mirolli, M., Gurney, K., Baldassarre, G.: Instrumental conditioning driven by neutral stimuli: A model tested with a simulated robotic rat. In: Proceedings of the Eight International Conference on Epigenetic Robotics, number 139, pp. 13–20. Lund University Cognitive Studies, Lund (2008)

Fuster, J.: The prefrontal cortex-an update: Time is of the essence. Neuron **2**, 319–333 (2001)

Geisler, S., Derst, C., Veh, R.W., Zahm, D.S.: Glutamatergic afferents of the ventral tegmental area in the rat. J. Neurosci. **27**(21), 5730–5743 (2007)

Grafton, S.T., Hamilton, A.: Evidence for a distributed hierarchy of action representation in the brain. Hum. Brain Mapp. Movement Sci. **26**(4), 590–616 (2007)

Graziano, M.: The organization of behavioral repertoire in motor cortex. Annu. Rev. Neurosci. **29**, 105–134 (2006)

Gurney, K., Lepora, N., Shah, A., Koene, A., Redgrave, P.: Action discovery and intrinsic motivation: A biologically constrained formalisation. In: Baldassarre, G., Mirolli, M. (eds.) Intrinsically Motivated Learning in Natural and Artificial Systems. Springer, Berlin (2012, this volume)

Gurney, K., Prescott, T.J., Redgrave, P.: A computational model of action selection in the basal ganglia I. A new functional anatomy. Biol. Cybern. **84**(6), 401–410 (2001)

Harlow, H.F.: Learning and satiation of response in intrinsically motivated complex puzzle performance by monkeys. J. Comp. Physiol. Psychol. **43**, 289–294 (1950)

Harlow, H.F., Harlow, M.K., Meyer, D.R.: Learning motivated by a manipulation drive. J. Exp. Psychol. **40**, 228–234 (1950)

Haruno, M., Wolpert, D., Kawato, M.: Mosaic model for sensorimotor learning and control. Neural Comput. **13**, 2201–2220 (2001)

Hebb, D.: Drives and the conceptual nervous system. Psychol. Rev. **62**, 243–254 (1955)

Heidbreder, C.A., Groenewegen, H.J.: The medial prefrontal cortex in the rat: Evidence for a dorso-ventral distinction based upon functional and anatomical characteristics. Neurosci. Biobehav. Rev. **27**(6), 555–579 (2003)

Hof, P.M., Scherer, C., Heuberger, P.S. (eds.): Model-Based Control: Bridging Rigorous Theory and Advanced Technology. Springer, Berlin (2009)

Horvitz, J.: Mesolimbocortical and nigrostriatal dopamine responses to salient non-reward events. Neuroscience **96**(4), 651–656 (2009)

Houk, J., Adams, J., Barto, A.: A model of how the basal ganglia generates and uses neural signals that predict reinforcement. In: Houk, J., Davis, J., Beiser, D. (eds.) Models of Information Processing in the Basal Ganglia, pp. 249–270. MIT, Cambridge (1995)

Huang, X., Weng, J.: Novelty and reinforcement learning in the value system of developmental robots. In: Proceedings Second International Workshop on Epigenetic Robotics, Edinburgh, pp. 47–55 (2002)

Hull, C.L.: Principles of Behavior. Appleton-Century-Crofts, New York (1943)

Hunt, H.: Intrinsic motivation and its role in psychological development. Nebraska Symp. Motiv. **13**, 189–282 (1965)

Joel, D., Niv, Y., Ruppin, E.: Actor-critic models of the basal ganglia: New anatomical and computational perspectives. Neural Netw. **15**(4), 535–547 (2002)

Joel, D., Weiner, I.: The organization of the basal ganglia-thalamocortical circuits: Open interconnected rather than closed segregated. Neuroscience **63**(2), 363–379 (1994)

Jonsson, A., Barto, A.: Causal graph based decomposition of factored mdps. J. Mach. Learn. Res. **7**, 2259–2301 (2006)

Jordan, M.I., Rumelhart, D.E.: Forward models: Supervised learning with a distal teacher. Cogn. Sci. **16**, 307–354 (1992)

Kagan, J.: Motives and development. J. Pers. Soc. Psychol. **22**, 51–66 (1972)

Kish, G.: Learning when the onset of illumination is used as the reinforcing stimulus. J. Comp. Physiol. Psychol. **48**(4), 261–264 (1955)

Kish, G., Antonitis, J.: Unconditioned operant behavior in two homozygous strains of mice. J. Genet. Psychol. Aging **88**(1), 121–129 (1956)

Konidaris, G.D., Barto, A.G.: Skill discovery in continuous reinforcement learning domains using skill chaining. In: Advances in Neural Information Processing Systems (NIPS 2009), pp. 1015–1023. Vancouver, B.C., Canada (2009)

Langton, C.G. (ed.): Artificial Life: The Proceedings of an Interdisciplinary Workshop on the Synthesis and Simulation of Living Systems. Addison-Wesley, Redwood City (1989)

Lee, R., Walker, R., Meeden, L., Marshall, J.: Category-based intrinsic motivation. In: Proceedings of the Ninth International Conference on Epigenetic Robotics, vol. 146, pp. 81–88. Lund University Cognitive Studies, Lund (2009)

Lisman, J.E., Grace, A.A.: The hippocampal-vta loop: Controlling the entry of information into long-term memory. Neuron **46**(5), 703–713 (2005)

Marshall, J., Blank, D., Meeden, L.: An emergent framework for self-motivation in developmental robotics. In: Proceedings of the Third International Conference on Development and Learning (ICDL 2004), La Jolla, pp. 104–111 (2004)

Merrick, K., Maher, M.L.: Motivated learning from interesting events: Adaptive, multitask learning agents for complex environments. Adap. Behav. **17**(1), 7–27 (2009)

Meunier, D., Lambiotte, R., Bullmore, E.T.: Modular and hierarchically modular organization of brain networks. Front. Neurosci. **4** (2010)

Meyer, J.-A., Wilson, S.W. (eds.): From Animals to Animats: Proceedings of the First International Conference on Simulation of Adaptive Behavior. MIT, Cambridge (1990)

Miller, E., Cohen, J.: An integrative theory of prefrontal cortex function. Annu. Rev. Neurosci. **24**, 167–202 (2001)

Mink, J.: The basal ganglia: Focused selection and inhibition of competing motor programs. Prog. Neurobiol. **50**(4), 381–425 (1996)

Mirolli, M., Santucci, V.G., Baldassarre, G.: Phasic dopamine as a prediction error of intrinsic and extrinsic reinforcements driving both action acquisition and reward maximization: A simulated robotic study. Neural Netw. (2012, submitted for publication)

Mitchell, T.M.: Mach. Learn.. McGraw-Hill, New York (1997)

Montgomery, K.: The role of exploratory drive in learning. J. Comp. Physiol. Psychol. **47**, 60–64 (1954)

Otmakova, N., Duzel, E., Deutch, A.Y., Lisman, J.E.: The hippocampal-vta loop: The role of novelty and motivation in controlling the entry of information into long-term memory. In: Baldassarre, G., Mirolli, M. (eds.) Intrinsically Motivated Learning in Natural and Artificial Systems. Springer, Berlin (2012, this volume)

Oudeyer, P.-Y., Kaplan, F.: What is intrinsic motivation? A typology of computational approaches. Front. Neurorobot. (2007)

Oudeyer, P.-Y., Kaplan, F., Hafner, V.V.: Intrinsic motivation systems for autonomous mental development. IEEE Trans. Evol. Comput. **11**(2), 265–286 (2007)

Parr, R., Russell, S.J.: Reinforcement learning with hierarchies of machines. In: Advances in Neural Information Processing Systems. MIT, Cambridge (1997)

Pfeifer, R., Scheier, C.: Understanding intelligence. MIT, Cambridge (1999)

Provost, J., Kuipers, B.J., Miikkulainen, R.: Developing navigation behavior through self-organizing distinctive state abstraction. Connect. Sci. **18**(2), 159–172 (2006)

Redgrave, P.: Basal ganglia. Scholarpedia **2**(6), 1825 (2007)

Redgrave, P., Gurney, K.: The short-latency dopamine signal: A role in discovering novel actions? Nat. Rev. Neurosci. **7**(12), 967–975 (2006)

Redgrave, P., Gurney, K., Stafford, T., Thirkettle, M., Lewis, J.: The role of the basal ganglia in discovering novel actions. In: Baldassarre, G., Mirolli, M. (eds.) Intrinsically Motivated Learning in Natural and Artificial Systems. Springer, Berlin (2012, this volume)

Redgrave, P., Prescott, T., Gurney, K.: The basal ganglia: A vertebrate solution to the selection problem? Neuroscience **89**, 1009–1023 (1999)

Reed, P., Mitchell, C., Nokes, T.: Intrinsic reinforcing properties of putatively neutral stimuli in an instrumental two-lever discrimination task. Anim. Learn. Behav. **24**, 38–45 (1996)

Reynolds, J.N., Wickens, J.R.: Dopamine-dependent plasticity of corticostriatal synapses. Neural Netw. **15**(4–6), 507–521 (2002)

Rizzolatti, G., Luppino, G.: The cortical motor system. Neuron **31**(6), 889–901 (2001)

Romanelli, P., Esposito, V., Schaal, D.W., Heit, G.: Somatotopy in the basal ganglia: Experimental and clinical evidence for segregated sensorimotor channels. Brain Res. Rev. **48**, 112–28 (2005)

Russell, S.J., Norvig, P.: Artificial Intelligence: A Modern Approach, 2nd edn. Prentice Hall, Upper Saddle River (2003)

Ryan, R., Deci, E.: Intrinsic and extrinsic motivations: Classic definitions and new directions. Contemp. Educ. Psychol. **25**, 54–67 (2000)

Santucci, V., Baldassarre, G., Mirolli, M.: Biological cumulative learning requires intrinsic motivations: A simulated robotic study on the development of visually-guided reaching. In: Proceedings of the Tenth International Conference on Epigenetic Robotics, vol. 149. Lund University Cognitive Studies, Lund (2010)

Saunders, R., Gero, J.: Curious agents and situated design evaluations. In: Gero, J., Brazier, F. (eds.) Agents in Design 2002, pp. 133–149. Key Centre of Design Computing and Cognition, University of Sydney, Sydney (2002)

Schembri, M., Mirolli, M., Baldassarre, G.: Evolution and learning in an intrinsically motivated reinforcement learning robot. In: Advances in Artificial Life. Proceedings of the 9th European Conference on Artificial Life, LNAI, vol. 4648, pp. 294–333. Springer, Berlin (2007a)

Schembri, M., Mirolli, M., Baldassarre, G.: Evolving childhood's length and learning parameters in an intrinsically motivated reinforcement learning robot. In: Proceedings of the Seventh International Conference on Epigenetic Robotics, pp. 141–148. Lund University Cognitive Studies, Lund (2007b)

Schembri, M., Mirolli, M., Baldassarre, G.: Evolving internal reinforcers for an intrinsically motivated reinforcement-learning robot. In: Proceedings of the 6th International Conference on Development and Learning, pp. E1–E6. Imperial College, London (2007c)

Schmidhuber, J.: Curious model-building control systems. In: Proceedings of the International Joint Conference on Neural Networks, vol. 2, pp. 1458–1463. IEEE, Singapore (1991a)

Schmidhuber, J.: A possibility for implementing curiosity and boredom in model-building neural controllers. In: From Animals to Animats: Proceedings of the First International Conference on Simulation of Adaptive Behavior, pp. 222–227. MIT, Cambridge (1991b)

Schmidhuber, J.: Exploring the predictable. In: Ghosh, S., Tsutsui, T. (eds.) Advances in Evolutionary Computing, pp. 579–612. Springer, Berlin (2002)

Schmidhuber, J.: Maximizing fun by creating data with easily reducible subjective complexity. In: Baldassarre, G., Mirolli, M. (eds.) Intrinsically Motivated Learning in Natural and Artificial Systems. Springer, Berlin (2012, this volume)

Schultz, W.: Predictive reward signal of dopamine neurons. J. Neurophysiol. **80**(1), 1–27 (1998)

Schultz, W., Dayan, P., Montague, P.: A neural substrate of prediction and reward. Science **275**, 1593–1599 (1997)

Schultz, W., Dickinson, A.: Neuronal coding of prediction errors. Annu. Rev. Neurosci. **23**, 473–500 (2000)

Simon, H.A.: The Sciences of the Artificial, 3rd edn. MIT, Cambridge (1996)

Singh, S.P.: Transfer of learning by composing solutions of elemental sequential tasks. Mach. Learn. **8**, 323–339 (1992)

Sirois, S., Mareschal, D.: An interacting systems model of infant habituation. J. Cogn. Neurosci. **16**(8), 1352–1362 (2004)

Storck, J., Hochreiter, S., Schmidhuber, J.: Reinforcement-driven information acquisition in non-deterministic environments. In: Proceedings of ICANN'95, vol. 2, pp. 159–164, Paris (1995)

Stout, A., Barto, A.G.: Competence progress intrinsic motivation. In: Proceedings of the 9th International Conference on Development and Learning (ICDL 2010), pp. 257–262. Ann Arbor, USA (2010)

Stout, A., Konidaris, G.D., Barto, A.G.: Intrinsically motivated reinforcement learning: A promising framework for developmental robot learning. In: Proceedings of the AAAI Spring Symposium on Developmental Robotics, Stanford (2005)

Sutton, R., Barto, A.: Reinforcement Learning: An Introduction. MIT, Cambridge (1998)

Sutton, R., Precup, D., Singh, S.: Between mdps and semi-mdps: A framework for temporal abstraction in reinforcement learning. Artif. Intell. **112**, 181–211 (1999)

Sutton, R.S.: Learning to predict by the methods of temporal differences. Mach. Learn. **3**, 9–44 (1988)

Taber, M., Das, S., Fibiger, H.: Cortical regulation of subcortical dopamine release: Mediation via the ventral tegmental area. J. Neurochem. **65**(3), 1407–1410 (1995)

Tani, J., Nishimoto, R., Paine, R.: Achieving 'organic compositionality' through self-organization: Reviews on brain-inspired robotics experiments. Neural Netw. **21**, 584–603 (2008)

Tani, J., Nolfi, S.: Learning to perceive the world as articulated: An approach for hierarchical learning in sensory-motor systems. Neural Netw. **12**, 1131–1141 (1999)

Vigorito, C., Barto, A.: Intrinsically motivated hierarchical skill learning in structured environments. IEEE Trans. Auton. Mental Dev. **2**(2), 83–90 (2010)

Weng, J., McClelland, J., Pentland, A., Sporns, O., Stockman, I., Sur, M., Thelen, E.: Autonomous mental development by robots and animals. Science **291**, 599–600 (2001)

White, R.W.: Motivation reconsidered: The concept of competence. Psychol. Rev. **66**, 297–333 (1959)

Wiering, M., Schmidhuber, J.: Hq-learning. Adap. Behav. **6**, 219–246 (1997)

Yamashita, Y., Tani, J.: Emergence of functional hierarchy in a multiple timescale neural network model: A humanoid robot experiment. PLoS Comput. Biol. **4**(11), e1000220 (2008)

Yin, H.H., Knowlton, B.J.: The role of the basal ganglia in habit formation. Nat. Rev. Neurosci. **7**, 464–476 (2006)

Exploration from Generalization Mediated by Multiple Controllers

Peter Dayan

Abstract Intrinsic motivation involves internally governed drives for exploration, curiosity, and play. These shape subjects over the course of development and beyond to explore to learn and expand the actions they are capable of performing and to acquire skills that can be useful in future domains. We adopt a utilitarian view of this learning process, treating it in terms of exploration bonuses that arise from distributions over the structure of the world that imply potential benefits from generalizing knowledge and skills to subsequent environments. We discuss how functionally and architecturally different controllers may realize these bonuses in different ways.

1 Introduction

The Gittins index (Berry and Fristedt 1985; Gittins 1989) is a famous pinnacle of the analytical analysis of the trade-off between exploration and exploitation. Although it applies slightly more generally, it is often treated in the most straightforward case of an infinite horizon, exponentially discounted, multiarmed bandit problem with appropriate known prior distributions for the payoffs of the arms. Under these circumstances, the index quantifies precisely an exploration bonus (Dayan and Sejnowski 1996; Kakade and Dayan 2002; Ng et al. 1999; Sutton 1990) for choosing (i.e., exploring) an arm whose payoff is incompletely known. This bonus arises because if, when *explored,* the arm is found to be better than expected, then it can be *exploited* in all future choices.

An exactly equivalent way of thinking about the Gittins index is in terms of generalization. Under the conditions above, there is perfect generalization over time

P. Dayan (✉)
University College London, Gatsby Computational Neuroscience Unit, London, UK
e-mail: dayan@gatsby.ucl.ac.uk

G. Baldassarre and M. Mirolli (eds.), *Intrinsically Motivated Learning in Natural and Artificial Systems*, DOI 10.1007/978-3-642-32375-1_4,

for each arm of the bandit. That is, an arm does not change its character—what is learned at one time is exactly appropriate at subsequent times also. Thus, what might typically be considered as intrinsically motivated actions such as playing with, exploring, and engaging with an uncertain arm in order to gain the skill of valuing it are useful, since this skill can be directly generalized to future choices. The exploration bonus (which is formally the difference between the Gittins index for an arm and its mean, certainty-equivalent, worth) translates the uncertainty into units of value (a sort of information value; Howard 1966) and thus quantifies the potential motivational worth of the actions concerned. This worth is intrinsic to the extent that it depends on intrinsic expectations about the possibilities for generalization. This account applies equally to more complex Markov decision problems, as in non-myopic, Bayesian reinforcement learning (RL; e.g., Duff 2000; Poupart et al. 2006; Şimşek and Barto 2006; Wang et al. 2005).

This redescription emphasizes two well-understood points. First, skills are useful because of the possibility of generalization. This is amply discussed in the framework of both hierarchical and multitask RL (e.g., Barto and Mahadevan 2003; Botvinick et al. 2009; Caruana 1997; Dayan and Hinton 1993; Dietterich 1998, 2000; Parr and Russell 1998; Ring 1997, 2005; Singh 1992; Sutton et al. 1999; Tanaka and Yamamura 2003; Wilson et al. 2007). Second, these potential generalization benefits of skill acquisition can be quantified directly in terms of expected value in the overall lifelong experience (Schmidhuber 2006) of the agent concerned.

In this chapter, we consider the resulting view of intrinsic motivation in the context of the multifaceted nature of neural control. That is, we examine aspects of intrinsic motivation that can be understood as arising from generalizability and how the prospect and fact of generalization may be realized in the brain. In order to do this, we depend critically on the concepts and ideas of RL (see Barto 2012). We attempt to put together two sets of issues. First is the statistical structure of the environment that underpins the possibility of generalization (Acuna and Schrater 2009; Wilson et al. 2007; Wingate et al. 2011) and thus formally justifies exploration. Second is the complex architecture underlying decision-making, which involves multiple different controllers based on contrasting functional principles (Daw and Doya 2006; Daw et al. 2005; Dickinson and Balleine 2002; Killcross and Coutureau 2003; Sutton and Barto 1998; Tricomi et al. 2009; Valentin et al. 2007) that embody distinct trade-offs between the computational and statistical complexities of learning and inference. These separate controllers can absorb different information about the structure of the environment and express individual exploration bonuses based on their own capacities. These bonuses, which underpin intrinsically motivated actions, will approximate their normative, Bayesian ideal values.

We first briefly outline this architecture of control. We then discuss environmental priors and generalization and bonus-generating approximations associated with the different controllers. Generalization is a large and complex topic—we discuss just a few of the issues relevant to transfer. Among others, we use as an example the rather saturnine case of learned helplessness (Huys and Dayan 2009; Maier and

Watkins 2005). It is our hope that it will ultimately be possible to interpret the internal rewards underlying intrinsic motivation (Barto et al. 2004; Blank et al. 2005; Huang and Weng 2007; Oudeyer et al. 2007; Schembri et al. 2007; Schmidhuber 1991; Şimşek and Barto 2006; Singh et al. 2005) with which this volume is mostly concerned—i.e., the ectopic constructs such as curiosity, entropy reduction, and novelty—through the lens of approximations embodied in the different controllers.

2 Multiple Controllers

A fierce battle raged in the middle half of the twentieth century between two groups of psychologists. Members of one group, represented prominently by Tolman, were convinced that animals build models of their environments (a form of cognitive mapping) and use them to plan their actions (Tolman 1948). The other group appealed to simpler policies which map stimuli that represent states of the environments directly to responses or actions (Guthrie 1952; Thorndike 1911). These would be learned through reinforcement. In the end, a long series of ingenious experiments into the effects of motivational manipulations (see, e.g., Dickinson and Balleine 2002; Holland 1998) suggested that animals can exhibit both sorts of control (and indeed others) under appropriate circumstances. Discussing these separate controllers might seem like a diversion in the context of a chapter on intrinsic motivation. However, their principles are so radically different that it is essential to understand them to comprehend the different ways that generalization-based exploration can work.

The hallmark of control via an environmental model is its ready sensitivity to changes in contingencies or outcomes that only a model can readily register. That is, consider the example case that the syllogism underpinning the behavior of lever pressing to a light stimulus puts together the premises that presses lead to cheese, and cheese is valuable. If the subject is then shown that the cheese is actually poisonous, then it should be less willing to press the lever by integrating the nature and current worth of the expected outcome. Its actions are then said to be goal directed. In RL terms (Sutton and Barto 1998), this sort of control can be interpreted (Daw et al. 2005) as a form of model-based RL, with the generative model of the domain (the premises of the syllogism) being inverted to give rise to the policy (to press or not to press). More complex problems with multiple steps, such as mazes, can be solved in the same way, but with much more extensive trees of actions and successive likely outcomes.

To preview later material, model-based RL can potentially absorb rather rich information about the prior and generalization structure of environments. Were it computationally tractable, it could therefore lead to sophisticated exploration bonuses, and thus sophisticated intrinsically motivated behavior.

Conversely, the response of lever pressing could have been stamped in by its success in leading to a valued outcome, namely, the cheese, but without the nature of the outcome itself being explicitly represented at all. There are at least two different knowledge structures that could underpin this, both of which can be considered as forms of model-free RL (Sutton and Barto 1998). One is indirect: a form of Q-value (Watkins 1989) for the action of pressing. The other is direct: a mere propensity to press, as in the actor portion of the actor-critic architecture (Barto et al. 1983). Although propensities can be trained by values, they themselves are divorced from particular notions of worth. In either of these cases, poisoning the cheese would have no immediate impact on behavior, since there would be no representation of the now-devalued outcome (the cheese) in the realization of the value or propensity. This behavior is called habitual. Model-free methods such as Q-learning and the actor-critic can famously acquire optimal policies in temporally extended environments such as mazes without building a model (Sutton 1988; Watkins 1989). They do this by a form of bootstrapping implied by the Bellman equation (Bellman 1957), eliminating inconsistencies in the values at successive nodes in the tree.

Model-free RL lacks the informational structure to absorb specific information about the prior or generalization structure of an environment. However, it can reflect general characteristics, for instance, in the form of an optimism bias. That is, consider the case that the subject is optimistic, and so awards a significant positive value to all possible states. As it visits states, it will likely ultimately learn that they are worse than this optimistic guess and will thus be motivated to continue exploring states that it knows less well, and so remains optimistic about. Optimism biases can generate exploration bonuses and thus forms of intrinsically motivated behavior.

The experiments mentioned above (Dickinson and Balleine 2002; Holland 1998) show that the effect of a manipulation such as devaluing the cheese can sometimes be significant, notably after limited training, but sometimes nugatory, e.g., after extended training, consistent with the notion of the progressive formation of habits. Exactly the same has been shown in humans (Tricomi et al. 2009). Further experiments involving reversible inactivation of regions of medial prefrontal cortex in rats showed that both sorts of control are simultaneously acquired and that either can be made to dominate (Killcross and Coutureau 2003) even in circumstances under which their effect would normally be suppressed. These, and other studies, comprise substantial evidence of the separate neural structures underpinning these forms of control, with prefrontal cortex and dorsomedial striatum associated with goal-directed influences and the dorsolateral striatum and, at least for appetitive outcomes, the neuromodulator dopamine, with habits (Balleine 2005; Barto 1995; Montague et al. 1996; Suri and Schultz 1999). The striatum and its dopaminergic input are discussed in Mirolli and Baldassarre (2012) and Redgrave et al. (2012), albeit from a somewhat different perspective. Roles have also been suggested for another neuromodulator, serotonin, in aversive aspects of model-free control (Daw et al. 2002; Dayan and Huys 2009; Deakin and Graeff 1991; Doya 2002). Neuromodulators such as dopamine and serotonin are signaling molecules that can regulate and control plasticity (their putative role in neural RL) and also influence the functional structure of networks.

Daw et al. (2005) interpreted this broad collection of results as suggesting that animals have access to information arising from both model-free and model-based RL. Choice between the two systems could be on the basis of their relative uncertainties. In many cases, the generative model underlying model-based RL can be acquired in a statistically efficient manner, since it requires little more than storing the statistics of immediate experience. Thus, the model can readily be as accurate as possible. However, inverting the generative model of a temporally extended environment to infer an optimal policy by building the tree of options and outcomes can be computationally tricky, potentially requiring substantial calculations and intermediate storage. Any infelicity in doing these would lead to inaccurate answers. Conversely, acquisition in model-free RL methods such as Q-learning or the actor-critic is hard, because of the reliance on bootstrapping (since, early on in learning, one set of potentially incorrect, estimated, values is used to teach another set). However, they more or less directly parametrize the inverse model of the environment and so only require simple or even trivial calculations to imply policies. Thus, Daw et al. (2005) suggested that the progressive development of behavioral habits arises when the calculational uncertainty of the model-based answer outweighs the learning uncertainty of the model-free one. Of course, it is the learning uncertainties that underlie exploration bonuses.

Model-based and model-free controllers are called instrumental, since the actions they suggest are instrumental for the acquisition of desired outcomes or escaping from undesirable ones. However, it could be very costly for an organism to have to learn for itself what to do in all circumstances—this is particularly true in the aversive domain of danger and threats. Thus, along with these instrumental controllers, there is evidence for evolutionary preprogrammed or hard-wired responses which are automatically elicited by the existence of, and critically also predictions of, reinforcing outcomes (Dickinson 1980; Mackintosh 1983). This controller is sometimes called Pavlovian. Responses elicited by predictions of rewarding outcomes are typically fairly simple, such as engagement, approach, and seeking (Berridge 2004; Panksepp 1998). However, for aversive outcomes, there is a wonderfully specific set of species-typical defensive fight-flight-freeze and inhibitory responses (Blanchard and Blanchard 1988; Bolles 1970; Gray and McNaughton 2003; McNaughton and Corr 2004), partly orchestrated by the periaqueductal gray (Bandler and Shipley 1994; Keay and Bandler 2001). Behavioral inhibition is a general Pavlovian response to predictions of future aversive outcomes and is putatively realized partly as an effect of serotonin (Soubrié 1986). The nucleus accumbens, which is the ventral part of the striatum, also plays a key role in controlling and coordinating the elicitation and nature of appetitive and aversive Pavlovian responses (Reynolds and Berridge 2001, 2002, 2008).

Critically, Pavlovian responses can compete with instrumental ones. That is, in experimental circumstances such as negative automaintenance (Sheffield 1965; Williams and Williams 1969) in which the automatic Pavlovian response of approaching a predictor of an appetitive outcome leads to the undesirable consequence that outcome is denied, animals are often unable to stop themselves from approaching. Many more florid examples of such misbehavior are also known (Breland and Breland 1961; Dayan et al. 2006; Hershberger 1986). We know rather less about the nature of the calculation of Pavlovian predictions (although it could presumably follow model-based and model-free lines) or the rules governing the competition between Pavlovian and instrumental responses.

Instrumental and Pavlovian controllers likely share the description of state in the world necessary for both learning and planning. One part of this state comes from the hierarchical representation of input realized in the areally layered architecture of sensory processing cortices that itself is believed to arise over the course of development and learning (Rao et al. 2002). In fact, such hierarchical state representations are themselves a key substrate for generalization within and between environments. A second part comes from the possibility of short-term storage and recall of information about recent past states in working memory (Dayan 2007; Hazy et al. 2007; O'Reilly and Frank 2006; Vasilaki et al. 2009), and possibly in other structures such as medium-term synaptic traces (Hempel et al. 2000; Mongillo et al. 2008) or the hippocampus. These play the particularly critical role of making tasks appear to have Markovian dynamics, in which the full state comprising external and internal representations is a sufficient statistic to determine the distribution over next states and rewards. Of course, the broader problem, including inference about environmental structures, typically remains non-Markovian.

Stepping back, there is an analogy between the interaction of instrumental and Pavlovian control and that between extrinsic and intrinsic motivation, with the evolutionary preprogramming in the latter being of environmental priors or their consequences for bonuses rather than actions appropriate to particular appetitive or aversive outcomes or predictions. Indeed, a similar sort of competition also applies—spending time learning skills can be detrimental in environments that afford no generalization; just failing to run away from sources of food is inappropriate in environments in which the food would then approach. Sadly, very few experiments have considered explicitly opportunities for generalization across environments.

To summarize, we have seen that there are multiple controllers, with different functional properties, located in at least partly separate loci in the brain. These controllers represent and process different information about the environment and so will therefore express different expectations about the nature and consequences of uncertainty about the present and possible future environments. Thus, they will exhibit different exploration bonuses and thus different forms of intrinsically motivated behavior.

3 Theory

As mentioned, the basic premise of this chapter is that skills are useful if they can be expected to generalize or transfer and that quantifying the benefits of potential generalization leads to a normative underpinning of exploration and ultimately intrinsic motivation. We discuss the catastrophic computational complexity of this and approximations in the next section; here we consider what can actually generalize between tasks.

At least four different sorts of generalization have been studied in the literature: specific generalization associated with either (a) model-free or (b) model-based RL, (c) broader facets of the (perhaps temporally local) prior distribution over environments such as controllability, and finally (d) representational generalization.

Much of the original work on generalization concerned cases in which agents had to solve many different tasks in what was almost the same Markov decision problem (MDP). Consider, for instance the famous taxicab problem, involving navigation in a maze between many, or indeed all, points (e.g., Dietterich 1998; Singh 1992; Thrun and Schwartz 1995). Here, the dynamics of the world (the effect of actions, the barriers in the maze) remain the same, but the reward function changes on a case by case basis. The idea has often been to learn some form of hierarchically structured policy or representation of the value function, including components that could be reused between different tasks. These quantities are broadly associated with model-free RL (Sutton and Barto 1998). It was also pointed out that such hierarchical structures can also aid the process of learning in a single, complex MDP with a unique value function, by making exploration more efficient. One of the more comprehensive hierarchical notions is that of an option (Sutton et al. 1999), which allows selection of an extended sequence of actions. However, work on understanding model-free generalization more broadly, outside the confines of a task such as this, is still in its early days (Konidaris and Barto 2007, 2009). Hierarchical RL as a whole is described, for instance, in Botvinick et al. (2009), Samejima et al. (2003), and Sutton et al. (1999).

More recently, model-based RL (Sutton and Barto 1998) has gained greater prominence, particularly because of the finer control it offers over the balance between exploration and exploitation (Asmuth et al. 2009; Brafman and Tennenholtz 2003; Dearden et al. 1999; Kearns and Singh 2002; Poupart et al. 2006; Strens 2000; Wiering and Schmidhuber 1998). Further, powerful new methods have been introduced for capturing hierarchical statistical structures, many centered around nonparametric Bayesian notions such as Dirichlet process mixtures (Beal et al. 2002; Neal 2000; Teh et al. 2006). These have been used to capture intra- and potentially inter-task transfer, arguing, for instance, that the transition matrices and possibly reward functions associated with different states might be shared in one of a number of ways (Acuna and Schrater 2009; Wilson et al. 2007; Wingate et al. 2011). Unfortunately, they come with potentially severe costs of inference.

One advantage of the nonparametric methods is they permit an agnosticism about the degree of sharing between different states (and also different tasks), since they allow essentially arbitrary numbers of components that can be shared. Another advantage is that they allow a more formal specification of the nature of generalization—by indicating exactly what potentially couples tasks. However, perhaps because of the notorious computational complexities concerned, the relationship between ideas of intrinsic motivational quantities such as uncertainty and curiosity and non-myopic Bayesian RL has seemingly not been extensively explored. Further, the methods have been developed in the face of much more limited generalization than is often conceived under intrinsic motivation—failing, for instance, to encompass much of the value of abstractions such as skill learning.

These forms of model-based and model-free generalization depend on a rather fine-grain relationship between environments. However, coarser relationships may also exist which can be expressed via a different parametrization of the hierarchical statistical model of domains. This can also have an important influence on exploration.

One excellent example comes from the literature on learned helplessness and the lack of controllability in depression (Huys and Dayan 2009; Maier and Watkins 2005; Seligman 1975). A standard experiment on learned helplessness involves two groups of subjects: master and yoked. The master subjects receive a punishment such as a mild electric shock, which they can terminate by executing one particular action in their environment (for instance, turning a running wheel). The yoked subjects experience the same environment as the master subjects and receive *exactly* the same shocks as them. However, there is no action they can take to terminate the shocks. The yoked subjects learn that they lack control in this environment and are deemed helpless. The consequences of learned helplessness training are typically probed in a different environment, i.e., via generalization (a point explicitly examined in Maier and Watkins 2005). Both groups, along with a third, untreated, group that did not experience the initial training, are tested according to various measures, such as the speed of learning to avoid an avoidable shock or exploratory drive. The master subjects, who had control over their original aversive learning experience, closely resemble the untreated rats. By comparison, the yoked subjects learn much more slowly and fail to explore. Rats can also become helpless for rewards if they do not earn them appropriately (Goodkin 1976).

From the perspective of model-based RL, the subjects may be building a causal description of the original environment (Courville et al. 2004; Gershman et al. 2010b; Tenenbaum et al. 2006) indicating what could and could not be responsible for their dismal fate. However, the details of the tasks used to assess the degree of learned helplessness are quite different from the original, and it is hard to see that anything as specific as a transition structure from a state could generalize.

Rather, Huys and Dayan (2009) and Huys (2007) argued that the subjects would acquire information about a "meta-statistic" of the environment in the form of its degree of controllability. Unfortunately, there is no unique definition of controllability (Skinner 1996), and existing experiments do not pin down exactly how it should be quantified. Indeed, some of the notions discussed in Mirolli and Baldassarre (2012) to do with competence-based notions of intrinsic motivation such as self-determination and autonomy (Deci and Ryan 1985; Ryan and Deci 2000) could be related. One of the simpler constructions is in the hierarchical Bayesian terms of the prior distribution over the entropy of the reinforcing outcomes (and/or state transitions) consequent on executing an action. If the distribution over outcomes has low entropy, then doing the action twice should have a good chance of leading to the same outcome, a consequence consistent with a high degree of controllability. Conversely, if the distribution has high entropy, then it would be impossible to arrange one outcome to occur reliably, which would be a form of low controllability.

Huys and Dayan (2009) formalized the evaluation and generalization of this form of entropy. They showed that one effect of the generalization was to structure the balance between exploration and exploitation in the new environment. In the face of low controllability, or helplessness, there is little point in exploring to find an action which leads to a good outcome, since this outcome would likely not reliably recur. However, Huys and Dayan (2009) did not take the next step we are discussing here and consider the benefits of taking actions in the first environment that would provide information about controllability that would be beneficial in the second one. Rather, they employed the myopic strategy (in fact a common approximate approach to the computational challenge of Bayesian RL; Asmuth et al. 2009; Brafman and Tennenholtz 2003; Wang et al. 2005) of just using in an appropriate fashion the experience gained in the pursuit of the optimal course of action in the first environment.

One interesting consequence of a prior that the outcome distribution should have a low entropy (i.e., high controllability) is that subjects should be motivated to find ways of eliminating apparently excess variability. For instance, they might deploy controlled working memory (Dayan 2007; Hazy et al. 2007; O'Reilly and Frank 2006; Vasilaki et al. 2009) to store aspects of the previous sensory input, in order to disambiguate outcomes that seem inexplicably stochastic. Indeed, anecdotally, this is quite common in human experiments involving stochastic rewards; subjects construct florid, higher-order Markovian explanations for what is just the output of a (pseudo-)random number generator.

Learned helplessness thus suggests that animals may indeed generalize aspects of structure between environments, with a direct effect on exploratory behavior, and thus intrinsically motivated actions.

The final approach to generalization involves the representation of problem and state. Representation is a ubiquitous part of any learning or inference problem and therefore hard to pin down specifically. However, conventional forms of unsupervised learning are based on the notion that the whole gamut of natural sensory inputs (say for vision) occupies a manifold or space that is very low dimensional compared with the space of all possible inputs. Unsupervised learning finds representations that act as a coordinate system for this low dimensional space so that all natural inputs can be described in terms of these underlying structures (e.g., visual objects and lighting) rather than the full input (i.e., all pixel values) (Hinton and Ghahramani 1997; Rao et al. 2002). If the re-representation can do this, then it should support broad and effective generalization to new inputs. For instance, consider the appropriate response to the image of a lion. If this response is acquired based on the pixel values, then a lion in a slightly different setting, for instance in the green of a forest rather than the yellow of a desert, might not engender the same response. If, however, the re-representation captures the underlying objects in the scene, including the lion, in an explicit fashion, then generalization can be immediate. Most such representations are, at least conceptually, hierarchical, capturing more abstract and therefore more general structure in successive layers

(Hinton et al. 1995; Hinton and Salakhutdinov 2006). Representations can also be hierarchical in time, as in the case discussed above of the use of controlled working memory.

The issue of representation is very similar for decision problems (e.g., Dayan 2007; Foster and Dayan 2002; Gershman et al. 2010a). That is, we have been discussing the natural ensemble of tasks and environments. It is the statistical structure and regularities in this ensemble that licenses generalization in the first place. A representational scheme for such problems that reflects the underlying structure could then support ready generalization itself. Some work along these lines has been attempted in simple multitask cases such as all-to-all navigation in a maze (Foster and Dayan 2002) or as a form of selective attention in which dimensions of the actual input are eliminated (Gershman et al. 2010a). However, as for most of the other forms of generalization, this has proceeded in a state of hapless myopia. The benefits of taking actions in one domain that reduce the uncertainty associated with the representational scheme that applies across tasks, and that would therefore speed learning in a new task, have yet to be considered.

4 Practicality

Unfortunately, although fully Bayesian methods for representing uncertainty using such devices as hierarchical nonparametric models are becoming relatively commonplace (Beal et al. 2002; Neal 2000; Teh et al. 2006; Thibaux and Jordan 2007), doing long-run planning in the face of these uncertainties is known to be radically intractable (Kaelbling et al. 1998; Madani et al. 2003; Papadimitriou and Tsitsiklis 1987). That is, it will not be possible to solve exactly for the true exploration bonuses associated with these various forms of generalization, even if we did have a statistical model of tasks of the forms we discussed above. Approximations will therefore be necessary. Key tasks for the future include inventing, characterizing, and analyzing approximations employed by the different controllers—we hope that many existing formalizations of intrinsic motivation (Barto et al. 2004; Blank et al. 2005; Huang and Weng 2007; Oudeyer et al. 2007; Schembri et al. 2007; Schmidhuber 1991; Şimşek and Barto 2006; Singh et al. 2005) may ultimately be seen in this light.

We cannot yet make completely formal a tie between classical views of intrinsic motivation and these concepts of generalization or indeed demonstrate extensions. However, we can consider how the different controllers outlined above can be manipulated away from pure, single-task reinforcement learning, together with some of the issues that arise. The model-based controller should enjoy the richest relationship with these concepts of statistical models of tasks and generalization. This is because, as mentioned above, the relationship among environments is most readily described in terms of models of the domain. Indeed, it was for just this reason that we suggested that the refined notion of controllability in depression that we discussed above would only be captured by this controller (Huys and Dayan 2009).

The model-based controller has also been considered to embody a model of its own uncertainty (Daw et al. 2005), which is a key substrate for both exact and approximate bonuses. However, although there is certainly evidence that prefrontal regions are involved in representing forms of uncertainty (Behrens et al. 2007; Daw et al. 2006; Rushworth and Behrens 2008; Yoshida and Ishii 2006), how refined this uncertainty is and how this controller copes with the calculational complexities concerned are not clear. In fact, there are some conflicting results in the literature. For instance, it has been noted that the rate of learning in a human behavioral experiment is appropriately sensitive to the degree of uncertainty engendered by environmental change, as in a Kalman filter. Furthermore, this learning rate is represented in a neural structure (the anterior cingulate cortex) that is likely involved in model-based control (Behrens et al. 2007). However, an explicit test of subjects' willingness to employ an uncertainty-sensitive exploration bonus in a restless four-armed bandit task found no evidence for this, rather subjects' behavior was best fit by a form of certainty-equivalent softmax control (Daw et al. 2006).

The model-free controller lacks the obvious informational substrate for sophisticated assessments of the nature and benefits of generalization, since it does not have any formal model of a single environment, let alone the relationship among multiple ones. Therefore, simple heuristics must play an even greater role in the way that model-free control can incorporate exploration bonuses. Some of these heuristics may involve the influence of model-based over model-free control, for instance via the neuromodulatory systems that mediate model-free learning (Aston-Jones and Cohen 2005; Doya et al. 2002; Ishii et al. 2002; Yu and Dayan 2005).

One example of these interactions is also seen in learned helplessness (discussed in Huys and Dayan 2009). A key effect of the shocks in the initial environment is to sensitize serotonergic neurons (appropriately, given their putative role of being involved in aversively motivated behavior; Boureau and Dayan 2011; Daw et al. 2002). Excess activation, which leads to the sequalæ of helplessness in the second environment putatively via the model-free system (Daw et al. 2002; Dayan and Huys 2009), is known to be opposed by a net effect of an area of the brain called the medial prefrontal cortex only in the case that the shocks are controllable (Maier et al. 2006). We can interpret the sensitization itself as a crude form of generalization—that the unpleasantness of the first environment is deemed to continue, changes the set point for the serotonergic system. The opposing force from the medial prefrontal cortex might then be a countermanding signal providing a more sophisticated, model-based evaluation that future environments should in fact be suitably exploitable.

One could well imagine a similar influence over the dopamine system, but in the appetitive rather than aversive domain. This could reflect a model-based estimate of the potential for controllable rewards, which would then inspire model-free exploration. Indeed, various theories of intrinsic motivation have been influenced by the fact that novel, salient objects likely inspire a phasic dopaminergic signal (Horvitz 2000; Horvitz et al. 1997; Redgrave et al. 1999; see Redgrave et al. 2012), which has been interpreted as an exploration or shaping bonus (Kakade and Dayan 2002) leading to engagement with the stimulus or situation concerned. Just as in the case of learned helplessness, there could be a coarse model-free heuristic, such as always increasing exploration bonuses when the reward rate increases, that would be tempered by model-based meta-statistics such as controllability. There could also be a role in this for norepinephrine, another neuromodulator like dopamine and serotonin, but that has a particular association with salience (Aston-Jones and Cohen 2005; Doya et al. 2002).

There are also quite some additional interactions between model-based, model-free, and Pavlovian controllers that could bear on exploration bonuses. First, model-free values may provide a grounding for model-based computations by providing approximate values at the leaves of the search tree (a maneuver standard in RL models of games playing since the earliest work; Samuel 1959). Second, Pavlovian biases such as inhibition in the face of predictions of aversion (Soubrié 1986) might influence the processes of model-based evaluation (Dayan and Huys 2008), in this case pruning out certain parts of the search tree. Something similar might happen via dopamine in the face of predictions of reward, but to opposite effect (Smith et al. 2006). Both of these could lead to the same sort of optimism that is typical in invigorating exploration.

A further difficult computation for the model-free controller concerns the stability-plasticity dilemma (Carpenter and Grossberg 1988) associated with protecting newly learned skills from being overwritten by subsequent tasks and allowing them to be appropriately reused in different combinations. As we mentioned above, the model-based controller can (at least conceptually, rather than neurally) easily achieve this using variants of the hierarchical Dirichlet process mixture (Acuna and Schrater 2009; Gershman and Niv 2010; Wingate et al. 2011), by allocating new structures to tasks that do not fit existing categories and protecting old structures. There are also mixture model methods for achieving this that predate the adoption of Dirichlet processes (Wolpert and Kawato 1998). However, doing this in a model-free manner, with only a policy, has proved somewhat tricky (Krueger and Dayan 2009; Singh 1992; the work of Collins 2010 is also closely related), and the neural substrate of protection and reuse remain mysterious.

5 Discussion

This chapter had two goals. The more modest one was to lay out current views of the neural architecture of decision-making to help understand how intrinsic motivation might be embedded. The architecture involves multiple systems, particularly model-based and model-free controllers, which have been anticipated both in behavioral psychology (Thorndike 1911; Tolman 1948) and reinforcement learning (Sutton and Barto 1998). These controllers, along with a couple of others, compete and cooperate, possibly according to their relative uncertainties, to influence action. Very roughly, the model-free controller can represent and act upon what we might see as scalar aspects of intrinsic motivation—e.g., boosting exploration in the face of high rates of reward. The model-based controller can capture much more sophisticated aspects of the statistical structure of domains, and thus intrinsic motivation, and can also influence the model-free controller. In turn, it is also influenced in ways that are not well understood. Both model-free and model-based controllers can take advantage of rich representational learning mechanisms, along with internally directed actions such as storing and retrieving disambiguating sensory information from working memory.

The rather more ambitious and distinctly less complete goal is to support attempts to bring intrinsic motivational concepts such as curiosity and uncertainty back under the fold of conventional control in terms of sophisticated exploration bonuses (Şimşek and Barto 2006). We did this by focusing on the notion of generalization that underpins the benefits of skill learning. We discussed various aspects of generalization in the different controllers and in representation formation. Of course, the infamous fly in the ointment is the radical intractability of deriving exploration bonuses in interestingly complicated domains. Thus, we might see intrinsic motivational ideas as heuristics, in just the same way that adding some function of the standard deviation of the uncertainty about the worth of an arm of a bandit to its estimated mean is a heuristic approximation to the Gittins index for the arm.

We should also note that there are other, less Bayesian, ways of linking intrinsic motivation more formally to generalization. These particularly include the extensive investigations of Hutter (2005) and Schmidhuber (2009) into very general problem solvers, which subsume Bayesian reinforcement learning as special cases. The prospect of rich links between these formal methods and intrinsic motivational concepts such as curiosity from the same group (e.g., Schmidhuber 2006) is enticing.

One of the more striking discoveries in the field of bandits is that of non-Bayesian methods, such as those associated with regret bounds. These are computationally vastly better behaved, are almost as rewarding as Bayesian methods when the latter apply, and also work well in a much wider range of settings, even against adversarial opponents (Auer et al. 2002a,b). These ideas had a significant influence over work on the trade-off between exploration and exploitation in single-task MDPs, leading to concepts such as knownness (Asmuth et al. 2009; Nouri and Littman 2009) that are close to intrinsic motivational ideas. It would be most interesting to adapt variants of these to the current, generalizing multitask setting.

Given the view in this chapter of intrinsic motivation in the context of actual animal behavior, what are the main challenges ahead? As will be evident from the preceding sections, there is a whole wealth of open problems. Perhaps the most important of these is to characterize the statistical structure of environments. This forms the basis of the information that underpins intrinsic motivation according to our account. It governs generalization and thus the benefits (and indeed costs) of exploration and skill learning. We speculated (indeed along with other chapters in the book) that this statistical structure is hierarchical, the full consequences of which are not clear.

Next comes the question of justifiable approximations to the Bayesian ideals that are embodied in the normative picture we have painted. We expect there to be a range of approximations at different levels of complexity and scale and indeed appropriate to the differing informational structures of model-based and model-free controllers. It would be important to analyze existing suggestions for formalizing intrinsic motivation in terms of approximations—as well as generating new approximations that might be beneficial in classes of environment. Heuristics that focus as much on the competence of the learner as the affordances of the environment, such as those based on the dynamics of ongoing prediction errors over the course of learning (discussed in various chapters in this book), or optimal level theories (see Barto 2012) merit particular attention. Finally is the most interesting possibility that existing intrinsic motivational concepts do not fit into this scheme and so demand new theoretical concepts and ideas.

Acknowledgements I am very grateful to Andrew Barto, the editors, and two anonymous reviewers for their comments on this chapter. My work is funded by the Gatsby Charitable Foundation.

References

Acuna, D., Schrater, P.: Improving bayesian reinforcement learning using transition abstraction. In: ICML/UAI/COLT Workshop on Abstraction in Reinforcement Learning. Montreal, Canada (2009)

Asmuth, J., Li, L., Littman, M., Nouri, A., Wingate, D.: A bayesian sampling approach to exploration in reinforcement learning. In: UAI, Montreal, Canada (2009)

Aston-Jones, G., Cohen, J.D.: An integrative theory of locus coeruleus-norepinephrine function: Adaptive gain and optimal performance. Annu. Rev. Neurosci. **28**, 403–450 (2005)

Auer, P., Cesa-Bianchi, N., Fischer, P.: Finite-time analysis of the multiarmed bandit problem. Mach. Learn. **47**(2), 235–256 (2002a)

Auer, P., Cesa-Bianchi, N., Freund, Y., Schapire, R.: The nonstochastic multiarmed bandit problem. SIAM J. Comput. **32**(1), 48–77 (2002b)

Balleine, B.W.: Neural bases of food-seeking: Affect, arousal and reward in corticostriatolimbic circuits. Physiol. Behav. **86**(5), 717–730 (2005)

Bandler, R., Shipley, M.T.: Columnar organization in the midbrain periaqueductal gray: Modules for emotional expression? Trends Neurosci. **17**(9), 379–389 (1994)

Barto, A.: Adaptive critics and the basal ganglia. In: Houk, J., Davis, J., Beiser, D. (eds.) Models of Information Processing in the Basal Ganglia, pp. 215–232. MIT, Cambridge (1995)

Barto, A., Mahadevan, S.: Recent advances in hierarchical reinforcement learning. Discr. Event Dyn. Syst. **13**(4), 341–379 (2003)

Barto, A., Singh, S., Chentanez, N.: Intrinsically motivated learning of hierarchical collections of skills. In: ICDL 2004, La Jolla, CA (2004)

Barto, A., Sutton, R., Anderson, C.: Neuronlike elements that can solve difficult learning control problems. IEEE Trans. Syst. Man Cybern. **13**(5), 834–846 (1983)

Barto, A.G.: Intrinsic motivation and reinforcement learning. In: Baldassarre, G., Mirolli, M. (eds.) Intrinsically Motivated Learning in Natural and Artificial Systems, pp. 17–47. Springer, Berlin (2012)

Beal, M., Ghahramani, Z., Rasmussen, C.: The infinite hidden Markov model. In: NIPS, pp. 577–584, Vancouver, Canada (2002)

Behrens, T.E.J., Woolrich, M.W., Walton, M.E., Rushworth, M.F.S.: Learning the value of information in an uncertain world. Nat. Neurosci. **10**(9), 1214–1221 (2007)
Bellman, R.E.: Dynamic Programming. Princeton University Press, Princeton (1957)
Berridge, K.C.: Motivation concepts in behavioral neuroscience. Physiol. Behav. **81**, 179–209 (2004)
Berry, D.A., Fristedt, B.: Bandit Problems: Sequential Allocation of Experiments. Springer, Berlin (1985)
Blanchard, D.C., Blanchard, R.J.: Ethoexperimental approaches to the biology of emotion. Annu. Rev. Psychol. **39**, 43–68 (1988)
Blank, D., Kumar, D., Meeden, L., Marshall, J.: Bringing up robot: Fundamental mechanisms for creating a self-motivated, self-organizing architecture. Cybern. Syst. **36**(2), 125–150 (2005)
Bolles, R.C.: Species-specific defense reactions and avoidance learning. Psychol. Rev. **77**, 32–48 (1970)
Botvinick, M.M., Niv, Y., Barto, A.C.: Hierarchically organized behavior and its neural foundations: A reinforcement learning perspective. Cognition **113**(3), 262–280 (2009)
Boureau, Y.-L., Dayan, P.: Opponency revisited: Competition and cooperation between dopamine and serotonin. Neuropsychopharmacology **36**(1), 74–97 (2011)
Brafman, R., Tennenholtz, M.: R-max-a general polynomial time algorithm for near-optimal reinforcement learning. J. Mach. Learn. Res. **3**, 213–231 (2003)
Breland, K., Breland, M.: The misbehavior of organisms. Am. Psychol. **16**(9), 681–84 (1961)
Carpenter, G., Grossberg, S.: The ART of adaptive pattern recognition by a self-organizing neural network. Computer **21**, 77–88 (1988)
Caruana, R.: Multitask learning. Mach. Learn. **28**(1), 41–75 (1997)
Collins, A.: Apprentissage et Contrôle Cognitif: Une Théorie de la Fonction Executive Préfrontale Humaine. Ph.D. Thesis, Université Pierre et Marie Curie, Paris (2010)
Courville, A., Daw, N., Touretzky, D.: Similarity and discrimination in classical conditioning: A latent variable account. In: NIPS, pp. 313–320, Vancouver, Canada (2004)
Daw, N.D., Doya, K.: The computational neurobiology of learning and reward. Curr. Opin. Neurobiol. **16**(2), 199–204 (2006)
Daw, N.D., Kakade, S., Dayan, P.: Opponent interactions between serotonin and dopamine. Neural Netw. **15**, 603–16 (2002)
Daw, N.D., Niv, Y., Dayan, P.: Uncertainty-based competition between prefrontal and dorsolateral striatal systems for behavioral control. Nat. Neurosci. **8**(12), 1704–1711 (2005)
Daw, N.D., O'Doherty, J.P., Dayan, P., Seymour, B., Dolan, R.J.: Cortical substrates for exploratory decisions in humans. Nature **441**(7095), 876–879 (2006)
Dayan, P.: Bilinearity, rules, and prefrontal cortex. Front. Comput. Neurosci. **1**, 1 (2007)
Dayan, P., Hinton, G.: Feudal reinforcement learning. In: Hanson, S.J., Cowan, J.D., Giles, C.L. (eds.) Advances in Neural Information Processing Systems (NIPS) 5. MIT, Cambridge (1993)
Dayan, P., Huys, Q.J.M.: Serotonin, inhibition, and negative mood. PLoS Comput. Biol. **4**(2), e4 (2008)
Dayan, P., Huys, Q.J.M.: Serotonin in affective control. Annu. Rev. Neurosci. **32**, 95–126 (2009)
Dayan, P., Niv, Y., Seymour, B., Daw, N.D.: The misbehavior of value and the discipline of the will. Neural Netw. **19**(8), 1153–1160 (2006)
Dayan, P., Sejnowski, T.: Exploration bonuses and dual control. Mach. Learn. **25**(1), 5–22 (1996)
Deakin, J.F.W., Graeff, F.G.: 5-HT and mechanisms of defence. J. Psychopharmacol. **5**, 305–316 (1991)
Dearden, R., Friedman, N., Andre, D.: Model based Bayesian exploration. In: UAI, Stockholm, Sweden pp. 150–159 (1999)
Deci, E., Ryan, R.: Intrinsic motivation and self-determination in human behavior. Plenum, New York (1985)
Dickinson, A.: Contemporary animal learning theory. Cambridge University Press, Cambridge (1980)
Dickinson, A., Balleine, B.: The role of learning in motivation. In: Gallistel, C. (ed.) Stevens' Handbook of Experimental Psychology, vol. 3, pp. 497–533. Wiley, New York (2002)

Dietterich, T.: The MAXQ method for hierarchical reinforcement learning. In: ICML, pp. 118–126, Madison, Wisconsin, (1998)

Dietterich, T.: Hierarchical reinforcement learning with the MAXQ value function decomposition. J. Artif. Intell. Res. **13**(1), 227–303 (2000)

Doya, K.: Metalearning and neuromodulation. Neural Netw. **15**(4–6), 495–506 (2002)

Doya, K., Samejima, K., ichi Katagiri, K., Kawato, M.: Multiple model-based reinforcement learning. Neural Comput. **14**(6), 1347–1369 (2002)

Duff, M.: Optimal Learning: Computational approaches for Bayes-adaptive Markov decision processes. Ph.D. Thesis, Computer Science Department, University of Massachusetts, Amherst (2000)

Foster, D., Dayan, P.: Structure in the space of value functions. Mach. Learn. **49**(2), 325–346 (2002)

Gershman, S., Cohen, J., Niv, Y.: Learning to selectively attend. In: Proceedings of the 32nd Annual Conference of the Cognitive Science Society, Portland, Oregon (2010a)

Gershman, S., Niv, Y.: Learning latent structure: Carving nature at its joints. Curr. Opin. Neurobiol. (2010)

Gershman, S.J., Blei, D.M., Niv, Y.: Context, learning, and extinction. Psychol. Rev. **117**(1), 197–209 (2010b)

Gittins, J.C.: Multi-Armed Bandit Allocation Indices. Wiley, New York (1989)

Goodkin, F.: Rats learn the relationship between responding and environmental events: An expansion of the learned helplessness hypothesis. Learn. Motiv. **7**, 382–393 (1976)

Gray, J.A., McNaughton, N.: The Neuropsychology of Anxiety, 2nd edn. OUP, Oxford (2003)

Guthrie, E.: The Psychology of Learning. Harper & Row, New York (1952)

Hazy, T.E., Frank, M.J., O'reilly, R.C.: Towards an executive without a homunculus: Computational models of the prefrontal cortex/basal ganglia system. Philos. Trans. R. Soc. Lond. B Biol. Sci. **362**(1485), 1601–1613 (2007)

Hempel, C.M., Hartman, K.H., Wang, X.J., Turrigiano, G.G., Nelson, S.B.: Multiple forms of short-term plasticity at excitatory synapses in rat medial prefrontal cortex. J. Neurophysiol. **83**(5), 3031–3041 (2000)

Hershberger, W.A.: An approach through the looking-glass. Anim. Learn. Behav. **14**, 443–51 (1986)

Hinton, G.E., Dayan, P., Frey, B.J., Neal, R.M.: The "wake-sleep" algorithm for unsupervised neural networks. Science **268**(5214), 1158–1161 (1995)

Hinton, G.E., Ghahramani, Z.: Generative models for discovering sparse distributed representations. Philos. Trans. R. Soc. Lond. B Biol. Sci. **352**(1358), 1177–1190 (1997)

Hinton, G.E., Salakhutdinov, R.R.: Reducing the dimensionality of data with neural networks. Science **313**(5786), 504–507 (2006)

Holland, P.: Amount of training affects associatively-activated event representation. Neuropharmacology **37**(4–5), 461–469 (1998)

Horvitz, J.C.: Mesolimbocortical and nigrostriatal dopamine responses to salient non-reward events. Neuroscience **96**(4), 651–656 (2000)

Horvitz, J.C., Stewart, T., Jacobs, B.L.: Burst activity of ventral tegmental dopamine neurons is elicited by sensory stimuli in the awake cat. Brain Res. **759**(2), 251–258 (1997)

Howard, R.: Information value theory. IEEE Trans. Syst. Sci. Cybern. **2**(1), 22–26 (1966)

Huang, X., Weng, J.: Inherent value systems for autonomous mental development. Int. J. Human. Robot. **4**, 407–433 (2007)

Hutter, M.: Universal Artificial Intelligence: Sequential Decisions Based on Algorithmic Probability. Springer, Berlin (2005)

Huys, Q.: Reinforcers and control. Towards a computational ætiology of depression. Ph.D. Thesis, Gatsby Computational Neuroscience Unit, UCL (2007)

Huys, Q.J.M., Dayan, P.: A Bayesian formulation of behavioral control. Cognition **113**, 314–328 (2009)

Ishii, S., Yoshida, W., Yoshimoto, J.: Control of exploitation-exploration meta-parameter in reinforcement learning. Neural Netw. **15**(4–6), 665–687 (2002)

Kaelbling, L., Littman, M., Cassandra, A.: Planning and acting in partially observable stochastic domains. Artif. Intell. **101**(1–2), 99–134 (1998)
Kakade, S., Dayan, P.: Dopamine: Generalization and bonuses. Neural Netw. **15**(4–6), 549–559 (2002)
Kearns, M., Singh, S.: Near-optimal reinforcement learning in polynomial time. Mach. Learn. **49**(2), 209–232 (2002)
Keay, K.A., Bandler, R.: Parallel circuits mediating distinct emotional coping reactions to different types of stress. Neurosci. Biobehav. Rev. **25**(7–8), 669–678 (2001)
Killcross, S., Coutureau, E.: Coordination of actions and habits in the medial prefrontal cortex of rats. Cereb. Cortex **13**(4), 400–408 (2003)
Konidaris, G., Barto, A.: Building portable options: Skill transfer in reinforcement learning. In: IJCAI, pp. 895–900, Hyderabad, India (2007)
Konidaris, G., Barto, A.: Efficient skill learning using abstraction selection. In: IJCAI, pp. 1107–1112, Pasadena, California (2009)
Krueger, K.A., Dayan, P.: Flexible shaping: How learning in small steps helps. Cognition **110**(3), 380–394 (2009)
Mackintosh, N.J.: Conditioning and Associative Learning. Oxford University Press, Oxford (1983)
Madani, O., Hanks, S., Condon, A.: On the undecidability of probabilistic planning and related stochastic optimization problems. Artif. Intell. **147**(1–2), 5–34 (2003)
Maier, S.F., Amat, J., Baratta, M.V., Paul, E., Watkins, L.R.: Behavioral control, the medial prefrontal cortex, and resilience. Dialogues Clin. Neurosci. **8**(4), 397–406 (2006)
Maier, S.F., Watkins, L.R.: Stressor controllability and learned helplessness: The roles of the dorsal raphe nucleus, serotonin, and corticotropin-releasing factor. Neurosci. Biobehav. Rev. **29**(4–5), 829–841 (2005)
McNaughton, N., Corr, P.J.: A two-dimensional neuropsychology of defense: Fear/anxiety and defensive distance. Neurosci. Biobehav. Rev. **28**(3), 285–305 (2004)
Mirolli, M., Baldassarre, G.: Functions and mechanisms of intrinsic motivations: The knowledge versus competence distinction. In: Baldassarre, G., Mirolli, M. (eds.) Intrinsically Motivated Learning in Natural and Artificial Systems, pp. 49–72. Springer, Berlin (2012)
Mongillo, G., Barak, O., Tsodyks, M.: Synaptic theory of working memory. Science **319**(5869), 1543–1546 (2008)
Montague, P.R., Dayan, P., Sejnowski, T.J.: A framework for mesencephalic dopamine systems based on predictive hebbian learning. J. Neurosci. **16**(5), 1936–1947 (1996)
Neal, R.: Markov chain sampling methods for Dirichlet process mixture models. J. Comput. Graph. Stat. **9**(2), 249–265 (2000)
Ng, A., Harada, D., Russell, S.: Policy invariance under reward transformations: Theory and application to reward shaping. In: ICML, pp. 278–287, Bled, Slovenia (1999)
Nouri, A., Littman, M.: Multi-resolution exploration in continuous spaces. NIPS, pp. 1209–1216 (2009)
O'Reilly, R.C., Frank, M.J.: Making working memory work: A computational model of learning in the prefrontal cortex and basal ganglia. Neural Comput. **18**(2), 283–328 (2006)
Oudeyer, P., Kaplan, F., Hafner, V.: Intrinsic motivation systems for autonomous mental development. IEEE Trans. Evol. Comput. **11**(2), 265–286 (2007)
Panksepp, J.: Affective Neuroscience. OUP, New York (1998)
Papadimitriou, C., Tsitsiklis, J.: The complexity of Markov decision processes. Math. Oper. Res. **12**(3), 441–450 (1987)
Parr, R., Russell, S.: Reinforcement learning with hierarchies of machines. In: NIPS, pp. 1043–1049, Denver, Colorado (1998)
Poupart, P., Vlassis, N., Hoey, J., Regan, K.: An analytic solution to discrete bayesian reinforcement learning. In: ICML, pp. 697–704, Pittsburgh, Pennslyvania (2006)
Rao, R.P.N., Olshausen, B.A., Lewicki, M.S. (eds.): Probabilistic Models of the Brain: Perception and Neural Function. MIT, Cambridge (2002)

Redgrave, P., Gurney, K., Stafford, T., Thirkettle, M., Lewis, J.: The role of the basal ganglia in discovering novel actions. In: Baldassarre, G., Mirolli, M. (eds.) Intrinsically Motivated Learning in Natural and Artificial Systems, pp. 129–149. Springer, Berlin (2012)
Redgrave, P., Prescott, T.J., Gurney, K.: Is the short-latency dopamine response too short to signal reward error? Trends Neurosci. **22**(4), 146–151 (1999)
Reynolds, S.M., Berridge, K.C. (2001): Fear and feeding in the nucleus accumbens shell: Rostrocaudal segregation of GABA-elicited defensive behavior versus eating behavior. J. Neurosci. **21**(9), 3261–3270 (1999)
Reynolds, S.M., Berridge, K.C.: Positive and negative motivation in nucleus accumbens shell: Bivalent rostrocaudal gradients for GABA-elicited eating, taste "liking"/"disliking" reactions, place preference/avoidance, and fear. J. Neurosci. **22**(16), 7308–7320 (2002)
Reynolds, S.M., Berridge, K.C.: Emotional environments retune the valence of appetitive versus fearful functions in nucleus accumbens. Nat. Neurosci. **11**(4), 423–425 (2008)
Ring, M.: CHILD: A first step towards continual learning. Mach. Learn. **28**(1), 77–104 (1997)
Ring, M.: Toward a formal framework for continual learning. In: NIPS Workshop on Inductive Transfer, Whistler, Canada (2005)
Rushworth, M.F.S., Behrens, T.E.J.: Choice, uncertainty and value in prefrontal and cingulate cortex. Nat. Neurosci. **11**(4), 389–397 (2008)
Ryan, R., Deci, E.: Intrinsic and extrinsic motivations: Classic definitions and new directions. Contemp. Educ. Psychol. **25**(1), 54–67 (2000)
Samejima, K., Doya, K., Kawato, M.: Inter-module credit assignment in modular reinforcement learning. Neural Netw. **16**(7), 985–994 (2003)
Samuel, A.: Some studies in machine learning using the game of checkers. IBM J. Res. Dev. **3**, 210–229 (1959)
Schembri, M., Mirolli, M., Baldassarre, G.: Evolving childhood's length and learning parameters in an intrinsically motivated reinforcement learning robot. In: Proceedings of the Seventh International Conference on Epigenetic Robotics, pp. 141–148, Piscataway, New Jersey (2007)
Schmidhuber, J.: Curious model-building control systems. In: IJCNN, pp. 1458–1463, Seattle, Washington State IEEE (1991)
Schmidhuber, J.: Gödel machines: Fully self-referential optimal universal self-improvers. Artif. Gen. Intell., pp. 199–226 (2006)
Schmidhuber, J.: Ultimate cognition à la gödel. Cogn. Comput. **1**, 117–193 (2009)
Seligman, M.: Helplessness: On Depression, Development, and Death. WH Freeman, San Francisco (1975)
Sheffield, F.: Relation between classical conditioning and instrumental learning. In: Prokasy, W. (ed.) Classical Conditioning, pp. 302–322. Appelton-Century-Crofts, New York (1965)
Şimşek, Ö., Barto, A.G.: An intrinsic reward mechanism for efficient exploration. In: ICML, pp. 833–840, Pittsburgh, Pennsylvania (2006)
Singh, S.: Transfer of learning by composing solutions of elemental sequential tasks. Mach. Learn. **8**(3), 323–339 (1992)
Singh, S., Barto, A., Chentanez, N.: Intrinsically motivated reinforcement learning. In: NIPS, pp. 1281–1288, Vancouver, Canada (2005)
Skinner, E.A.: A guide to constructs of control. J. Pers. Soc. Psychol. **71**(3), 549–570 (1996)
Smith, A., Li, M., Becker, S., Kapur, S.: Dopamine, prediction error and associative learning: A model-based account. Network **17**(1), 61–84 (2006)
Soubrié, P.: Reconciling the role of central serotonin neurons in human and animal behaviour. Behav. Brain Sci. **9**, 319–364 (1986)
Strens, M.: A Bayesian framework for reinforcement learning. In: ICML, pp. 943–950, Stanford, California (2000)

Suri, R.E., Schultz, W.: A neural network model with dopamine-like reinforcement signal that learns a spatial delayed response task. Neuroscience **91**(3), 871–890 (1999)
Sutton, R.: Learning to predict by the methods of temporal differences. Mach. Learn. **3**(1), 9–44 (1988)
Sutton, R.: Integrated architectures for learning, planning, and reacting based on approximating dynamic programming. ICML Austin, Texas **216**, 224 (1990)
Sutton, R., Precup, D., Singh, S.: Between MDPs and semi-MDPs: A framework for temporal abstraction in reinforcement learning. Artif. Intell. **112**(1), 181–211 (1999)
Sutton, R.S., Barto, A.G.: Reinforcement Learning: An Introduction (Adaptive Computation and Machine Learning). MIT, Cambridge (1998)
Tanaka, F., Yamamura, M.: Multitask reinforcement learning on the distribution of MDPs. IEEJ Trans. Electron. Inform. Syst. C **123**(5), 1004–1011 (2003)
Teh, Y., Jordan, M., Beal, M., Blei, D.: Hierarchical dirichlet processes. J. Am. Stat. Assoc. **101**(476), 1566–1581 (2006)
Tenenbaum, J., Griffiths, T., Kemp, C.: Theory-based Bayesian models of inductive learning and reasoning. Trends Cogn. Sci. **10**(7), 309–318 (2006)
Thibaux, R., Jordan, M.: Hierarchical beta processes and the Indian buffet process. In: AIStats, pp. 564–571, San Juan, Puerto Rico (2007)
Thorndike, E.: Animal Intelligence. MacMillan, New York (1911)
Thrun, S., Schwartz, A.: Finding structure in reinforcement learning. In: NIPS, pp. 385–392, Denver, Colorado (1995)
Tolman, E.C.: Cognitive maps in rats and men. Psychol. Rev. **55**(4), 189–208 (1948)
Tricomi, E., Balleine, B.W., O'Doherty, J.P.: A specific role for posterior dorsolateral striatum in human habit learning. Eur. J. Neurosci. **29**(11), 2225–2232 (2009)
Valentin, V.V., Dickinson, A., O'Doherty, J.P.: Determining the neural substrates of goal-directed learning in the human brain. J. Neurosci. **27**(15), 4019–4026 (2007)
Vasilaki, E., Fusi, S., Wang, X.-J., Senn, W. (2009): Learning flexible sensori-motor mappings in a complex network. Biol. Cybern. **100**(2), 147–158 (2007)
Wang, T., Lizotte, D., Bowling, M., Schuurmans, D.: Bayesian sparse sampling for on-line reward optimization. In: ICML, pp. 956–963, Bonn, Germany (2005)
Watkins, C. (1989): Learning from delayed rewards. Ph.D. Thesis, University of Cambridge (2005)
Wiering, M., Schmidhuber, J.: Efficient model-based exploration. In: Simulation of Adaptive Behavior, pp. 223–228, Zurich, Switzerland (1998)
Williams, D.R., Williams, H.: Auto-maintenance in the pigeon: Sustained pecking despite contingent non-reinforcement. J. Exp. Anal. Behav. **12**(4), 511–520 (1969)
Wilson, A., Fern, A., Ray, S., Tadepalli, P.: Multi-task reinforcement learning: A hierarchical bayesian approach. In: ICML, pp. 1015–1022, Corvallis, Oregon (2007)
Wingate, D., Goodman, N.D., Roy, D.M., Kaelbling, L.P., Tenenbaum, J.B.: Bayesian policy search with policy priors. In: Proceedings of the Twenty-Second International Joint Conference on Artificial Intelligence-Volume, vol. 2, pp. 1565–1570. AAAI Press, Menlo Park (2011)
Wolpert, D.M., Kawato, M.: Multiple paired forward and inverse models for motor control. Neural Netw. **11**(7–8), 1317–1329 (1998)
Yoshida, W., Ishii, S.: Resolution of uncertainty in prefrontal cortex. Neuron **50**(5), 781–789 (2006)
Yu, A.J., Dayan, P.: Uncertainty, neuromodulation, and attention. Neuron **46**(4), 681–692 (2005)

Part II
Prediction-Based Intrinsic Motivation Mechanisms

Maximizing Fun by Creating Data with Easily Reducible Subjective Complexity

Jürgen Schmidhuber

Abstract The *Formal Theory of Fun and Creativity* (1990–2010) [Schmidhuber, J.: Formal theory of creativity, fun, and intrinsic motivation (1990–2010). IEEE Trans. Auton. Mental Dev. **2**(3), 230–247 (2010b)] describes principles of a curious and creative agent that never stops generating nontrivial and novel and surprising tasks and data. Two modules are needed: a data encoder and a data creator. The former encodes the growing history of sensory data as the agent is interacting with its environment; the latter executes actions shaping the history. Both learn. The encoder continually tries to encode the created data more efficiently, by discovering new regularities in it. Its *learning progress* is the *wow-effect* or *fun* or intrinsic reward of the creator, which maximizes future expected reward, being motivated to invent skills leading to interesting data that the encoder does not yet know but can easily learn with little computational effort. I have argued that this simple formal principle explains science and art and music and humor.

Note: This overview heavily draws on previous publications since 1990, especially Schmidhuber (2010b), parts of which are reprinted with friendly permission by IEEE.

1 Introduction

"All life is problem solving," wrote Popper (1999). To solve existential problems such as avoiding hunger or heat, a baby has to learn how the initially unknown environment responds to its actions. Even when there is no immediate need to satisfy

J. Schmidhuber (✉)
IDSIA, Galleria 2, 6928 Manno-Lugano, Switzerland

University of Lugano & SUPSI, Manno-Lugano, Switzerland
e-mail: juergen@idsia.ch

G. Baldassarre and M. Mirolli (eds.), *Intrinsically Motivated Learning in Natural and Artificial Systems*, DOI 10.1007/978-3-642-32375-1_5,

thirst or other built-in primitive drives, the baby does not run idle. Instead it actively conducts experiments: what sensory feedback do I get if I move my eyes or my fingers or my tongue just like that? Being able to predict effects of actions will later make it easier to plan control sequences leading to desirable states, such as those where heat and hunger sensors are switched off.

The growing infant quickly gets bored by things it already understands well, but also by those it does not understand at all, always searching for new effects exhibiting some yet unexplained but *easily learnable* regularity. It acquires more and more complex behaviors building on previously acquired, simpler behaviors. Eventually it might become a physicist discovering previously unknown physical laws, or an artist creating new eye-opening artworks, or a comedian coming up with novel jokes.

For a long time I have been arguing, using various wordings, that all this behavior is driven by a very simple algorithmic mechanism that uses more or less general reinforcement learning (RL) methods (Hutter 2005; Kaelbling et al. 1996; Schmidhuber 1991d, 2009e; Sutton and Barto 1998) to maximize internal *wow-effects* or *fun* or *intrinsic reward* through reductions of subjective data complexity. To make this more precise, consider two modules: a data encoder and a data creator. The former encodes the growing history of sensory data (tactile, auditory, visual, etc.) as the agent is interacting with its environment; the latter executes actions influencing and shaping the history. The encoder uses some learning algorithm to encode the data more efficiently, trying to discover new regularities that allow for saving storage space or computation time. The encoder's *progress* (the improvement through learning) is the *fun* of the creator, which uses RL to maximize future expected fun, being motivated to invent behaviors leading to interesting data that the encoder does not yet know but can easily learn.

Since 1990, agents were built that implement this idea (Schmidhuber 2010b). They may be viewed as simple artificial scientists or artists with an intrinsic desire to create experiments for building a better model of the world and of what can be done in it (Schmidhuber 1990a, 1991a,b,c, 1997c, 2002a, 2006a, 2007c, 2008, 2009a,c,d, 2010a,b, 2012; Storck et al. 1995). Crucial ingredients are the following:

1. An adaptive world model, essentially an encoder or predictor or compressor of the continually growing history of actions/events/sensory inputs, reflecting what is currently known about how the world works.
2. A learning algorithm that continually improves the encoder (detecting novel, initially surprising spatiotemporal patterns that subsequently become known patterns).
3. Intrinsic rewards measuring the encoder's improvements (first derivative of learning progress) due to the learning algorithm (thus measuring the *degree* of subjective novelty and surprise).
4. A separate reward optimizer or reinforcement learner, which translates those rewards into action sequences or behaviors expected to optimize future reward.

A simple example may help to see that it is really possible to learn from intrinsic reward signals *à la* Item **3** that one can learn even more in places never visited before. In an environment with red and blue boxes, whenever the learning agent opens a red box, it will find an easily learnable novel geometric pattern (that is, its encoder will make progress and thus generate intrinsic reward), while all blue boxes contain a generator of unpredictable, incompressible white noise. That is, all the RL creator has to learn is a simple policy: open the next unopened red box.

Ignoring issues of computation time, it is possible to devise mathematically optimal, *universal* RL methods for such systems (Schmidhuber 2006a, 2007c, 2009c,d) (2006–2009). More about this in Sect. 2. However, the practical implementations so far (Schmidhuber 1991a,b, 1997c, 2002a; Storck et al. 1995) were nonuniversal and made approximative assumptions. Among the many ways of combining algorithms for **1–4** the following variants were implemented:

A. Nontraditional RL for partially observable Markov decision processes (POMDPs without restrictive traditional assumptions (Schmidhuber 1991d)) based on an adaptive recurrent neural network as a predictive data encoder (Schmidhuber 1990b) is used to maximize intrinsic reward for the creator in proportion to the model's prediction errors (1990) (Schmidhuber 1990a, 1991c).

B. Traditional RL (Kaelbling et al. 1996; Sutton and Barto 1998) is used to maximize intrinsic reward created in proportion to *improvements* (first derivatives) of prediction error (1991) (Schmidhuber 1991a,b).

C. Traditional RL maximizes intrinsic reward created in proportion to relative entropies between the learning agent's priors and posteriors (1995) (Storck et al. 1995).

D. Nontraditional RL (Schmidhuber et al. 1997) (without restrictive Markovian assumptions) learns probabilistic, hierarchical programs and skills through zero-sum intrinsic reward games of two players, each trying to out-predict or surprise the other, taking into account the computational costs of learning, and learning *when* to learn and *what* to learn (1997–2002) (Schmidhuber 1997c, 2002a).

B–D. (1991–2002) also showed experimentally how intrinsic rewards can substantially accelerate goal-directed learning and *external* reward intake.

Outline. Section 2 will summarize the formal theory of creativity in a nutshell, laying out a mathematically rigorous but not necessarily practical framework. Section 3 will then discuss previous concrete implementations of the nonoptimal but currently still more practical variants **A–D** mentioned above and their limitations. Section 4 will discuss relations to work by others and show how the theory greatly extends the traditional field of active learning and how it formalizes and extends previous informal ideas of developmental psychology and aesthetics theory. Section 5 will offer a natural typology of computational intrinsic motivation (IM), and Sect. 6 will briefly explain how the theory is indeed sufficiently general to explain all kinds of creative behavior, from the discovery of new physical laws through active design of experiments to the invention of jokes and works of art.

2 Formal Details of the Theory of Creativity

The theory formulates essential principles behind numerous intrinsically motivated *creative* behaviors of biological or artificial agents embedded in a possibly unknown environment. The corresponding algorithmic framework uses general RL (Sect. 2.6; Hutter 2005; Schmidhuber 2009e) to maximize not only external reward for achieving goals such as the satisfaction of hunger and thirst but also *intrinsic* reward or *wow-effect* reward for learning a better data encoder or model, by creating/discovering/learning novel patterns in the growing history of actions and sensory inputs, where the theory formally specifies what exactly is a *pattern*, what exactly is *novel* or surprising, and what exactly it means to incrementally *learn* novel skills, leading to more novel patterns.

2.1 *The Creative Agent and Its Improving Data Encoder*

Let us consider a learning agent whose single life consists of discrete cycles or time steps $t = 1, 2, \ldots, T$. Its complete lifetime T may or may not be known in advance. In what follows, the value of any time-varying variable Q at time t $(1 \leq t \leq T)$ will be denoted by $Q(t)$, the ordered sequence of values $Q(1), \ldots, Q(t)$ by $Q(\leq t)$, and the (possibly empty) sequence $Q(1), \ldots, Q(t-1)$ by $Q(<t)$. At any given t, the agent receives a real-valued input $x(t)$ from the environment and executes a real-valued action $y(t)$ which may affect future inputs. At times $t < T$, its goal is to maximize future success or *utility*

$$u(t) = E_{\mu}\left[\sum_{\tau=t+1}^{T} r(\tau) \;\middle|\; h(\leq t)\right], \tag{1}$$

where the reward $r(t)$ is a special real-valued input (vector) at time t, $h(t)$ the ordered triple $[x(t), y(t), r(t)]$ (hence $h(\leq t)$ is the known history up to t), and $E_{\mu}(\cdot \mid \cdot)$ denotes the conditional expectation operator with respect to some possibly unknown distribution μ from a set $\mathcal{M}$ of possible distributions. Here $\mathcal{M}$ reflects whatever is known about the possibly probabilistic reactions of the environment. As a very general example, $\mathcal{M}$ may contain all computable distributions (Hutter 2005; Li and Vitányi 1997; Solomonoff 1978). This essentially includes all environments one could write scientific papers about. There is just one life, no need for predefined repeatable trials, no restriction to Markovian interfaces between sensors and environment (Schmidhuber 1991d). (Note that traditional Markovian RL (Sutton and Barto 1998) typically is too limited as it assumes the current input tells the agents everything it needs to know and does not work in realistic scenarios where robots have to learn to memorize previous relevant inputs in the form of appropriate internal representations.) The utility function implicitly takes into account the expected remaining lifespan $E_\mu(T \mid h(\leq t))$ and thus the possibility to extend the lifespan through appropriate actions (Schmidhuber 2005a, 2009e). Note that mathematical analysis is *not* simplified by discounting future rewards like in traditional RL theory (Sutton and Barto 1998)—one should avoid such distortions of real rewards whenever possible.

To maximize $u(t)$, the agent may profit from an adaptive, predictive *model p* of the consequences of its possible interactions with the environment. At any time t $(1 \leq t < T)$, the model $p(t)$ will depend on the observed history so far, $h(\leq t)$. It may be viewed as the current explanation or description of $h(\leq t)$ and may help to predict future events, including rewards. Let $C(p, h)$ denote some given model p's quality or performance evaluated on a given history h. Natural quality measures taking into account storage space and computation time will be discussed in Sect. 2.2.

To encourage the agent to actively create data leading to easily learnable improvements of p (Schmidhuber 1991b,c, 2002a, 2006a, 2007c, 2009a,c,d, 2010a,b; Storck et al. 1995), the reward signal $r(t)$ is simply split into two scalar real-valued components: $r(t) = g(r_{\text{ext}}(t), r_{\text{int}}(t))$, where g maps pairs of real values to real values, for example, $g(a, b) = a + b$. Here $r_{\text{ext}}(t)$ denotes traditional *external* reward provided by the environment, such as negative reward in response to bumping against a wall or positive reward in response to reaching some teacher-given goal state. The formal theory of creativity, however, is especially interested in $r_{\text{int}}(t)$, the internal or *intrinsic* reward, which is provided whenever the data encoder's quality improves—for *purely creative* agents $r_{\text{ext}}(t) = 0$ for all valid t:

> The current *fun* $r_{\text{int}}(t)$ of the action selector is measured by the *improvements* of the data encoder p at time t.

Formally, the intrinsic reward in response to the encoder's progress (due to some application-dependent model improvement algorithm) between times t and $t + 1$ is

$$r_{\text{int}}(t + 1) = f[C(p(t), h(\leq t + 1)), C(p(t + 1), h(\leq t + 1))], \tag{2}$$

where f maps pairs of real values to real values. Various alternative progress measures are possible; most obvious is $f(a, b) = a - b$. This corresponds to a discrete time version of maximizing the first derivative of the encoder's quality. *Note that both the old and the new encoder have to be tested on the same data, namely, the history so far.* So progress between times t and $t + 1$ is defined based on two encoders of $h(<= t + 1)$, where the old one is trained only on $h(<= t)$ and the new one also gets to see $h(t <= t + 1)$. This is like $p(t)$ predicting data of time $t + 1$, then observing it, then learning something, and then becoming a measurably better encoder $p(t + 1)$.

The above description of the agent's motivation conceptually separates the goal (finding or creating data that can be modeled better or faster than before) from the means of achieving the goal. Let the creator's RL mechanism figure out how to translate such rewards into action sequences that allow the given encoder improvement algorithm to find and exploit previously unknown types of regularities. It is the task of the RL algorithm to trade off long-term versus short-term intrinsic rewards of this kind, taking into account all costs of action sequences (Schmidhuber 1991b,c, 2002a, 2006a, 2007c, 2009a,c,d, 2010a,b; Storck et al. 1995). The universal RL methods of Sect. 2.6 as well as RNN-based RL (Sect. 3.1) and SSA-based RL (Sect. 3.4) can in principle learn useful internal states containing memories of relevant previous events; less powerful RL methods (Sects. 3.2 and 3.3) cannot.

2.2 How to Measure Encoder Quality Under Time Constraints

In theory $C(p, h(\leq t))$ should take the entire history of actions and perceptions into account (Schmidhuber 2006a), like the following performance measure C_{xry}:

$$C_{xry}(p, h(\leq t)) = \sum_{\tau=1}^{t} || \, pred(p, x(\tau)) - x(\tau) \, ||^2 + || \, pred(p, r(\tau)) - r(\tau) \, ||^2 + || \, pred(p, y(\tau)) - y(\tau) \, ||^2 \tag{3}$$

where $pred(p, q)$ is p's prediction of event q from earlier parts of the history (Schmidhuber 2006a).

C_{xry} ignores the danger of overfitting through a p that just stores the entire history without compactly representing its regularities, if any. The principle of minimum description length (MDL) (Kolmogorov 1965; Li and Vitányi 1997; Rissanen 1978; Solomonoff 1978; Wallace and Boulton 1968; Wallace and Freeman 1987), however, also takes into account the description size of p, viewing p as a compressor program of the data $h(\leq t)$. This program p should be able to deal with any prefix of the growing history, computing an output starting with $h(\leq t)$ for any time t ($1 \leq t < T$). (A program that wants to halt after t steps can easily be fixed/augmented by the trivial method that simply stores any raw additional data coming in after the halt.)

$C_l(p, h(\leq t))$ denotes p's compression performance on $h(\leq t)$: the number of bits needed to specify both the encoder and the deviations of the sensory history from its predictions, in the sense of loss-free compression. The smaller the C_l, the more regularity and compressibility and predictability and lawfulness in the observations so far.

For example, suppose p uses a small encoder that correctly predicts many $x(\tau)$ for $1 \leq \tau \leq t$. This can be used to encode $x(\leq t)$ compactly: given the predictor, only the wrongly predicted $x(\tau)$ plus information about the corresponding time steps τ are necessary to reconstruct input history $x(\leq t)$, for example (Schmidhuber 1992). Similarly, a predictor that learns a probability distribution on the possible next events, given previous events, can be used to efficiently encode observations with high (respectively low) predicted probability by few (respectively many) bits (Sect. 3.3; (Huffman 1952; Schmidhuber and Heil 1996)), thus achieving a compressed history representation.

Alternatively, p could also make use of a 3D world model or simulation. The corresponding MDL-based quality measure $C_{3D}(p, h(\leq t))$ is the number of bits needed to specify all polygons and surface textures in the 3D simulation plus the number of bits needed to encode deviations of $h(\leq t)$ from the predictions of the simulation. Improving the 3D model by adding or removing polygons may reduce the total number of bits required.

The ultimate limit for $C_l(p, h(\leq t))$ would be $K^*(h(\leq t))$, a variant of the Kolmogorov complexity of $h(\leq t)$, namely, the length of the shortest program (for the given hardware) that computes an output starting with $h(\leq t)$ (Kolmogorov 1965; Li and Vitányi 1997; Schmidhuber 2002b; Solomonoff 1978). Here there is no need to worry about the fact that $K^*(h(\leq t))$ in general cannot be computed exactly, only approximated from above (indeed, for most practical predictors, the approximation will be crude). This just means that some patterns will be hard to detect by the limited encoder of choice, that is, the reward maximizer will get discouraged from spending too much effort on creating those patterns.

$C_l(p, h(\leq t))$ does not take into account the time $\tau(p, h(\leq t))$ spent by p on computing $h(\leq t)$. A runtime-dependent performance measure inspired by concepts of optimal universal search (Levin 1973; Schmidhuber 2002c, 2004, 2006a, 2009c, 2010a) is

$$C_{l\tau}(p, h(\leq t)) = C_l(p, h(\leq t)) + \log \tau(p, h(\leq t)). \tag{4}$$

Here compression by one bit is worth as much as runtime reduction by a factor of $\frac{1}{2}$. From an asymptotic optimality-oriented point of view, this is one of the best ways of trading off storage and computation time (Levin 1973; Schmidhuber 2002c, 2004).

In practical applications (Sect. 3), the encoder of the continually growing data typically will have to calculate its output online, that is, it will be able to use only a constant number of computational instructions per second to predict/compress new data. The goal of the possibly much slower learning algorithm must then be to improve the encoder such that it keeps operating online within those time limits, while encoding better than before. The costs of computing $C_{xry}(p, h(\leq t))$ and $C_l(p, h(\leq t))$ and similar performance measures are linear in t, assuming p consumes equal amounts of computation time for each single prediction. Therefore, online evaluations of learning progress on the full history so far generally cannot take place as frequently as the continually ongoing online predictions.

At least some of the learning and its progress evaluations may take place during occasional "sleep" phases (Schmidhuber 2006a, 2009c). But practical implementations so far have looked only at parts of the history for efficiency reasons: the systems described in Sects. 3 and 3.1–3.4 (Schmidhuber 1991b,c, 2002a; Storck et al. 1995) used online settings (one prediction per time step and constant computational effort per prediction), nonuniversal adaptive encoders, and approximative evaluations of learning progress, each consuming only constant time despite the continual growth of the history.

2.3 *Optimal Predictors Versus Optimal Compressors*

For the theoretically inclined, there is a deep connection between optimal prediction and optimal compression. Consider Solomonoff's theoretically optimal, universal way of predicting the future (Hutter 2005; Li and Vitányi 1997; Solomonoff 1964, 1978). Given an observation sequence $q(\leq t)$, the Bayes formula is used to predict the probability of the next possible $q(t+1)$. The only assumption is that there exists a computer program that can take any $q(\leq t)$ as an input and compute its a priori probability according to the μ prior. (This assumption is extremely general, essentially including all environments one can write scientific papers about, as mentioned above.) In general this program is unknown; hence, a mixture prior is used instead to predict:

$$\xi(q(\leq t)) = \sum_i w_i \mu_i(q(\leq t)), \tag{5}$$

a weighted sum of *all* distributions $\mu_i \in \mathcal{M}$, $i = 1, 2, \ldots$, where the sum of the constant positive weights satisfies $\sum_i w_i \leq 1$. This is indeed the best one can possibly do, in a very general sense (Hutter 2005; Solomonoff 1978). The drawback of the scheme is its incomputability, since $\mathcal{M}$ contains infinitely many distributions. One may increase the theoretical power of the scheme by augmenting $\mathcal{M}$ by certain non-enumerable but limit-computable distributions (Schmidhuber 2002b) or restrict it such that it becomes computable, for example, by assuming the world is computed by some unknown but deterministic computer program sampled from the speed prior (Schmidhuber 2002c) which assigns low probability to environments that are hard to compute by any method.

Remarkably, under very general conditions, both universal inductive inference (Li and Vitányi 1997; Solomonoff 1964, 1978) and the compression-oriented MDL approach (Kolmogorov 1965; Li and Vitányi 1997; Rissanen 1978; Wallace and Boulton 1968; Wallace and Freeman 1987) converge to the correct predictions in the limit (Poland and Hutter 2005). It should be mentioned, however, that the former converges faster.

2.4 *Discrete Asynchronous Framework for Maximizing Fun*

Let $p(t)$ denote the agent's current encoder program at time t, $s(t)$ its current creator, and **DO:**

Creator: At any time t $(1 \leq t < T)$ do:

1. Let $s(t)$ use (parts of) history $h(\leq t)$ to select and execute $y(t+1)$.
2. Observe $x(t+1)$.
3. Check if there is nonzero intrinsic reward $r_{\text{int}}(t+1)$ provided by the asynchronously running improvement algorithm of the encoder (see below). If not, set $r_{\text{int}}(t+1) = 0$.

4. Let the creator's RL algorithm use $h(\leq t+1)$ including $r_{\text{int}}(t+1)$ (and possibly also the latest available compressed version of the observed data—see below) to obtain a new creator $s(t+1)$, in line with objective (1). Note that some actions may actually trigger learning algorithms that compute changes of the encoder and the creator's policy, such as in Sect. 3.4 (Schmidhuber 2002a). That is, the computational cost of learning can be taken into account by the reward optimizer, and the decision when and what to learn can be learned as well (Schmidhuber 2002a).

Encoder: Set p_{new} equal to the initial data encoder. Starting at time 1, repeat forever until interrupted by death at time T:

1. Set $p_{\text{old}} = p_{\text{new}}$, get current time step t, and set $h_{\text{old}} = h(\leq t)$.
2. Evaluate p_{old} on h_{old} to obtain performance measure $C(p_{\text{old}}, h_{\text{old}})$. This may take many time steps.
3. Let some (possibly application-dependent) encoder improvement algorithm (such as a learning algorithm for an adaptive neural network predictor, possibly triggered by a creator action) use h_{old} to obtain a hopefully better encoder p_{new} (such as a neural net with the same size and the same constant computational effort per prediction but with improved predictive power and therefore improved compression performance (Schmidhuber and Heil 1996)). Although this may take many time steps (and could be partially performed off-line during "sleep" (Schmidhuber 2006a, 2009c)), p_{new} may not be optimal due to limitations of the learning algorithm, for example, local maxima. (To inform the creator about beginnings of encoder evaluation processes, etc., augment its input by unique representations of such events.)
4. Evaluate p_{new} on h_{old} to obtain $C(p_{\text{new}}, h_{\text{old}})$. This may take many time steps.
5. Get current time step τ and generate fun

$$r_{\text{int}}(\tau) = f[C(p_{\text{old}}, h_{\text{old}}), C(p_{\text{new}}, h_{\text{old}})], \tag{6}$$

for example, $f(a,b) = a - b$. [Here the τ replaces the $t+1$ of Eq. (2).]

This asynchronous scheme (Schmidhuber 2006a, 2007c, 2009c) may cause long temporal delays between creator actions and corresponding rewards or fun events and may impose a heavy burden on the creator's RL algorithm whose task is to assign credit to past actions. Nevertheless, Sect. 2.6 will discuss RL algorithms for this purpose which are theoretically optimal in various senses (Schmidhuber 2006a, 2007c, 2009c,d).

2.5 Continuous Time Formulation

In continuous time, $O(t)$ denotes the state of subjective observer O at time t. The subjective computational complexity $Complexity(D, O(t))$ of a sequence of observations and/or actions is a measure of the effort required to encode/decode D, given $O(t)$'s current limited prior knowledge and limited encoding method. The time-dependent and observer-dependent subjective $Fun(D, O(t))$ is

$$Fun(D, O(t)) \sim \frac{\partial Complexity(D, O(t))}{\partial t}, \tag{7}$$

the *first derivative* of subjective complexity or simplicity: as O improves its encoder, formerly apparently random data parts become subjectively more regular/elegant/beautiful, requiring fewer bits (or less time) for their encoding.

There are at least two ways of having fun: execute a learning algorithm that improves the compression of the already known data (in online settings, without increasing computational needs of the encoder) or execute actions that generate more data, then learn to better encode this new data.

2.6 Optimal Creativity, Given the Encoder's Limitations

The previous sections discussed how to measure encoder improvements and how to translate them into intrinsic reward signals, but did not say much about the RL method used to maximize expected future reward. The chosen encoder class typically will have certain computational limitations. In the absence of any external rewards, one may define *optimal pure curiosity behavior* relative to these limitations: at discrete time step t, this behavior would select the action that maximizes

$$u(t) = E_{\mu}\left[\sum_{\tau=t+1}^{T} r_{\text{int}}(\tau) \;\middle|\; h(\leq t)\right]. \tag{8}$$

Since the true, world-governing probability distribution μ is unknown, the resulting task of the creator's RL algorithm may be a formidable one. As the system is revisiting previously incompressible parts of the environment, some of those will tend to become more subjectively compressible, and the corresponding curiosity rewards will decrease over time. A good RL algorithm must somehow detect and then *predict* this decrease and act accordingly. Traditional RL algorithms (Kaelbling et al. 1996), however, do not provide any theoretical guarantee of optimality for such situations.

Is there a best possible RL algorithm that comes as close as any other computable one to maximizing objective (8)? Indeed, there is. Its drawback, however, is that it is not computable in finite time. Nevertheless, it serves as a reference point for defining what is achievable at best, that is, what is *optimal* creativity.

How does it work? Optimal inductive inference as defined in Sect. 2.3 can be extended by formally including the effects of executed actions, to define an optimal action selector maximizing future expected reward. At any time t, Hutter's theoretically optimal (yet uncomputable) RL algorithm AIXI (Hutter 2005) uses such an extended version of Solomonoff's scheme to select those action sequences that promise maximal future reward up to some horizon T (e.g., twice the lifetime so far), given the current data $h(\leq t)$. That is, in cycle $t + 1$, AIXI selects as its next action the first action of an action sequence maximizing ξ-predicted reward up to the given horizon, appropriately generalizing Eq. (5). AIXI uses observations optimally (Hutter 2005): the Bayes-optimal policy p^{ξ} based on the mixture ξ is self-optimizing in the sense that its average utility value converges asymptotically for all $\mu \in \mathcal{M}$ to the optimal value achieved by the Bayes-optimal policy p^{μ} which knows μ in advance. The necessary and sufficient condition is that $\mathcal{M}$ admits self-optimizing policies. The policy p^{ξ} is also Pareto optimal in the sense that there is no other policy yielding higher or equal value in *all* environments $\nu \in \mathcal{M}$ and a strictly higher value in at least one (Hutter 2005).

AIXI as above needs unlimited computation time. Its computable variant AIXI*(t,l)* (Hutter 2005) has asymptotically optimal runtime but may suffer from a huge constant slowdown. To take the consumed computation time into account in a general, optimal way, one may use the recent Gödel machine s (Schmidhuber 2005a,b, 2006b, 2009e) instead. They represent the first class of mathematically rigorous, fully self-referential, self-improving, general, optimally efficient problem solvers and are applicable to the problem embodied by objective (8).

The initial software $\mathcal{S}$ of such a Gödel machine contains an initial problem solver, for example, some typically suboptimal RL method (Kaelbling et al. 1996). It also contains an asymptotically optimal initial proof searcher, typically based on an online variant of Levin's *universal search* (Levin 1973), which is used to run and test *proof techniques*. Proof techniques are programs written in a universal language implemented on the Gödel machine within $\mathcal{S}$. They are in principle able to compute proofs concerning the system's own future performance, based on an axiomatic system $\mathcal{A}$ encoded in $\mathcal{S}$. $\mathcal{A}$ describes the formal *utility* function, in the present case Eq. (8), the hardware properties, axioms of arithmetic and probability theory and data manipulation, etc., and $\mathcal{S}$ itself, which is possible without introducing circularity (Schmidhuber 2009e).

Inspired by Kurt Gödel's celebrated self-referential formulas (1931), the Gödel machine rewrites any part of its own code (including the proof searcher) through a self-generated executable program as soon as its *universal search* variant has found a proof that the rewrite is *useful* according to objective (8). According to the Global Optimality Theorem (Schmidhuber 2005a,b, 2006b, 2009e), such a self-rewrite is globally optimal—no local maxima possible!—since the self-referential code first had to prove that it is not useful to continue the search for alternative self-rewrites.

If there is no provably useful optimal way of rewriting $\mathcal{S}$ at all, then humans will not find one either. But if there is one, then $\mathcal{S}$ itself can find and exploit it. Unlike the previous *non*-self-referential methods based on hardwired proof searchers (Hutter 2005), Gödel machine s not only boast an optimal *order* of complexity but can optimally reduce (through self-changes) any slowdowns hidden by the $O()$-notation, provided the utility of such speedups is provable (Schmidhuber 2006c, 2007a,b).

Limitations of the "Universal" Approaches. The methods above are optimal in various ways, some of them not only computable but even optimally time efficient in the asymptotic limit. Nevertheless, they leave open an essential remaining practical question: If the agent can execute only a fixed number of computational instructions per unit time interval (say, 10 trillion elementary operations per second), what is the best way of using them to get as close as possible to the theoretical limits of universal AIs? Especially when external rewards are very rare, as is the case in many realistic environments? As long as there is no good answer to this question, one has to resort to approximations and heuristics when it comes to practical applications. The next section reviews what has been achieved so far along these lines, discussing our implementations of curiosity-driven creative agents from the 1990s; quite a few aspects of these concrete systems are still of relevance today.

3 Previous Implementations of Curious/Creative Agents: Pros and Cons

The above mathematically rigorous framework for optimal curiosity and creativity (2006–) was established *after* first approximations thereof were implemented (1991, 1995, 1997–2002). Sections 3.1–3.4 will discuss advantages and limitations of online learning systems described in the original publications on artificial intrinsic motivation (Schmidhuber 1991b,c, 1997c; Storck et al. 1995) which already can be viewed as example implementations of a compression progress drive or prediction progress drive that encourages the discovery or creation of novel, surprising patterns. Some elements of this earlier work are believed to remain essential for creating systems that are both theoretically sound and *practical*.

3.1 Intrinsic Reward for Coding Error (1990)

Early work (Schmidhuber 1990a, 1991c) describes a data encoder based on an adaptive world model implemented as a recurrent neural network (RNN) (in principle, a rather powerful computational device, even by today's machine learning standards), predicting sensory inputs including reward signals from the entire previous history of actions and inputs. A second RNN (the creator) uses the world model and gradient descent to search for a control policy or program maximizing the sum of future expected rewards according to the model. Some of the rewards are intrinsic curiosity rewards, which are proportional to the predictor's errors. So the same mechanism that is used for normal goal-directed learning is used for implementing creativity and curiosity and boredom—there is no need for a separate system aiming at improving the encoder.

This first description of a general, curious, world-exploring RL agent implicitly and optimistically assumes that the encoder will indeed improve by motivating the creator/controller to go to places where the prediction error is high. One drawback of the prediction error-based approach is that it encourages the creator to focus its search on those parts of the environment where there will always be high prediction errors due to noise or randomness or due to computational limitations of the encoder. This may *prevent* learning progress instead of promoting it and motivates the next subsection, whose basic ideas could be combined with the RL method of (Schmidhuber 1990a, 1991c), but this has not been done yet.

Another potential drawback is the nature of the particular RNN-based RL method. Although the latter has the potential to learn internal memories of previous relevant sensory inputs, and thus can deal with POMDPs as it is not limited to Markovian interfaces between agent and environment (Schmidhuber 1991d), like all gradient-based methods, it may suffer from local minima, as well as from potential problems of online learning, since gradients for the recurrent RL creator are computed with the help of the dynamically changing, online learning recurrent predictive encoder. Apart from this limitation, the RNN of back then were less powerful than today's LSTM RNN (Hochreiter and Schmidhuber 1997; Schmidhuber et al. 2011), which yielded state of the art performance in challenging applications such as connected handwriting recognition (Graves et al. 2009), and should be used instead.

3.2 *Intrinsic Reward for Encoder Improvements (1991)*

Follow-up work (Schmidhuber 1991a,b) points out that one should not focus on the errors of the encoder, but on its improvements. The basic principle can be formulated as follows: *Learn a mapping from actions (or action sequences) to the expectation of future performance improvement of the encoder. Encourage action sequences where this expectation is high.*

Two implementations were described: The first models the reliability of the predictions of the encoder/predictor by a separate, so-called confidence network. At any given time, reinforcement for the model-building control system is created in proportion to the current *change* or first derivative of the reliability of the adaptive predictor. The "curiosity goal" of the creator (it might have additional "pre-wired" external goals) is to maximize the expectation of the cumulative sum of future positive or negative changes in prediction reliability.

The second implementation replaces the confidence network by a network H which at every time step tries to predict the current *change* or first derivative of the model network's output (caused by its learning algorithm). H will learn approximations of the expectations of the changes (first derivatives) of the encoder's responses to given inputs. The *absolute value* of H's output is taken as the intrinsic reward.

While the neural predictor of the implementations is computationally less powerful than the recurrent one of Sect. 3.1 (Schmidhuber 1991c), there is a novelty, namely, an explicit (neural) adaptive model of the predictor's improvements, measured in terms of mean squared error (MSE). This model essentially learns to predict the encoder's changes (the prediction derivatives). For example, although noise is unpredictable and leads to wildly varying target signals for the predictor, in the long run, these signals do not change the adaptive encoder's parameters much, and the predictor of predictor changes is able to learn this. A variant of the standard RL algorithm Q-learning (Sutton and Barto 1998) is fed with curiosity reward signals proportional to the expected long-term predictor changes; thus, the agent is intrinsically motivated to make novel patterns within the given limitations. In fact, one may say that the system tries to maximize an approximation of the (discounted) sum of the expected first derivatives of the data's subjective predictability, thus also maximizing an approximation of the (discounted) sum of the expected changes of the data's subjective compressibility (the surprise or novelty).

Both variants avoid the theoretically desirable but impractical regular evaluations of the encoder on the entire history so far, as discussed in Sect. 2.2. Instead they monitor the recent effects of learning on the learning mechanism (a neural network in this case). Experiments illustrate the advantages of this type of directed, curious exploration over traditional random exploration.

One RL method-specific drawback is given by the limitations of standard Markovian RL (Schmidhuber 1991d), which assumes the current input tells the agent everything it needs to know and does not work well in realistic scenarios where it has to learn to memorize previous relevant inputs to select optimal actions. For general robot scenarios, more powerful RL methods are necessary, such as those mentioned in Sect. 3.1 and other parts of this chapter.

Any RL algorithm has to deal with the fact that intrinsic rewards vanish where the encoder becomes perfect. In the simple toy world (Schmidhuber 1991a,b),this is not a problem, since the creator continually updates its Q-values based on recent experience. But since the learning rate is chosen heuristically (as usual in RL applications), this approach lacks the theoretical justification of the general framework of Sect. 2.

For probabilistic worlds, there are prediction error measures that are more principled than MSE. This motivates research described next.

3.3 Fun Depending on the Relative Entropy Between Encoder's Prior and Posterior (1995)

Follow-up work (1995) describes an information theory-oriented variant of the approach in nondeterministic worlds (Storck et al. 1995). Here the intrinsic reward is proportional to the encoder's surprise/information gain (Fedorov 1972), measured as the Kullback–Leibler distance (Kullback 1959) between a learning predictor's subjective probability distributions before and after new observations—the relative entropy between its prior and posterior, essentially another measure of learning progress which does not take into account computation time. Again experiments show the advantages of this type of curious exploration over conventional random exploration.

Since this implementation also uses a traditional RL method (Sutton and Barto 1998) instead of a more general one, the discussion of RL method-specific drawbacks in previous subsections remains valid here as well.

Note the connection to Sect. 2: the concepts of Huffman coding (Huffman 1952) and relative entropy between prior and posterior immediately translate into a measure of learning progress reflecting the number of saved bits—a measure of improved data compression.

Note also, however, that the naive probabilistic approach to data compression is unable to discover more general types of *algorithmic* compressibility (Li and Vitányi 1997) as discussed in Sect. 2. For example, the decimal expansion of π looks random and incompressible but is not: there is a very short algorithm computing all of π, yet any finite sequence of digits will occur in π's expansion as frequently as expected if π were truly random, that is, no simple statistical learner will outperform random guessing at predicting the next digit from a limited time window of previous digits. More general *program* search techniques are necessary to extract the underlying algorithmic regularity. This motivates the universal approach discussed in Sect. 2 but also the research on a more general practical implementation described next.

3.4 Learning Better Encodings and Skills Through Zero-Sum Intrinsic Reward Games (1997–2002)

The universal variants of the principle of novel pattern creation of Sect. 2 focused on theoretically optimal ways of measuring encoder progress/surprise/novelty, as well as mathematically optimal ways of selecting action sequences or experiments within the framework of artificial curiosity and creativity (Schmidhuber 2006a, 2007c, 2009c,d, 2010b). These variants take the entire lifelong history of actions and observations into account and make minimal assumptions about the nature of the environment, such as the following: the (unknown) probabilities of possible event histories are at least enumerable. The resulting systems exhibit "mathematically optimal curiosity and creativity" and provide a yardstick against which all less universal intrinsically motivated systems can be measured. However, most of them ignore important issues of time constraints in online settings. For example, in practical applications, one cannot frequently measure encoder improvements by testing encoder performance on the entire history so far. The costs of learning and testing have to be taken into account. This insight drove the research discussed next.

To address the computational costs of learning and the costs of measuring learning progress, computationally powerful encoders and creators (Schmidhuber 1997c, 2002a) were implemented as two very general, coevolving, symmetric, opposing modules called the *right brain* and the *left brain*, both able to construct self-modifying probabilistic programs written in a universal programming language (1997–2002). An internal storage for temporary computational results of the programs is viewed as part of the changing environment. Each module can suggest experiments in the form of probabilistic algorithms to be executed and make predictions about their effects, *betting intrinsic reward* on their outcomes. The opposing module may accept such a bet in a zero-sum game by making a contrary prediction or reject it. In case of acceptance, the winner is determined by executing the algorithmic experiment and checking its outcome; the intrinsic reward for wow-effects eventually gets transferred from the surprised loser to the confirmed winner. Both modules try to maximize reward using a rather general RL algorithm [the so-called success-story algorithm SSA (Schmidhuber et al. 1997)] designed for complex stochastic policies—alternative RL algorithms could be plugged in as well. Thus, both modules are motivated to discover *truly novel* algorithmic patterns/compressibility, where the subjective baseline for novelty is given by what the opponent already knows about the (external or internal) world's repetitive patterns. Since the execution of any computational or physical action costs something (as it will reduce the cumulative reward per time ratio), both modules are motivated to focus on those parts of the dynamic world that currently make learning progress *easy*, to minimize the costs of identifying promising experiments and executing them. The system learns a partly hierarchical structure of more and more complex skills or programs necessary to solve the growing sequence of self-generated tasks, reusing previously acquired simpler skills where this is beneficial. Experimental studies exhibit several sequential stages of emergent developmental sequences, with and without external reward.

Many ingredients of this system may be just what one needs to build *practical yet sound* curious and creative systems that never stop expanding their knowledge about what can be done in a given world, although future reimplementations should probably use alternative reward optimizers that are more general and powerful than SSA (Schmidhuber et al. 1997), such as variants of the Optimal Ordered Problem Solver (Schmidhuber 2004).

3.5 Recent Implementations

More recently implemented variants deal with applications to vision-based reinforcement learning/evolutionary search (Cuccu et al. 2011; Luciw et al. 2011), active learning of currently easily learnable functions (Ngo et al. 2011), black-box optimization (Schaul et al. 2011b), and detection of "interesting" sequences of Wikipedia articles (Schaul et al. 2011a).

3.6 Improving Real Reward Intake (1991–)

References above demonstrated through several experiments that the presence of intrinsic reward or curiosity reward can actually speed up the collection of *external* reward. However, the previous papers also pointed out that it is always possible to design environments where the bias toward regularities introduced through artificial curiosity can lead to worse performance—curiosity can indeed kill the cat.

4 Relation to Work by Others

4.1 Beyond Traditional Information Theory and Active Learning

How does the notion of surprise in the theory of creativity differ from the notion of surprise in traditional information theory? Consider two extreme examples of uninteresting, unsurprising, boring data: a vision-based agent that always stays in the dark will experience an extremely compressible, soon totally predictable history of unchanging visual inputs. In front of a screen full of white noise conveying a lot of information and "novelty" and "surprise" in the traditional sense of Boltzmann and Shannon (Shannon 1948), however, it will experience highly unpredictable and fundamentally incompressible data. According to the theory of creativity, in both cases, the data is not *surprising* but *boring* (Schmidhuber 2002a, 2007c) as it does not allow for further encoding progress—there is no novel pattern. Therefore, the traditional notion of surprise is rejected. Neither the arbitrary nor the fully predictable is *truly* novel or surprising. Only data with still *unknown* algorithmic regularities are (Schmidhuber 1991b,c, 2002a, 2006a, 2007c, 2009c,d; Storck et al. 1995), for example, a previously unknown song containing a subjectively novel harmonic pattern. That is why one really has to measure the *progress of the learning encoder* to compute the degree of surprise. (Compare Sect. 4.4.2 for a related discussion on what is aesthetically pleasing.)

How does the theory generalize the related traditional field of *active learning*, for example (Fedorov 1972)? To optimize a function may require expensive data evaluations. Original active learning is limited to supervised classification tasks, for example (Balcan et al. 2009; Cohn 1994; Fedorov 1972; Hwang et al. 1991; MacKay 1992; Plutowski et al. 1994; Seung et al. 1992), asking which data points to evaluate next to maximize information gain, typically (but not necessarily) using one step look-ahead, assuming all data point evaluations are equally costly. The objective (improve classification error) is given externally; there is no explicit intrinsic reward in the sense discussed in this chapter. The more general framework of creativity theory also takes formally into account:

1. Reinforcement learning agents embedded in an environment where there may be arbitrary delays between experimental actions and corresponding information gains, for example (Schmidhuber 1991b; Storck et al. 1995)
2. The highly environment-dependent costs of obtaining or creating not just individual data points but data *sequences* of *a priori* unknown size

3. Arbitrary algorithmic or statistical dependencies in sequences of actions and sensory inputs, for example (Schmidhuber 2002a, 2006a)
4. The computational cost of learning new skills, for example (Schmidhuber 2002a)

While others recently have started to study active RL as well, for example, Brafman and Tennenholtz [R-max algorithm (Brafman and Tennenholtz 2002)] and Li et al. [KWIK-framework (Li et al. 2008)] (Strehl et al. 2010), our more general systems measure and maximize *algorithmic* (Kolmogorov 1965; Li and Vitányi 1997; Schmidhuber 2002b; Solomonoff 1978) novelty (learnable but previously unknown compressibility or predictability) of self-generated spatiotemporal patterns in the history of data and actions (Schmidhuber 2006a, 2007c, 2009c,d).

4.2 Relation to Handcrafted Interestingness

Lenat's discovery system EURISKO (Lenat 1983) has a preprogrammed interestingness measure which was observed to become more and more inappropriate ("stagnation" problem) as EURISKO creates new concepts from old ones with the help of human intervention. Unsupervised systems based on creativity theory, however, continually redefine what is interesting based on what is currently easy to learn, in addition to what is already known.

4.3 Related Implementations Since 2005

In 2005, Baldi and Itti demonstrated experimentally that the method of 1995 (Sect. 3.3, Storck et al. 1995) explains certain patterns of human visual attention better than certain previous approaches (Itti and Baldi 2005).

Klyubin et al.'s seemingly related approach to intrinsic motivation (Klyubin et al. 2005) of 2005 tries to maximize *empowerment* by maximizing the information an agent could potentially "inject" into its future sensory inputs via a sequence of actions. The authors assume a good world model is already given or at least learned before *empowerment* is measured (D. Polani, personal communication, 2010). For example, using one step look-ahead in a deterministic and well-modeled world, their agent will prefer states where the execution of alternative actions will make a lot of difference in the immediate sensory inputs, according to the reliable world model. Generally speaking, however, it might prefer actions leading to high-entropy, random inputs over others—compare Sect. 3.1.

In 2005, Singh et al. (Singh et al. 2005) also used intrinsic rewards proportional to prediction errors as in Sect. 3.1 (Schmidhuber 1991c), employing a different type of reward maximizer based on the option framework which can be used to specify subgoals. As pointed out earlier, it is useful to make the conceptual distinction between the objective and the means of reaching the objective: the latter is shared by the approaches of (Singh et al. 2005) and of Sect. 3.1; the reward maximizer is different.

In related work, Schembri et al. address the problem of learning to compose skills, assuming different skills are learned by different RL modules. They speed up skill learning by rewarding a top-level, module-selecting RL agent in proportion to the TD error of the selected module (Schembri et al. 2007).

Other researchers in the nascent field of developmental robotics (Blank and Meeden 2006; Gold and Scassellati 2006; Hart 2009; Hart et al. 2008; Kuipers et al. 2006; Olsson et al. 2006; Oudeyer and Kaplan 2006; Provost et al. 2006; Schlesinger 2006; Stronger and Stone 2006) and intrinsic reward also followed the line of basic ideas presented here, in particular, Oudeyer et al. (Oudeyer et al. 2007).

Friston et al. (2010) also propose an approach which at first glance seems similar to ours, based on free energy minimization and predictive coding. Predictive coding is a special case of compression, for example, (Schmidhuber and Heil 1996), and free energy is another approximative measure of algorithmic compressibility/algorithmic information (Li and Vitányi 1997); the latter concept is more general though. As Friston et al. write, *"Under simplifying assumptions free energy is just the amount of prediction error,"* like in the 1991 paper (Schmidhuber 1991c) discussed in Sect. 3.1. Under slightly less simplifying assumptions, it is the Kullback–Leibler divergence between probabilistic world model and probabilistic world, like in the 1995 paper (Storck et al. 1995) (which looks at the learning model before and after new observations; see Sect. 3.3). Despite these similarities, however, what Friston et al. do is to select actions that *minimize* free energy. In other words, their agents like to visit highly predictable states. Hence, their approach does *not* describe a system intrinsically motivated to learn new, previously unknown things; instead their agents really want to stabilize and make everything predictable. Friston et al. are well aware of potential objections: *"At this point, most (astute) people say: but that means I should retire to a dark room and cover my ears."* This pretty much sums up the expected criticism. In contrast, the theory of creativity has no problem whatsoever with dark rooms—the latter get boring as soon as they are predictable; then there are no wow-effects and learning progresses no more, that is, the first derivative of subjective data encodability is zero, that is, the intrinsic reward is zero, that is, the reward-maximizing agent is motivated to leave the room to find or make additional rewarding, nonrandom, learnable, novel patterns.

4.4 Previous, Less Formal Work in Aesthetics Theory and Psychology

Two millennia ago, Cicero already called curiosity a "passion for learning." In the recent millennium's final century, art theorists and developmental psychologists extended this view. In its final decade, the concept eventually became sufficiently formal to permit the computer implementations discussed in Sect. 3.

4.4.1 Developmental Psychology

In the 1950s, psychologists revisited the idea of curiosity as the motivation for exploratory behavior (Berlyne 1950, 1960), emphasizing the importance of novelty (Berlyne 1950) and non-homeostatic drives (Harlow et al. 1950). Piaget (1955) explained explorative learning behavior in infants through his informal concepts of assimilation (new inputs are embedded in old schemas—this may be viewed as a type of compression) and accommodation (adapting an old schema to a new input—this may be viewed as a type of compression improvement). Unlike Sect. 2, however, these ideas did not provide sufficient formal details to permit the construction of artificial curious and creative agents.

4.4.2 Aesthetics Theory

The closely related field of aesthetics theory (Bense 1969; Birkhoff 1933; Frank 1964; Franke 1979; Moles 1968; Nake 1974) emerged even earlier in the 1930s. Why are humans somehow intrinsically motivated to observe or make certain novel patterns, such as aesthetically pleasing works of art, even when this seems irrelevant for solving typical frequently recurring problems such as hunger and even when the action of observation requires a serious effort, such as spending hours to get to the museum? Since the days of Plato and Aristotle, many have written about aesthetics and taste, trying to explain why some behaviors or objects are more interesting or aesthetically rewarding than others, for example (Collingwood 1938; Goodman 1968; Kant 1781). However, they did not have or use the mathematical tools necessary to provide formal answers to the questions above. What about more formal theories of aesthetic perception from the 1930s (Birkhoff 1933) and especially the 1960s (Bense 1969; Frank 1964; Franke 1979; Moles 1968; Nake 1974)? Some of the previous attempts at explaining aesthetic experience in the context of information theory (Bense 1969; Frank 1964; Franke 1979; Moles 1968; Nake 1974) tried to quantify the intrinsic aesthetic reward through an *"ideal"* ratio between expected and unexpected information conveyed by some aesthetic object (its *"order"* vs. its *"complexity"*). The basic idea was that aesthetic objects should neither be too simple nor too complex, as reflected by the *Wundt curve* (Wundt 1874), which assigns maximal interestingness to data whose complexity is somewhere in between the extremes. Using certain measures based on information theory (Shannon 1948), Bense (1969) argued for an ideal ratio of $1/e \sim 37\,\%$. However, these approaches were not detailed and formal enough to construct artificial, intrinsically motivated agents with a built-in desire to create aesthetically pleasing works of art.

Our formal theory of creativity does not have to postulate any objective ideal ratio of this kind. Unlike previous works emphasizing the significance of the subjective observer (Frank 1964; Frank and Franke 2002; Franke 1979), its dynamic formal definition of fun reflects the *change* in the computational resources required to encode artistic and other objects, explicitly taking into account the subjective observer's growing knowledge as well as the limitations of its learning algorithm (or compression *improvement* algorithm). For example, random noise is always novel in the sense that it is unpredictable. But it is not rewarding since it has no pattern. It cannot be compactly encoded at all; there is no way of learning to encode it better than by storing the raw data. On the other hand, a given pattern may not be novel to a given observer at a given point in his life, because he already perfectly understands it—again there may be no way of learning to encode it even more efficiently. The value of an aesthetic experience (the fun of a creative or curious maker or observer of art) is not defined by the created or observed object per se, but by the algorithmic encoding *progress* of the subjective, learning observer.

Why did not early pioneers of aesthetic information theory put forward similar views? Perhaps because back then, the fields of algorithmic information theory and machine learning were still in their infancy?

5 Simple Typology of Intrinsic Motivation

By definition, intrinsic reward is something that is independent of external reward, although it may sometimes help to accelerate the latter as discussed in Sect. 3.6 (Schmidhuber 1991b, 2002a; Storck et al. 1995). So far, most if not all intrinsically motivated computational systems had the following:

1. A more or less limited adaptive encoder/predictor/compressor/model of the history of sensory inputs, internal states, reinforcement signals, and actions.
2. Some sort of real-valued intrinsic reward indicative of the learning progress of **(1)**.
3. A more or less limited reinforcement learner able to maximize future expected reward.

Hence, the typology just needs to classify previous systems with respect to properties and limitations of their specific instances of **(1–3)**. The few (if any) implementations of intrinsic motivation that do *not* fit this typology can be treated as outliers, at least until their significance/number grows, if ever. The typology actually realizes the MDL principle: find a compact model (in this case: a typology) of the data (in this case: various approaches to IM). To minimize the description length of the set of all IM approaches, minimize the description size of the typology *plus* the description size of badly modeled outliers. How? By identifying what the majority of the previous IM approaches have in common. Outliers do not fit and thus cost more extra bits, but that is ok as they are rare, since they are outliers.

(1) Includes many subtypes characterized by the answers to the following questions:

1. What exactly can the encoder encode (or the predictor predict or the compressor compress)?

(a) All sensory inputs as in Sect. 3.1 (Schmidhuber 1991c)? A preprocessed subset of the sensory inputs? For example, features indicating synchronicity of certain processes (Oudeyer and Kaplan 2006)? The latter may be of interest for certain limited types of IM-based learning.
(b) Reinforcement signals as in Sect. 3.1 (Schmidhuber 1991c)? (Even traditional RL agents without IM do this.)
(c) Creator actions as in Sect. 2 (Schmidhuber 2002a, 2006a, 2007c, 2009c,d)? Then even in absence of sensory feedback, curious and creative agents will be motivated to learn new motor patterns, such as previously unknown dances.
(d) Results of internal computations through sequences of internal actions as in Sect. 3.4 (Schmidhuber 2002a)? This will motivate a curious agent to create novel patterns not only in the space of sensory inputs but also in the space of abstract input transformations, such as an earlier-learned mapping from all images of cars to an internal symbol "car." The agent will also be motivated to create purely "mental" novel patterns independent of external inputs, such as number sequences obeying previously unknown mathematical laws (corresponding to mathematical discoveries).
(e) Some combination of the above? All of the above as in Sect. 3.4 (Schmidhuber 2002a)? The latter should be the default for artificial general intelligences (AGIs).

2. Is the encoder deterministic as in Sect. 3.1 (Schmidhuber 1991c), or does it predict probability distributions on possible events as in Sect. 3.3 (Storck et al. 1995)?
3. How are the encoder and its learning algorithm implemented?

(a) Is the encoder actually a continually changing, growing 3D model or simulation of the agent in the environment, used to predict future visual or tactile inputs, given agent actions (Sect. 2.2)?
(b) Is it a traditional machine learning model? A feedforward neural network mapping pairs of actions and observations to predictions of the next observation as in Sect. 3.2 (Schmidhuber 1991b)? A recurrent neural network that is in principle able to deal with event histories of arbitrary size as in Sect. 3.1 (Schmidhuber 1991c)? A Gaussian process? A support vector machine? A hidden Markov model? etc.

(2) Includes many subtypes characterized by the answers to the following questions:

1. Is the entire history used to evaluate the encoder's performance as in Sect. 2 (Schmidhuber 2006a, 2007c, 2009c,d) (in theory the correct thing to do, but sometimes impractical)? Or only recent data, for example, the one acquired at the present time step as in Sect. 3.2 (Schmidhuber 1991b) or in a limited time window of recent inputs? (If so, a performance decline on earlier parts of the history may go unnoticed.)
2. Which measure is used to indicate learning progress and create intrinsic reward?

(a) Mean squared prediction error or similar measures as in Sect. 3.1 (Barto et al. 2004; Klyubin et al. 2005; Schmidhuber 1991c; Singh et al. 2005)? This may fail whenever high prediction errors do not imply expected prediction progress, for example, in noisy environments, but also when the limitations of the predictor's learning algorithm prevent learning progress even in deterministic worlds.
(b) Improvements (first derivatives) of prediction error as in Sect. 3.2 (Oudeyer and Kaplan 2006; Schmidhuber 1991b)? This properly deals with both noisy/nondeterministic worlds and the computational limitations of the encoder.
(c) The information-theoretic Kullback–Leibler divergence (a.k.a. relative entropy) (Kullback 1959) between belief distributions before and after learning steps, as in Sect. 3.3 (Itti and Baldi 2005; Storck et al. 1995)? This makes sense under the assumption that all potential statistical dependencies between inputs can indeed be modeled by the given probabilistic model, which in previous implementations (Sect. 3.3) was limited to singular events (Itti and Baldi 2005; Storck et al. 1995) as opposed to arbitrary event sequences, for efficiency reasons.
(d) Minimum description length (MDL)-based measures (Rissanen 1978; Solomonoff 1964, 1978; Wallace and Boulton 1968; Wallace and Freeman 1987) comparing the number of bits required to encode the observation history before and after learning steps, as in Sect. 2 (Schmidhuber 2006a, 2007c, 2009c,d, 2010b)? Unlike the methods above, this approach automatically punishes unnecessarily complex encoders that overfit the data and can easily deal with long event sequences instead of simple one step events. For example, if the encoder uses a 3D world model or simulation, the MDL approach will ask (Sect. 2.2): how many bits are currently needed to specify all polygons in the simulation and how many bits are needed to encode deviations of the sensory history from the predictions of the 3D simulation? Adding or removing polygons may reduce the total number of bits (and decrease future prediction errors).

3. Is the computational effort of the encoder and its learning algorithm taken into account when measuring its performance, as in Sect. 2.2 (Schmidhuber 1997c, 2002a, 2006a)? The only implementation of this (Sect. 3.3; Schmidhuber 1997c, 2002a) still lacks theoretical optimality guarantees.
4. Which are the relative weights of external and intrinsic reward? This is of importance as long as the latter does not vanish in environments where after some time *nothing new* can be learned anymore.

(3) Includes many subtypes characterized by the answers to the following questions:

1. Which is the action repertoire of the creator?

   (a) Can it produce only external motor actions, as in Sect. 3.2 (Schmidhuber 1991b; Storck et al. 1995)?

(b) Can it also manipulate an internal mental state through internal actions as in Sect. 3.4 (Schmidhuber 1997c, 2002a), thus being able to deal not only with raw sensory inputs but also with internal abstractions thereof and to create/discover novel purely mathematical patterns, like certain theoreticians who sometimes do not care much about the external world?

(c) Can it trigger learning processes by itself, by executing appropriate actions as in Sect. 3.4 (Schmidhuber 1997c, 2002a)? This is important for learning when to learn and what to learn, trading off the costs of learning versus the expected benefits in terms of intrinsic and extrinsic rewards.

2. Which are the perceptive abilities of the creator?

   (a) Can it choose at any time to see any element of the entire history (Schmidhuber 2006a) of all sensory inputs, rewards, executed actions, and internal states? Or only a subset thereof, possibly a recent one, as in Sect. 3.2 (Schmidhuber 1991b)? The former should be the default for AGIs.

   (b) Does it have access to the parameters and internal state of the encoder, like in Sect. 3.4 (Schmidhuber 2002a)? Or just a subset thereof? Such introspective abilities are important to predict future intrinsic rewards which depend on the already existing knowledge encoded in the encoder.

3. Which optimizer of expected intrinsic and extrinsic reward is used?

   (a) A traditional Q-learner (Watkins and Dayan 1992) able to deal with delayed rewards as long as the environment is fully observable, like in Sect. 3.2? A more limited 1-step look-ahead learner (Oudeyer and Kaplan 2006) that will break down in presence of delayed intrinsic rewards? A more sophisticated RL algorithm for delayed rewards in partially observable environments (Kaelbling et al. 1996; Schmidhuber 1991d), like in Sect. 3.1? A hierarchical, subgoal-learning RL algorithm (Bakker and Schmidhuber 2004; Ring 1991, 1994; Schmidhuber and Wahnsiedler 1992; Wiering and Schmidhuber 1998a) or perhaps other hierarchical methods that do not learn to create subgoals by themselves (Barto et al. 2004; Dayan and Hinton 1993; Singh et al. 2005)?

   (b) An action planner using a 3D simulation of the world to generate reward-promising trajectories (see MDL example in Sect. 2.2)?

   (c) An evolutionary algorithm (Gomez et al. 2008; Holland 1975; Rechenberg 1971; Schwefel 1974) applied to recurrent neural networks (Gomez et al. 2008) or other devices that compute action sequences (Cuccu et al. 2011; Luciw et al. 2011; Schaul et al. 2011b)? Or a policy gradient method (Rückstieß et al. 2010; Sehnke et al. 2010; Sutton et al. 1999; Wierstra et al. 2008)?

   (d) One of the recent universal, mathematically optimal RL algorithms (Hutter 2005; Schmidhuber 2009e), like in Sect. 2.6? Variants of universal search (Levin 1973) or its incremental extension, the Optimal Ordered Problem Solver (Schmidhuber 2004)?

   (e) Something else? Obviously lots of alternative search methods can be plugged in here.

4. How does the system deal with problems of online learning?
   (a) Action sequences producing patterns that used to be novel do not get rewarded anymore once the patterns are known. Can the practical reward optimizer reliably deal with this problem of vanishing rewards, like the theoretically optimal systems of Sect. 2.6?
   (b) Can the reward optimizer actually use the continually improving predictive world model to improve or speed up the search for a better policy? This is automatically done by the above-mentioned action planner using a continually improving 3D world simulation and also by the RNN-based world model of the system in Sect. 3.1 (Schmidhuber 1991c). Does the changing model cause problems of online learning? Are those problems dealt with in a heuristic way (e.g., small learning rates) or in a theoretically sound way as in Sect. 2.6?

Each node or leaf of the typology above can be further expanded, thus becoming the root of additional straightforward refinements. But let us now address some of the recent confusion surrounding the concept of intrinsic motivation and clarify what it is *not*.

5.1 What IM Is Not

5.1.1 Secondary Reward as an Orthogonal Issue

Reward propagation procedures of traditional RL such as Q-learning (Watkins and Dayan 1992) or RL economies and bucket brigade systems (Holland 1985; Schmidhuber 1989a,b; Wilson 1994) may be viewed as translating *rare* external rewards for achieving some goal into *frequent* internal rewards for earlier actions setting the stage. Should one call these internal "secondary" rewards intrinsic rewards? Of course not. They are just internal by-products of the method used to maximize *external* reward, which remains the only measure of overall success.

5.1.2 Speeding Up RL as an Orthogonal Issue

Many methods have been proposed to speed up traditional RL. Some Q-learning accelerators simply update pairs of actions and states with currently quickly changing Q-values more frequently than others (that is, Q-values with high first derivatives are favored). Others postpone updates until needed (Wiering and Schmidhuber 1998b). Again one should resist the temptation to confuse such types of secondary reward modulation with intrinsic reward, because the only thing important to such methods is the *external* reward. [Otherwise one would also have to call intrinsic reward many of the things that could be invented by any (possibly universal; Hutter 2005; Schmidhuber 2009e) RL method whose only goal is to maximize expected *external* reward.]

5.1.3 Subgoal Learning as an Orthogonal Issue

Some goal-seeking RL systems search a space of possible subgoal combinations, internally rewarding subsystems whose policies learn to achieve those subgoals (Bakker and Schmidhuber 2004; Ring 1994; Schmidhuber and Wahnsiedler 1992; Wiering and Schmidhuber 1998a). External reward (for reaching a final goal) is used to measure the quality of subgoal combinations: good ones survive; others are discarded. Again the internal reward for the subsystems should not be called intrinsic reward, as it is totally driven and justified by *external* reward.

5.1.4 Evolution of Reward Functions as an Orthogonal Issue

Essentially the same argument holds for methods that search a space of reward functions until they find one that helps a given RL method to achieve more reward more quickly, for example (Littman and Ackley 1991; Singh et al. 2009) [in many ways such methods are like the subgoal evolvers (Wiering and Schmidhuber 1998a) mentioned above]. One should not call this intrinsic reward, since once more the only thing that counts here is the *external* reward; the rest is just implementation details of the external reward maximizer.

But did not humans evolve to have this intrinsic reward component? Sure, they did, but now it is there, and now it is independent of external reward, otherwise it would not be intrinsic reward, by definition. Scientific papers on intrinsic reward should start from there. It is a different issue to analyze how and why evolution or another search process *invented* intrinsic rewards to facilitate satisfaction of *external* goals (such as survival).

6 How the Theory Explains Art, Science, and Humor

How does the encoding progress drive explain *humor*? Consider the following statement by comedian Bob Monkhouse:

> People laughed when I said I'd become a comedian. Well, they're not laughing now.

Some subjective observers who read this for the first time think it is funny. Why? As the eyes are sequentially scanning the text the brain receives a complex visual input stream. The latter is subjectively partially compressible as it relates to the observer's previous knowledge about letters and words. That is, given the reader's current knowledge and current encoder, the raw data can be encoded by fewer bits than required to store random data of the same size. But the punch line is unexpected for those who did not know it. Initially this failed expectation results in suboptimal data compression—storage of expected events does not cost anything, but deviations from predictions require extra bits to encode them. The encoder, however, does not stay the same forever: within a short time interval, its learning algorithm improves its performance on the data seen so far, by discovering the nonrandom, nonarbitrary, and therefore compressible pattern relating the punch line to previous text and previous knowledge about comedians. This saves a few bits of storage. The number of saved bits (or a similar measure of learning progress) becomes the observer's intrinsic reward, possibly strong enough to motivate him to read on in search for more reward through additional yet unknown patterns.

While most previous attempts at explaining humor (e.g., Raskin 1985) also focus on the element of surprise, they lack the essential concept of *novel pattern detection* measured by compression *progress* due to learning. This progress is zero whenever the unexpected is just random white noise, and thus no fun at all. Applications of the new theory of humor can be found in recent videos (Schmidhuber 2009b).

How does the theory informally explain the motivation to create or perceive *art and music* (Schmidhuber 1997a,b, 2006a, 2007c, 2009a,c,d, 2012)? For example, why are some melodies more interesting or aesthetically rewarding than others? Not the one the listener (composer) just heard (played) twenty times in a row. It became too subjectively predictable in the process. Nor the weird one with completely unfamiliar rhythm and tonality. It seems too irregular and contain too much arbitrariness and subjective noise. The observer (creator) of the data is interested in melodies that are unfamiliar enough to contain somewhat unexpected harmonies or beats, etc., but familiar enough to allow for quickly recognizing the presence of a new learnable regularity or compressibility in the sound stream: a novel pattern! Sure, it will get boring over time, but not yet. All of this perfectly fits the principle: The current encoder of the observer or data creator tries to compress his history of acoustic and other inputs where possible. The action selector tries to find history-influencing actions such that the continually growing historic data allows for improving the encoder's performance. The interesting or aesthetically rewarding musical and other subsequences are precisely those with previously unknown yet learnable types of regularities, because they lead to encoder improvements. The boring patterns are those that are either already perfectly known or arbitrary or random or whose structure seems too hard to understand.

Similar statements hold not only for other dynamic art including film and dance (take into account the compressibility of action sequences) but also for "static" art such as painting and sculpture, created through action sequences of the artist and perceived as dynamic spatiotemporal patterns through active attention shifts of the observer. When not occupied with optimizing *external* reward, artists and observers of art are just following their encoding progress drive!

The previous computer programs discussed in Sect. 3 already incorporated (approximations of) the basic creativity principle. But do they really deserve to be viewed as rudimentary artists and scientists? The patterns they create are novel with respect to their own limited encoders and prior knowledge, but not necessarily relative to the knowledge of sophisticated adults. The main difference to human artists/scientists, however, may be only quantitative by nature, not qualitative. Current computational limitations of artificial artists do not prevent us from already using the basic principle in human–computer interaction to create art appreciable by humans—see example applications in references (Schmidhuber 1997b, 2006a, 2007c, 2009a,c,d, 2012).

How does the theory explain the nature of *inductive sciences such as physics*? If the history of the entire universe were computable and there is no evidence against this possibility (Schmidhuber 2006d), then its simplest explanation would be the shortest program that computes it. Unfortunately there is no general way of finding the shortest program computing any given data (Li and Vitányi 1997). Therefore, physicists have traditionally proceeded incrementally, analyzing just a small aspect of the world at any given time, trying to find simple laws that allow for describing their limited observations better than the best previously known law, essentially trying to find a program that encode the observed data better than the best previously known program. An unusually large encoding breakthrough deserves the name *discovery*. For example, Newton's law of gravity can be formulated as a short piece of code which allows for substantially compressing many observation sequences involving falling apples and other objects. Although its predictive power is limited—for example, it does not explain quantum fluctuations of apple atoms—it still allows for greatly reducing the number of bits required to encode the data stream, by assigning short codes to events that are predictable with high probability (Huffman 1952) under the assumption that the law holds. Einstein's general relativity theory yields additional compression progress as it compactly explains many previously unexplained deviations from Newton's predictions. Most physicists believe there is still room for further advances, and this is what is driving them to invent new experiments unveiling novel, previously unpublished patterns (Schmidhuber 2009a,c,d, 2012). When not occupied with optimizing *external* reward, physicists are also just following their encoding progress drive! All of this is compatible with Kuhn's vision of scientific revolutions (Kuhn 1962): plateaus in the evolution of a given scientific field may correspond to yet uncompressed observations that call for a new predictor or paradigm.

7 Concluding Remarks and Outlook

It was pointed out that systems described in the first publications on artificial curiosity and creativity (Schmidhuber 1991b,c, 2002a; Storck et al. 1995) (Sect. 3) already can be viewed as examples of implementations of a subjective data encoding progress drive that encourages the discovery or creation of novel and surprising patterns, resulting in artificial scientists or artists with various types of computational limitations, as discussed in the typology of Sect. 5. To improve previous implementations of the basic ingredients of the creativity framework and to build a continually growing, mostly unsupervised AGI, one should evaluate additional combinations of novel, advanced RL algorithms and adaptive compressors and test them on humanoid robots such as the iCub. In particular:

1. One should study better practical adaptive data encoders, such as the recent, novel artificial recurrent neural networks (RNN) (Hochreiter and Schmidhuber 1997; Schmidhuber et al. 2011) and other general yet practically feasible methods for making predictions.

2. One should reimplement the intrinsically motivated system of Sect. 3.4 (Schmidhuber 2002a) (which can learn when to learn and what to learn) with more recent, alternative, more powerful reward optimizers, such as variants of the Optimal Ordered Problem Solver (Schmidhuber 2004).
3. One should investigate under which conditions learning progress measures can be computed both accurately and efficiently, without frequent expensive compressor performance evaluations on the entire history so far.
4. Recently there has been substantial progress for a class of RL algorithms that are not quite as general as the universal ones (Hutter 2005; Schmidhuber 2002c, 2009e), but nevertheless capable of learning very general, program-like behavior in partially observable environments. One should study the applicability of recent improved RL techniques in the fields of artificial evolution (Gomez et al. 2008), policy gradients (Rückstieß et al. 2010; Sehnke et al. 2010; Sutton et al. 1999; Wierstra et al. 2008, and others).

Acknowledgements Thanks to Benjamin Kuipers, Herbert W. Franke, Marcus Hutter, Andy Barto, Jonathan Lansey, Michael Littman, Julian Togelius, Faustino J. Gomez, Giovanni Pezzulo, Gianluca Baldassarre, Martin Butz, Moshe Looks, Mark Ring, and several anonymous reviewers for useful comments that helped to improve this chapter or earlier papers on this subject. This research has received funds from the European Commission 7th Framework Programme (FP7/2007–2013), "Challenge 2: Cognitive Systems, Interaction, Robotics," Grant Agreement No. ICT-IP-231722, Project "IM-CLeVeR: Intrinsically Motivated Cumulative Learning Versatile Robots."

References

Bakker, B., Schmidhuber, J.: Hierarchical reinforcement learning based on subgoal discovery and subpolicy specialization. In: Groen, F., Amato, N., Bonarini, A., Yoshida, E., and Kröse, B. (eds.) Proceedings of the 8th Conference on Intelligent Autonomous Systems IAS-8, pp. 438–445. IOS Press, Amsterdam (2004)

Balcan, M., .Beygelzimer, A., Langford, J.: Agnostic active learning. J. Comput. Syst. Sci. **75**(1), 78–89 (2009)

Barto, A.G., Singh, S., Chentanez, N.: Intrinsically motivated learning of hierarchical collections of skills. In: Proceedings of International Conference on Developmental Learning (ICDL). MIT, Cambridge (2004)

Bense, M.: Einführung in die informationstheoretische Ästhetik. Grundlegung und Anwendung in der Texttheorie (Introduction to Information-Theoretical Aesthetics. Foundation and Application to Text Theory). Rowohlt Taschenbuch Verlag (1969)

Berlyne, D.E.: Novelty and curiosity as determinants of exploratory behavior. Br. J. Psychol. **41**, 68–80 (1950)

Berlyne, D.E.: Conflict, Arousal, and Curiosity. McGraw Hill, New York (1960)

Birkhoff, G.D.: Aesthetic Measure. Harvard University Press, Cambridge (1933)

Blank, D., Meeden, L.: Introduction to the special issue on developmental robotics. Connect. Sci. **18**(2) (2006)

Brafman, R.I., Tennenholtz, M.: R-MAX—a general polynomial time algorithm for near-optimal reinforcement learning. J. Mach. Learn. Res. **3**, 213–231 (2002)

Cohn, D.A.: Neural network exploration using optimal experiment design. In: Cowan, J., Tesauro, G., Alspector, J. (eds.) Advances in Neural Information Processing Systems 6, pp. 679–686. Morgan Kaufmann, San Francisco (1994)

Collingwood, R.G.: The Principles of Art. Oxford University Press, London (1938)

Cuccu, G., Luciw, M., Schmidhuber, J., Gomez, F.: Intrinsically motivated evolutionary search for vision-based reinforcement learning. In: Proceedings of the 2011 IEEE Conference on Development and Learning and Epigenetic Robotics IEEE-ICDL-EPIROB. IEEE (2011)

Dayan, P., Hinton, G.: Feudal reinforcement learning. In: Lippman, D.S., Moody, J.E., Touretzky, D.S. (eds.) Advances in Neural Information Processing Systems 5, pp. 271–278. Morgan Kaufmann, San Francisco (1993)

Fedorov, V.V.: Theory of Optimal Experiments. Academic, New York (1972)

Frank, H.G.: Kybernetische Analysen subjektiver Sachverhalte. Verlag Schnelle, Quickborn (1964)

Frank, H.G., Franke, H.W.: Ästhetische Information. Estetika informacio. Eine Einführung in die kybernetische Ästhetik. Kopäd Verlag (2002)

Franke, H.W.: Kybernetische Ästhetik. Phänomen Kunst, 3rd edn. Ernst Reinhardt Verlag, Munich (1979)

Friston, K.J., Daunizeau, J., Kilner, J., Kiebel, S.J.: Action and behavior: A free-energy formulation. Biol. Cybern. **102**(3), 227–260 (2010)

Gold, K., Scassellati, B.: Learning acceptable windows of contingency. Connect. Sci. **18**(2) (2006)

Gomez, F.J., Schmidhuber, J., Miikkulainen, R.: Efficient non-linear control through neuroevolution. J. Mach. Learn. Res. **9**, 937–965 (2008)

Goodman, N.: Languages of Art: An Approach to a Theory of Symbols. The Bobbs-Merrill Company, Indianapolis (1968)

Graves, A., Liwicki, M., Fernandez, S., Bertolami, R., Bunke, H., Schmidhuber, J.: A novel connectionist system for improved unconstrained handwriting recognition. IEEE Trans. Pattern Anal. Mach. Intell. **31**(5) (2009)

Harlow, H.F., Harlow, M.K., Meyer, D.R.: Novelty and curiosity as determinants of exploratory behavior. J. Exp. Psychol. **41**, 68–80 (1950)

Hart, S.: The Development of Hierarchical Knowledge in Robot Systems. Ph.D. Thesis, Department of Computer Science, University of Massachusetts Amherst (2009)

Hart, S., Sen, S., Grupen, R.: Intrinsically motivated hierarchical manipulation. In: Proceedings of the 2008 IEEE Conference on Robots and Automation (ICRA), Pasadena (2008)

Hochreiter, S., Schmidhuber, J.: Long short-term memory. Neural Comput. **9**(8), 1735–1780 (1997)

Holland, J.H.: Adaptation in Natural and Artificial Systems. University of Michigan Press, Ann Arbor (1975)

Holland, J.H.: Properties of the bucket brigade. In: Proceedings of an International Conference on Genetic Algorithms. Lawrence Erlbaum, Hillsdale (1985)

Huffman, D.A.: A method for construction of minimum-redundancy codes. Proc. IRE **40**, 1098–1101 (1952)

Hutter, M.: Universal Artificial Intelligence: Sequential Decisions based on Algorithmic Probability. Springer, Berlin (2005). (On J. Schmidhuber's SNF grant 20-61847)

Hwang, J., Choi, J., Oh, S., II, R.J.M.: Query-based learning applied to partially trained multilayer perceptrons. IEEE Trans. Neural Netw. **2**(1), 131–136 (1991)

Itti, L., Baldi, P.F.: Bayesian surprise attracts human attention. In: Advances in Neural Information Processing Systems 19, pp. 547–554. MIT, Cambridge (2005)

Kaelbling, L.P., Littman, M.L., Moore, A.W.: Reinforcement learning: A survey. J. AI Res. **4**, 237–285 (1996)

Kant, I.: Critik der reinen Vernunft (1781)

Klyubin, A.S., Polani, D., Nehaniv, C.L.: Empowerment: A universal agent-centric measure of control. In: Congress on Evolutionary Ccomputation (CEC-05), IEEE (2005)

Kolmogorov, A.N.: Three approaches to the quantitative definition of information. Prob. Inform. Transm. **1**, 1–11 (1965)

Kuhn, T.: The Structure of Scientific Revolutions. University of Chicago Press, Chicago (1962)

Kuipers, B., Beeson, P., Modayil, J., Provost, J.: Bootstrap learning of foundational representations. Connect. Sci. **18**(2) (2006)

Kullback, S.: Statistics and Information Theory. Wiley, New York (1959)

Lenat, D.B.: Theory formation by heuristic search. Mach. Learn. **21** (1983)

Levin, L.A.: Universal sequential search problems. Prob. Inform. Transm. **9**(3), 265–266 (1973)

Li, L., Littman, M.L., Walsh, T.J.: Knows what it knows: A framework for self-aware learning. In: Proceedings of the Twenty-Fifth International Conference on Machine Learning (ICML-08) (2008)

Li, M., Vitányi, P.M.B.: An Introduction to Kolmogorov Complexity and Its Applications, 2nd edn. Springer, Berlin (1997)

Littman, M.L., Ackley, D.H.: Adaptation in constant utility non-stationary environments. In: Belew, R.K., Booker, L. (eds.) Proceedings of the Fourth International Conference on Genetic Algorithms, pp. 136–142. Morgan Kaufmann, San Mateo (1991)

Luciw, M., Graziano, V., Ring, M., Schmidhuber, J.: Artificial curiosity with planning for autonomous perceptual and cognitive development. In: Proceedings of the First Joint Conference on Development Learning and on Epigenetic Robotics ICDL-EPIROB, Frankfurt (2011)

MacKay, D.J.C.: Information-based objective functions for active data selection. Neural Comput. **4**(2), 550–604 (1992)

Moles, A.: Information Theory and Esthetic Perception. University of Illinois Press, Illinois (1968)

Nake, F.: Ästhetik als Informationsverarbeitung. Springer, Berlin (1974)

Ngo, H., Ring, M., Schmidhuber, J.: Compression progress-based curiosity drive for developmental learning. In: Proceedings of the 2011 IEEE Conference on Development and Learning and Epigenetic Robotics IEEE-ICDL-EPIROB. IEEE (2011)

Olsson, L., Nehaniv, C.L., Polani, D.: From unknown sensors and actuators to actions grounded in sensorimotor perceptions. Connect. Sci. **18**(2) (2006)

Oudeyer, P.-Y., Kaplan, F.: What is intrinsic motivation? a typology of computational approaches. Front. Neurorobot. **1** (2006)

Oudeyer, P.-Y., Kaplan, F., Hafner, V.F.: Intrinsic motivation systems for autonomous mental development. IEEE Trans. Evol. Comput. **11**(2), 265–286 (2007)

Piaget, J.: The Child's Construction of Reality. Routledge and Kegan Paul, London (1955)

Plutowski, M., Cottrell, G., White, H.: Learning Mackey-Glass from 25 examples, plus or minus 2. In: Cowan, J., Tesauro, G., Alspector, J. (eds.) Advances in Neural Information Processing Systems, vol. 6, pp. 1135–1142. Morgan Kaufmann, San Francisco (1994)

Poland, J., Hutter, M.: Strong asymptotic assertions for discrete MDL in regression and classification. In: Annual Machine Learning Conference of Belgium and the Netherlands (Benelearn-2005), Enschede (2005)

Popper, K.R.: All Life Is Problem Solving. Routledge, London (1999)

Provost, J., Kuipers, B.J., Miikkulainen, R.: Developing navigation behavior through self-organizing distinctive state abstraction. Connect. Sci. **18**(2) (2006)

Raskin, V.: Semantic Mechanisms of Humor. Dordrecht/Boston/Lancaster (1985)

Rechenberg, I.: Evolutionsstrategie - Optimierung technischer Systeme nach Prinzipien der biologischen Evolution. Dissertation. Published 1973 by Fromman-Holzboog (1971)

Ring, M.B.: Incremental development of complex behaviors through automatic construction of sensory-motor hierarchies. In: Birnbaum, L., Collins, G. (eds.) Machine Learning: Proceedings of the Eighth International Workshop, pp. 343–347. Morgan Kaufmann, San Francisco (1991)

Ring, M.B.: Continual Learning in Reinforcement Environments. Ph.D. Thesis, University of Texas at Austin, Austin (1994)

Rissanen, J.: Modeling by shortest data description. Automatica **14**, 465–471 (1978)

Rückstieß, T., Sehnke, F., Schaul, T., Wierstra, D., Yi, S., Schmidhuber, J.: Exploring parameter space in reinforcement learning. Paladyn J. Behav. Robot. **1**(1), 14–24 (2010)

Schaul, T., Pape, L., Glasmachers, T., Graziano, V., Schmidhuber, J.: Coherence Progress: A Measure of Interestingness Based on Fixed Compressors. In: Fourth Conference on Artificial General Intelligence (AGI) (2011a)

Schaul, T., Sun, Y., Wierstra, D., Gomez, F., Schmidhuber, J.: Curiosity-Driven Optimization. In: IEEE Congress on Evolutionary Computation (CEC), New Orleans (2011b)

Schembri, M., Mirolli, M., Baldassarre, G.: Evolving internal reinforcers for an intrinsically motivated reinforcement-learning robot. In: Demiris, Y., Scassellati, B., Mareschal, D. (eds.) The 6th IEEE International Conference on Development and Learning (ICDL2007), pp. 282–287. Imperial College, London. IEEE Catalog Number: 07EX1740C, Library of Congress: 2007922394 (2007)

Schlesinger, M.: Decomposing infants' object representations: A dual-route processing account. Connect. Sci. **18**(2) (2006)

Schmidhuber, J.: A local learning algorithm for dynamic feedforward and recurrent networks. Connect. Sci. **1**(4), 403–412 (1989a)

Schmidhuber, J.: The neural bucket brigade. In: Pfeifer, R., Schreter, Z., Fogelman, Z., Steels, L. (eds.) Connectionism in Perspective, pp. 439–446. Elsevier, North-Holland, Amsterdam (1989b)

Schmidhuber, J.: Dynamische neuronale Netze und das fundamentale raumzeitliche Lernproblem. Dissertation, Institut für Informatik, Technische Universität München (1990a)

Schmidhuber, J.: An on-line algorithm for dynamic reinforcement learning and planning in reactive environments. In: Proceedings of the IEEE/INNS International Joint Conference on Neural Networks, San Diego, vol. 2, pp. 253–258 (1990b)

Schmidhuber, J.: Adaptive curiosity and adaptive confidence. Technical Report FKI-149-91, Institut für Informatik, Technische Universität München. See also Schmidhuber (1991b) (1991a)

Schmidhuber, J.: Curious model-building control systems. In: Proceedings of the International Joint Conference on Neural Networks, Singapore, vol. 2, pp. 1458–1463. IEEE (1991b)

Schmidhuber, J.: A possibility for implementing curiosity and boredom in model-building neural controllers. In: Meyer, J.A., Wilson, S.W. (eds.) Proceedings of the of the International Conference on Simulation of Adaptive Behavior: From Animals to Animats, pp. 222–227. MIT/Bradford Books (1991c)

Schmidhuber, J.: Reinforcement learning in Markovian and non-Markovian environments. In: Lippman, D.S., Moody, J.E., Touretzky, D.S. (eds.) Advances in Neural Information Processing Systems 3 (NIPS 3), pp. 500–506. Morgan Kaufmann, San Francisco (1991d)

Schmidhuber, J.: Learning complex, extended sequences using the principle of history compression. Neural Comput. **4**(2), 234–242 (1992)

Schmidhuber, J.: Femmes fractales. Report IDSIA-99-97, IDSIA, Switzerland, (1997)

Schmidhuber, J.: Low-complexity art. Leonardo, J. Int. Soc. Arts Sci. Technol. **30**(2), 97–103 (1997b)

Schmidhuber, J.: What's interesting? Technical Report IDSIA-35-97, IDSIA (1997c). ftp://ftp.idsia.ch/pub/juergen/interest.ps.gz; extended abstract in Proc. Snowbird'98, Utah, 1998; see also Schmidhuber (2002a)

Schmidhuber, J.: Exploring the predictable. In: Ghosh, A., Tsuitsui, S. (eds.) Advances in Evolutionary Computing, pp. 579–612. Springer, Berlin (2002a)

Schmidhuber, J.: Hierarchies of generalized Kolmogorov complexities and nonenumerable universal measures computable in the limit. Int. J. Found. Comput. Sci. **13**(4), 587–612 (2002b)

Schmidhuber, J.: The Speed Prior: a new simplicity measure yielding near-optimal computable predictions. In: Kivinen, J., Sloan, R.H. (eds.) Proceedings of the 15th Annual Conference on Computational Learning Theory (COLT 2002), Lecture Notes in Artificial Intelligence, pp. 216–228. Springer, Sydney (2002c)

Schmidhuber, J.: Optimal ordered problem solver. Mach. Learn. **54**, 211–254 (2004)

Schmidhuber, J.: Completely self-referential optimal reinforcement learners. In: Duch, W., Kacprzyk, J., Oja, E., Zadrozny, S. (eds.) Artificial Neural Networks: Biological Inspirations - ICANN 2005, LNCS 3697, pp. 223–233. Springer (2005a). Plenary talk

Schmidhuber, J.: Gödel machines: Towards a technical justification of consciousness. In: Kudenko, D., Kazakov, D., Alonso, E. (eds.) Adaptive Agents and Multi-Agent Systems III (LNCS 3394), pp. 1–23. Springer, Berlin (2005b)

Schmidhuber, J.: Developmental robotics, optimal artificial curiosity, creativity, music, and the fine arts. Connect. Sci. **18**(2), 173–187 (2006a)

Schmidhuber, J.: Gödel machines: Fully self-referential optimal universal self-improvers. In: Goertzel, B., Pennachin, C. (eds.) Artificial General Intelligence, pp. 199–226. Springer, Berlin (2006b). Variant available as arXiv:cs.LO/0309048

Schmidhuber, J.: The new AI: General & sound & relevant for physics. In: Goertzel, B., Pennachin, C. (eds.) Artificial General Intelligence, pp. 175–198. Springer, Berlin (2006c). Also available as TR IDSIA-04-03, arXiv:cs.AI/0302012

Schmidhuber, J.: Randomness in physics. Nature **439**(3), 392 (2006d). Correspondence

Schmidhuber, J.: 2006: Celebrating 75 years of AI - history and outlook: The next 25 years. In: Lungarella, M., Iida, F., Bongard, J., Pfeifer, R. (eds.) 50 Years of Artificial Intelligence, LNAI, vol. 4850, pp. 29–41. Springer, Berlin (2007a). Preprint available as arXiv:0708.4311

Schmidhuber, J.: New millennium AI and the convergence of history. In: Duch, W., Mandziuk, J. (eds.) Challenges to Computational Intelligence, vol. 63, pp. 15–36. Studies in Computational Intelligence, Springer, Berlin (2007b). Also available as arXiv:cs.AI/0606081

Schmidhuber, J.: Simple algorithmic principles of discovery, subjective beauty, selective attention, curiosity & creativity. In: Proceedings of the 10th International Conf. on Discovery Science (DS 2007), LNAI, vol. 4755, pp. 26–38. Springer, Berlin. Joint invited lecture for ALT 2007 and DS 2007, Sendai, Japan, 2007 (2007c)

Schmidhuber, J.: Driven by compression progress. In: Lovrek, I., Howlett, R.J., Jain, L.C. (eds.) Knowledge-Based Intelligent Information and Engineering Systems KES-2008, Lecture Notes in Computer Science, vol. 5177, Part I, p. 11. Springer, Berlin. Abstract of invited keynote (2008)

Schmidhuber, J.: Art & science as by-products of the search for novel patterns, or data compressible in unknown yet learnable ways. In: Botta, M. (ed.) Multiple ways to design research. Research cases that reshape the design discipline, Swiss Design Network - Et al. Edizioni, pp. 98–112. Springer, Berelin (2009a)

Schmidhuber, J.: Compression progress: The algorithmic principle behind curiosity and creativity (with applications of the theory of humor). 40 min video of invited talk at Singularity Summit 2009, New York City (2009b). http://www.vimeo.com/7441291. 10 min excerpts: http://www.youtube.com/watch?v=Ipomu0MLFaI.

Schmidhuber, J.: Driven by compression progress: A simple principle explains essential aspects of subjective beauty, novelty, surprise, interestingness, attention, curiosity, creativity, art, science, music, jokes. In: Pezzulo, G., Butz, M.V., Sigaud, O., Baldassarre, G. (eds.) Anticipatory Behavior in Adaptive Learning Systems. From Psychological Theories to Artificial Cognitive Systems, LNCS, vol. 5499, pp. 48–76. Springer, Berlin (2009c)

Schmidhuber, J.: Simple algorithmic theory of subjective beauty, novelty, surprise, interestingness, attention, curiosity, creativity, art, science, music, jokes. J. Soc. Instrum. Control Eng. **48**(1), 21–32 (2009d)

Schmidhuber, J.: Ultimate cognition à la Gödel. Cogn. Comput. **1**(2), 177–193 (2009e)

Schmidhuber, J.: Artificial scientists & artists based on the formal theory of creativity. In: Eric, B., Marcus, H., Emanuel, K. (eds.) Artificial General Intelligence. Springer, Berlin (2010a)

Schmidhuber, J.: Formal theory of creativity, fun, and intrinsic motivation (1990–2010): IEEE Trans. Auton. Mental Dev. **2**(3), 230–247 (2010b)

Schmidhuber, J.: A formal theory of creativity to model the creation of art. In: McCormack, J., d'Inverno, M. (eds.) Computational Creativity. MIT, Cambridge (2012)

Schmidhuber, J., Gomez, F., Graves, A.: Sequence Learning with Artificial Recurrent Neural Networks. Cambridge University Press, Cambridge (2012) (in preparation)

Schmidhuber, J., Heil, S.: Sequential neural text compression. IEEE Trans. Neural Netw. **7**(1), 142–146 (1996)

Schmidhuber, J., Wahnsiedler, R.: Planning simple trajectories using neural subgoal generators. In: Meyer, J.A., Roitblat, H.L., Wilson, S.W. (eds.) Proc. of the 2nd International Conference on Simulation of Adaptive Behavior, pp. 196–202. MIT, Cambridge (1992)

Schmidhuber, J., Zhao, J., Wiering, M.: Shifting inductive bias with success-story algorithm, adaptive Levin search, and incremental self-improvement. Mach. Learn. **28**, 105–130 (1997)

Schwefel, H.P.: Numerische Optimierung von Computer-Modellen. Dissertation. Published 1977 by Birkhäuser, Basel (1974)

Sehnke, F., Osendorfer, C., Rückstieß, T., Graves, A., Peters, J., Schmidhuber, J.: Parameter-exploring policy gradients. Neural Netw. **23**(4), 551–559 (2010)

Seung, H.S., Opper, M., Sompolinsky, H.: Query by committee. In: COLT '92: Proceedings of the Fifth Annual Workshop on Computational Learning Theory, pp. 287–294. ACM, New York (1992)

Shannon, C.E.: A mathematical theory of communication (parts I and II): Bell Syst. Techn. J. **XXVII**, 379–423 (1948)

Singh, S., Barto, A.G., Chentanez, N.: Intrinsically motivated reinforcement learning. In: Advances in Neural Information Processing Systems 17 (NIPS). MIT, Cambridge (2005)

Singh, S., Lewis, R.L., Barto, A.G.: Where do rewards come from? In: Taatgen, N., van Rijn, H. (eds.) Proceedings of the 31st Annual Conference of the Cognitive Science Society. Austin (2009)

Solomonoff, R.J.: A formal theory of inductive inference. Part I. Inform. Control **7**, 1–22 (1964)

Solomonoff, R.J.: Complexity-based induction systems. IEEE Trans. Inform. Theory **IT-24**(5), 422–432 (1978)

Storck, J., Hochreiter, S., Schmidhuber, J.: Reinforcement driven information acquisition in non-deterministic environments. In: Proceedings of the International Conference on Artificial Neural Networks, Paris, vol. 2, pp. 159–164. EC2 & Cie (1995)

Strehl, A., Langford, J., Kakade, S.: Learning from logged implicit exploration data. Technical Report arXiv:1003.0120 (2010)

Stronger, D., Stone, P.: Towards autonomous sensor and actuator model induction on a mobile robot. Connect. Sci. **18**(2) (2006)

Sutton, R., Barto, A.: Reinforcement Learning: An Introduction. MIT, Cambridge (1998)

Sutton, R.S., McAllester, D.A., Singh, S.P., Mansour, Y.: Policy gradient methods for reinforcement learning with function approximation. ü In: Solla, S.A., Leen, T.K., Müller, K.-R. (eds.) Advances in Neural Information Processing Systems 12 [NIPS Conference, Denver, Colorado, USA, November 29 – December 4(1999)], pp. 1057–1063. MIT, Cambridge (1999)

Wallace, C.S., Boulton, D.M.: An information theoretic measure for classification. Comput. J. **11**(2), 185–194 (1968)

Wallace, C.S., Freeman, P.R.: Estimation and inference by compact coding. J. R. Stat. Soc. B **49**(3), 240–265 (1987)

Watkins, C., Dayan, P.: Q-learning. Mach. Learn. **8**(3/4), 279–292 (1992)

Wiering, M., Schmidhuber, J.: HQ-learning. Adap. Behav. **6**(2), 219–246 (1998a)

Wiering, M.A., Schmidhuber, J.: Fast online Q(λ): Mach. Learn. **33**(1), 105–116 (1998b)

Wierstra, D., Schaul, T., Peters, J., Schmidhuber, J.: Fitness expectation maximization. In: Proceedings of Parallel Problem Solving from Nature (PPSN 2008) (2008)

Wilson, S.: ZCS: A zeroth level classifier system. Evol. Comput. **2**, 1–18 (1994)

Wundt, W.M.: Grundzüge der Phvsiologischen Psychologie. Engelmann, Leipzig (1874)

The Role of the Basal Ganglia in Discovering Novel Actions

Peter Redgrave, Kevin Gurney, Tom Stafford, Martin Thirkcttlc, and Jen Lewis

Abstract Our interest is in the neural circuitry which supports the discovery and encoding of novel actions. We discuss the significant existing literature which identifies the basal ganglia, a complex of subcortical nuclei, as important in both the selection of actions and in reinforcement learning. We discuss the complementarity of these problems of action selection and action learning. Two basic mechanisms of biasing action selection are identified: (a) adjusting the relative strengths of competing inputs and (b) adjusting the relative sensitivity of the receiver of reinforced inputs. We discuss the particular importance of the phasic dopamine signal in the basal ganglia and its proposed role in conveying a reward prediction error. Temporal constraints of this signal limit the information it can convey to immediately surprising sensory events, thus—we argue—making it inappropriate to convey information regarding the economic value of actions (as proposed by the reward prediction error hypothesis). Rather, we suggest this signal is ideal to support the identification of novel actions and their encoding via the biasing of future action selection.

1 Introduction

This chapter will consider the brain mechanisms that support the discovery of novel actions. Action acquisition is viewed as a fundamental competence on which much of the intrinsically motivated cumulative learning by robots will rest. Given that most animals are born without detailed instructions of how to behave in any given circumstance, yet in comparatively short times develop numerous actions

P. Redgrave (✉) · K. Gurney · T. Stafford · M. Thirkettle · J. Lewis
Adaptive Behaviour Research Group, Department of Psychology, University of Sheffield, Sheffield, UK
e-mail: p.redgrave@sheffield.ac.uk; k.gurney@sheffield.ac.uk; t.stafford@sheffield.ac.uk; m.thirkettle@sheffield.ac.uk; j.m.lewis@sheffield.ac.uk

G. Baldassarre and M. Mirolli (eds.), *Intrinsically Motivated Learning in Natural and Artificial Systems*, DOI 10.1007/978-3-642-32375-1_6,

and patterns of adaptive behaviour, our approach is to learn as much as we can from action development in biological systems. In the contemporary neuroscience literature, a recurring theme is that one of the brain's fundamental processing units, the basal ganglia, is associated with action selection (Grillner et al. 2005; Hikosaka 2007; Humphries et al. 2006; Mink 1996; Prescott et al. 2006; Redgrave 2007; Redgrave et al. 1999b) and reinforcement learning (Berridge 2007; Houk 2005; Salamone and Correa 2002; Schultz 1998, 2006; Wickens 1993; Wickens et al. 2003; Wise 2004). It appears likely that it is within the circuits of the basal ganglia and associated structures that behavioural output is related to outcome. This document will therefore (a) identify selection as a fundamental problem faced by all multifunctional agents, (b) indicate how the architecture of the basal ganglia can provide a generic solution to a variety of selection problems, (c) discuss how the selection architecture of the basal ganglia can be influenced by reinforcement learning and (d) identify phasic dopamine signalling as the reinforcement signal. We will conclude by showing how basal ganglia circuitry could provide a substrate for the learning of novel actions and thus can provide an inspiration for those hoping to design mechanisms of action-outcome learning in autonomous agents.

2 Selection: A Fundamental Problem

Despite numerous suggestions implicating the basal ganglia in a wide range of functions including perception, learning, memory, attention, many aspects of motor function and even analgesia and seizure suppression, accumulating evidence points to them having a fundamental role in basic selection processes (Grillner et al. 2005; Hikosaka 2007; Humphries et al. 2006; Mink 1996; Prescott et al. 2006; Redgrave 2007; Redgrave et al. 1999b). Basic selection problems are common to all multifunctional systems and have been discussed in detail elsewhere (Prescott et al. 1999; Redgrave et al. 1999a). Briefly, one of the basic problems that must be solved is to resolve which functional system, at any point in time, should be permitted to direct "the final common motor path", i.e. determine behavioural output. The macro-architecture of the basal ganglia (Fig. 1a) may be seen as providing a potential solution to this selection problem (Redgrave et al. 1999b). The critical components involved in selection are the parallel-looped components that originate from and return to diverse cortically and subcortically based functional systems (Alexander et al. 1986; McHaffie et al. 2005). Afferent projections to the basal ganglia convey excitatory signals which, according to the "selection" view, are seen as competing bids or options for behavioural output. In a computational model of the basal ganglia and related circuitry (Gurney et al. 2001a,b; Humphries et al. 2006), intrinsic processing, which is responsive to the comparative magnitudes or "saliences" of competing inputs, generates patterns of output in which the external structure(s)/representation(s) providing the most "salient" input(s) is selectively disinhibited (Chevalier and Deniau 1990). In the absence of any consideration of biological systems, a conceptually similar control architecture was developed to

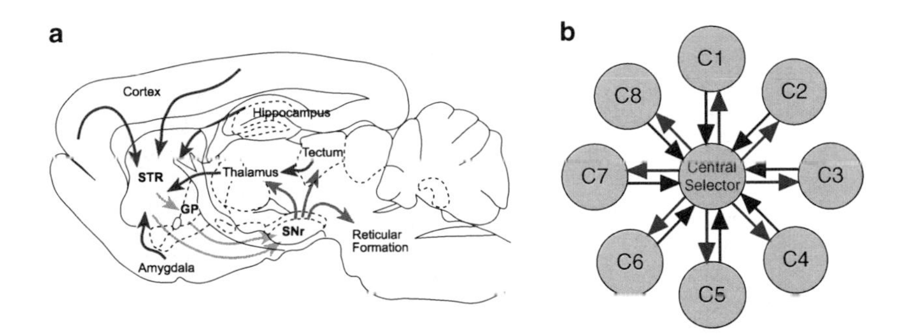

Fig. 1 Biological and artificial selection architectures. (**a**) Principle input and output connections of the mammalian basal ganglia. Phasic excitatory inputs (*red arrows*) are directed to the striatum (STR) from subcortical structures via the thalamus, cerebral cortex and limbic structures (amygdala and hippocampus). The main output nuclei are the substantia nigra pars reticulata (SNr) and the internal globus pallidus nucleus (not shown). Tonically active inhibitory connections (*bright blue arrows*) are indirectly relayed back to the cerebral cortex (via the thalamus) and directly back to midbrain (tectum) and brainstem structures. *Dull-blue arrows* represent intrinsic inhibitory connections. (**b**) A schematic illustration of the artificial selection architecture proposed by Snaith and Holland (1990) in which competing behavioural systems (C1–C8) provide phasically active excitatory input to and receive tonically active inhibitory outputs from a central selection mechanism

select the actions of an autonomous mobile robot (Fig. 1b) (Snaith and Holland 1990). Subsequently, it has been confirmed that sequences of actions that allow a mobile robot to forage when "hungry" and hide when "frightened" can be selected appropriately by a biologically constrained model of basal ganglia architecture (Prescott et al. 2006). In the present context, the term "salience" is used to denote the "common-currency" parameter against which the competing inputs to the basal ganglia are evaluated. Use of the term in this way has large overlap with the concept of "value" in the reinforcement learning literature since it is the parameter according to which selections are made. In biological systems the relative "salience values" of particular competing input signals to the basal ganglia can be determined by evolution (the timid wolf and the aggressive rabbit have not done well) and by individual experience—reinforcement learning. We will now consider why the topic of reinforcement learning should be so intimately associated with that of the nature of any generic selection mechanism.

3 Reinforcement Learning

The basal ganglia have long been associated with reinforcement learning, in particular, with instrumental conditioning (Berridge 2007; Schultz 2006; Wise 2004). In his famous law of effect, Thorndike (1911) declared that "any act which in a given situation produces satisfaction becomes associated with that situation so

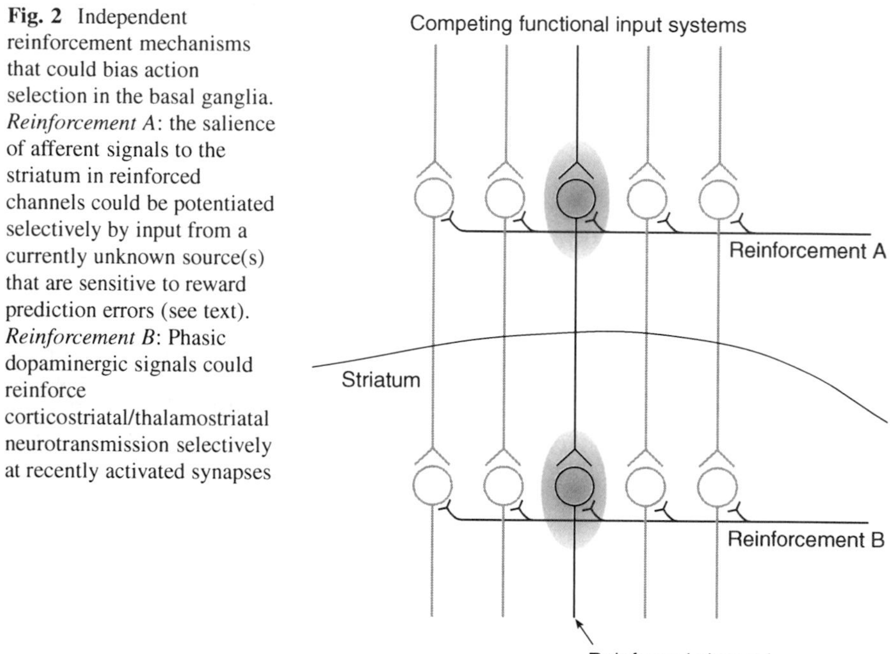

Fig. 2 Independent reinforcement mechanisms that could bias action selection in the basal ganglia. *Reinforcement A*: the salience of afferent signals to the striatum in reinforced channels could be potentiated selectively by input from a currently unknown source(s) that are sensitive to reward prediction errors (see text). *Reinforcement B*: Phasic dopaminergic signals could reinforce corticostriatal/thalamostriatal neurotransmission selectively at recently activated synapses

that when the situation recurs the act is more likely than before to recur also". Using slightly different language, Thorndike is stating that in a given context, an action that is associated with reinforcement is more likely to be selected in the future when the same or similar contexts are encountered. Therefore, in essence, reinforcement learning can be seen as a process for biasing the operation of a selection machine. The question we will now address is how a reinforcer could bias the operation of a central selection mechanism of the kind represented in the macro-architecture of basal ganglia described above? There are several possibilities but two in particular stand out.

3.1 How Reinforcement Could Bias Selection, 1: Adjust the Relative Strengths of Competing Inputs (Fig. 2a)

Theoretically, selection could be biased simply by increasing the input salience of competing systems associated with a reinforcer. Since the proposed selection process works by assessing the relative magnitudes of input saliences in competing channels (Gurney et al. 2001a,b; Humphries et al. 2006), reinforcement-related boosting of a particular channel's input would increase the probability of it being selected in any future competition. Much evidence in the biological literature indicates that when a particular stimulus is associated with reward, its representation in afferent structures projecting to the basal ganglia is enhanced (Ding and Hikosaka 2006; Ikeda and Hikosaka 2003; Kobayashi et al. 2002, 2006; Schultz 2000; Watanabe et al. 2002). Although the origin of these reinforcement signals is currently unknown, there are reasons to believe they originate from structures that are sensitive to detailed post-saccadic estimates of outcome value (Padoa-Schioppa and Assad 2006; Potts et al. 2006).

3.2 How Reinforcement Could Bias Selection, 2: Change the Relative Sensitivity of the Receiver to Reinforced Inputs (Fig. 2b)

A different way to bias selection would be to adjust the sensitivity of basal ganglia intrinsic circuitry by enhancing its responses, specifically to reinforced inputs. Increased activity associated with reinforced inputs could be combined with corresponding reductions in sensitivity to non-reinforced or punished inputs. This version of biasing action selection has received most attention in analyses of the basal ganglia's role in reinforcement learning (Arbuthnott and Wickens 2007; Everitt and Robbins 2005; Reynolds and Wickens 2002; Schultz 1998, 2006; Wickens 1993; Wickens et al. 2003; Wise 2004). Selectivity is achieved by restricting the effects of reinforcement to specific subsets of recently or concurrently active inputs based on comparative signal timing (Arbuthnott and Wickens 2007). In most contemporary models, reward-related actions are thought to be specific inputs from the cerebral cortex that are reinforced by signals from DA neurones in the ventral midbrain (Schultz 2006). While it is clear that DA neurotransmission operates in a range of different modes (Fiorillo et al. 2003; Floresco et al. 2003; Grace 1995; Heien et al. 2005; Roitman et al. 2004; Schultz 2007; Venton and Wightman 2007), the responses linked most often with reinforcement learning are the short-latency phasic responses which are widely accepted as signalling reward prediction errors (Schultz 1998).

4 Phasic DA Signalling

In most species the unexpected presentation of a primary reward, or a neutral stimulus previously associated with primary rewards, normally evokes a stereotypic phasic DA response (Freeman et al. 1985; Guarraci and Kapp 1999; Horvitz et al. 1997; Schultz 1998). It is characterised by a short-latency (70–100 ms), short-duration (100–200 ms) burst of activity (Schultz 1998) (Fig. 3b). However, it is the adaptive nature of phasic DA responses when experimental conditions are altered that has attracted most interest (Bayer and Glimcher 2005; Nakahara et al. 2004; Satoh et al. 2003; Schultz 1998, 2006). The properties of phasic DA signalling on which most contemporary theories are based can be itemised as

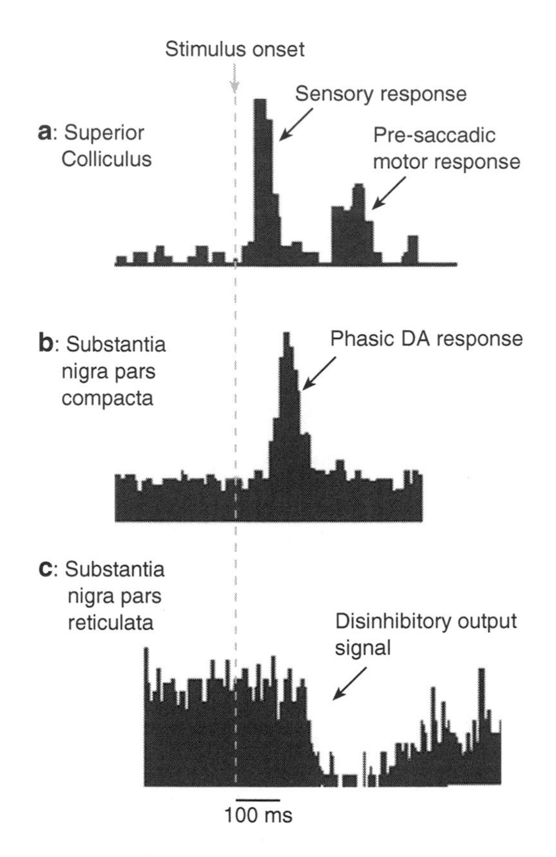

Fig. 3 A latency constraint associated with visual input to DA neurones. Typical examples show the relative timing of responses evoked by an unexpected visual stimulus in the superior colliculus, substantia nigra pars compacta and substantia nigra pars reticulata. Peri-stimulus histograms from different publications are aligned on stimulus onset. (**a**) Activity in the superior colliculus is characterised by an early sensory response (latency ~40 ms) followed by a later motor response (latency ~200 ms). The latter is responsible for driving the orienting gaze shift to bring the stimulus onto the fovea (modified with permission from Jay and Sparks 1987). (**b**) The phasic dopaminergic response (latency ~70 ms) (modified with permission from Schultz 1998) occurs after the collicular sensory response but prior to its pre-saccadic motor response. (**c**) Phasic dopaminergic activity also occurs prior to the output signal from substantia nigra pars reticulata that disinhibits the motor-related activity of target neurones in the superior colliculus (modified with permission from Hikosaka and Wurtz 1983)

follows: (a) while neutral sensory events also initially elicit phasic DA responses, they habituate rapidly if not associated with reward (Ljungberg et al. 1992). (b) If an habituated neutral stimulus is subsequently associated with a primary reward, its capacity to evoke a phasic DA response is re-established (Ljungberg et al. 1992). (c) As a primary reward becomes increasingly predicted by a prior event, its capacity to evoke a phasic DA response diminishes (Pan et al. 2005; Schultz 1998). (d) If a reward is predicted and fails to occur, DA neurones exhibit a brief pause about the time of expected reward delivery (Schultz et al. 1997). These seminal observations have been interpreted as indicating that DA neurones signal events that are "better" or "worse" than expected (i.e. reward prediction errors; Montague et al. 1996). Because behavioural experiments have established that unpredicted reward, rather than reward per se, is critical for learning (see Schultz 2006, for a review), the phasic response properties of DA neurones have captured the imagination of both the biological (BarGad et al. 2003; Bayer and Glimcher 2005; Morris et al. 2004; O'Doherty et al. 2003; Schultz 1998; Ungless 2004) and computational neuroscience communities (Dayan and Balleine 2002; Montague et al. 1996, 2004; Singh et al. 2005; Sutton and Barto 1998). Indeed, the reward prediction error hypothesis of phasic DA signalling has become one of the widely accepted tenets of contemporary neuroscience. However, there is a body of evidence that does not easily fit with this view (Horvitz 2000; Redgrave and Gurney 2006; Redgrave et al. 2008, 1999a).

5 Inconvenient Observations

(a) DA neurones exhibit robust phasic responses to unexpected neutral stimuli that are novel and elicit orienting, but have no reinforcement consequences (Horvitz 2000). Counterclaims that such stimuli must therefore be rewarding are circular. (b) Phasic DA neuronal responses are remarkably stereotyped (~100 ms latency, ~100 ms duration) across species, numerous experimental paradigms, and are largely independent of sensory modality or perceptual complexity of eliciting events (Schultz 1998). (c) The latencies of phasic, sensory-evoked DA responses (~100 ms, Schultz 1998) are typically shorter than those of the gaze shift (~150–200 ms) that brings the eliciting event onto the fovea for examination (Jay and Sparks 1987; compare Fig. 3a and b). Therefore, under most natural circumstances, both the identity and conscious appreciation of the event have yet to be established at the time of DA signalling (Stoerig 2006). (d) Pre-saccadic visual input to DA neurones derives largely, if not exclusively, from the midbrain superior colliculus (Comoli et al. 2003; Dommett et al. 2005). Note that short-latency visual input from the superior colliculus may influence DA neurones either directly via the tectonigral projection or indirectly via other routes including the pedunculopontine tegmental nucleus (Pan et al. 2005) and the subthalamic nucleus (Coizet et al. 2009). However, the important point is that while collicular neurones are exquisitely sensitive to the location of luminance changes, they are largely insensitive to colour, static contrast and high spatial frequency (Grantyn 1988; Sparks 1986; Stein and Meredith 1993; Wurtz and Albano 1980). Note also that collicular neurones are responsive at short-latency to multisensory stimuli (visual, auditory and somatosensory; Stein and Meredith 1993); however, the extent to which nonvisual activity in the superior colliculus can influence DA neurones is currently unknown. However, in the absence of specific training in highly constrained environments, pre-saccadic visual processing in the superior colliculus is particularly ill equipped to determine the identity and hence the value of an unexpected event. (e) Despite numerous reports of DA neurones effectively discriminating complex characteristics of visual stimuli used to signal reward magnitude and probability (Schultz 2006), it must be noted that, with few exceptions (Morris et al. 2004), relevant experiments contain a confound based on numerous (typically 1,000s, sometimes 10s of 1,000s) prior associations between the location of stimulus presentation (encoded within collicular retinocentric maps; Wurtz and Albano 1980) and stimulus value. While such procedures may not easily generalise to natural environments (where evolution "designed" relevant neural systems to operate), they may have the ability to differentially sensitise "rewarded" regions of the retinotopic collicular response field (Ikeda and Hikosaka 2003), thereby giving the impression that the colliculus, and hence DA neurones, can discriminate stimulus value at pre-saccadic latencies.

6 The Reinforcing Function of Phasic DA

Most versions of the reward prediction error hypothesis assume that phasic DA activity is reward-related and reinforces the selection of behaviour that will maximise the future acquisition of reward (Dayan and Balleine 2002; Schultz 2006). Here, a reward prediction error represents a difference between the predicted and actual utility value of the current state/event. Unfortunately, when an event is both temporally and spatially unpredictable (i.e. most natural situations), subcortical afferent sensory processing would be in a position to report only preliminary estimates of stimulus valence (Dean et al. 1989). In contrast, after a foveating gaze shift, the event can be analysed by more sophisticated cortical perceptual processing and its identity established (Thorpe and Fabre-Thorpe 2001). Insofar as an accurate determination of value depends on knowing what the stimulus is, it seems that post-gaze-shift stimulus identification may be a necessary precondition for calculating genuine errors of "reward prediction". Accumulating evidence suggests that such calculations can be performed by neurones in prefrontal cortex (Padoa-Schioppa and Assad 2006; Potts et al. 2006; Rolls 2000). However, to date we know of no evidence suggesting that DA neurones can be activated phasically by the appreciation of an unexpected reward determined on the basis of post-gaze-shift analyses of stimulus identity. Consequently, although there is doubt that early subcortical sensory processing in real-world situations can provide DA neurones with sufficient information to signal reward prediction errors (Redgrave et al. 1999a), evidence that phasic DA is performing an essential reinforcing function is substantially stronger. Thus, biologically significant events (classified by early sensory processing as "not immediately harmful"; Dean et al. 1989) evoke positive DA responses (Horvitz 2000; Schultz 1998), while noxious stimuli (Coizet et al. 2006; Ungless et al. 2004) or the failure of predicted salient events (Schultz 1998) evoke predominantly negative responses (however, note the recent paper by Matsumoto and Hikosaka 2009, reporting DA neurones that are activated by both positive and negative prediction errors). Since DA neurones seem to be made aware that something has happened, rather than what has happened, perhaps it would be safer to regard phasic DA activity as reporting “sensory prediction errors” rather than “reward prediction errors”. However, this leaves open the important question of what is being reinforced.

7 An Alternative Proposal

Relying on what is known of the sensory properties of the superior colliculus (Boehnke and Munoz 2008; Stein and Meredith 1993; Wurtz and Albano 1980), we assume that DA neurones are likely to be informed that a biologically significant event has occurred. Typically, if neutral stimuli are not reinforced, their capacity to evoke a sensory response in the superior colliculus habituates rapidly (Grantyn 1988; Horn and Hill 1966; Sprague et al. 1968). Consequently, in the present context, biological significance is defined in terms of the magnitude of a non-habituated sensory response in the superior colliculus (Boehnke and Munoz 2008). In addition, simple stimulus characteristics, such as size, speed and direction of movement (especially loom), would enable the colliculus to assess whether or not a novel event is likely to be immediately harmful (Dean et al. 1989). It is likely, therefore, that short-latency afferent sensory information originating from the superior colliculus contains preliminary estimates of both biological salience (Boehnke and Munoz 2008) and potential harm (Dean et al. 1989). With this point in mind, we proposed recently (Redgrave and Gurney 2006; Redgrave et al. 2008) that rather than reinforcing actions that maximise future reward, afferent information from the superior colliculus may be more suitable for reinforcing assessments of agency (i.e. when some aspect of the agent's behaviour is the cause of an initially unpredicted event), and hence this circuitry may be pivotal in the discovery of novel actions. A novel action would be acquired when the agent identifies which particular aspects of its behaviour are the critical cause. The definition of an action in this context would therefore be a specific set of movements that accurately predicts a particular outcome. Such learning would make notably less stringent demands of early sensory processing than envisaged by the reward prediction error hypothesis and is more likely to be within the scope of subcortical sensory systems (Boehnke and Munoz 2008; Comoli et al. 2003; Dommett et al. 2005). The important point here is that our suggestion subdivides the overall process of operant or instrumental conditioning into two subcomponents: (a) intrinsically motivated computations required to determine agency and discover novel actions, and (b) extrinsically motivated computations to bias future action selection on the basis of outcome utility.

8 A Neural Network for Determining Agency

The agency hypothesis (Redgrave and Gurney 2006; Redgrave et al. 2008) proposes that the basal ganglia appear ideally configured to determine whether the agent is the likely cause of the unpredicted event. It proposed that DA-related repetition and neural plasticity underlie the discovery of the causal components of behavioural output and that these components are encoded as novel actions. This proposal is based on an analysis of the functional architecture of the basal ganglia and considerations of signal timing. (Note that we use the general term "agent" to accommodate biomimetic architectures used to control robot behaviour (Prescott et al. 2006) as well as the neural systems in the brains of animals that control their behaviour.) For example, the relatively invariant pre-gaze-shift timing of the phasic DA response (Schultz 1998) highlights the importance of considering the signals that are also likely to be present in targeted structures at the time of phasic DA release, because it is with these signals that DA is most likely to interact. For the purpose of this analysis, we will continue to restrict ourselves primarily to signal processing in the striatum which is the principal target of ascending DA systems (Gerfen and Wilson 1996; Lindvall and Björklund 1974). A review of relevant literature (Redgrave and Gurney 2006; Redgrave et al. 2008) suggests there will be at least three additional afferent signals present in the striatum at the time of phasic DA release (Fig. 4a). (a) Sensory: many tectonigral axons that innervate substantia nigra pars compacta have collateral projections that terminate in regions of the thalamus that provide direct input to the striatum (Coizet et al. 2007). This branched architecture would ensure that a separate short-latency sensory representation of the unexpected event that triggered the phasic DA signal would also elicit a corresponding phasic glutamatergic input to the striatum from the thalamus (Lacey et al. 2007; Smith et al. 2004). The known timing of these two afferent signals (Dommett et al. 2005; Schulz et al. 2008) suggests they have the potential to converge. (b) Contextual: striatal neurones are influenced by contextual variables related to the general sensory, metabolic and cognitive state of the animal (Hikosaka et al. 1989; Schultz 2000). Such inputs are likely to originate in cortical, limbic and subcortical (thalamic) structures (Gerfen and Wilson 1996). (c) Motor copy: anatomical and physiological data suggest that copies of motor commands from both cortical and subcortical sensorimotor structures to the brainstem are also relayed to the striatum via collaterals of fibres that contact motor and premotor neurones in the medulla and spinal cord (Bickford and Hall 1989; Crutcher and DeLong 1984; Lévesque et al. 1996; McHaffie et al. 2005; Mink 1996; Reiner et al. 2003). These efference copy signals of action decisions and motor commands may be seen as providing the striatum with a running record of ongoing behavioural output.

9 Signal Timing and the Determination of Agency

The combination of potentially convergent signals identified in Fig. 4a could permit the agent to determine whether any aspect of its behavioural output (motor copy) was related to the onset of a biologically significant sensory event. In cases where the agent is causally responsible, a representation of the critical movement will most often be embedded in the immediately preceding record of motor output

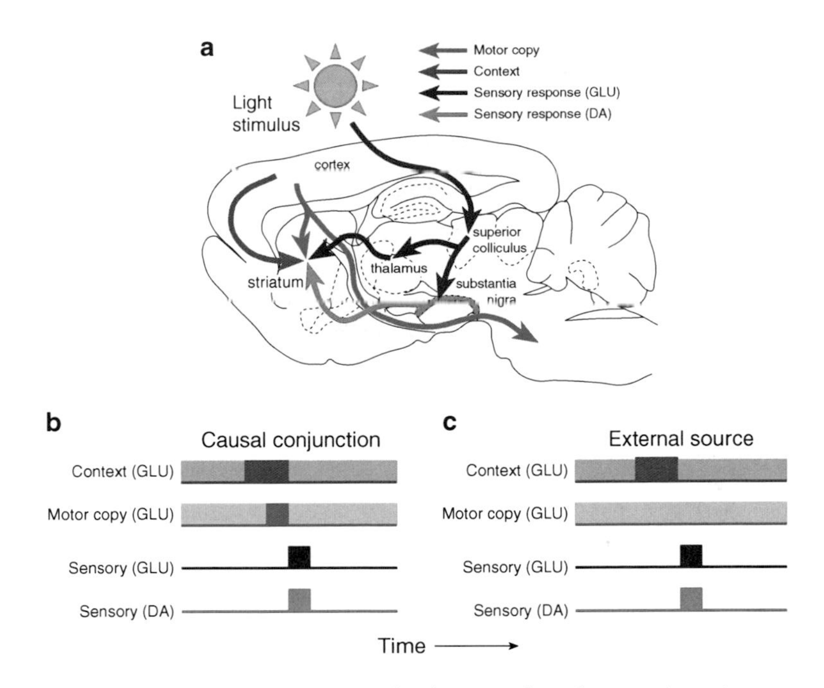

Fig. 4 Potential interaction between converging inputs to the striatum to determine agency. (**a**) Four classes of anatomically and physiologically identified afferent signals to the striatum: (1) efference motor copy via branched pathways from motor cortex and subcortical sensorimotor structures (e.g. superior colliculus) reaches the striatum directly (cortex) or indirectly via the thalamus (subcortical structures) (*green arrows*); (2) striatal neurones are sensitive to experimental context (see text for references) (*blue arrows*); and (3) a sequence of retino-tecto-thalamostriatal projections conveys a short-latency glutamatergic version of unpredicted visual events (*red arrows*); (4) retino-tecto-nigro-striatal projections convey a short-latency dopaminergic version of unpredicted visual events (*red and orange arrows*). (**b**) Event caused by agent. Whenever the agent is the cause of the unpredicted event, relevant components of the multidimensional contextual (*blue*) and motor efference copy (*green*) inputs will directly precede short-latency glutamatergic sensory input from the thalamus (*red*) and the phasic dopaminergic input from substantia nigra (*orange*). (**c**) Event caused by external source. When no relevant motor-copy inputs precede the phasic sensory inputs (glutamatergic and dopaminergic), the unpredicted event is likely to have been caused by an external source. The colour coding of the functional inputs to the striatum in (**b**) and (**c**) is maintained from (**a**). This figure was modified with permission from the artwork that appeared in Redgrave and Gurney (2006)

(Fig. 4b), while if the event was caused by an external source (i.e. not the agent), then nothing in the preceding motor record would correlate (Fig. 4c). How might such a mechanism operate? A clue to DA's reinforcing role is given by the observation that high levels of DA receptor activation cause segments of behaviour to be repeated, e.g. pharmacologically induced stereotypies (Robbins and Sahakian 1981). Consequently, we suppose that sensory-evoked phasic DA release reinforces the reselection of any immediately preceding behavioural output. In other words, the selection mechanisms within the basal ganglia are biased towards repeating the just-performed action. This effect could perhaps be considered a special case of DA-induced "wanting" (Berridge 2007), in this case making the agent want to do again what it has just done. Thus, if the agent is the cause of the sensory event and prior behaviour is repeated, then the event will occur again; if not, it will not. At a mechanistic level, we suppose the phasic DA signal causes a form of plasticity that adjusts the "sensitivity of the receiver" to bias the reselection of causal behavioural output (i.e. Reinforcement B in Fig. 2). However, this comparatively simple story entails a major computational problem—how is the agent/reinforcement system to know, or be able to identify, which aspects of its prior behaviour are causal? In most circumstances, the contextual and motor record will be multidimensional and, at the beginning, possibly with few components causally related to the sensory event. However, if the phasic release of DA promotes repetition of prior behavioural selections with some variability (i.e. where not all components are included in each iteration), then by facilitating/potentiating recently active channels when the event occurs, and suppressing active channels when it fails, the system should converge on the causal/relevant components of contextual and behavioural output. This repetition-bias hypothesis would ensure that increasingly refined representations of the critical aspects of behavioural output and the consequent sensory outcome will occur more frequently in brain areas external to the basal ganglia which have the capacity to develop and store associative links between action and outcome (Corbit and Balleine 2003). At the end of this process when critical causal components of behavioural output have been identified and refined, and the sensory consequences of enactment fully predicted, a new action channel would have developed within the basal ganglia and a novel action-outcome pairing stored externally (Singh et al. 2005). At this point, an entirely new action/response would have been developed which was not previously in the agent's repertoire. An interesting consequence of this analysis is that the definition of "action" becomes clear—an action is a movement or sequence of movements that has a predicted outcome. The fact that the outcome is always predicted means that it is appropriate to view actions as "purposive". This definition applies to actions initiated either by goal-directed or habitual control mechanisms. So far so good, but what happens if the unexpected sensory event caused by the agent is bad? Thus far, we have considered almost exclusively the role of positive DA neuronal responses in promoting action-outcome learning. We will now turn our attention to the issue of phasic suppressions of DA neuronal activity.

10 Aversive Stimuli and Failures of Predicted Reward

If a caused event was aversive or detrimental, discovering causative aspects of behaviour through repetitions promoted by phasic DA responses would be ill-advised, if not dangerous. In such cases, the adaptive option would be to suppress any tendency to repeat immediately prior behaviour and avoid the context(s) in which the event occurred. It is significant, therefore, that noxious stimuli can elicit a short-latency phasic inhibition of significant numbers of ventral midbrain DA neurones that generally lasts for the duration of the noxious event (Coizet et al. 2006; Ungless et al. 2004). If positive DA responses are thought to promote behavioural repetitions, it would be natural to suggest that negative DA signals act to reduce the likelihood of reselecting immediately preceding behaviour. To initiate negative DA, responses would require afferent sensory processing to discriminate, at short latency, potentially harmful events and by some means direct inhibitory afferent signals to DA neurones. Recent experimental evidence shows that the parabrachial nucleus, a major target of afferent nociceptive pathways from the spinal cord (Klop et al. 2005), provides direct projections to ventral midbrain regions containing DA neurones (Klop et al. 2005; Overton et al. 2005). The mechanism by which these inputs suppress the activity of DA neurones remains to be determined. Similarly, additional work will be required to determine the precise consequences of a population pause in DA neuronal activity on striatal neurotransmission.

A further detrimental situation where agency could be important is when a well-predicted reward fails to occur. Perhaps it was something the agent did that was responsible for the predicted event failing. If so, the adaptive option would also be to suppress any tendency to repeat immediately prior behavioural selections. Under such circumstances, it is well established that DA neurones typically exhibit a short pause/negative response about the time of the failed reward delivery (Schultz 1998). Thus, failures of predicted reward may have similar effects in structures targeted by DA, to those elicited by noxious stimuli (Coizet et al. 2006; Ungless et al. 2004). The source(s) of the afferent inhibitory signals that suppress DA activity when a predicted event fails is currently unknown; however, very recent evidence is pointing in the direction of the habenula (Matsumoto and Hikosaka 2009). A final point is that, as with positive phasic DA signals (Schultz 1998), negative phasic responses of DA neurones occur at very short latencies following noxious stimulus onset (Coizet et al. 2006) or following the failure of a predicted reward (Schultz 1998). We will now consider why this might be.

11 Why Are Short-Latency DA Reinforcement Signals So Short?

Anatomical studies indicated that early sensory input to DA neurones in the ventral midbrain comes mainly, if not exclusively, from the comparatively primitive sensory systems of the brainstem (Comoli et al. 2003; Dommett et al. 2005; Omelchenko and Sesack 2007; Overton et al. 2005). Viewed from the perspective of the reward prediction error hypothesis, it is difficult to understand why the sensory information indicating “current state” that used to generate a reward prediction error should be based on such limited and preliminary sensory processing. There seem manifest advantages of waiting just an additional few hundred milliseconds for cortical systems to identify the stimulus and provide incomparably better estimates of utility. However, if instead DA neurones are signalling sensory prediction errors that are used to determine agency and discover novel actions, largely independent of immediate outcome value (Redgrave and Gurney 2006; Redgrave et al. 2008), pre-saccadic latencies of DA responses are an advantage, not a problem. Indeed, the agency view of phasic DA signalling provides a potential explanation of why the reinforcement signal should occur before any behaviour elicited by the onset of an unpredicted biologically significant event, i.e. the initial orienting/approach or defensive/withdrawal movements (Dean et al. 1989; Grantyn 1988; Sparks 1986; Stein and Meredith 1993; Wurtz and Albano 1980). In the proposed basal ganglia circuitry, a critical component is the record of behavioural output relayed to the striatum by collateral projections from sensorimotor regions to motor effector systems in the brainstem (Bickford and Hall 1989; Crutcher and DeLong 1984; Lévesque et al. 1996; McHaffie et al. 2005; Mink 1996; Reiner et al. 2003) (Fig. 4). Assuming some aspect of the agent's behaviour causes an initially unpredicted event, and reinforcement is delayed until after the event has been properly investigated and identified—which may require combinations of eye, head and body movements associated with orienting gaze shifts, inspection, etc.—the record of behavioural output would immediately be contaminated by movements elicited by the event itself, but unrelated to its cause. The overall system would then be faced with a drastically more difficult task of identifying and then reinforcing critical causative components of behaviour embedded somewhere further back in the past motor record. This has been recognised as an important general element of the credit-assignment problem (Izhikevich 2007; Sutton and Barto 1998). On the other hand, if an agent is the proximal cause of a phasic sensory event, it is its immediately preceding behaviour that is most likely to be responsible. Having a DA reinforcement signal (positive or negative) delivered before any event-elicited behavioural reactions would greatly simplify the credit-assignment problem and ensure reinforcement was directed to the most likely cause. This mechanism could explain the profound detrimental effect of delaying reinforcement by just a few seconds on acquisition rates in associative learning (Black et al. 1985; Dickinson 2001; Elsner and Hommel 2004; Schultz 2006). For example, in the case of instrumental conditioning, the longer the delay between causal component of behaviour (e.g. lever press) and sensory reinforcement (the delivery of reward), the more likely the record of "motor output" in the striatum will be contaminated with irrelevant behavioural output which, inadvertently, would be reinforced by the sensory-evoked DA response when reward is delivered. This problem would be exacerbated if the active inputs representing copies of behavioural (motivational, affective, cognitive and sensorimotor) selections establish a temporary "eligibility trace" (that decays over seconds) that sensitises the recently active striatal neurones to subsequent DA-related reinforcement (see Arbuthnott and Wickens 2007, for an alternative articulation of the same idea). The processes by which synaptic efficacies are adjusted following reinforcement-related phasic DA receptor activation (Greengard et al. 1999), and how long they remain in an altered state, will necessarily extend well beyond the duration of the phasic DA response (100–200 ms). Presumably it is this arrangement that permits a discrete "trigger" event (a phasic DA response measured in ms) to produce selective and lasting adjustments (measured in minutes) to an action selection mechanism that biases subsequent selections towards (positive DA) or away from (negative DA) what the agent has just done.

12 Conclusions and Open Challenges

This document is an elaboration of the recent proposal that short-latency sensory-driven DA responses provide the reinforcement signals that enable the brain to discriminate the non-harmful sensory events for which it is responsible (Redgrave and Gurney 2006). As part of this process, new responses required in specific circumstances to make events happen are discovered. In the brain these basic functions rely on combining the selective and adaptive properties of basal ganglia neural processing. Quick and dirty sensory analysis is sufficient to generate the necessary reinforcing signals, with the system needing to know only if a sensory event is likely to be immediately detrimental, so appropriate (positive or negative) DA reinforcement signals can be generated. We have made a clear distinction between this "sensory prediction error" system and systems driven by "reward prediction errors" which require outcomes to be identified so useful estimates of utility can be made to guide the choice of future actions. The latter system is thought to be associated with processing in the prefrontal cortex (Padoa-Schioppa and Assad 2006; Potts et al. 2006); however, a major open research issue concerns the mechanism(s) by which genuine errors in reward prediction are used to adjust the magnitude of representations of reward-related stimuli in structures with afferent projections to the basal ganglia (Ding and Hikosaka 2006; Ikeda and Hikosaka 2003; Kobayashi et al. 2002, 2006; Pleger et al. 2008; Watanabe et al. 2002) (Reinforcement A in Fig. 2) which remains to be determined.

12.1 Challenges for Biology

From the perspective of brain biology, the above material reviews important strands of empirical evidence for particular elements of a proposed network; however, as with most large system-level hypotheses, much work is needed to determine whether individual components and hypothesised sub-functions work together in the prescribed manner. Several important challenges can be identified.

First, it will be necessary to develop an experimental paradigm in which action acquisition can best be investigated. Such a paradigm would require that the learning agent has to discover what aspects of its behaviour are responsible for evoking a salient sensory event. We have devised several versions of a joystick task (which is the principal topic of Stafford et al. 2012) which satisfy this requirement. Briefly, this task can be performed by a wide range of species from mouse to man, also by robots. It can be used to study independently the different aspects of action acquisition, including "where" a response has to be made, "what" the response should be, "when" it should be performed and also "how fast" the movement should be. Given that different neural architectures located within different parts of the brain may be required to produce different action characteristics, a major future challenge will be to resolve how activities in the different networks are "bound" together to produce a coherent behavioural output. This can be viewed as a motor version of the "binding problem" which is an important issue in the area of sensory perception. As research into sensory binding is further advanced, a good place to start will be to examine in detail the data and hypotheses in the perceptual literature.

A second important feature of the joystick task is that it can support repeated measures experimental designs. For example, when the agent has discovered that a movement made to a specific location, or forming a particular gesture, or any movement made at a particular time or speed is causal in eliciting a sensory reinforcer, the criteria can be changed, thereby requiring novel actions to be discovered. This can be done repeatedly and will be important for investigating brain mechanisms contributing to action discovery. The option of determining performance before and after experimental treatments in the same subject will add considerable power to the design. For example, one of the major issues to be addressed is the extent to which phasic dopamine acts as the reinforcing agent for novel action acquisition. In the present programme, this will be addressed through the investigation of action acquisition in patients with Parkinson's disease. In these subjects, dopaminergic neurones have degenerated, and their consequent loss of dopamine is ameliorated by the therapeutic administration of L-DOPA. While the systemic application of this drug reinstates tonic levels of dopaminergic neurotransmission in the basal ganglia, hence the ability to operate in selection mode is recovered, phasic dopaminergic activity remains dysfunctional, and hence the reinforcement learning aspect of basal ganglia function should remain impaired. These predictions will be evaluated experimentally. A further important question will be to determine the sources of sensory input which can elicit a phasic dopamine response. This issue is particularly important because it will shed light on the quality of the sensory processing that can elicit reinforcement in this system. The question to be addressed is whether the comparatively crude subcortical sensory processing is solely responsible for phasic dopamine responses or whether this can be supplemented by early sensory processing from the cerebral cortex. This is important because a range of more sophisticated perceptual competencies would be afforded by cortical sensory networks. These questions will be addressed, first, by using reinforcing stimuli that can be discriminated only by cortical sensory processing, e.g. determinations of colour and high spatial frequencies, and second by the use of masking paradigms which block conscious cortical analysis of sensory events while leaving subcortical sensory processing intact.

12.2 Challenges for the Construction of Artificial Systems

An important aspect of this work is the extent to which biological solutions to fundamental computational issues in behavioural control can provide insights or be used to inform the construction of artificial systems. We would expect significant advantage to be gained by exploiting our analysis of the biological mechanisms responsible for intrinsically motivated determination of agency and acquisition of novel actions. The issue of whether an event in the world results from something an artificial agent did, or derived from an external source, is fundamental for the execution of effective purposive behaviour. Equally important is the discovery of exactly what aspect of behavioural output is causal. Our analysis of the potential role of basal ganglia architecture in contributing to the solution of these problems would be an excellent starting point for the design of artificial systems. Important insights would be (a) that the primary role of selection is an emergent property of the looped architecture by which the basal ganglia are connected to external structures. That is, the comparative value of input saliences is used to determine the release of "selected" target structures from tonic inhibitory control while maintaining inhibitory control over nonselected channels. (b) "Attention" can therefore be viewed as a property of this architecture and defined simply as "the currently selected channel". (c) Important questions arise immediately concerning how the aspects of competing inputs, which contribute to the evaluation of salience on which the selective processes are based, are determined. (d) Given that reinforcement learning is a process that biases selection, it is unsurprising that a biological architecture that can select (the basal ganglia) should also be closely associated with reinforcement learning. The different mechanisms whereby these biasing processes can occur were outlined above (Fig. 2). In any design of an artificial behavioural control system, it could be important to consider the advantages of having reinforcement learning mechanisms responsible for the determination of agency/action discovery separate from those ensuring that action-outcome options responsible for maximising future reward are selected more frequently. Specifically, the reinforcement mechanism of the former should make crude assessments of valence and be activated prior to any responses elicited by the unpredicted sensory reinforcer to simplify the credit-assignment problem. The latter should be based on accurate determinations of stimulus identity and consequent utility following closer inspection. These issues will be addressed in detail in Gurney et al. (2012).

Acknowledgements Written while the authors were in receipt of research funding from The Wellcome Trust, BBSRC and EPSRC, this research has also received funds from the European Commission 7th Framework Programme (FP7/2007-2013), "Challenge 2—Cognitive Systems, Interaction, Robotics", Grant Agreement No. ICT-IP-231722 and Project "IM-CLeVeR—Intrinsically Motivated Cumulative Learning Versatile Robots".

References

Alexander, G., DeLong, M., Strick, P.: Parallel organization of functionally segregated circuits linking basal ganglia and cortex. Annu. Rev. Neurosci. **9**, 357–381 (1986)

Arbuthnott, G.W., Wickens, J.: Space, time and dopamine. Trends Neurosci. **30**(2), 62–69 (2007)

BarGad, I., Morris, G., Bergman, H.: Information processing, dimensionality reduction and reinforcement learning in the basal ganglia. Prog. Neurobiol. **71**(6), 439–473 (2003)

Bayer, H.M., Glimcher, P.W.: Midbrain dopamine neurons encode a quantitative reward prediction error signal. Neuron **47**(1), 129–141 (2005)

Berridge, K.C.: The debate over dopamine's role in reward: The case for incentive salience. Psychopharmacology **191**(3), 391–431 (2007)

Bickford, M., Hall, W.: Collateral projections of predorsal bundle cells of the superior colliculus in the rat. J. Comp. Neurol. **283**, 86–106 (1989)

Black, J., Belluzzi, J.D., Stein, L.: Reinforcement delay of one second severely impairs acquisition of brain self-stimulation. Brain Res. **359**(1–2), 113–119 (1985)

Boehnke, S.E., Munoz, D.P.: On the importance of the transient visual response in the superior colliculus. Curr. Opin. Neurobiol. **18**(6), 544–551 (2008)

Chevalier, G., Deniau, J.: Disinhibition as a basic process in the expression of striatal functions. Trends Neurosci. **13**(7), 277–280 (1990)

Coizet, V., Dommett, E.J., Redgrave, P., Overton, P.G.: Nociceptive responses of midbrain dopaminergic neurones are modulated by the superior colliculus in the rat. Neuroscience **139**(4), 1479–1493 (2006)

Coizet, V., Graham, J.H., Moss, J., Bolam, J.P., Savasta, M., McHaffie, J.G., Redgrave, P., Overton, P.G.: Short-latency visual input to the subthalamic nucleus is provided by the midbrain superior colliculus. J. Neurosci. **29**(17), 5701–5709 (2009)

Coizet, V., Overton, P.G., Redgrave, P.: Collateralization of the tectonigral projection with other major output pathways of superior colliculus in the rat. J. Comp. Neurol. **500**(6), 1034–1049 (2007)

Comoli, E., Coizet, V., Boyes, J., Bolam, J.P., Canteras, N.S., Quirk, R.H., Overton, P.G., Redgrave, P.: A direct projection from superior colliculus to substantia nigra for detecting salient visual events. Nat. Neurosci. **6**(9), 974–980 (2003)

Corbit, L., Balleine, B.: The role of prelimbic cortex in instrumental conditioning. Behav. Brain Res. **146**(1–2), 145–157 (2003)

Crutcher, M.D., DeLong, M.R.: Single cell studies of the primate putamen. II. Relations to direction of movement and pattern of muscular activity. Exp. Brain Res. **53**(2), 244–258 (1984)

Dayan, P., Balleine, B.: Reward, motivation, and reinforcement learning. Neuron **36**(2), 285–298 (2002)

Dean, P., Redgrave, P., Westby, G.: Event or emergency? two response systems in the mammalian superior colliculus. Trends Neurosci. **12**(4), 137–147 (1989)

Dickinson, A.: The 28th bartlett memorial lecture causal learning: An associative analysis. Quart. J. Exp. Psych. B Comp. Phys. P **54**(1), 3–25 (2001)

Ding, L., Hikosaka, O.: Comparison of reward modulation in the frontal eye field and caudate of the macaque. J. Neurosci. **26**(25), 6695–6703 (2006)

Dommett, E., Coizet, V., Blaha, C.D., Martindale, J., Lefebvre, V., Walton, N., Mayhew, J.E., Overton, P.G., Redgrave, P.: How visual stimuli activate dopaminergic neurons at short latency. Science **307**(5714), 1476–1479 (2005)

Elsner, B., Hommel, B.: Contiguity and contingency in action-effect learning. Psychol. Res. **68**(2–3), 138–154 (2004)

Everitt, B.J., Robbins, T.W.: Neural systems of reinforcement for drug addiction: From actions to habits to compulsion. Nat. Neurosci. **8**(11), 1481–1489 (2005)

Fiorillo, C., Tobler, P., Schultz, W.: Discrete coding of reward probability and uncertainty by dopamine neurons. Science **299**(5614), 1898–1902 (2003)

Floresco, S., West, A., Ash, B., Moore, H., Grace, A.: Afferent modulation of dopamine neuron firing differentially regulates tonic and phasic dopamine transmission. Nat. Neurosci. **6**(9), 968–973 (2003)

Freeman, A.S., Meltzer, L.T., Bunney, B.S.: Firing properties of substantia nigra dopaminergic neurons in freely moving rats. Life Sci. **36**(20), 1983–1994 (1985)

Gerfen, C., Wilson, C.: The basal ganglia. In: Swanson, L., Bjorklund, A., Hokfelt, T. (eds.) Handbook of Chemical Neuroanatomy, vol 12: Integrated Systems of the CNS, Part III., pp. 371–468. Elsevier, Amsterdam (1996)

Grace, A.A.: The tonic/phasic model of dopamine system regulation: Its relevance for understanding how stimulant abuse can alter basal ganglia function. Drug Alcohol Depend. **37**, 111–129 (1995)

Grantyn, R.: Gaze control through superior colliculus: Structure and function. In: Buttner-Ennever, J. (ed.) Neuroanatomy of the Oculomotor System, pp. 273–333. Elsevier, Amsterdam (1988)

Greengard, P., Allen, P.B., Nairn, A.C.: Beyond the dopamine receptor: The darpp-32/protein phosphatase-1 cascade. Neuron **23**(3), 435–447 (1999)

Grillner, S., Helligren, J., Ménard, A., Saitoh, K., Wikström, M.A.: Mechanisms for selection of basic motor programs - roles for the striatum and pallidum. Trends Neurosci. **28**(7), 364–370 (2005)

Guarraci, F., Kapp, B.: An electrophysiological characterization of ventral tegmental area dopaminergic neurons during differential pavlovian fear conditioning in the awake rabbit. Behav. Brain Res. **99**(2), 169–179 (1999)

Gurney, K., Lepora, N., Shah, A., Koene, A., Redgrave, P.: Action discovery and intrinsic motivation: A biologically constrained formalisation. In: Baldassarre, G., Mirolli, M. (eds.) Intrinsically Motivated Learning in Natural and Artificial Systems, pp. 151–181. Springer, Berlin (2012)

Gurney, K., Prescott, T., Redgrave, P.: A computational model of action selection in the basal ganglia. I. A new functional anatomy. Biol. Cybern. **84**(6), 401–410 (2001a)

Gurney, K., Prescott, T., Redgrave, P.: A computational model of action selection in the basal ganglia. II. Analysis and simulation of behaviour. Biol. Cybern. **84**(6), 411–423 (2001b)

Heien, M., Khan, A.S., Ariansen, J.L., Cheer, J.F., Phillips, P.E.M., Wassum, K.M., Wightman, R.M.: Real-time measurement of dopamine fluctuations after cocaine in the brain of behaving rats. Proc. Natl. Acad. Sci. U. S. A. **102**(29), 10023–10028 (2005)

Hikosaka, O.: GABAergic output of the basal ganglia. Prog. Brain Res. **160**, 209–226 (2007)

Hikosaka, O., Sakamoto, M., Usui, S.: Functional properties of monkey caudate neurons III. Activities related to expectation of target and reward. J. Neurophysiol. **61**(4), 814–832 (1989)

Hikosaka, O., Wurtz, R.: Visual and oculomotor function of monkey substantia nigra pars reticulata. I. Relation of visual and auditory responses to saccades. J. Neurophysiol. **49**(5), 1230–1253 (1983)

Horn, G., Hill, R.M.: Effect of removing the neocortex on the response to repeated sensory stimulation of neurones in the mid-brain. Nature **211**, 754–755 (1966)

Horvitz, J.: Mesolimbocortical and nigrostriatal dopamine responses to salient non-reward events. Neuroscience **96**(4), 651–656 (2000)

Horvitz, J., Stewart, T., Jacobs, B.: Burst activity of ventral tegmental dopamine neurons is elicited by sensory stimuli in the awake cat. Brain Res. **759**(2), 251–258 (1997)

Houk, J.C.: Agents of the mind. Biol. Cybern. **92**(6), 427–437 (2005)

Humphries, M.D., Stewart, R.D., Gurney, K.N.: A physiologically plausible model of action selection and oscillatory activity in the basal ganglia. J. Neurosci. **26**(50), 12921–12942 (2006)

Ikeda, T., Hikosaka, O.: Reward-dependent gain and bias of visual responses in primate superior colliculus. Neuron **39**(4), 693–700 (2003)

Izhikevich, E.M.: Solving the Distal Reward Problem through linkage of STDP and dopamine signaling. Cereb. Cortex **17**(10), 2443–2452 (2007)

Jay, M., Sparks, D.: Sensorimotor integration in the primate superior colliculus. I. Motor convergence. J. Neurophysiol. **57**(1), 22–34 (1987)

Klop, E.M., Mouton, L.J., Hulsebosch, R., Boers, J., Holstege, G.: In cat four times as many lamina I neurons project to the parabrachial nuclei and twice as many to the periaqueductal gray as to the thalamus. Neuroscience **134**(1), 189–197 (2005)

Kobayashi, S., Lauwereyns, J., Koizumi, M., Sakagami, M., Hikosaka, O.: Influence of reward expectation on visuospatial processing in macaque lateral prefrontal cortex. J. Neurophysiol. **87**(3), 1488–1498 (2002)

Kobayashi, S., Nomoto, K., Watanabe, M., Hikosaka, O., Schultz, W., Sakagami, M.: Influences of rewarding and aversive outcomes on activity in macaque lateral prefrontal cortex. Neuron **51**(6), 861–870 (2006)

Lacey, C.J., Bolam, J.P., Magill, P.J.: Novel and distinct operational principles of intralaminar thalamic neurons and their striatal projections. J. Neurosci. **27**(16), 4374–4384 (2007)

Lévesque, M., Charara, A., Gagnon, S., Parent, A., Deschênes, M.: Corticostriatal projections from layer V cells in rat are collaterals of long-range corticofugal axons. Brain Res. **709**(2), 311–315 (1996)

Lindvall, O., Björklund, A.: The organization of the ascending catcholamine neuron systems in the rat brain as revealed by the glyoxylic acid fluoresence method. Acta Physiol. Scand. Suppl. **412**, 1–48 (1974)

Ljungberg, T., Apicella, P., Schultz, W.: Responses of monkey dopamine neurons during learning of behavioural reactions. J. Neurophysiol. **67**(1), 145–163 (1992)

Matsumoto, M., Hikosaka, O.: Representation of negative motivational value in the primate lateral habenula. Nat. Neurosci. **12**(1), 77–84 (2009)

McHaffie, J.G., Stanford, T.R., Stein, B.E., Coizet, V., Redgrave, P.: Subcortical loops through the basal ganglia. Trends Neurosci. **28**(8), 401–407 (2005)

Mink, J.: The basal ganglia: Focused selection and inhibition of competing motor programs. Prog. Neurobiol. **50**(4), 381–425 (1996)

Montague, P.R., Dayan, P., Sejnowski, T.J.: A framework for mesencephalic dopamine systems based on predictive hebbian learning. J. Neurosci. **16**(5), 1936–1947 (1996)

Montague, P.R., Hyman, S.E., Cohen, J.D.: Computational roles for dopamine in behavioural control. Nature **431**(7010), 760–767 (2004)

Morris, G., Arkadir, D., Nevet, A., Vaadia, E., Bergman, H.: Coincident but distinct messages of midbrain dopamine and striatal tonically active neurons. Neuron **43**(1), 133–143 (2004)

Nakahara, H., Itoh, H., Kawagoe, R., Takikawa, Y., Hikosaka, O.: Dopamine neurons can represent context-dependent prediction error. Neuron **41**(2), 269–280 (2004)

O'Doherty, J., Dayan, P., Friston, K., Critchley, H., Dolan, R.: Temporal difference models and reward-related learning in the human brain. Neuron **38**(2), 329–337 (2003)

Omelchenko, N., Sesack, S.R.: Glutamate synaptic inputs to ventral tegmental area neurons in the rat derive primarily from subcortical sources. Neuroscience **146**(3), 1259–1274 (2007)

Overton, P.G., Coizet, V., Dommett, E., Redgrave, P.: The parabrachial nucleus is a source of short latency nociceptive input to midbrain dopaminergic neurones in rat. Program No. 301.5, Neuroscience 2005 Abstracts. Society for Neuroscience, Washington. Online (2005)

Padoa-Schioppa, C., Assad, J.A.: Neurons in the orbitofrontal cortex encode economic value. Nature **441**(7090), 223–226 (2006)

Pan, W.X., Schmidt, R., Wickens, J.R, Hyland, B.I.: Dopamine cells respond to predicted events during classical conditioning: Evidence for eligibility traces in the reward-learning network. J. Neurosci. **25**(26), 6235–6242 (2005)

Pleger, B., Blankenburg, F., Ruff, C.C., Driver, J., Dolan, R.J.: Reward facilitates tactile judgments and modulates hemodynamic responses in human primary somatosensory cortex. J. Neurosci. **28**(33), 8161–8168 (2008)

Potts, G.F., Martin, L.E., Burton, P., Montague, P.R.: When things are better or worse than expected: The medial frontal cortex and the allocation of processing resources. J. Cogn. Neurosci. **18**(7), 1112–1119 (2006)

Prescott, T.J., Montes González, F.M., Gurney, K., Humphries, M.D., Redgrave, P.: A robot model of the basal ganglia: Behavior and intrinsic processing. Neural Netw. **19**(1), 31–61 (2006)

Prescott, T.J., Redgrave, P., Gurney, K.: Layered control architectures in robots and vertebrates. Adap. Behav. **7**(1), 99–127 (1999)

Redgrave, P.: Basal ganglia. Scholarpedia **2**(6), 1825 (2007)

Redgrave, P., Gurney, K.: The short-latency dopamine signal: A role in discovering novel actions? Nat. Rev. Neurosci. **7**(12), 967–975 (2006)

Redgrave, P., Gurney, K., Reynolds, J.: What is reinforced by phasic dopamine signals? Brain Res. Rev. **58**(2), 322–339 (2008)

Redgrave, P., Prescott, T., Gurney, K.: The basal ganglia: A vertebrate solution to the selection problem? Neuroscience **89**(4), 1009–1023 (1999a)
Redgrave, P., Prescott, T., Gurney, K.: Is the short latency dopamine response too short to signal reward error? Trends Neurosci. **22**(4), 146–151 (1999b)
Reiner, A., Jiao, Y., Del Mar, N., Laverghetta, A., Lei, W.: Differential morphology of pyramidal tract-type and intratelencephalically projecting-type corticostriatal neurons and their intrastriatal terminals in rats. J. Comp. Neurol. **457**, 420–440 (2003)
Reynolds, J.N., Wickens, J.R.: Dopamine-dependent plasticity of corticostriatal synapses. Neural Netw. **15**(4–6), 507–521 (2002)
Robbins, T., Sahakian, B.: Behavioral and neurochemical determinants of drug-induced stereotypy. In: Rose, F. (ed.) Metabolic Disorders of the Nervous System, pp. 244–291. Pitman Pr., London (1981)
Roitman, M., Stuber, G., Phillips, P., Wightman, R., Carelli, R.: Dopamine operates as a subsecond modulator of food seeking. J. Neurosci. **24**(6), 1265–1271 (2004)
Rolls, E.T.: The orbitofrontal cortex and reward. Cereb. Cortex **10**(3), 284–294 (2000)
Salamone, J., Correa, M.: Motivational views of reinforcement: Implications for understanding the behavioral functions of nucleus accumbens dopamine. Behav. Brain Res. **137**(1–2), 3–25 (2002)
Satoh, T., Nakai, S., Sato, T., Kimura, M.: Correlated coding of motivation and outcome of decision by dopamine neurons. J. Neurosci. **23**(30), 9913–9923 (2003)
Schultz, W.: Predictive reward signal of dopamine neurons. J. Neurophysiol. **80**(1), 1–27 (1998)
Schultz, W.: Multiple reward signals in the brain. Nat. Rev. Neurosci. **1**(3), 199–207 (2000)
Schultz, W.: Behavioral theories and the neurophysiology of reward. Annu. Rev. Psychol. **57**, 87–115 (2006)
Schultz, W.: Multiple dopamine functions at different time courses. Annu. Rev. Neurosci. **30**, 259–288 (2007)
Schultz, W., Dayan, P., Montague, P.: A neural substrate of prediction and reward. Science **275**(5306), 1593–1599 (1997)
Schulz, J., Redgrave, P., Clements, K., Reynolds, J.: Short latency activation of striatal spiny neurons via subcortical visual pathways. Program No. 180.2, 2008 Neuroscience Meeting Planner. Society for Neuroscience, Washington. Online (2008)
Singh, S., Barto, A., Chentanez, N.: Intrinsically motivated reinforcement learning. In: Saul, K., Weiss, Y., Bottou, L. (eds.) Advances in Neural Information Processing Systems **17**, pp. 1281–1288 (2005)
Smith, Y., Raju, D.V., Pare, J.F., Sidibe, M.: The thalamostriatal system: A highly specific network of the basal ganglia circuitry. Trends Neurosci. **27**(9), 520–527 (2004)
Snaith, S., Holland, O.: An investigation of two mediation strategies suitable for behavioural control in animals and animats. In: Meyer, J.-A., Wilson, S. (eds.) From Animals to Animats: Proceedings of the First International Conference on the Simulation of Adaptive Behaviour, pp. 255–262. MIT, Cambridge (1990)
Sparks, D.: Translation of sensory signals into commands for control of saccadic eye movements: Role of the primate superior colliculus. Physiol. Rev. **66**(1), 118–171 (1986)
Sprague, J.M., Marchiafava, P.L., Rixxolatti, G.: Unit responses to visual stimuli in the superior colliculus of the unanesthetized, mid-pontine cat. Arch. Ital. Biol. **106**(3), 169–193 (1968)
Stafford, T., Walton, T., Hetherington, L., Thirkettle, M., Gurney, K., Redgrave, P.: A novel behavioural task for researching intrinsic motivation. In: Baldassarre, G., Mirolli, M. (eds.) Intrinsically Motivated Learning in Natural and Artificial Systems, pp. 395–410. Springer, Berlin (2012)
Stein, B., Meredith, M.: The Merging of the Senses. MIT, Cambridge (1993)
Stoerig, P.: Blindsight, conscious vision, and the role of primary visual cortex. Prog. Brain Res. **155B**, 217–234 (2006)
Sutton, R., Barto, A.: Reinforcement Learning: An Introduction. MIT, Cambridge (1998)
Thorndike, E.: Animal Intelligence. Macmillan, New York (1911)
Thorpe, S., Fabre-Thorpe, M.: Seeking categories in the brain. Science **291**(5502), 260–263 (2001)
Ungless, M.: Dopamine: The salient issue. Trends Neurosci. **27**(12), 702–706 (2004)

Ungless, M., Magill, P., Bolam, J.: Uniform inhibition of dopamine neurons in the ventral tegmental area by aversive stimuli. Science **303**(5666), 2040–2042 (2004)

Venton, B.J., Wightman, R.M.: Pharmacologically induced, subsecond dopamine transients in the caudate-putamen of the anesthetized rat. Synapse **61**(1), 37–39 (2007)

Watanabe, M., Hikosaka, K., Sakagami, M., Shirakawa, S.: Coding and monitoring of motivational context in the primate prefrontal cortex. J. Neurosci. **22**(6), 2391–2400 (2002)

Wickens, J.: A theory of the striatum. Pergamon, Oxford (1993)

Wickens, J., Reynolds, J., Hyland, B.: Neural mechanisms of reward-related motor learning. Curr. Opin. Neurobiol. **13**(6), 685–690 (2003)

Wise, R.: Dopamine, learning and motivation. Nat. Rev. Neurosci. **5**(6), 483–494 (2004)

Wurtz, R., Albano, J.: Visual-motor function of the primate superior colliculus. Annu. Rev. Neurosci. **3**, 189–226 (1980)

Action Discovery and Intrinsic Motivation: A Biologically Constrained Formalisation

Kevin Gurney, Nathan Lepora, Ashvin Shah, Ansgar Koene, and Peter Redgrave

Abstract We introduce a biologically motivated, formal framework or "ontology" for dealing with many aspects of action discovery which we argue is an example of intrinsically motivated behaviour (as such, this chapter is a companion to that by Redgrave et al. in this volume). We argue that action discovery requires an interplay between separate internal forward models of prediction and inverse models mapping outcomes to actions. The process of learning actions is driven by transient changes in the animal's policy (repetition bias) which is, in turn, a result of unpredicted, phasic sensory information ("surprise"). The notion of salience as value is introduced and broken down into contributions from novelty (or surprise), immediate reward acquisition, or general task/goal attainment. Many other aspects of biological action discovery emerge naturally in our framework which aims to guide future modelling efforts in this domain.

1 Introduction

As described in detail elsewhere in this volume, there are several reasons why behaviour can be described as "intrinsically motivated" and why intrinsically motivated behaviour is useful. Common to many accounts is the idea that intrinsically motivated behaviour allows us to gain competence in achieving goals in

K. Gurney (✉) · N. Lepora · A. Shah · P. Redgrave
Adaptive Behaviour Research Group, Department of Psychology, University of Sheffield, Sheffield, UK
e-mail: k.gurney@sheffield.ac.uk; n.lepora@sheffield.ac.uk; a.shah@sheffield.ac.uk; p.redgrave@sheffield.ac.uk

A. Koene
Laboratory for Integrated Theoretical Neuroscience, RIKEN Brain Science Institute, Saitama, Japan
e-mail: a.r.koene@bham.ac.uk

G. Baldassarre and M. Mirolli (eds.), *Intrinsically Motivated Learning in Natural and Artificial Systems*, DOI 10.1007/978-3-642-32375-1_7,

an environment by developing skills for, and knowledge of, our interaction with that environment (see, e.g. Barto et al. 2004). In addition, intrinsically motivated behaviour of this kind usually results in the development of internal models of the action-outcome causality or "know-how" (Oudeyer and Kaplan 2007). Such competences allow us to accomplish subsequent tasks and goals more effectively.

In this chapter we focus on how intrinsic motivation helps an animal determine action-outcome causality. Recently we have developed the first steps in a biologically plausible account of this process (Redgrave and Gurney 2006; Redgrave et al. 2008). These ideas are also described in Redgrave et al. (2012) and summarised in Sect. 2. The focus of that work was on an analysis of the physiological and anatomical evidence that implicates short latency phasic (transient) changes in the levels of the neurotransmitter dopamine in learning causality and, in particular, its role as a signal of sensory prediction error.

In the tradition of Marr and Poggio (1976), we have therefore proposed a computational rationale for phasic dopamine. Thus, in brief, phasic dopamine causes the animal to repeat any movements it may have made immediately prior to a surprising event. By repeatedly executing those movements, the animal can determine agency—did the animal's movement cause the surprising event? It can also determine exactly what movements and under what circumstances they must be executed to provide the outcome. The acquisition of this knowledge is the discovery of a novel action—analogous in many respects to a skill or an "option" (Barto et al. 2004)—that can be used to interact with the environment.

In Marr's analysis, the next step is to determine *how* the computation (of action discovery) is performed. In our scheme, we propose that the repetition of movement execution repeatedly generates representations of those movements, their circumstances, and the outcome. These representations are then presented to associative networks in the brain responsible for building internal models of action-outcome contingency. However, in attempting to articulate this process in detail, several ideas such as "prediction", "prediction error", "habituation", "salience" and "sensory context" play a prominent role. Some of them may be characterised as representations in the brain; others are putative processes manipulating these signals. In any case, their definitions are often somewhat nebulous, and they all remain to be formally defined. Since much of this chapter is aimed at remedying this, it is important to understand the importance of such a project.

Many times in the cognitive sciences, debates (sometimes rather heated!) occur about the meaning, interpretation and status of concepts, terms and definitions. One pertinent example is that of "reward". This has a more specific interpretation in biology (being confined to appetitive stimuli such as food and liquid) than it does in computational reinforcement learning theory (e.g. see Sutton and Barto 1998), where it is semantically neutral and is defined implicitly by its symbolic occurrence in learning algorithms. An understanding of this situation lies at the heart of our recent analysis of the role of dopamine in reinforcement learning (Redgrave and Gurney 2006). A lack of precision in conceptualisation can lead to lack of collaboration, wasted effort and missed opportunities for advancement of the subject.

A similar set of problems occurred in artificial intelligence (AI) during attempts in the 1980s to capture, precisely, knowledge in a specific domain so that it could be manipulated in AI programmes like "expert systems". This culminated in the formulation of the notion of a domain-specific *ontology*. According to Gruber (1992) "[an ontology is] a specification of a conceptualisation... a description (like a formal specification of a programme) of the concepts and relationships that can formally exist for an agent or a community of agents...". The requirement of such an ontology, as used by computer scientists, is that it is specified in a formal ontology language. However, the bioinformatics community has made real progress with ontology-like tools with more relaxed frameworks. The Gene Ontology (Gene Ontology Consortium 2001) is a tool for the representation and processing of information about gene products and functions. According to the Gene Ontology Consortium, "The exponential growth in the volume of accessible biological information has generated a confusion of voices surrounding the annotation of molecular information about genes and their products. The Gene Ontology (GO) project seeks to provide *a set of structured vocabularies* for specific biological domains..." [our italics]. By helping to dispel the "confusion of voices" in its subject domain, GO has materially facilitated the progress of genetics science. We argue that cognitive science and robotics can avoid a similar cacophony by using an appropriate "structured vocabulary" for their discourse, defined using the relevant formal methods.

In this chapter, we therefore attempt to provide a formalisation of some terms in the vocabulary of action selection and action discovery, which will also be applicable in discussions of behaviour and intrinsically motivated learning in general. In defining an ontology of action discovery, it is essential to understand what is being done: it is *not* the case that we are seeking to establish the "truth" that the normal language label L "really is" given by the formal definition D (e.g. "action" really means D_1 rather than D_2). Rather, we are proposing that *defining* label L to mean D is *useful* because D is useful for our purposes, and D is *plausibly* assigned the label L. Other mappings may also be plausible, but at least we should try and be clear which mapping we are using. Disagreement about such mappings should not take priority over establishing a formalism that is self-consistent, comprehensive, and useful in formulating new theories and models.

The outcome of a programme such as that presented here is that we sharpen the computational hypothesis of agency being proposed here. In addition, it helps us to develop key functional architectural components for action discovery. Finally, the interpretation of alternative hypotheses in the same framework will facilitate a comparison of hypotheses. We start by describing the behavioural and neurobiological paradigm we are attempting to formalise.

2 The Action-Outcome Paradigm

We first outline the situation we have in mind in functional terms; many of the terms such as "action" and "context", which we define more precisely later, occur informally here. We imagine an animal interacting with its environment and trying to discover causal relations between itself and the environment, that is, developing a sense of "agency", in which events caused by the agent are discovered and the causal components of behavioural output determined. This is supposed to occur through an exploration of the animal's environment in a way that is governed by the unpredictability of the outcome associated with the action(s) performed.

In much of our exposition elsewhere, we have used the term "novelty" in a very general sense to mean this unpredictability. Here we will find it useful to distinguish between the unpredictability of simple phasic outcomes (such as a luminance change) and the more general case that might require evaluation of complex aspects of the environment (e.g. new objects or old ones in new situations). We will refer to the former as *surprise* and the general case as *novelty*. Thus, we conceive of surprise as a special (limited) instance of novelty and will use "novelty" where a general interpretation suffices, and only specialise to "surprise" where necessary. These definitions are formalised in Sect. 3.3. Much of our exposition will focus on surprise, which is sufficient to cause phasic dopamine release (Schultz et al. 1997).

In the action-outcome paradigm, post-action, unpredicted change may, or may not, be caused by the animal's behaviour; it might be purely coincidental and noncorrelated with behaviour. The animal is therefore attempting to discover whether there is, in fact, a causal link between any aspect of its behaviour and the outcome. In any case, if the post-action environment is unexpected, there is a sensory prediction error between what is anticipated and what actually occurs.

While the outcome is surprising, the animal continues to explore possibilities for causal relations between its actions and the environment. During this exploratory phase, we suppose the animal will have its action-selection policy biased to repeat those actions which most recently preceded unpredicted outcomes; we refer to this process as *repetition bias*. As well as being surprising, these outcomes may contain other novel elements requiring rich sensory representations. Repetition bias allows the reliable presentation of such representations, together with relevant contextual and motor (action-related) signals, to associative networks in the brain, thereby allowing establishment of internal models of causal relations.

In the process of "latent learning" (Tolman 1948), animals which have *sufficient exposure* to an environment are able to learn a model of that environment (including action-outcome contingencies) which may be recruited at a later stage for goal-directed behaviour. One view of repetition bias in our scenario, therefore, is that it is a means of ensuring rapid and plentiful exposure to the correct stimuli for learning of action-outcome contingencies for later deployment.

We now detail some neurobiological specifics which act as constraints on our thinking. We propose that the ability for a surprising outcome to effect policy change (repetition bias) is critically dependent on it being able to elicit short latency phasic (transient) changes in levels of the neurotransmitter dopamine. This, in turn, works by facilitating synaptic plasticity between cortex and the basal ganglia—a set of subcortical structures which are believed to be a key locus for implementing the action policy. Details of how this synaptic plasticity causes policy change and the role of the basal ganglia in our paradigm are provided in the companion chapter.

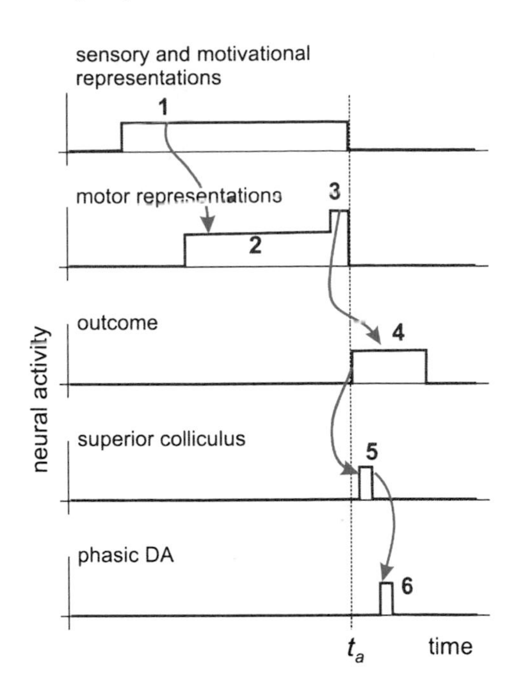

Fig. 1 Neural representations and causality in the action-outcome learning scheme. *Red traces* are activity levels in various neural representations. *Green arrows* show causal relation between representations

For our purposes here, it is enough to summarise the supposed sequence of neural events after an action with an unpredicted causal outcome (numbers refer to items in Fig. 1).

Cortical representations of sensory and motivational information (1) initiate representations of motor *preparation* (2). For example, in the case of reaching, this preparatory activity is encoded in areas of posterior parietal cortex (PPC) (Snyder et al. 1997). Of all possible actions being initiated, usually only one will be selected for execution by the basal ganglia.

In Fig. 1, the action is supposed to occur prior to time t_a and has motor representation (3) (shown with signal level elevated with respect to that for preparatory motor representations). The basis for this selection is that highly active or *salient* representations in cortex are able to dominate competitive mechanisms in basal ganglia, thereby enabling their behavioural enactment. Salience may be influenced by task-, goal- or reward-related information.

It is important to note that the neural signals have been shown for only one motor act. In addition, behaviour is assumed continuous, and so similar sets of signals will be in various stages of development at any time. This scheme is similar to that of Cisek (2007) and Cisek and Kalaska (2010) who stress the intimate relation between partial action specification (preparation) and action selection. Thus, the environment offers a continuous stream of possible actions or *affordances* which generate an associated stream of contextual and preparatory activity for each action. These activities are then run in a continuous competition to yield a single behavioural action. This idea is formalised in our notion of *action request* (Sect. 4.1). The gradual transition from perceptual to action-based representation also has resonance with the notion that perception exists *for* action, not passive evaluation of the environment (Allport et al. 1987).

The action will cause a phasic change in the environment which leads to a perceptual representation of that outcome (4). In particular, there will be a signal in superior colliculus (a midbrain structure) that responds simply to the phasic onset of the outcome, and a gaze shift is initiated. The collicular signal will also elicit a phasic response in dopamine neurons via their direct innervation (Comoli et al. 2003; Dommett et al. 2005). The phasic dopamine facilitates cortico-striatal plasticity which makes the repetition of the action more likely in the current situation. Finally, after the gaze shift and after more sophisticated cortical sensory processing, more complex representations of the structural features of the outcome will occur in cortex.

As an example, consider the sensory information provided by the animal being near a light switch constituted by a long toggle or lever. If the animal does not know the specific action required to operate the switch, several motor preparatory representations might be elicited (pushing up or down, rotating the toggle, etc). Eventually an action is selected and some outcome ensues. If it turns on the light, there will be a phasic response in the colliculus due to a change in luminance, and subsequently, a specific light will be identified as the outcome with accompanying nuances of light levels, shadows cast, etc. In a more extreme scenario, the animal will not have acted intentionally with the toggle, but will have accidentally switched it on while pursuing other behaviours. More exploration is required in this case to discover causality, but the principles of action discovery we outline here are supposed to apply quite generally.

Other relevant process at work here include habituation and sensitisation. Habituation of sensory representations refers to a decline in response when the perceptual features are no longer surprising or novel *and* do not have any rewarding consequences (Sokolov 1963). In the example, once the causal relation between the switch and the light onset has been discovered, we expect the colliculus response to decline (if the light onset has no rewarding consequences). In contrast, sensitisation (elevated response) occurs if the caused event is a reward or reward predictor (Ikeda and Hikosaka 2003; Wurtz and Albano 1980). These phenomena will form a key part of our narrative.

3 Formalisation

3.1 The Environment and Its Internal Representation

The Environment

Our basic objects are dynamically evolving environmental or "world" states, which are experienced by the animal or agent, and corresponding internal states or neural representations, which are constituted by patterns of activity over populations of neurons. Thus, we suppose that, at any time t_s, the external world is in some state $\boldsymbol{\gamma}(t_s) \in \Gamma_S$, where Γ_S is the set of all possible world states and t_s is the time at which the state occurs. The use of bold symbols to represent states implies they are some kind of *vector*.[1] The evolution of the world in time through this state space then defines a vector-valued function,[2] its trajectory or *world path* $\boldsymbol{\gamma}$, through Γ_S:

$$\boldsymbol{\gamma} : \mathbb{R} \to \Gamma_S , \qquad \boldsymbol{\gamma} \in \Gamma ,$$

where the space of possible world paths is denoted by Γ. While there is no technical limit on the time domain, pragmatically, we may choose to limit time around some relevant epoch in the animal's history with consequent limiting of Γ.

The use of dynamic trajectories in *function* space as the grounding for our ideas, rather than instantaneously defined *states*, allows a more flexible and realistic interpretation of perception, its relation to action and the use of prediction. It encompasses, as a special case, the use of states defined at single times, even if these are defined over a continuous time domain (as, e.g. in the work of Oudeyer and Kaplan 2007). The approach is inspired by the use of functional methods in physics for studying dynamics and, while it lacks the superficial simplicity of discrete, state-based views, we contend that because animal behaviour is at least as complex as that of inanimate systems, the functional approach will ultimately facilitate a simpler analysis when we confront the complexities of behaviour head on.

Representations of the Environment

Corresponding to states in the world, we suppose there are internal states of the agent or brain states in some set N_S. We will refer to the components of the vectors in N_S as the *neural features* of the state (which might, e.g. be the activity of a population of neurons).

Then, in line with our continuous, dynamic approach, we define the space of time-dependent *neural representations* N_Γ which are vector-valued functions, $\boldsymbol{y}$, of time

$$\boldsymbol{y} : \mathbb{R} \to N_S , \qquad \boldsymbol{y} \in N_\Gamma .$$

Representations are supposed to arise in the brain via sensory processes perceiving the environment as a stimulus. Although the exact trajectory of $\boldsymbol{y}$ may also depend on the history of the agent and its internal states, we will refer to

[1] We use the term "vector", but in the sense adopted in computer science to mean a 1D-array or n-tuple; there is no implication that these n-tuples form a true vector space. Indeed, if we use only positive-valued components (a natural choice to indicate presence of a feature), the space does not have an additive inverse.

[2] We use the normal convention that y denotes a function and $y(t)$ its value at time t.

a transformation from world trajectories to their neural correlates as a *sensory transformation* $\mathcal{S}$; it is a mapping from the space of world paths Γ to representations N_Γ

$$\mathcal{S} : \Gamma \to N_\Gamma \qquad \text{with} \qquad y = \mathcal{S}[\boldsymbol{\gamma}] \tag{1}$$

(where the notation $\mathcal{T}[\cdot]$ denotes a mapping from one function space to another). At this stage, $\boldsymbol{y}$ includes all internal state information about the agent; we do not distinguish between "sensory" and "motor" representations, although this will prove useful later. Note that we may be interested in a variety of different sensory transformations with different levels of complexity, making use of more or less limited representation spaces. However, we will avoid a proliferation of such spaces as far as possible and refer to relations in (1) in a generic sense.

It is also natural to seek a mapping between neural representations and the world, a feature which will be particularly useful in dealing with prediction. In general, we assume that the world is richer than our mental representations of it. For example, visual perception is acknowledged to be an ill-posed problem (Poggio and Koch 1985) in which multiple world states give rise to the same visual percept, and more broadly, perceptual neural representations generalise across stimuli (small nuances of the world are often lost unless we have a special reason to encode them). There is, in general therefore, an equivalence class of world paths $\tilde{\boldsymbol{\gamma}}$, which all have the same neural representation $\boldsymbol{y}$, and we define the inverse mapping from representations to the set of world path equivalence classes $\tilde{\Gamma}$:

$$\mathcal{S}^{-1} : N_\Gamma \to \tilde{\Gamma} \qquad \text{with} \qquad \mathcal{S}^{-1}[\boldsymbol{y}] = \tilde{\boldsymbol{\gamma}} \ . \tag{2}$$

Contexts and Outcomes

In the action-outcome situation we consider, much hinges around comparing representations either side of some critical time (t_a in Fig. 1). It is therefore convenient to define subsegments of $\boldsymbol{\gamma}$ with respect to the current time t_s. From the animal's point of view, that part of $\boldsymbol{\gamma}$ in the past constitutes its *context* $\boldsymbol{\gamma}^-$. Thus, if the time domain is $T^- = (-\infty, t_\mathrm{s}]$,

$$\boldsymbol{\gamma}^- : T^- \to \Gamma_\mathrm{S} \qquad \text{with} \qquad \boldsymbol{\gamma}^-(t) = \boldsymbol{\gamma}(t) \ , \qquad t \in T^- \ .$$

In a similar way, we define the *outcome* as the future trajectory, so with time domain $T^+ = [t_\mathrm{s}, \infty)$,

$$\boldsymbol{\gamma}^+ : T^+ \to \Gamma_\mathrm{S} \qquad \text{with} \qquad \boldsymbol{\gamma}^+(t) = \boldsymbol{\gamma}(t) \ , \qquad t \in T^+ \ .$$

The context has a corresponding neural representation $\boldsymbol{y}^-$, where

$$\boldsymbol{y}^- = \mathcal{S}[\boldsymbol{\gamma}^-] \ ,$$

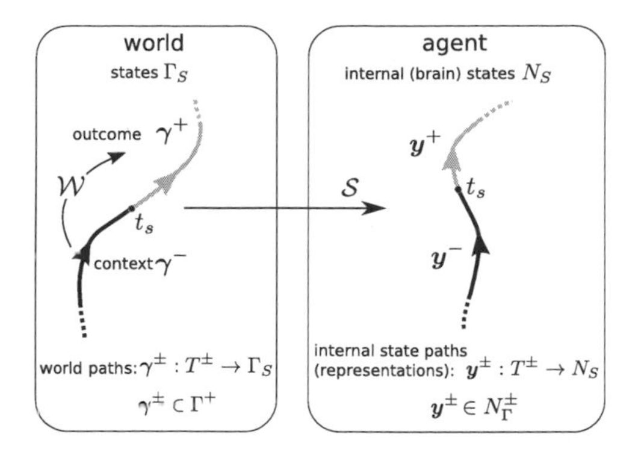

Fig. 2 Graphic depiction of the formalisation thus far. The world (or environment) is described by spaces of vector-valued states (Γ_S, N_S, respectively). However, the emphasis is on vector-valued functions of time which define "trajectories" or "paths" through these state spaces. It is convenient to consider the trajectory referenced to some time marker t_s so that prior/subsequent events constitute a *context/outcome*, respectively. This will usually apply to some phasic event at t_s, but this is not a requirement. Internal representations are derived by *sensory transforms* like $\mathcal{S}$ occurring within the agent

and the functions $\boldsymbol{\gamma}^-$ and $\boldsymbol{y}^-$ reside in spaces Γ^- and N_Γ^-, respectively. These spaces are simply suitable temporal restrictions of Γ and N_Γ and will be useful in introducing notions of prediction. The outcome also has representation $\boldsymbol{y}^+ = \mathcal{S}[\boldsymbol{\gamma}^+]$ with associated spaces N_Γ^+, Γ^+.

The physics of the world dictate how contexts are transformed into outcomes, and we define a *world transform* $\mathcal{W}$:

$$\mathcal{W} : \Gamma^- \to \Gamma^+ \qquad \text{where} \qquad \boldsymbol{\gamma}^+ = \mathcal{W}[\boldsymbol{\gamma}^-] \,. \tag{3}$$

Reference to this kind of transform will serve to highlight the contrast between the way contexts get transformed into outcomes in the world and the way their representational counterparts get transformed in the agent. The formalism described so far is summarised in Fig. 2. Notice that, while we will normally regard the context/outcome boundary as some pivotal, operantly defined time $t_s = t_a$ (see Fig. 1), this is not necessary, and the formalism holds for an arbitrary partition of time.

3.2 Behaviour and Action

Behaviour

Behaviour is defined in an analogous way to the environment as an evolving trajectory of *externally observable* states that the agent or animal can take. Formally, we suppose that at each time t_s, the physical pose of the animal is described by a vector $\beta(t_s)$ with $\beta(t_s) \in B_S$. Behaviour is defined as the trajectory given by the vector-valued function:

$$\boldsymbol{\beta} : \mathbb{R} \rightarrow B_S \ .$$

Since the animal can observe itself, B_S is a subspace of the world states Γ_S; that is, the animal's body is part of its environment.[3] This approach enables us to subsume the effects of action into the existing framework, since behaviour is then just a part of the world's trajectory; that is, $\boldsymbol{\beta}$ is a suitable restriction of $\boldsymbol{\gamma}$ so that its range or codomain is B_S.

Action

Actions are conceived of as discrete blocks of behaviour defined over finite time intervals. In particular, we are interested in intervals just prior to operantly relevant times t_a. Thus, if $T_{act} = \{t : t_a - \Delta t < t \leq t_a\}$, for any finite Δt, we define the action

$$\boldsymbol{\alpha} : T_{act} \rightarrow B_S \qquad \text{with} \qquad \boldsymbol{\alpha}(t) = \boldsymbol{\beta}(t) \ , \quad t \in T_{act} \ .$$

The functional definition of action is quite general, with no constraint on its temporal extent or ethological semantics. This generality is a useful starting point because it is notoriously non-trivial to segment behaviour in a meaningful way into discrete actions (Schleidt and Kien 1997).

Representations of Behaviour and Action

We now turn to the neural representations of behaviour and action; the approach here mirrors that of the environment. Behaviour will elicit sensory representation of the agent's own body, but more importantly for us here, behaviour is associated with internal *motor states* in a subspace $N_M \subset N_S$, in which features in N_M are responsible for eliciting the behaviour. In a similar way, then, to the treatment of world trajectories and behaviour, we define a motor neural representation of behaviour, $\boldsymbol{b}$, that is a restriction of $\boldsymbol{y}$ to a function with codomain N_M. These ideas are shown in Fig. 3.

Note that the designation of internal state features as "motor" (defined by their being in N_M) has no agenda about what constitutes a motor signal; indeed, different settings and models may require different selections of N_M. However, while neural representations are often allowed to have sensory and motor aspects, it is useful to be able to refer to the complementary space $N_{S \backslash M}$, of N_M with respect to N_S, as

[3]Throughout this chapter, we use the expression "A is a subspace of B" (or $A \subset B$) to mean that A is defined over a subset of the features in B. Also, note that B is supposed to be upper case Greek β in keeping with the notation that Greek and Roman symbols refer to the external world and neural representations, respectively.

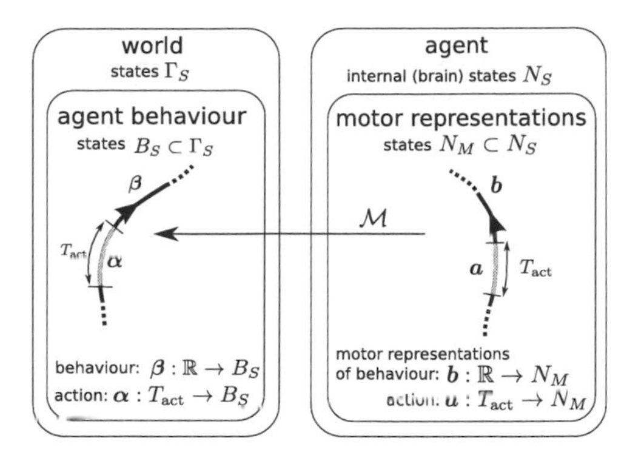

Fig. 3 Graphic depiction of the formalisation of behaviour and action. Behaviour is described with respect to a subspace of the world states $B_S \subset \Gamma_S$ via trajectories $\boldsymbol{\beta}$ through B_S. Corresponding motor representations $\boldsymbol{b}$ are defined through a subspace $N_M \subset N_S$ of internal states. Actions are defined as behaviour over a small time segment T_{act} with associated representations $\boldsymbol{a}$. *Motor transforms* like $\mathcal{M}$ occur within the agent

"sensory" neural states.[4] The sensory states give rise to sensory representations $\boldsymbol{c}$ so that the entire internal representation $\boldsymbol{y}$ is defined by the pair $[\boldsymbol{b}, \boldsymbol{c}]$.

Actions are represented by a suitable temporal restriction of $\boldsymbol{b}$. The neural representation of action $\boldsymbol{\alpha}$ will be denoted $\boldsymbol{a}$. Behaviour may be divided into contextual and outcome phases with respect to some specific time, t_a, and we will usually consider an action as occurring in the contextual period (that is, T_{act} terminates at t_a—see above). The context therefore has motor and sensory representations grounded in N_M and $N_{S \setminus M}$ respectively.

From Representation to Behaviour

We define a *motor transformation* $\boldsymbol{\beta} = \mathcal{M}[\boldsymbol{b}]$ or its action equivalent $\boldsymbol{\alpha} = \mathcal{M}[\boldsymbol{a}]$ which shows how the internal state of the agent elicits behaviour.

Minimal and Efficient Action

The definition of action so far is quite general; behaviour is unsegmented agent activity, and actions, while time delimited, have no ethological definition as yet. However, we want to consider 'strongly' causal models of the world, and it may be helpful, on occasion, to be specific about which actions we are considering. Consider the light switch toggle example described earlier. There are a multitude of actions which will "do the job": operating the toggle while waving the other

[4] $N_{S \setminus M}$ is defined over the features in N_S which are *not* contained in N_M.

hand/paw in the air or walking in a circle before pressing the toggle—all are effective actions in the sense defined above. However, learning that such actions are necessary for a particular outcome amounts to developing "superstitious" behaviour (Timberlake and Lucas 1985). What is needed is the notion of a *minimal* or most *efficient* action.

Consider first the elimination of spurious components of action ("hand or paw waving"). Elimination of action components amounts to defining behaviour using proper subspaces $B_i \subset B_S$. Then, let B_I be the intersection of all such B_i rich enough to define actions that can cause a given outcome.

Elimination of spurious prior actions amounts to considering the smallest T_{act} for which a biologically realisable action exists that can yield the given outcome. This minimisation has to be done with both world and animal in mind, for whereas the world is only concerned about the action $\boldsymbol{\alpha}(t_a)$ *at* time t_a, (e.g. required force on the toggle), it is not possible for the animal to generate $\boldsymbol{\alpha}(t_a)$ without a prior action trajectory (start moving the paw and increase speed) which may be subject to a range of dynamic and kinematic constraints (Körding and Wolpert 2006).

With these issues in mind, we define a *minimal action* $\boldsymbol{\alpha}$ for a given outcome, as that defined by B_I, and the correspondingly smallest T_{act}. A key part of the process of *action discovery* then may be the establishing of a minimal action for a given outcome.[5]

3.3 Prediction

The notion of prediction is pervasive throughout much theoretical neuroscience: it is a key idea in computational reinforcement learning (Sutton and Barto 1998) (where it occurs as estimates of future reward), and Friston (2005) has elevated prediction to the central pillar of any theoretical account of the brain. This is not an unreasonable stance for, if an animal can predict its environment and the result of its actions, it can generate integrated, goal-directed behaviour in an efficient manner.

Prediction is a result of the animal having some kind of *internal model* of the world. In our framework, an internal model can be used to allow neural representations derived from *context* to influence future sensory representations of *outcome*, where these terms are used in the sense defined in Sect. 3.1. We have in mind here that processes, like habituation, sensitisation from reward or "priming" of sensory systems via task information, all result from signals becoming manifest via internal models of one kind or another and that they all modify sensory representations.

Internal models, as we envision them, have several important characteristics in addition to their general role as predictors. First, they result from structural

[5]Other notions of action efficiency/optimality could have been used (e.g. minimal energy expenditure), but temporal optimality and action simplicity seem most appropriate in the context of action discovery.

parameters within the brain architecture of networks of neurons and the strengths of the connections therein. Second, the internal model may be viewed as performing a form of data compression or abstraction on the input: "raw" input is transformed into key abstract features, and it is these features that are used to generate predictions. For example, a red ball is represented not as a multitude of independent red "pixels", but rather as the abstract concept of a sphere parameterised by colour and size. In addition, as a result of the data compression, the model generalises so that it makes similar predictions from a variety of related inputs. The data compression characteristic of an internal model enables us to make contact with theories of novelty and intrinsic motivation that are related to information compression (Schmidhuber 2009). Third, while the model is structurally encoded in a network architecture, the model only becomes "expressed" or "manifest" when it elicits output signals; that is, it generates neural activity that represents predicted sensory information (such as the appearance of a red ball within the visual field of the agent).

As an example to illustrate these ideas, consider a feedforward neural network with "hidden" units, conceived of as a statistical model of some data. One interpretation of its operation is that, given a pattern of "context" at the input layer, the network delivers a "prediction" at the output layer. The model is encoded in the network connection strengths, but the prediction is made manifest only when the net delivers its output signals. The network may be viewed as performing a data compression on the input because the hidden layers extract only key features of the data (especially if the number of hidden units is less than that of the inputs). As a result of the data compression, the network generalises and will make similar "predictions" from a wide variety of inputs.

Representation of Predictions

The *internal* representations of predictions elicited by an internal model will, in general, be trajectories of internal states denoted $\mathbf{y}^*$. These constitute a class of internal representations, and since we want predictions to interact with sensory-derived representations—typically in some process of comparison—we identify the space of $\mathbf{y}^*$ with N_Γ. While a sensory prediction y^* is *developed* during the contextual period (if it is to reliably influence representations in the outcome, y^+), they are *deployed* during the outcome when they are compared with y^+. We therefore consider the space of trajectories $y^* \in N_\Gamma^+$.

Internal Prediction Models

An internal prediction model $\mathcal{I}_\mathrm{P}$ is a map from representations of context to those of outcome, generating an internal prediction y^*:

$$\mathcal{I}_\mathrm{P} : N_\Gamma^- \to N_\Gamma^+ \qquad \text{with} \qquad y^* = \mathcal{I}_\mathrm{P}[y^-] \,. \tag{4}$$

We also refer to $\mathcal{I}_{\mathrm{P}}$ as a feedforward model to distinguish it from inverse models defined later. In practice, the trajectories will be defined over a suitable subspace of N_{S} since the entire brain state is not usually required to generate a prediction. The paths $\boldsymbol{y}^*, \boldsymbol{y}^-$ are then suitable restrictions defined over this subspace.

Phasic Events and their Predictions

A phasic event is defined by a segment of world path, $\boldsymbol{\gamma}_{\phi}$, restricted to only a short time interval $T_{\phi} = [t_{\phi}, t_{\phi} + \Delta t]$; that is, $\boldsymbol{\gamma}_{\phi} : T_{\phi} \rightarrow \Gamma_{\mathrm{S}}$. Under a sensory transform, there will be a corresponding short-lived representation of the event, $\boldsymbol{y}_{\phi} = \mathcal{S}[\boldsymbol{\gamma}_{\phi}]$. We will denote the associated internal representations of predictions with their event suffix $\boldsymbol{y}^*_{\phi}$ where the intention is that $\boldsymbol{y}^*_{\phi}$ is active for a time of the order of Δt centred around T_{ϕ}.

Predictions in the World

We have emphasised prediction as something occurring internally to the agent. However, we also speak of predictions as being grounded in the world—simply saying "the light will come on" refers to the world, not our internal state. This aspect of prediction is addressed through an inverse mapping such as (2), in which the predicted sensory representation $\mathbf{y}^*$ can be transformed to an equivalence class of world trajectories, $\mathcal{S}^{-1}[\boldsymbol{y}^*] = \tilde{\boldsymbol{\gamma}}$.

Sensory Error Functions

Predictions only become useful if they are used to make comparisons with representations of reality, derived directly from sensory transforms of the environment, that is $\boldsymbol{y}^+$. This is accomplished using an error function $\mathcal{E}[\boldsymbol{y}^*, \boldsymbol{y}^+]$ to derive error signals e. Such functions may or may not be true metrics or divergences, and several may be needed to capture all relevant aspects of the contrast between prediction and percept. Error signals may then be used to drive adjustment of the prediction models $\mathcal{I}_{\mathrm{P}}$ so that they become increasingly accurate and are able to deliver better predictions (in the sense of minimising e).

Novelty and Surprise

Novelty and surprise have been discussed in computational terms in a variety of ways by other authors (see, e.g. Baldi and Itti 2010; Oudeyer and Kaplan 2007; Ranganath and Rainer 2003). Our interpretation was noted in Sect. 2 and we formalise it here. Thus, we take surprise to mean an error defined over a phasic

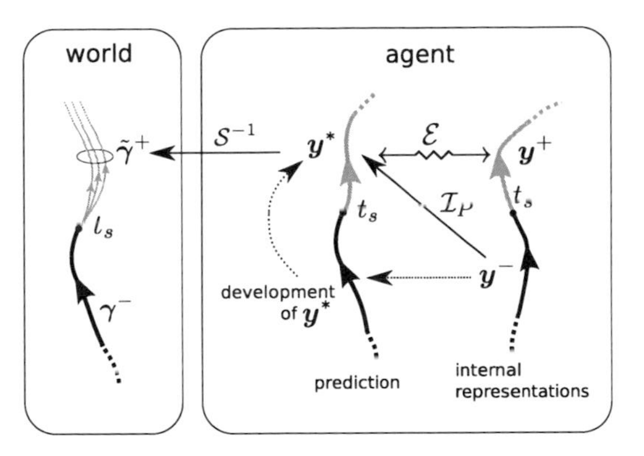

Fig. 4 Graphic depiction of the formalisation of prediction. Internal representations $\boldsymbol{y}^{-}$ prior to some time t_s (differentiating context from outcome) start to cause predictions to occur ("development of $\boldsymbol{y}^{*}$"). These continue to evolve beyond t_s and are deployed after t_s. Error signals are obtained by comparing $\boldsymbol{y}^{+}$ and $\boldsymbol{y}^{*}$ using an error function $\mathcal{E}$ (a metric or divergence between pairs of functions in the space N_{Γ}^{+}). The model $\mathcal{I}_{\mathrm{P}}$ is defined as function which maps $\boldsymbol{y}^{-}$ to $\boldsymbol{y}^{*} \in N_{\Gamma}^{+}$. Internal predictions like $\boldsymbol{y}^{*}$ are associated (via inverse sensory maps like $\mathcal{S}^{-1}$) with nonunique world paths which collectively form equivalence classes like $\tilde{\boldsymbol{\gamma}}^{+}$

outcome and its prediction, which makes use of only a single feature y_{ϕ}^{+} (e.g. luminance change). That is,

$$\text{surprise} : \mathcal{E}(y_{\phi}^{+}, y_{\phi}^{*}) \, . \tag{5}$$

The prediction model which gives rise to y_{ϕ}^{*} is denoted $\mathcal{I}_{\mathrm{P}_{\phi}}$. Any error measure which is more general than this (i.e. with non-phasic features or vector-valued representations in general) will necessarily require the use of the term "novelty".

$$\text{novelty} : \mathcal{E}(\boldsymbol{y}^{+}, \boldsymbol{y}^{*}) \, . \tag{6}$$

Such an error will be associated with the general prediction model $\mathcal{I}_{\mathrm{P}}$. The definition in (6) subsumes that in (5) as a special case, and this is reflected in our use of terminology; we will use "novelty" where a general interpretation suffices, and only specialise to "surprise" where necessary.

The ideas of this section are illustrated in Fig. 4. We now investigate a particularly important representation—that of *salience*—and how it is implicated in several important prediction processes.

4 Salience and Action Selection

In our previous work on action selection, we introduced the notion of the *salience* of sensorimotor representations that contribute to the selection of actions (see companion chapter and Redgrave et al. 1999). Roughly speaking, salience represents the urgency of, or degree of demand for, an action, as encoded in the strength of signals afferent to basal ganglia.

For example, a strong local luminance change will, in many cases, elicit an orienting movement to the locus of that change. The stimulus gives strong activity in the corresponding areas of the brain that respond to these stimuli (such as superior colliculus and frontal eye fields). The locus of the activity in the neural tissue is often topographic with respect to spatial location of the stimulus, suggesting spatially defined "features" in the neural representation of salience. This localised activity elicits the orienting movement (saccade or head movement) with an "urgency" contingent on its overall "strength" or the salience level.

4.1 Formalising Salience

Salience is referenced to a collection of sensorimotor features, suggesting a vector, but, at the same time, has an overall (scalar) "strength". The vector aspect chimes with our definition of neural representations since the supporting space (N_S and its subspaces) contain vectors. Thus, we may write $\boldsymbol{y} = (y_1, y_2, \ldots)$, where individual component functions y_f or features have been articulated. The function y_f may signal the presence of a particular kind of object or *world feature*, which is, in turn, described by several components of the world trajectory $\boldsymbol{\gamma}$. To simplify notation, we will use the index f to refer to the object or world feature signalled by y_f. We will also use the shorter term "feature" to refer to the "world feature" where the context is clear.

Salience Maps

We now suppose there is a particular class of internal representations $\boldsymbol{s} \in N_\Gamma$ which is deployed in action-selection policy formation. We have in mind here that $\boldsymbol{s}$ are signals afferent to basal ganglia and will call this vector the *salience map* (this reference is inspired by the common occurrence of topography of $\boldsymbol{s}$ in the brain). The scope of $\boldsymbol{s}$ is supposed to be large enough to encompass selection of all actions of interest.

Action Requests

Consider now a single action $\boldsymbol{\alpha}$ occurring prior to time t_a which defines a context/outcome partition. Let $N_\alpha \subset N_\Gamma^-$ be a subspace of representations containing just sufficient features of the salience map to elicit $\boldsymbol{\alpha}$. Let $\boldsymbol{s}^{(a)}$ be the restriction of $\boldsymbol{s}$ to N_α, then we refer to $\boldsymbol{s}^{(a)}$ as the *action request* for $\boldsymbol{\alpha}$.

Two Kinds of Action Discovery

In terms of the preceding framework, a key part of the problem of action discovery is to learn how to partition the salience map into sets N_α defining action requests for minimal actions. There are two interesting special cases of action discovery to consider here. First, the action itself (e.g. lever pressing) may be well-learned, and so any motor components of the request are well established, but the sensory contextual components are not (the lever is in a novel situation with novel outcome). The action discovery may then have the behavioural appearance of *purposeful investigative behaviour* (repeated skilful lever pressing). In a second case, both the sensory context *and* the action have to be established. Here, there will be *wide-ranging, exploratory behaviour* (discovering how to interact with levers efficiently) and will involve learning a minimal or efficient action (Sect. 3.1).

Salience as Strength of Action Request

The scalar strength or *salience*, S_α of the action request is supposed to be captured by some measure of its overall level of activity. If we interpret the component features as representative of neural activity, then they are all positive, and we can write

$$S_\alpha = \sum_f s_f^{(a)} , \tag{7}$$

where the sum is over features in the space N_α.

4.2 Salience and Value

We now turn to an interpretation of the salience map that allows us to make closer contact with intrinsically motivated learning and concepts from machine learning. If an action is urgently requested (and assuming a well-trained animal), it is reasonable to suppose that the action is of high "value" to the animal. We use the term "value" in a loose sense here, but for goal-directed behaviours, we suggest that the salience of an action request is, or at least is influenced by, the estimated "action value" as used in machine learning. In action discovery, while the feature sets (defined via $N_\alpha \subset N_\Gamma$) are being determined, the value estimates are being refined. We are now naturally led to the question: what is it about an action that endows it with value?

While our arguments are valid for any sensory modality and class of actions, we draw examples from orienting movements in response to visual stimuli. Thus, consider the topographic maps of salience for visual orienting in colliculus or cortical areas devoted to gaze control such as frontal eye fields. We now suggest there are three broad reasons why a "hotspot" of salience may have developed in the salience maps for orienting (with ensuing redirection of gaze). First, features in the visual field are unpredicted, and so objects at that location in space are "interesting" (surprising or novel). This results in action discovery via intrinsically motivated behaviour. Second, the animal may have associated the object with primary reward (food, drink, etc.) and can direct behaviour immediately to that reward. Third, the object may have been identified as task relevant and, while not known to deliver reward immediately, is believed to be useful in guiding behaviour towards reward as a distal goal.

There is a fourth possibility which, perforce, implies a lack of a correspondence between salience and value. Thus, in the above situations, it is assumed that behaviour is goal directed, in the sense that it is *not* habitual (Balleine and Dickinson 1998; Gurney et al. 2009b). Habitual actions are not contingent on the value of the current goal and are evoked instead by sensory context alone. For habits, therefore, we suppose that action selection is not conducted with reference to internal models of the world and prediction. However, since these concepts are our main concern, we limit ourselves henceforth to goal-directed behaviour and now go on to explore the three components of salience discussed above.

4.2.1 Novelty and Habituation

The first component of value defined above refers to unpredicted sensory features. We make links with the notion of habituation (a decline in response to a feature when that feature is no longer novel and has no rewarding consequences (Sokolov 1963)) and identify the need to consider two kinds of prediction error: failure to predict correctly the occurrence of a feature and failure to predict correctly its absence.

To simplify the arguments, we restrict ourselves at first to a single feature f and consider evaluation over intervals during which the representations may be considered approximately constant. In this case, the feature outcome is represented by a scalar y^+ and the prediction by another scalar y^*. One possible measure of the discrepancy, or error, s_P resulting from the prediction is

$$s_P = |y^+ - y^*| \,. \tag{8}$$

The notation s_P is supposed to suggest that this is a salience signal derived from a prediction. Poor prediction results in a larger value for s_P, and there is then surprise or novelty, according to whether the feature f is (respectively) a phasic event or more continuously available. As the prediction becomes more accurate, s_P becomes smaller, and the detection of the feature habituates. Habituation is therefore viewed as a consequence of development of the internal model responsible for y^*.

The right-hand side of (8) is symmetric with respect to sign$(y^+ - y^*)$. There is, however, a profound contrast in interpretation under sign change. For if $y^+ > y^*$, this signifies novelty through a failure to adequately predict a feature's *presence*. However, if $y^+ < y^*$, this signifies novelty because of failure to predict an *absence* of the feature. Mechanistically, if we assume one of y^+, y^* supplies inhibitory and the other excitatory signals to a neural novelty detector, then it is not clear how the neuron can be excited by a net negative activity (if, say $y^+ < y^*$).

It is therefore more natural to split the salience due to novelty across two kinds of detectors: one which signals presence of unpredicted features, $s_{P\wedge}$, and one which signals absence of predicted features, $s_{P\vee}$.

$$\begin{aligned} s_{P\wedge} &= [y^+ - y^*]_{\geq 0} \\ s_{P\vee} &= [y^* - y^+]_{\geq 0} , \end{aligned} \tag{9}$$

where $[x]_{\geq 0}$ is a half-wave rectification function ($[x]_{\geq 0} = x$, if $x \geq 0$, and is 0 otherwise).[6] Their separation makes sense, not just from a mechanistic point of view, but because different actions may be required according to whether novelty is determined via the absence or presence of a feature.

The existence of "absence detectors" like $s_{P\vee}$ is more than just a theoretical possibility. In our account of prediction errors in Sect. 5, we will introduce the idea that the lateral habenula may encode such signals (Matsumoto and Hikosaka 2007). In the meantime, we will focus on those like $s_{P\wedge}$, which we suppose are the norm. Our exposition has focussed on a single feature, and if that feature refers to a phasic outcome, the error measure denotes surprise. In all other cases, we are dealing with a salience map from novelty which will, in general, be a vector-valued function of time $\mathbf{s}_P$, obtained by considering all features and their time evolution. This may not simultaneously contain "feature present" and "feature absent" forms, but we can write, in general,

$$\mathbf{s}_P = \mathbf{s}_{P\wedge} + \mathbf{s}_{P\vee} . \tag{10}$$

We now move on to consider other contributions to salience features which are intimately linked to goal-directed behaviour. Essentially, our hypothesis is that behaviour directed at obtaining reward, or achieving goal-directed outcomes, occurs because the requests for the pertinent actions are generated by "inverse models" from goals/rewards to action requests. Specifically, action requests are produced via a process of *sensitisation* of representations of salience features via top-down signals derived from the internal models.

4.2.2 Reward and Salience

We start by considering behaviour (such as orienting, reach and approach) which may be directly driven by reward-related stimuli comprising high-level visual features or objects. Let $x_R(t)$ be the motivational level for seeking reward of type R (e.g. food). Then we suppose there is a learned, *inverse* or "top-down" internal

[6] This is equivalent to $xH(x)$ where $H(x)$ is the Heaviside function, but the notation in the text is more expedient here.

model[7] $\mathcal{I}_{\mathrm{R}}$ which causes x_{R} to sensitise representations of features $\boldsymbol{y}_{\mathrm{R}} \in N_{\Gamma}$, related to objects that carry reward R (Ikeda and Hikosaka 2003; Wurtz and Albano 1980). Another term often used here is that the features have been *conditioned* through learning about the contingencies associated with the reward. This process is indeed one of "sensitisation" of pre-existing representations derived through perception, rather than initiation of new ones (otherwise, the agent would be hallucinating the presence of the associated features and objects). This is captured by putting $\mathcal{I}_{\mathrm{R}}(\boldsymbol{y}_{\mathrm{R}}, x_{\mathrm{R}}) = \boldsymbol{y}_{\mathrm{R}} f(x_{\mathrm{R}})$, where $f(x_{\mathrm{R}})$ is a positive scalar, and supposing that the sensitised feature representation $\hat{\boldsymbol{y}}_{\mathrm{R}}$ is given by

$$\begin{aligned} \hat{\boldsymbol{y}}_{\mathrm{R}} &= \boldsymbol{y}_{\mathrm{R}} + \mathcal{I}_{\mathrm{R}}(\boldsymbol{y}_{\mathrm{R}}, x_{\mathrm{R}}) \\ &= \boldsymbol{y}_{\mathrm{R}}(1 + f(x_{\mathrm{R}})) \, . \end{aligned} \tag{11}$$

If the sensitisation is transmitted to salience for action, it therefore contributes an amount

$$\boldsymbol{s}_{\mathrm{R}} = \mathcal{I}_{\mathrm{R}}(\boldsymbol{y}_{\mathrm{R}}, x_{\mathrm{R}}) = \boldsymbol{y}_{\mathrm{R}} f(x_{\mathrm{R}}) \tag{12}$$

to that salience.

Often this process may take place in two stages. First, spatially invariant representations of entire objects are sensitised; this kind of learning may take place at any time in the agent's lifetime. Then, second, these representations are transformed to topographic representations of salience that request actions such as visual orienting, reach and approach (Connor et al. 2004; Cope et al. 2009; Thompson et al. 2005). These transforms might be an integral part of the sensorimotor system and are acquired in early development of the animal.

4.2.3 Goal or Outcome-Based Salience

We now turn to models that go to the heart of our exposition: those dealing with the relation between learned actions and outcomes. In this case, we want top-down information about desired outcomes or goals to become manifest at the level of motor action selection. Each such outcome may be a stage on the way to some final goal (acquiring food may require going outside, making a car journey, going shopping, etc.), but we will refer to each subtask as a goal in its own right.

The argument proceeds in an analogous way to that for reward, but our starting point here are representations of goal $\boldsymbol{y}_{\mathrm{G}} \in N_{\Gamma}$. These may include features about objects, whole scenes, and spatial relationships. In any case, we suppose there are inverse models $\mathcal{I}_{\mathrm{G}}$ providing contributions $\boldsymbol{s}_{\mathrm{G}}$ to action salience via mappings of the form

$$\mathcal{I}_{\mathrm{G}}[\boldsymbol{y}_{\mathrm{G}}] = \boldsymbol{s}_{\mathrm{G}} \, . \tag{13}$$

---

[7] Some researchers call this a *competence* model 3.

Once again (just as for $\mathcal{I}_R$), $\mathcal{I}_G$ may be composed of multiple stages; from "high-level" representations of outcome situations to objects to salience maps for motoric acts such as reach and gaze. However, we also admit the possibility that some instances of $\mathcal{I}_R$ map one high-level representation to another in generating sequence behaviour, in which one task outcome generates the next desired outcome. These high-level representations, occurring in limbic and associative structures, may also be subject to selection under basal ganglia control (Yin and Knowlton 2006).

Notice that the action-outcome model $\mathcal{I}_G$ is a model of how the action for the outcome is invoked, that is, how a representation of the desired outcome in y_G is transformed into an action request s_G. Thus, $\mathcal{I}_G$ is a model of *deployment*, not *prediction*, which is the role of forward models such as $\mathcal{I}_P$ described in Sect. 3.3. These two models may be intimately related. The prediction (e.g. my computer will wake from sleep) derived from a context (sat at the computer and pressed the space bar) under $\mathcal{I}_P$ may, itself, correspond to a desired outcome. Thus, under a related model $\mathcal{I}_G$, this outcome (computer waking from sleep) must elicit an action request (press space bar) which was part of the original context for $\mathcal{I}_P$. It is in this sense that one model is the inverse of the other. The main point to note is that two distinct models are required for action-outcome learning.

4.3 *Combining Salience Contributions*

We now synthesise the results of the previous subsections on the definition of salience contributions to define the overall salience s for goal-directed action. We assume that salience, within a particular salience map or brain structure, is additive with respect to its various contributions components s_P, s_R, s_G defined via (10), (12) and (13), respectively.

$$\begin{aligned} s &= \mathcal{E} \text{ using } \mathcal{I}_P + \mathcal{I}_R(y_R, x_R) + \mathcal{I}_G[y_G] \\ s &= \underset{\text{novelty and surprise}}{s_P} + \underset{\text{immediate reward}}{s_R} + \underset{\text{goal/outcome}}{s_G}, \end{aligned} \tag{14}$$

where the first equation indicates the internal models used and the second, the notation we use for salience.

5 Sensory Prediction Errors

Errors initiated by surprise at phasic events are at the centre of our exegesis of the role played by phasic dopamine. Here, we build on the work in Sect. 4.2.1 to develop a more detailed account of such errors. The implications for habituating to, and prediction of, these phasic events is described, but the full implications for learning internal models is deferred until Sect. 6.1.

Sensory Prediction Errors and Their Implementation in the Brain

It is often useful to allow error signals for learning to take positive and negative values so that they can force increments and decrements, respectively, in model parameters. In our current context, the target is what actually transpires in the form of the outcome $\mathbf{y}^+$, and the prediction is $\mathbf{y}^*$. That is, we define a *sensory prediction error* Δ by

$$\Delta = \mathbf{y}^+ - \mathbf{y}^* . \tag{15}$$

We now specialise to the case based on surprise, where the outcome is encoded by a single feature y_ϕ^+ of a phasic event and the scalar prediction y_ϕ^* is a result of a prediction model $\mathcal{I}_{\mathrm{P}_\phi}$ (see Sect. 3.3). Then (15) becomes

$$\Delta_\phi = y_\phi^+ - y_\phi^* . \tag{16}$$

A brain structure which has been implicated in such processing is the superior colliculus (SC) (Wurtz and Albano 1980). However, the SC cannot encode Δ_ϕ itself since it delivers only non-negative salience signals $s_{\mathrm{P}\wedge}$:

$$s_{\mathrm{P}\wedge} = [y_\phi^+ - y_\phi^*]_{\geq 0} , \tag{17}$$

where we have used the notation (9) to indicate this is a detection of surprise through detection of unpredicted features. In order to compute Δ_ϕ and make use of existing resources such as SC, we require a complementary signal

$$s_{\mathrm{P}\vee} = [y_\phi^* - y_\phi^+]_{\geq 0} , \tag{18}$$

for then

$$\Delta_\phi = s_{\mathrm{P}\wedge} - s_{\mathrm{P}\vee} . \tag{19}$$

Our hypothesis (discussed in detail in Redgrave et al. 2012) is that phasic dopamine encodes Δ_ϕ in Eqs. (16) and (19). Thus, positive phasic changes in dopamine indicate a failure to predict the occurrence of the feature signalled by y_ϕ^+, whereas negative changes ("dips") in dopamine signal the absence of the feature when it was predicted. Physiologically, it will require the combination of an excitatory signal $s_{\mathrm{P}\wedge}$ and an inhibitory one $s_{\mathrm{P}\vee}$. We have argued that SC generates $s_{\mathrm{P}\wedge}$, and there is now evidence that SC directly excites midbrain dopamine neurons (Comoli et al. 2003; Dommett et al. 2005). Recent work by Matsumoto and Hikosaka (2007) has shown that the lateral habenula is able to signal negative prediction errors in the phasic dopamine signal and that it acts on dopamine neurons in an inhibitory way. It is therefore a candidate for encoding $s_{\mathrm{P}\vee}$.

Reward Sensitisation of Sensory Prediction

In spite of our interpretation of phasic dopamine in terms of a sensory prediction error, there is evidence that the strength of the phasic dopamine signal can, under certain circumstances, be modulated by the precise reward value supplied by a stimulus (for review, see Schultz 2010). In particular, Fiorillo et al. (2003) and Tobler et al. (2005) have shown that, with well-trained animals, graded reward probabilities associated with unpredictable phasic events produced phasic dopamine responses which reflected the expected amount of reward. This is often cited as strong evidence that phasic dopamine is signalling reward-prediction error. However, we think the situation is rather subtle and can be incorporated into our scheme as follows.

We take account of reward by supposing that the sensory error is given by a sensitised version of its original value (16). Using ideas leading to (11) and (12), we put

$$\Delta_\phi = (y_\phi^+ - y_\phi^*)(1 + f(x_R)) \,. \tag{20}$$

The term with the difference between the internal representations of stimulus and prediction ensures we retain the requirement that the phasic dopamine signal is suppressed when the stimulus is predicted.

Further, we note that superior colliculus may be sensitised by reward, thereby overcoming habituation to a predicted stimulus in the presence of reward association with that stimulus (Ikeda and Hikosaka 2003). Therefore, using (11) we write the collicular response to the stimulus $s_{P\wedge}$ as

$$s_{P\wedge} = [y_\phi^+(1 + f(x_R)) - y_\phi^*]_{\geq 0} \,. \tag{21}$$

We now require an expression for a complementary inhibitory signal $s_{P\vee}$ so that, just as in (19), the sensory error—this time given by (20)—can be written $\Delta_\phi = s_{P\wedge} - s_{P\vee}$. In line with our neural interpretation thus far, we seek a simple form for $s_{P\vee}$ as a rectified version of its input. While there is no such expression for $s_{P\vee}$ that makes $s_{P\wedge} - s_{P\vee}$ exactly equal to the right-hand side of (20), putting

$$s_{P\vee} = [y_\phi^*(1 + f(x_R)) - y_\phi^+]_{\geq 0} \tag{22}$$

ensures a good approximation. In particular, $s_{P\wedge} - s_{P\vee}$ is a symmetric function of y_ϕ^*, y_ϕ^+, which is zero if $y_\phi^* = y_\phi^+$. Further, we are able to maintain the interpretation of $s_{P\vee}$ as originating in the lateral habenula, as the new form is still positive if the outcome y_ϕ^+ fails to occur (Matsumoto and Hikosaka 2007). We therefore take (20)–(22) as a more complete account of the dopamine signal including reward modulation.

Notice that Δ_ϕ is still a *sensory* prediction error—there is no mention of a difference between observed *reward* as such and its prediction. It is true that y_ϕ^+ has been sensitised or "tagged" with reward (if the term $f(x_\mathrm{R})$ is non-zero) and so is, itself, a predictor of reward—but the basic signals here are a sensory feature representation, y_{ϕ}^{+}, and its prediction y_{ϕ}^{*}. Moreover, the development of sensitisation via $f(x_{\mathrm{R}})$ requires learning (under a model $\mathcal{I}_{\mathrm{R}}$) which may require massive exposure to the reward stimulus and (simultaneously) the feature y_{ϕ}^{+}. This is a hallmark of many laboratory experiments but not so in many natural situations in which we may therefore expect $f(x_{\mathrm{R}}) \approx 0$ (Redgrave et al. 2008). In these cases, Δ_{ϕ} is most certainly a sensory (only) prediction error, and so we argue that the emphasis on sensory encoding/error-production is more general. However, the fact that reward should find a role in action discovery is not surprising; it is reasonable to suppose that actions delivering reward should be learned more quickly and/or reliably.

6 A Framework for Intrinsically Motivated Learning

Here we bring together the threads we have developed to give an account of action discovery as intrinsically motivated learning driving the development of internal models of prediction and action-outcome contingencies.

Learning to "Listen" to Action Requests

The first process we consider is one in which basal ganglia learns to encode the new action. In (7), salience was defined via an action request—a representation $\boldsymbol{s}^{(a)}$, with components $s_f^{(a)}$, for an action $\boldsymbol{\alpha}$. In the brain, this request is first "filtered" by neurons in striatum[8] before taking part in a selection process in the basal ganglia for behavioural expression. The neuronal response in striatum $\hat{S}_{\alpha}(t)$ is given by

$$\hat{S}_{\alpha} = \sum_{f} w_f s_f^{(a)} , \tag{23}$$

where w_f are the synaptic weights on striatal neurons receiving cortical inputs $s_f^{(a)}$. The notion of filtering here is inspired by the formal equivalence of (23) and the convolution sums defining finite impulse response (FIR) filters. Here, the cortico-striatal weights w_f play the role of filter coefficients acting on signals $s_f^{(a)}$. This view highlights the fact that a key part of biological action discovery is the adjustment or "tuning" of the striatal filter (i.e. the weights) so that basal ganglia can "listen" effectively to the action request.

In vector terms, if $\boldsymbol{w}$ is the weight vector comprising components w_f, the right-hand side of (23) is the inner product $\boldsymbol{w} \cdot \boldsymbol{s}^{(a)}$ which takes its maximal value when both vectors are in the same "direction". Striatal tuning in action discovery is therefore one of "weight vector rotation".

[8]The striatum is the main input nucleus of the basal ganglia.

Dopamine is known to modulate cortico-striatal plasticity using learning rules that are otherwise broadly Hebb-like (Reynolds and Wickens 2002). Now suppose that the most recently selected action $\boldsymbol{\alpha}$ (associated with $\hat{S}_\alpha$) causes a sensory prediction error Δ_ϕ due to unexpected phasic change in the environment. The resultant phasic dopamine is able to reinforce the match between $\mathbf{w}$ and $\mathbf{s}^{(a)}$ as long as the pattern of neural activity in $\boldsymbol{s}^{(a)}$ does not decline substantially before delivery of the dopamine signal.[9]

Repetition Bias

The increased match between $\boldsymbol{w}$ and $\boldsymbol{s}^{(a)}$ promoted by phasic dopamine will cause an increase in $\hat{S}_\alpha$, as long as the relevant context contributing to the action request is maintained. This will, in turn, be reflected in a change in the animal's policy as an increase in the probability $\pi(\boldsymbol{\alpha})$ of selecting $\boldsymbol{\alpha}$. Eventually, any contextual salience that may have sustained $\boldsymbol{s}^{(a)}$ will decline as habituation occurs to the contextual features in the action request. The striatal response $\hat{S}_\alpha$ becomes small again and so too, therefore, does $\pi(\boldsymbol{\alpha})$. We refer to the temporary increase in $\pi(\boldsymbol{\alpha})$ as *repetition bias*.

6.1 Learning Internal Models

Action-outcome discovery would appear to involve establishing two internal models: a (forward) prediction model $\mathcal{I}_\mathrm{P}$ and a (inverse) deployment model $\mathcal{I}_\mathrm{G}$. Furthermore we have postulated a division of prediction so that $\mathcal{I}_\mathrm{P}$ is a combination of a model $\mathcal{I}_{\mathrm{P}_\phi}$, based on surprise, and another dealing with the remaining structural complexity of outcome (see equations (5,6)). How does the animal learn these models? As described below, repetition bias is a key driver for these processes.

Action-Outcome Pairings

During action discovery, the increase in the probability $\pi(\boldsymbol{\alpha})$ for action $\boldsymbol{\alpha}$ causes representations of context $\boldsymbol{y}^-$ (containing $\boldsymbol{a}$) and its consequent outcome $\boldsymbol{y}^+$, to be present with an increased probability. The sustained presence of such representations will induce plasticity in the relevant brain areas responsible for learning the associations implied in $\mathcal{I}_\mathrm{P}$ and $\mathcal{I}_\mathrm{G}$.

The dynamics of repetition bias are governed by learning of models like $\mathcal{I}_{\mathrm{P}_\phi}$. However, learning in the other models may not necessarily follow an identical

[9] Additionally, this may be supported by some kind of *eligibility trace* associated with $s^{(a)}$ which dopamine acts upon (Gurney et al. 2009a).

time course, which poses the possibility of incomplete learning of all required models. This problem may be overcome during further behaviour by the animal in ways which rely on the relationship between model representations. Suppose, for example, that the inverse model $\mathcal{I}_{\mathrm{G}}$ has been inadequately learned, resulting in performance errors for the action involved in this model. This will cause unexpected phasic outcomes which will, in turn, incur sensory prediction errors. These will drive a further round of repetition bias resulting in action-discovery refinement.

Models Without Action Contingency

We now consider the learning of models $\mathcal{I}_{\mathrm{P}}$ which do not contain phasic-related components. These are non-operant models which might, for example, concern the representation of environmental elements in relation to each other. Novelty (not simply surprise) may then arise if new elements are found where they are unexpected ("why is there a football shirt in my office!?") or there is an absence of expected elements ("where has my computer gone!?"). The novelty in these situations will induce high salience for investigative behaviours directed at the novel elements (or the space they previously occupied). Two possibilities can now occur. First, there is no unexpected causal outcome associated with the investigative behaviour (picking up the football shirt does not, e.g. turn the room lights on). In this case, novelty is reduced by developing explanatory accounts of the situation which might predict how the situation arose. Second, there *is* an unexpected outcome upon investigation, in which case we are now back in the action-outcome scenario described above. That is, a new prediction model presents itself for learning which *does* have a phasic component of the form $\mathcal{I}_{\mathrm{P}_\phi}$. Note that this new model is separate from the non-operant, non-phasic model which induced the investigative behaviour in the first place.

The Need for Distinct Prediction and Inverse Models

One question which arises here is why the animal needs an inverse model $\mathcal{I}_{\mathrm{G}}$ for deploying the learned action-outcome element *and* a prediction model? First, acquisition of the sub-model of prediction $\mathcal{I}_{\mathrm{P}_\phi}$ instigates repetition bias; phasic sensory prediction error is a trigger for learning the other models, and just as important, a lack of error (through prediction) terminates learning. Second, suppose the full prediction model $\mathcal{I}_{\mathrm{P}}$ was not completely developed. This would give rise to a constant stream of salience due to (general) novelty, and the agent would be continually drawn to stimuli that it had seen countless times. This would make it difficult for the animal to engage in purposeful behaviours driven, not by novelty, but by salience derived from $\mathcal{I}_{\mathrm{G}}$ and $\mathcal{I}_{\mathrm{R}}$. Prediction therefore prevents "attentional deficit" behaviour which would constitute a continuous stream of exploration without pursuit of specific goals.

7 Discussion

7.1 Summary of Main Ideas

We have introduced a formal framework for considering the relationships between animals, their environment, their internal neural representations of that environment and their behaviour. In particular, we define relations between a context, an action in that context and a causally related outcome. This framework is a functional one, considering entire path histories or trajectories of state variables.

Our notion of prediction is based on internal neural models of causal relations which become manifest ("make predictions") by expressing signals at their output. The resulting neural representations interact with sensory processes to drive habituation and sensitisation.

Salience maps were defined via the components of sensorimotor representations defining action policy, and action requests comprise a subset of features in a salience map. Salience (as a scalar value) is defined as the sum of feature values in an action request. We made the hypothesis that (for non-habitual actions) salience may be indicative of the value of an action and that salience comprises three components: feature novelty, sensitisation due to reward, and task-driven (outcome) priming. Sensitisation is driven by inverse models of reward conditioning and action-outcome contingency like $\mathcal{I}_{\mathrm{R}}$ and $\mathcal{I}_{\mathrm{G}}$ in (12) and (13), respectively.

An analysis of novelty with a simple example led to the idea that habituation comprises inhibition of the sensory representation by the prediction. The example also led naturally to the existence of two opponent novelty detectors (for feature presence and absence). A sensory prediction error was defined as the difference between the opponent novelty detectors [see Eq. (19)]. For the special case of surprise detection, we putatively identified the feature presence/absence detectors as superior colliculus and lateral habenula, respectively. Phasic dopamine was then identified as the sensory prediction error corresponding to surprise. In addition, the ability of reward to sensitise the colliculus and habenula led to the idea that phasic dopamine can be modulated by reward (as observed experimentally), but remains best described as a sensory prediction error.

Finally we have shown how learning of the internal models may proceed under temporary changes in policy—repetition bias—and that this learning could be robust via continued interaction with the environment.

7.2 Implications for Intrinsic Motivation

We started by noting that action-outcome skill acquisition is a hallmark of many formulations of what constitutes intrinsically motivated learning. In this sense, our framework lies at the heart of the field. However, in the survey of Oudeyer and Kaplan (2007), they admit the possibility that some intrinsically motivated learning deals with "passive" observation of the environment and learning intra-world contingencies rather than agent–environment ones. This process was discussed in Sect. 6.1 ("Models without action contingency"). We therefore agree that the learning of novelty-driven prediction models, without associated inverse models, is a suitable candidate for the tag of "intrinsically motivated learning". The common ground here is that the learning is promoted by novelty (taken to subsume surprise as a special case). More specifically, we might argue that it is a successful *reduction* in novelty, through information compression in prediction-model construction, which is the key characteristic. This idea has been explored more fully by Schmidhuber (2009).

If novelty-induced behaviour is a hallmark of intrinsically motivated learning, our framework suggests a quantitative formal definition. Thus, we *could* define the level of intrinsic motivation according to the relative contribution of novelty salience, $\boldsymbol{s}_{\mathrm{P}}^{(a)}$, in the action request, $\boldsymbol{s}^{(a)}$, for the current action; use the dissection of $\boldsymbol{s}^{(a)}$ given in (14); and compute $||\boldsymbol{s}_{\mathrm{P}}^{(a)}||/||\boldsymbol{s}^{(a)}||$. This definition is given in the spirit of ontology construction (see the Introduction)—it is a *plausible* formal definition of "intrinsic motivation" without laying claim to be a "truth".

While this formal definition of intrinsic motivation is plausible, it may not satisfy other interpretations. Intrinsically motivated behaviour has also been described as "doing something for its inherent satisfactions rather than for some separable consequence" (Ryan and Deci 2000). We take "separable consequences" here to mean external primary rewards. The action-discovery scenario, driven as it is (in general) by biologically neutral events caused by the agent, is therefore intrinsically motivated from this perspective too. It might be claimed that the unexpected outcomes observed during action discovery constitute such external rewards but, as we have argued elsewhere (Redgrave and Gurney 2006), this does not adhere to conventional notions of biologically defined primary reward. Further, while it is difficult to determine whether action discovery is being conducted subjectively "for its own sake", we know from experience that this is, indeed, often the case with accompanying feelings of "curiosity" and "satisfaction". Finally, we argue that, irrespective of any experience of "curiosity", the brain mechanisms invoked during internal model building of causality, contingent on unexpected outcomes, will be substantially the same as those deployed when "curiosity" might be established as a causative factor. We therefore contend that a mechanistic account of action discovery can shed light on intrinsically motivated learning in general.

7.3 Prospectus

The ideas presented here do not specify any particular detailed model of intrinsically motivated learning. Rather, they provide a framework for computational modelling work. Our thinking here was informed by neurobiological relevance, and so we would hope that this will facilitate the future construction of biologically plausible models. The processes and mappings demonstrated here, when concatenated together, may also help specify future ground plans for functional brain architectures. The specific formalism of action-discovery ontology presented here may be incomplete, and some features remain less well-defined than others. More radically, others may disagree altogether with our approach and demand an alternative formalism, but we would welcome this if it engages with the effort of building an ontology of action selection and discovery and, more widely, of intrinsically motivated learning.

Notwithstanding the general scope of this work, we have dealt with an analysis of sensory prediction errors and phasic dopamine at a level which makes contact with specific neural functions—see Eqs. (21)–(22). Establishing the accuracy of these putative functions offers an immediate programme of work for modelling the colliculus, habenula and midbrain dopamine circuits.

Acknowledgements Written while the authors were in receipt of research funding from The Wellcome Trust, BBSRC and EPSRC.

This research has also received funds from the European Commission 7th Framework Programme (FP7/2007-2013), "Challenge 2 - Cognitive Systems, Interaction, Robotics", Grant Agreement No. ICT-IP-231722, Project "IM-CLeVeR—Intrinsically Motivated Cumulative Learning Versatile Robots". (NL was partially supported by EU Framework project EFAA (ICT-270490))

References

Allport, A., Sanders, H., Heuer, A.: Selection for action: Some behavioural and neurophysiological considerations of attention and action. In: Perspectives on Perception and Action. Lawrence Erlbaum Associates Inc., Hillsdale (1987)

Baldi, P., Itti, L.: Of bits and wows: A bayesian theory of surprise with applications to attention. Neural Netw. **23**(5), 649–666 (2010)

Balleine, B.W., Dickinson, A.: Goal-directed instrumental action: Contingency and incentive learning and their cortical substrates. Neuropharmacology **37**(4–5), 407–419 (1998)

Barto, A., Singh, S., Chentanez, N.: Intrinsically motivated reinforcement learning. In: 18th Annual Conference on Neural Information Processing Systems (NIPS). Vancouver (2004)

Cisek, P.: Cortical mechanisms of action selection: The affordance competition hypothesis. Philos.Trans. R. Soc. Lond B Biol. Sci. **362**(1485), 1585–1599 (2007)

Cisek, P., Kalaska, J.: Neural mechanisms for interacting with a world full of action choices. Annu. Rev. Neurosci. **33**, 269–298 (2010)

Comoli, E., Coizet, V., Boyes, J., Bolam, J., Canteras, N., Quirk, R., Overton, P, Redgrave, P.: A direct projection from superior colliculus to substantia nigra for detecting salient visual events. Nat. Neurosci. **6**(9), 974–980 (2003)

Connor, C.E., Egeth, H.E., Yantis, S.: Visual attention: Bottom-Up versus Top-Down. Curr. Biol. **14**(19), R850–R852 (2004)

Cope, A., Chambers, J., Gurney, K.: Object-based biasing for attentional control of gaze: A comparison of biologically plausible mechanisms. BMC Neurosci. **10**(Suppl. 1), P19 (2009)

Dommett, E., Coizet, V., Blaha, C., Martindale, J., Lefebvre, V., Walton, N., Mayhew, J., Overton, P., Redgrave, P.: How visual stimuli activate dopaminergic neurons at short latency. Science **307**(5714), 1476–1479 (2005)

Fiorillo, C.D., Tobler, P.N., Schultz, W.: Discrete coding of reward probability and uncertainty by dopamine neurons. Science **299**(5614), 1898 (2003)

Friston, K.: A theory of cortical responses. Philos. Trans. R. Soc. B Biol. Sci. **360**(1456), 815–836 (2005)

Gene Ontology Consortium: Creating the gene ontology resource: Design and implementation. Genome Res. **11**(8), 1425–1433 (2001)

Gruber, T.: A translation approach to portable ontology specification. http://www-ksl.stanford.edu/kst/what-is-an-ontology.html (1992)

Gurney, K., Humphries, M., Redgrave, P.: Cortico-striatal plasticity for action-outcome learning using spike timing dependent eligibility. BMC Neurosci. **10**(Suppl. 1), P135 (2009a)

Gurney, K., Hussain, A., Chambers, J., Abdullah, R.: Controlled and automatic processing in animals and machines with application to autonomous vehicle control. In: Controlled and Automatic Processing in Animals and Machines with Application to Autonomous Vehicle Control, Lecture Notes in Computer Science, vol. 5768, pp. 198–207. Springer, Berlin (2009b)

Ikeda, T., Hikosaka, O.: Reward-dependent gain and bias of visual responses in primate superior colliculus. Neuron **39**(4), 693–700 (2003)

Körding, K.P., Wolpert, D.M.: Bayesian decision theory in sensorimotor control. Trends Cogn. Sci. **10**(7), 319–326 (2006)

Marr, D., Poggio, T.: From understanding computation to understanding neural circuitry. Technical report, MIT AI Laboratory (1976)

Matsumoto, M., Hikosaka, O.: Lateral habenula as a source of negative reward signals in dopamine neurons. Nature **447**(7148), 1111–1115 (2007)

Oudeyer, P., Kaplan, F.: What is intrinsic motivation? a typology of computational approaches. Front. Neurorobot. **1**, 6 (2007). PMID 18958277

Poggio, T., Koch, C.: Ill-posed problems in early vision: From computational theory to analogue networks. Proc. R. Soc. Lond. B. Biol. Sci. **226**(1244), 303 (1985)

Ranganath, C., Rainer, G.: Neural mechanisms for detecting and remembering novel events. Nat. Rev. Neurosci. **4**(3), 193–202 (2003)

Redgrave, P., Gurney, K.: The short-latency dopamine signal: A role in discovering novel actions? Nat. Rev. Neurosci. **7**(12) (2006)

Redgrave, P., Gurney, K., Reynolds, J.: What is reinforced by phasic dopamine signals? Brain Res. Rev. **58**(2), 322–339 (2008)

Redgrave, P., Gurney, K., Stafford, T., Thirkettle, M., Lewis, J.: The role of the basal ganglia in discovering novel actions. In: Baldassarre, G., Mirolli, M. (eds.) Intrinsically Motivated Learning in Natural and Artificial Systems, pp. 129–149. Springer, Berlin (2012)

Redgrave, P., Prescott, T., Gurney, K.: The basal ganglia: A vertebrate solution to the selection problem? Neuroscience **89**, 1009–1023 (1999)

Reynolds, J.N.J., Wickens, J.R.: Dopamine-dependent plasticity of corticostriatal synapses. Neural Netw. **15**(4–6), 507–521 (2002)

Ryan, R.M., Deci, E.L.: Intrinsic and extrinsic motivations: Classic definitions and new directions. 1. Contemp. Educ. Psychol. **25**(1), 54–67 (2000)

Schleidt, M., Kien, J.: Segmentation in behavior and what it can tell us about brain function. Hum. Nat. **8**(1), 77–111 (1997)

Schmidhuber, J.: Driven by compression progress: A simple principle explains essential aspects of subjective beauty, novelty, surprise, interestingness, attention, curiosity, creativity, art, science, music, jokes. In: Anticipatory Behavior in Adaptive Learning Systems, pp. 48–76 (2009)

Schultz, W.: Dopamine signals for reward value and risk: Basic and recent data. Behav. Brain Funct. **6**(1), 24 (2010)

Schultz, W., Dayan, P., Montague, P.: A neural substrate of prediction and reward. Science **275**, 1593–1599 (1997)

Snyder, L.H., Batista, A.P., Andersen, R.A.: Coding of intention in the posterior parietal cortex. Nature **386**(6621), 167–170 (1997)

Sokolov, E.N.: Higher nervous functions: The orienting reflex. Annu. Rev. Physiol. **25**(1), 545–580 (1963)

Sutton, R., Barto, A.: Reinforcement Learning : An Introduction. MIT, Cambridge (1998)

Thompson, K.G., Bichot, N.P., Sato, T.R.: Frontal eye field activity before visual search errors reveals the integration of Bottom-Up and Top-Down salience. J. Neurophysiol. **93**(1), 337–351 (2005)

Timberlake, W., Lucas, G.A.: The basis of superstitious behavior: Chance contingency, stimulus substitution, or appetitive behavior? J. Exp. Anal. Behav. **44**(3), 279 (1985)

Tobler, P., Fiorillo, C., Schultz, W.: Adaptive coding of reward value by dopamine neurons. Science **307**(5715), 1642 (2005)

Tolman, E.: Cognitive maps in rats and men. Psychol. Rev. **55**(4), 189 (1948)

Wurtz, R.H., Albano, J.E.: Visual-motor function of the primate superior colliculus. Annu. Rev. Neurosci. **3**(1), 189–226 (1980)

Yin, H.H., Knowlton, B.J.: The role of the basal ganglia in habit formation. Nat. Rev. Neurosci. **7**(6), 464–476 (2006)

Part III
Novelty-Based Intrinsic Motivation Mechanisms

Novelty Detection as an Intrinsic Motivation for Cumulative Learning Robots

Ulrich Nehmzow, Yiannis Gatsoulis, Emmett Kerr, Joan Condell, Nazmul Siddique, and T. Martin McGinnity

Abstract Novelty detection is an inherent part of intrinsic motivations and constitutes an important research issue for the effective and long-term operation of intelligent robots designed to learn, act and make decisions based on their cumulative knowledge and experience. Our approach to novelty detection is from the perspective that the robot ignores perceptions that are already known, but is able to identify anything different. This is achieved by developing biologically inspired novelty detectors based on habituation. Habituation is a type of non-associative learning used to describe the behavioural phenomenon of decreased responsiveness of a cognitive organism to a recently and frequently presented stimulus, and it has been observed in a number of biological organisms. This chapter first considers the relationship between intrinsic motivations and novelty detection and outlines some works on intrinsic motivations. It then presents a critical review of the methods of novelty detection published by the authors. A brief summary of some key recent surveys in the field is then provided. Finally, key open challenges that need to be considered in the design of novelty detection filters for cumulative learning tasks are discussed.

1 Introduction

Novelty detection is an important factor for the effective and long-term operation of intelligent robots designed to explore, evolve and make decisions based on their cumulative knowledge and experience. Novelty detection and intrinsic motivations are tightly coupled and play an important role in the cumulative learning process. Although there is no strict definition of novelty detection, it is

U. Nehmzow · Y. Gatsoulis (✉) · E. Kerr · J. Condell · N. Siddique · T.M. McGinnity
Intelligent Systems Research Centre, University of Ulster, Derry/Londonderry BT48 7JL, UK
e-mail: i.gatsoulis@ulster.ac.uk; ep.kerr@ulster.ac.uk; j.condell@ulster.ac.uk; nh.siddique@ulster.ac.uk; tm.mcginnity@ulster.ac.uk

G. Baldassarre and M. Mirolli (eds.), *Intrinsically Motivated Learning in Natural and Artificial Systems*, DOI 10.1007/978-3-642-32375-1_8,

widely regarded (Markou and Singh 2003a; Marsland 2003; Saunders and Gero 2000) as the process of identifying novel stimuli that are "different from anything known before; new, interesting and often seeming slightly strange"—definition of "novel" by Wehmeier (2005).

Based on this description, we approach novelty detection from the perspective that the robot ignores perceptions that are similar to those seen during training, but is able to highlight anything different. In this sense, novelty detection can be seen as a form of selective learning: examples are provided of those features that should not be detected, and the novelty filter aims to highlight anything that differs from the inputs used in training. As such, novelty detection is the ability to identify perceptions that have never been experienced before and constitutes an important component for the effective and long-term operation of intelligent robot systems allowing computationally efficient, unsupervised and incremental exploration and learning of new skills and environments (Baranes and Oudeyer 2009; Hart and Grupen 2011; Kaplan and Oudeyer 2007).

A number of novelty detection methods have been proposed in the literature, mainly focusing on detecting anomalies, that is, identifying patterns that do not conform to expected behaviour, in application domains such as diagnosing medical problems, detecting machine faults, network security, surveillance and fraud detection (Chandola et al. 2009; Hodge and Austin 2004). Typically for these problems, there is substantial data about the normal classes (e.g. healthy subjects, normal operation of a machine), but very little data displaying the features that should be detected. Hence, it is common to learn a model of the normal dataset and then attempt to detect deviations from this model. This means that a training set of normal data is sufficient for the effective operation of a system. If there is a need for further expansion, then this is easier done in batch processing, which also allows the retraining of the system from scratch.

Such an approach to novelty detection seems unsuitable for the application domain of cumulative learning, which is the focus in this chapter, for a number of reasons. First, a novelty response in the learning process depends on intrinsic motivation (Berlyne 1960; Oudeyer and Kaplan 1999; Oudeyer et al. 1999). Intrinsic motivations are motivations based on mechanisms that drive learning of skills and knowledge, and the exploitation and energisation of behaviours that facilitate this (Baldassare 2011). In the next section, we discuss the inherent relationship between intrinsic motivation and novelty. Second, offline learning might be inappropriate in cases where the learning task depends on a sequence of prior learnt actions; an online learning filter is then needed instead. Another reason is that ab-initio retraining is inefficient, undesirable and contrary to the whole concept of cumulative learning. Furthermore, the notion of normal data as expressed in anomaly detection is not the same in novelty detection, particularly in the domain of cumulative learning: a novelty is not necessarily an anomaly, and as such there is no initial training dataset that can be complete. From a practical point of view, a novelty detector must be able to reliably identify the novel perceptions that are distorted due to the noisy sensor readings of the robot, as well as operate online if an immediate response is required. In cases where a learnt action determines the next one, it is also necessary for the novelty detector to operate and learn online. Such a novelty detector requires learning architectures that support dynamic and incremental expansion of knowledge representation.

This chapter summarises the research work on novelty detection, with Sect. 2 discussing the relationship between intrinsic motivation and novelty, Sect. 3 presenting the authors' previous research on novelty detection and Sect. 4 discussing recent surveys on the field. Section 5 discusses key open challenges for the effective operation of a novelty detection filter in a cumulative learning task. Finally, Sect. 6 presents the conclusion of the chapter.

2 Intrinsic Motivations and Novelty Detection

The concept of intrinsic motivation has been developed by psychologists to explain some findings that could not be accounted for by the behaviourist theory of learning and drives, for example, the tendency of animals to explore complex, novel or surprising stimuli (Berlyne 1960; Hunt 1965; White 1959).

White (1959) argued that intrinsically motivated behaviour is essential for an organism to gain competences. Ample evidence exists that the opportunity to explore a novel environment can itself act as a reward. Moreover, not only exploration incited by novelty but also manipulation or just activity itself can be rewarding. Ryan and Deci (2000) defined intrinsic motivation as doing an activity for its inherent satisfaction rather than doing it for any reward or any other consequence. In terms of function, intrinsic motivations are drives that guide learning of skills and knowledge. Another view of intrinsic motivations links them to the drive to manipulate and explore features of intrinsic motivation (Harlow 1950). Some other researchers proposed different conceptualisations such as cognitive dissonance (Festinger 1957), which defines motivation as a process directed to minimise dissonance between internal structures of cognition and perceived situations. Hunt (1965) proposed the concept of optimal incongruity. He argued that interesting stimuli are those that differ from standard stimuli. Another group of researchers define intrinsic motivation as effectance (White 1959), personal causation (De Charms 1968) and competence with self-determination (Deci and Ryan 1985).

Within neuroscience, one of the most articulated and empirically well-supported theories (Redgrave and Gurney 2006)—see also chapter by Mirolli and Baldassare (2011) in this book—states that intrinsic motivations are related to the function of phasic dopamine (DA) caused by the activation of the superior colliculus located in the midbrain. The theory claims that phasic DA is a learning signal that is generated by the colliculus when the organism perceives sudden events (e.g. a sudden light going on) and that the signal ceases after the learning of the action causing the stimuli is complete. A second important theory on intrinsic motivations proposed within the neuroscientific literature has been proposed by Lisman and Grace (2005) and Otmakhova et al. (2011). This theory is particularly important for this chapter as it relates to mechanisms that might represent a possible biological correspondent of the computational novelty detection mechanisms presented here. This theory is focused on the hippocampus and surrounding brain areas: these have been shown to respond to novel stimuli, novel associations between familiar stimuli or familiar stimuli in novel contexts. The activation of these brain areas causes a learning DA signal that is proposed to drive the memorisation of the novel stimuli within the same areas. With learning the response of these areas progressively attenuates.

Some authors (Baldassare 2011; Mirolli and Baldassare 2011) have proposed an integrated view of these processes for which intrinsic motivations are based on mechanisms that measure the success of the acquisition of skills and knowledge. These mechanisms drive animals to continue to engage in an activity if their competence in achieving interesting outcomes is improving or if their capacity to predict, abstract or recognise perceptions is not yet good or is improving. Once the skills and knowledge are acquired, they can be used as readily available building blocks. The building blocks are used to learn and produce behaviours and actions invoked by extrinsic motivations or as a basis for new acquisitions influenced by intrinsic motivations ("cumulative learning").

There has been growing interest among researchers in the cognitive computing, machine learning and robotics communities in modelling and reproducing intrinsic motivations. A variety of computational models of intrinsic motivations have been reported in this area of research (Barto et al. 2004; Kaplan and Oudeyer 2007; Mirolli and Baldassare 2011; Oudeyer and Kaplan 1999; Oudeyer et al. 1999; Schembri et al. 2007; Schmidhuber 2010). These works used learning signals generated by intrinsic motivations to train reinforcement learning systems. A useful distinction between functions and mechanisms of intrinsic motivations and their computational models is reported in Mirolli and Baldassare (2011). An overview of a formal theory of intrinsic motivations based on prediction improvement and the exploitation of the resulting learning signal to train reinforcement learning systems is reported in Schmidhuber (2010, 2011).

From the above discussion and views, novelty is seen as a particular aspect of intrinsic motivation, which is the focus of this chapter. A number of computational models have been reported in the literature that implement novelty detection methods (Neto and Nehmzow 2007a,b) and machines that are intrinsically motivated (Kaplan and Oudeyer 2007). The widely known computational models of intrinsic motivations are:

- Competence-based models of intrinsic motivation: these models use reinforcement learning to learn new actions on the basis of intrinsic motivation (Barto et al. 2004; Schembri et al. 2007).
- Knowledge-based models of intrinsic motivation: these models use reinforcement learning to learn to perform actions based on prediction (Schmidhuber 1991a,b, 2010, 2011).
- Novelty-based models of intrinsic motivation: these models use novelty filters to detect novel stimuli (Lee et al. 2009; Marshall et al. 2004; Merrick 2011; Merrick and Maher 2009; Saunders and Gero 2002). In general, novelty filters are implemented using habituation neural networks. Different novelty detection models and algorithms reported in the literature are discussed in the following sections.

3 Authors' Related Work

The previous published work of the authors in the domain of novelty detection is discussed in this section. This is presented in chronological development order. The developed novelty detection filters are based on the following methods:

- Kohonen maps with habituated synapses (Sect. 3.1).
- Grow-when-required (GWR) networks (Sect. 3.2).
- GWR networks with a selective attention mechanism based on saliency maps (Sect. 3.3).
- Incremental principal component analysis (IPCA) with a selective attention mechanism based on saliency maps (Sect. 3.4).
- GWR networks and IPCA with selective attention mechanisms based on multi-scale Harris detectors (Sect. 3.5).

These methods are explained in more detail in the following sections.

3.1 Novelty Detection Based on Kohonen Maps with Habituated Synapses

Marsland et al. (2000) presented a novelty filter that has the purpose of learning to recognise known features and evaluate their novelty based on the frequency with which these input stimuli have been seen recently. It is based on a Kohonen map with habituated synapses linking the nodes of the network to an output node. The novelty filter is shown in Fig. 1. A habituated synapse decreases in strength as its input node fires and increases in strength when already known stimuli are not seen for some time. The behavioural phenomenon of habituation has its roots in biology, and as mentioned by Marsland et al. (2000), cross citing Thompson and Spencer (1966), it is thought to be one of the simplest forms of plasticity in the brain of a large number of organisms. Habituation has a long research history in cognitive organisms (Thompson 2009b) and has recently been revisited by a team of experts (Rankin 2009a,b).

Two sets of experiments were conducted to test the ability of the novelty filter to learn a representation model of an operational environment and to investigate the effects of the habituated synapses on novelty detection (Marsland et al. 2000). The experimental scenario consisted of a robot traversing a corridor. The robot was equipped with 16 sonar sensors that formulated the input vectors. Two further similar corridors were used as additional experimental environments.

In the first set of experiments the novelty filter was based only on the Kohonen map without any habituated synapses, and the aim was to demonstrate the ability of the novelty filter to learn a representation of an environment and recognise novel features in it. The experimental procedure was as follows: a number of learning and non-learning trials, succeeding each other in turn, were initially conducted

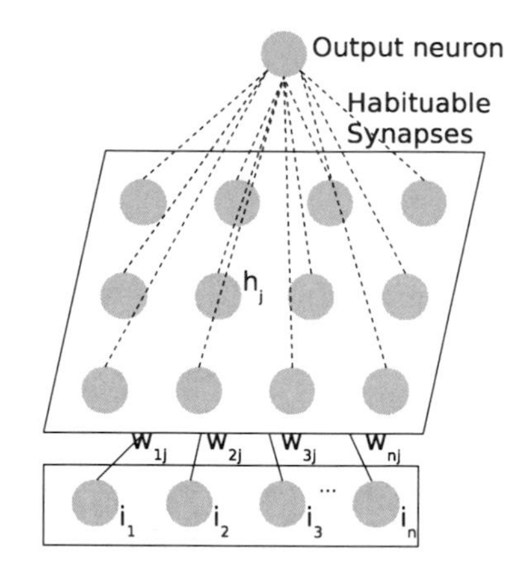

Fig. 1 Neural network with habituating synapses

in the first environment. The novelty filter was always active, even during the non-learning phase to better demonstrate what has been learnt in the previous learning trial. Once the first environment was learnt, as indicated by the lack of any novelties produced by the novelty filter, the robot was moved to another similar corridor where the current novelty filter was further trained using the same foregoing procedure. The experimental results showed that the system was able to firstly learn the first environment and then expand its knowledge to the second one. An interesting question would be to investigate the effect of further training in the second environment to what was already learnt in the first environment.

In the second set of experiments the effect of the habituated synapses was investigated, and the aim was to demonstrate the phenomenon of habituation and how stimuli that have not been observed for some time were being forgotten (dishabituation). Initially, only one environment was used, and features of it were deliberately altered between the trials. The experimental results confirmed that the model of habituation used was able to detect the novel items; the system was able to learn and habituate over the environment, but when a feature was changed and not observed for some time, then the novelty filter showed increasing levels of novelty over this feature. To further investigate the effect of habituation, the robot was moved to another similar corridor after being trained in the first corridor. A non-learning trial, but with the novelty filter still active, was conducted back in the first training environment after each learning trial in the second environment. The experimental results showed that the system exhibited increasing novelty levels in the first environment as its training progressed in the second environment. Such a behaviour was observed largely because of the dishabituated synapses. However, dishabituation might not be the only reason for explaining the increasing levels of novelty detection in this case. The further training received in the second environment had an influential impact on what has been already known, that is, on the representation of the first environment. This shows that further training is not necessarily beneficial in all cases; in fact it can prove to be destructive to already acquired data.

Although this form of habituation is beneficial since it promotes temporal exploration, it has its limitations, mainly because it assumes that the frequency of seeing a stimulus and the amount of time needed to forget it are always the same for all stimuli and for every individual. Furthermore, these frequency and time parameters are set subjectively by the system designer. A more sophisticated mechanism of habituation, such as one that takes into account other aspects of the environment and the task at hand, may be more effective. An approach that has been suggested that exists in biological organisms is to habituate the levels of habituation, so that perceptions that have been attended a number of times by the organism seem to be less interesting in the future unless they have very high levels of novelty (Rankin 2009b).

Another issue is the static structure of the Kohonen maps. They are capable of being trained only up to a certain amount of data, depending on their fixed size, which is set initially. This is a drawback for the use of Kohonen maps in the domain of cumulative learning as at some point they will become replete and incapable of further learning.

3.2 *Novelty Detection Based on Grow-When-Required Networks*

In order to address the drawbacks caused by the static structure of the Kohonen maps, Marsland et al. (2002b) proposed a dynamic network, called the "grow-when-required" (GWR) network, capable of expanding as necessary when it seems to become replete and unrepresentative of new data.

The GWR network consists of two important components: nodes with their associated weights and edges that separate clusters of nodes that represent similar perceptions. The edges are being updated using the competitive Hebbian learning method used by Fritzke (1995) and Martinetz and Schulten (1991). In brief, each edge has a counter that is incremented when the edge is connected to the winning node, and when a counter exceeds a threshold, it is deleted. When the deletion of edges leads to the creation of orphan nodes, these are removed, ensuring effective pruning and learning within the network. The GWR is explained in more detail in Marsland et al. (2002b).

The idea of a dynamically growing network is not novel—see Marsland et al. (2002b, Sect. 2) for related work. The originality of the GWR network lies in the way that new nodes are added to it and how it deals with a common issue of expandable networks, namely, the premature addition of a new node before giving an opportunity for the last added node to settle. To overcome this problem, many techniques allow a new node to be added after a certain number of steps (Fritzke 1994, 1995). In contrast to this method, the GWR network allows nodes to be added at any time. This is achieved as follows. A new node is added when the activation value of the best-matching unit is below a threshold set by the experimenter. To deal with the issue of premature creation of a node, the nodes of the GWR network have a variable that decreases exponentially from 1, signifying that the node has not fired often and it is a new untrained node, to 0, signifying that the node has fired often and it had time to be trained. This variable is resembling the phenomenon of habituation presented in Sect. 3.1. As such when the activation value of the best-matching unit is above an insertion threshold, then a new node is added if the unit is mature; otherwise, the network is further trained. The weights of the new node are initialised to the mean average of the weights of the best-matching node and the input so the new node lies between the best-matching node of the network and the input.

A set of experiments was carried out to test the effectiveness of the GWR network as a novelty filter (Marsland et al. 2002a). The experimental task involved a robot learning the representation of a set of corridors by exploring them through a wall-following behaviour. For each one of the environments, a separate GWR network/filter was trained. The effectiveness of the system was assessed based on whether it was able to select the correct network representing the environment in which it was located. This was achieved by keeping normalised values, called familiarity indices, which indicated how well each one of the filters represented the current environment. The familiarity index f_i of a filter i was computed according to Eq. (1), where n_i was the filter's output and c was a scaling constant. Each familiarity index was updated for the current perception, and then all of the familiarity indices were normalised so that their sum was equal to 1. The initial values of the familiarity indices were all the same and equal to $1/m$, where m was the number of filters.

$$f_i = f_i + c \times n_i \tag{1}$$

The experimental results demonstrated that the robot is capable of learning representations of all environments and in general of selecting the correct filter, although there were instances where a wrong filter was chosen. This was because the robot was performing classification based only on the current perception, and as such it was incapable of distinguishing between similar environments.

Crook et al. (2002) conducted a comparative study between the GWR-based filter and one based on the extended work of Bogacz et al. (1999) on Hopfield networks. The results showed that the GWR network has a better sensitivity and is more robust to noise than the Hopfield network, mainly due to the different way that each one of these methods encodes the data; the GWR network is able to deal with continuous data, while the Hopfield network can only work with binary representations. Crook et al. (2002, p. 3899) further explain this by saying that "the Hopfield network stores memories in such a way that parts of separately learnt perceptions can be recalled together, creating a spurious memory. A perception matching this spurious combination will be classified as familiar even though it is not. In contrast, the GWR network compares the distance between the input and network nodes that represent separate clusters of the previously seen inputs, thus a novel perception that is a combination of parts of previously perceived perceptions would still be found novel".

One of the main advantages of the GWR networks is their ability to expand as necessary. By eliminating the drawbacks of the Kohonen maps caused by their fixed size, GWR networks provide an attractive method for the domain of cumulative learning. Furthermore, like self-organising maps, GWR networks also make it easy for the system designer to assess their performance and the similarities between objects. On the other hand, the decision on when to add a new node is determined by a fixed threshold set by the designer. A better approach might be the use of a dynamically adjusted threshold (Thompson 2009a). A further issue with GWR networks is that they can be computationally expensive, particularly in problems of cumulative learning where there is no restriction on how much data can be learnt. These computational issues become apparent in the foregoing experiments, as in order to select the network that best resembles the current environment, all networks had to be assessed to find the best-matching unit, and in order to do so, for any individual network, its complete structure had to be traversed. Another issue highlighted by these experiments was that the incorrect novelty filter was selected in cases where the perception of the robot was similar to more than one of the networks that had been learnt. The system would select the correct filter when a distinct feature was perceived, but the problem still remains: as long as the robot performs this selection task based only on its current perception, then it will fail every time an observed input is similar to multiple known filters. One possible solution to this issue is to take into account the past history, for example, in some form of time-series data. Lastly careful consideration should be given to make sure that the trained networks do not overfit the data, and hence become inefficient and unable to effectively generalise beyond their training sets. Although the habituation component and the overall algorithmic approach of the GWR networks should be robust to data overfitting, long running experiments and in more complex environments would be needed to reach reliable conclusions. The problem is that long running experiments would never be able to simulate the true operational time and use of a real-world cumulative learning robot. For this reason, it might be necessary to investigate pruning algorithms and other organisational architectures for learning.

3.3 Visual Novelty Detection with Selective Attention Based on Saliency

The work presented in Sects. 3.1 and 3.2 involved experiments where the perception vector consisted of the readings of the sonar sensors of the robot. Although sonars are common in robotic systems, the information they can provide is limited in comparison to other popular sensors, such as cameras. For this reason, further work of the authors has focused on investigating novelty detection using cameras and machine vision.

Initial experiments were conducted with a monochrome camera in the same foregoing wall-following scenario and set-up (see Sect. 3.2 for details). The results showed that the GWR network was able to cope with more complex data than the sonar readings (Marsland et al. 2001, 2005).

However, in these first experiments, the robot's camera was positioned to solely acquire close-up images of the wall, restricting its field of view, implicitly constraining the visual features almost only to texture and as such limiting its overall usefulness for more general applications (Neto and Nehmzow 2004, 2007a). Furthermore, in order to resolve potential computational issues associated with robotic vision, Neto and Nehmzow (2007a) and Neto and Nehmzow (2004) proposed a model of selective visual attention based on a saliency map (Itti et al. 1998). This model is inspired by the neural architecture of the early primate visual system and consisted of multi-scale feature maps that allow the detection of local discontinuities in intensity, colour and orientation. The attention model selected raw image patches from the input image frame. The interesting property of this implementation of a saliency map is that the saliency points were robust to geometric transformations, contributing as such to the desired general robustness of the image encoding mechanism. The colour histograms of these local image patches were fed as inputs to a GWR network. The improving effect of the saliency component on the GWR network was demonstrated in a set of experiments, in which an orange ball and a grey box were added to an already known environment; the robot was then asked to identify these new objects (Nehmzow and Neto 2004; Neto and Nehmzow 2007a).

The experimental results showed that the novelty filter failed to detect the novelty caused by the new object when the novelty filter was working without the saliency map, that is, without an attention mechanism, forcing it to take into consideration the complete image. On the other hand, when the saliency component was added to the novelty filter, and as such the system was focussing its attention only to areas of interest, the area with the additional object was recognised as novel. One issue of concern in the initial experiments (Nehmzow and Neto 2004; Neto and Nehmzow 2004) was that the novelty filter never converged fully, as it was still detecting novelties in the unchanged environment even after training. The reason for this was that although the novelty filter examined was able to cope with geometrical translations of the novelties, it was affected by their scaling. Different feature encodings, tested in further experiments (Neto and Nehmzow 2007a,b), have led to some improvements with respect to these problems.

3.4 Visual Novelty Detection Based on Incremental Principal Component Analysis

To further explore potential methods for novelty detection, Neto and Nehmzow (2005a,b) investigated a novelty filter based on incremental principal component analysis (IPCA) (Artac et al. 2002). Principal component analysis (PCA) is a useful method for dimensionality reduction based on projecting the input data onto its principal axes. The drawback with PCA is that, in its standard form, it is unsuitable for online learning, as it operates in batch mode and requires the complete set of data. However, Artac et al. (2002) have proposed an incremental computation of

PCA by discarding the original data once the eigenspace is updated and keeping only the data projected onto it. In this way, online learning is feasible.

A comparative study was conducted to assess the effectiveness of the IPCA-based filter with that of GWR networks. The experiments were in the same arena and very similar to the ones described in the previous Sects. 3.2 and 3.3; the novelty filter had to detect new unseen objects (an orange ball and a grey box) that were placed at different locations in an environment on which the robot had already been trained. In order to minimise the computational costs associated with visual processing, the aforementioned selective attention mechanism based on saliency was used, thus selecting only potential areas of interest. One main difference from the previous implementation of saliency was that in this case normalised raw image patches were used, instead of colour histograms, so as to have a fair comparison between the two methods.

The experimental results showed that in some cases, both novelty detectors had similar performances, while in others one method outperformed the other method by a small difference. This finding is in agreement with the general view that there is no single optimal novelty method, but the solution depends on the task and the type of data (Chandola et al. 2007, 2009; Hodge and Austin 2004; Markou and Singh 2003a,b; Marsland 2003). The size of the GWR network was smaller than that of the IPCA in all experiments. This meant that the GWR-based novelty filter was computationally and resource-wise more efficient than the IPCA novelty filter, being able to perform twice as fast on average.

On the other hand, IPCA-based filters are able to deal better with dimensionality issues, associated with the use of the Euclidean distances as metrics of the similarity between the input and the learnt vectors; these are caused because a small difference between two high-dimensional vectors tends to be large in value, making it difficult to establish thresholds of similarity for high-dimensional spaces. In contrast to GWR networks, IPCA can easily integrate alternative methods (e.g. Mahalanobis distances) that do not suffer from such drawbacks. Another advantage of the IPCA-based filters over the GWR-based ones is their ability to reduce dimensionality automatically, allowing optimal reconstruction of the original input image patch from the inverse transformation of the corresponding projected vector. As such, the user can evaluate which parts of the environment were actually learnt by the system. However, the GWR networks have the advantage of building a topological map for the stored vectors, through connections between similar patterns, hence allowing the researcher to better visualise the relations between the stored patterns.

Overall, this comparative study showed that an IPCA-based novelty filter has a number of strengths and weaknesses and a performance which is comparable to that of a GWR-based method, therefore making it a promising approach to novelty detection.

3.5 Visual Novelty Detection with Automatic Scale Selection

One of the strengths of a saliency-based selective attention algorithm is its robustness with geometric transformations, as it is able to cope with translations of features within the image frame by centring areas of interest (image patches) on stable salient locations. However, other alterations in appearance such as changes in scale, rotations or affine transformations need more elaborated methods to be dealt with efficiently. In the work presented so far (Sects. 3.3 and 3.4), scaling generalisation was achieved by acquiring multiple image patches in different scales for the salient visual features found in the environment. The experimental results presented in Sect. 3.3 have shown that feature encodings that are robust to scaling issues have a positive influence on the performance of the novelty detector; however, they were incapable of eliminating the problem completely.

In order to resolve these scaling issues, Nehmzow and Neto (2006) and Neto and Nehmzow (2007b) suggested a technique, based on the work of Lindeberg (1998), which is able to select the size of the image patches automatically.

The experiments were similar to the ones described in the previous Sects. 3.3 and 3.4; the novelty filter had to detect new unseen objects (an orange ball and a grey box) which were placed at different locations in an environment on which the robot had already been trained. In addition to the saliency map, a multi-scale Harris Detector was also used as a visual attention mechanism, in order to acquire more data. The two novelty filters used were based again on a GWR network and the IPCA method.

Experimental results showed that the sizes of the models of normality were smaller by 26 %–40 % when using an automatic scale selection rather than a fixed-scale one. This means that an image encoding that is robust to changes in scale would improve the novelty filter's ability to generalise and also reduce the number of acquired concepts by the used learning mechanism.

On the other hand, performance was generally better when using a fixed-scale image encoding, particularly in the case of the inconspicuous grey box. The conclusion drawn was that a fixed scale should be used, unless the model size matters, in which case an automatic scale might be preferred.

3.6 Summary of the Section

The methods presented in this section have some advantages that make them good solutions for novelty detection in the domain of cumulative learning. First, their ability to expand as required is an important property of a novelty filter for the continual and long-term operation, adaptation and learning of a robot system. Moreover, their ability to operate and learn online is also another useful feature, because there are many cases where offline learning is not an option. These methods have also demonstrated some level of abstraction and tolerance to noisy data, an important issue as noise can make non-novel objects appear as novel. The mechanism of habituation, drawn from the psychological literature, has provided an effective way of dealing with the question of when to expand the knowledge network.

On the other hand, there are still many open research issues and improvements for the effective operation of novelty detectors based on habituation in real-world applications of cumulative learning robots. In more detail, although a model of saliency was used to reduce the high computational cost of machine vision, cumulative learning can lead to a large set of learnt data, which still results in computational power and performance problems. For example, in the experiments with selecting the correct filter described in Sect. 3.2, the total set of filters had to be searched before making a decision. Furthermore, complexity issues might have been reduced by taking into account only the current perception, but this has also resulted in cases where the novelty filters failed to function effectively as detailed in Sect. 3.2. Also, although the novelty filters presented here provide an easy and clear way of measuring the novelty of an object, they do so in a unidimensional way, neglecting that novelty (or its absence) can occur at different levels of abstraction. Finally, the tight integration of the novelty detector with the visual classifier makes it difficult to improve the system with current state of the art in machine vision, as well as update the current model with recent findings in the domain of habituation (Rankin 2009b).

4 Overview of Novelty Detection Methods

A comprehensive literature review of all novelty detection methods in this chapter is currently unnecessary, due to the number of extensive surveys that have been published recently (Chandola et al. 2007, 2009; Hodge and Austin 2004; Markou and Singh 2003a,b; Marsland 2003). This section summarises these published surveys as a general reference. The surveys presented here are recent general reviews of novelty detection methods over a broad range of application domains, rather than specific reviews focusing in one particular domain only (e.g. Agyemang et al. 2006; Bakar et al. 2006; Helali 2010; Patcha and Park 2007; Zhang et al. 2010). The emphasis is on the different categorisation schemes of novelty detection methods (see Table 1). Such a summary would allow an easier comparison of the strengths and weaknesses of each method. The surveys are grouped in reviews of methods for novelty detection, reviews of methods for outlier detection and reviews of methods for anomaly detection. Although there are fundamental differences between them (see Sect. 1), authors often use the terms novelty detection, outlier detection and anomaly detection interchangeably (Chandola et al. 2009; Hodge and Austin 2004; Marsland 2003), as the methods used are usually common.

Table 1 Categories of novelty detection methods according to the surveys presented

Categories	Markou and Singh (2003a)	Markou and Singh (2003b)	Marsland (2003)	Hodge and Austin (2004)	Chandola et al. (2009)
Classification based		✓	✓	✓	✓
Neural networks		✓	✓	✓	✓
Clustering based			✓	✓	✓
Nearest neighbour based			✓	✓	✓
Statistical	✓		✓	✓	✓
Information theoretic					✓
Spectral			✓		✓

Part of this table is adapted from Chandola et al. (2009)

4.1 Surveys in Novelty Detection

Markou and Singh (2003a,b) distinguish between two main categories of novelty detection methods: statistical approaches and neural network-based approaches. Statistical-based methods typically test whether the test samples come from the same distribution as the one learnt from the training data, for example, by measuring the distance of the sample from the mean of a distribution or by using density functions to model the data of known classes and then computing the probabilities that a sample belongs to one of these classes. Their main strength is that they are transparent methods, meaning they can be analysed easily using standard numerical methods. Their main drawback is that they make a number of assumptions; for example, parametric methods assume that the data distributions are Gaussian, which restrict their analytical power.

In contrast, neural network-based approaches make no prior assumptions on the form of the data distributions, requiring only the optimisation of a small number of training parameters (Markou and Singh 2003b). The work described in Sect. 3 provides examples of neural network-based approaches. A drawback of neural network-based approaches is that they cannot be as easily retrained as statistical models. This is not a major issue in cumulative learning problems, where adaptation and expandability of the learning structures are more important factors. Markou and Singh (2003b) identify three general algorithmic approaches: regularisation algorithms that optimise the weights of a neural network during training and do not change its initial size; pruning algorithms, which start with a large network size and remove nodes that are not active during training; and constructive algorithms, which start with a small network size and expand as necessary. Constructive algorithms are usually preferred, because they start with smaller networks that are faster to train and expand as necessary. Furthermore, it is more difficult to decide on how big the initial network should be with pruning algorithms. Two important issues that a designer has to deal with when working with constructive algorithms are (a) what is the most effective way of training method to enable integrating new units to the existing network and (b) when to stop adding new units.

Marsland (2003) provides another extensive summary of novelty detection methods. Although the paper is not structured in a manner that would allow an easy and structured comparison between the methods, as they are organised in specific categories based on their main algorithmic approach, rather than in general categories, the paper still offers a concise description of each of the methods it presents. Most importantly, some important issues with novelty detection are emphasised, these being how different a stimulus should be before it is classified as novel and how often a novel stimulus must be seen before it stops being novel, a question that the author has investigated in his earlier work (Marsland et al. 2000) and is summarised in Sect. 3.1.

4.2 *Surveys in Outlier Detection*

A similar yet not identical approach to novelty detection is outlier detection. Hodge and Austin (2004) treat outlier detection according to the definition given by Grubbs (1969)—"an outlying observation, or outlier, is one that appears to deviate markedly from other members of the sample in which it occurs"—and provide an extensive review of various methods used for outlier detection. They distinguish between three types of approaches. The first type includes methods where the outliers are determined without any prior knowledge of the data, this being analogous to unsupervised clustering. In the second type, both normal and abnormal cases are modelled; the authors say that such an approach is analogous to supervised classification and requires pre-labelled data tagged as normal or abnormal. Finally, methods of the third type mainly model normal cases together with a few abnormal cases also. Hodge and Austin (2004) mention that this third type is generally acknowledged as novelty detection or novelty recognition, and it is analogous to a semi-supervised detection/recognition task.

Like Markou and Singh (2003a,b), and Hodge and Austin (2004) also distinguish the methods used for novelty detection in statistical models and neural networks, and in addition to these two categories, they suggest another two, these being machine learning methods and hybrid methods. Their critique to the statistical and neural network-based approaches is similar to that of Markou and Singh (2003a,b); that is, statistical models are easy to deploy and transparent, but their computational demands increase if complex data transformations are needed before processing, while neural networks can generalise and learn complex class boundaries well, but they are opaque with respect to the underlying mechanisms and typically require longer training and tuning sessions. Because statistical-based approaches and neural networks typically require vectors consisting of at least ordinal data, the machine learning category was suggested to cover methods capable of also dealing with categorical data, such as the ones produced in rule-based systems, further clustering methods, decision trees and other tree-structure-based methods.

The hybrid category of outlier detection methods includes the most recent developments in the field and covers those methods that incorporate algorithms from the other three categories (statistical, neural networks and machine learning). This is done in order to gain the benefits of each one of the methods used while eliminating their limitations. It is for these reasons that hybrid methods appear attractive, but Hodge and Austin (2004) warn that the use of more than one classifier unless carefully designed can lead to the exhaustion of the available computational resources.

4.3 Surveys in Anomaly Detection

The most recent comprehensive survey on novelty detection methods was written by Chandola et al. (2009), which is an updated and shorter version of their previous survey paper, published as a technical report (Chandola et al. 2007). The focus is on anomaly detection, that is, "patterns in data that do not conform to a well defined notion of normal behaviour" (Chandola et al. 2007, p. 15). Although such a notion makes a clear distinction between normal and abnormal data, the authors acknowledge that anomaly detection is related to the domain of novelty detection, as methods used in one area are often used in the other area also, and vice versa. The authors group the different methods into six categories, these being the same four as the ones presented in Hodge and Austin (2004) and Agyemang et al. (2006), that is, classification-based methods, clustering-based methods, nearest neighbour-based methods and statistical methods, and two additional ones, these being information theoretic methods and spectral methods. An interesting suggestion is that anomalies can be classified in three categories. The first category includes point anomalies, which occur when an individual data instance is considered anomalous with respect to the rest of the data, for example, a robot guard of a post office seeing an unknown person. The second category is contextual anomalies, which include data instances that are considered anomalous in a particular context but not otherwise; this type of anomaly is often investigated in time-series data. An example of a contextual anomaly would be the robot guard of a post office seeing an unknown person in out-of-office hours, which might not be detected as an anomaly during working hours. Finally, collective anomalies consist of sets of data instances that are anomalous with respect to the entire dataset. A further agreement between the surveys of Hodge and Austin (2004) and Chandola et al. (2009) is on the general approaches of the detection methods, these being supervised, semi-supervised and unsupervised.

The authors identify a number of challenges that exist in anomaly detection, and two of them are of particular interest to novelty detection as well. First, there is the issue of the boundaries between normal data and anomalies or, in terms of novelty detection, the boundaries between known data and novelties, an issue acknowledged also by Marsland (2003). The second issue is that of noise in the data. As the authors mention, noise tends to generate data similar to actual anomalies, and hence it creates serious difficulties in identifying the true novelties.

5 Open Challenges

In the foregoing sections a number of issues and research questions have been identified for the effective operation of a cumulative learning system, with particular emphasis on novelty detection and hierarchical learning structures, two research topics that are closely related to each other.

Novelty detection plays an important role in a cumulative learning robot, as it is the cognitive component responsible for identifying perception and actions unknown to the system. However, the research question of novelty detection cannot be examined without also looking at the learning and knowledge representation structures. One of the key differences in the novelty detection methods described in this chapter is the different ways they represent data.

Dynamically expandable self-organising maps, called grow-when-required (GWR) networks, were used in various works (see Sect. 3). The experimental results have shown that GWR networks have performed satisfactorily when asked to identify previously seen inputs or to detect novelties (Sect. 3.2), and they generally result in fast small networks (Sect. 3.4).

The biologically inspired concept of habituation has also been shown to be very useful. Habituation controls when a GWR network should be further trained or when a new node should be added instead; this is achieved by looking if the frequency of a stimulus overcomes a threshold over a certain period of time. An issue related to this is that the parameters controlling the behaviour of the habituated GWR network are subjectively set by the user. A dynamic way of setting these values would be desirable (Thompson 2009a), particularly if they also take into account the individual characteristics of the agents, for example, in the form of intrinsic and extrinsic motivations and some other form of goal-oriented feedback. These solutions can also benefit of recent trends in habituation related to habituating the levels of habituation (Rankin 2009b).

Another issue that has been identified by the experiments conducted with the GWR networks was that of making a classification of the environment based on the current perception or taking into account prior history as well. Working only with the current perception has, in general, the benefit of reducing the processing complexity. However, the experiments that were conducted, aiming to assess the ability of the novelty filter in choosing the network that represents the currently perceiving and already known environment (Sect. 3.2), have shown that by relying only on the current perception and neglecting any prior history, the novelty filter was unable to choose the correct network among a set of similar networks. The notion of temporal abstraction in the form of time-series data signifying prior history could provide an improvement, although the research topic of temporal abstraction has a much wider scope. The challenge of temporal abstraction can be viewed informally as a type of generic interpretation task: "...given a set of time-stamped data, external events and abstraction goals, produce abstractions of the data that interpret past and present states and trends and that are relevant for the given set of goals" (Shahar 1996, p. 82). In this context, temporal abstraction involves creating context-sensitive interpretations of time-stamped data in terms of higher-level concepts and patterns that hold over time intervals; these interval-based abstractions are useful for planning and monitoring the execution of plans (Shahar and Cheng 2000) and for classifying perceptions and actions that are meaningful in a time coordinate system.

From a practical point of view, further challenges include how to fuse the information from the different sensors of the system and how to deal with noisy data. Clearly, relevant features in the environment need to be sensed and discriminated; otherwise, it would be impossible for the agent to respond appropriately. Therefore, the sensor modality used to generate the perceptual input plays an important role in the agent's performance for a given task or behaviour. Among the various sensors commonly available to a mobile robot, vision allows measurement and estimation of several environmental features and provides high-resolution readings in two dimensions, making the detection of small details of the environment more likely. Previous work carried out on camera sensors with novelty detection mechanisms (Neto and Nehmzow 2007a,b) will assist in investigating these complex issues. This work is also based on the GWR network. Although this has demonstrated good results, there is a need for taking advantage of recent developments in visual processing. However, the habituation concept is so tightly integrated that makes its use difficult with the current state of the art in visual processing. To address this limitation, a clear separation of habituation/novelty detection and a distinct framework for habituation are needed.

Lastly, all the work discussed in this chapter is focused on visual inspection and incremental learning of perceptions. In the research literature, there are a large number of papers discussing intrinsic motivation theories for action selection and skill acquisition from a neuroscience perspective. In addition, there are also proposed frameworks and experiments in intrinsically motivated learning robots. The theory of intrinsic motivation behind these studies is based on predictions and reinforcement learning, which typically require specific goals to be known a priori for the computation of the appropriate reward signals. Although these approaches have produced significant results, they explain and can be mainly used in task-oriented learning scenarios. On the other hand, novelty detection based on habituation does not require any type of reward and hence can be used in open learning systems without a specific task. If it was argued that the habituation and the dishabituation rates are similar to rewards depending on the amount known about the observation with the goal of minimising the error rate, then this argument is only partial; indeed, habituation, by definition, is also dependent on the frequency and the time period a stimulus is observed (Gurney et al. 2001a,b; Redgrave and Gurney 2006; Ryan and Deci 2000). Furthermore, habituation and reinforcement are very different concepts from a psychological point of view, explaining different types of cognitive processes. For example, infants may get engaged in activities that do not necessarily "make sense" to an adult, for example, picking an object from the floor and putting it into their mouth and trying to balance a ball on a traffic warning cone; however, they choose to engage and disengage in these activities through some kind of intrinsic motivation, which in some cases is habituation (Colombo and Mitchell 2009). The result of these superficially "meaningless" activities is to support the developmental process that can lead to the acquisition of new knowledge and skills that might be useful in a different context and time (Baldassare 2011; Mirolli and Baldassare 2011). As such, novelty detection based on the theories and models of habituation acts as an intrinsic motivation that guides an agent in areas of both specific and generic new knowledge and provides a mechanism where new behaviours can emerge. Whether these emergent behaviours are desirable and useful is a function of time and context, and a follow-up reinforcement learning module can be complimentary to the habituation module in these cases (Baranes and Oudeyer 2009; Barto et al. 2004; Schembri et al. 2007; Schmidhuber 1991a,b, 2010; Storck et al. 1995). For all these reasons, developing intrinsically motivated learning systems for skill acquisition based on novelty detection and habituation remains an open challenge.

6 Conclusions

In this chapter, we have provided a sample of the area of work under consideration. We consider the problem of novelty detection in autonomous cumulative learning robots as an instance of knowledge-based intrinsic motivation (Baldassare 2011; Mirolli and Baldassare 2011; Oudeyer and Kaplan 1999; Oudeyer et al. 1999). We approach the problem as one of novelty detection, so that the robot ignores perceptions that are similar to those seen during training, but is able to highlight anything different. Previous work by the authors and further literature have been presented and discussed extensively.

Recent surveys on the field of novelty detection have shown that there are a number of strengths and weaknesses associated with existing approaches and that there is no single universal method for novelty detection, rather than a suitable choice depends on the task. There are still many open challenges that need to be dealt with for the effective and long-term operation of a novelty detection filter in a cumulative learning robot. From the side of knowledge representation, dynamically expandable learning structures, able to cope with the demands of cumulative learning and prevent knowledge repletion, are needed. A related issue specific to dynamically expandable learning structures is the decision on whether to further train or expand when a new perception is misclassified. From a practical point of view, further challenges are having abstract representations able to generalise beyond the cases seen during training and the real-world issue of dealing with noisy data. An effective novelty detection filter should be able to provide multilevel and reliable measures of novelty. Previous work has shown that detecting novelty based only on the current perception is not always robust, and some form of temporal abstraction, where previous readings are also taken into account, is required. Finally, the computational costs, particularly associated with machine vision, cannot be neglected and are important issues that need to be tackled for the real-world operation of the system.

The methods presented here have some of the desired properties. First, their ability to expand as required is an important property of a novelty filter for the continual and long-term operation of a robot. Moreover, their ability to operate and learn online is also another useful feature, because there are a lot of cases where offline learning is not an option. Finally, they have demonstrated some level of abstraction and tolerance to noisy data; an important issue as noise can affect nonnovel objects to appear as novel. These key properties make these methods promising starting points for further research and meeting the specific requirements of novelty detection in the domain of cumulative learning. However, in order to take advantage of current state of the art in vision algorithms for improving the real-world effectiveness of the novelty detectors presented in this chapter, a new approach and redesign is needed that also takes into account recent findings in habituation (Rankin 2009b).

As a final conclusion, in this chapter, we have shown that a novelty detector based on habituation is a type of intrinsic motivation that is capable of driving the cumulative learning of autonomous robots, and we have also identified the open challenges that need to be resolved so that it can be effectively used in real-world applications.

Acknowledgements Professor Ulrich Nehmzow passed away in April 2010 during the IM-CLeVeR project implementation. While he did initiate the book chapter, he was unable due to illness to contribute to its completion. However, as this book chapter is mainly based on his pioneering ideas and works on novelty detection, we, his colleague researchers, dedicate it to his memory. This research has received funds from the European Commission 7th Framework Programme (FP7/2007-2013), "Challenge 2—Cognitive Systems, Interaction, Robotics", Grant Agreement No. ICT-IP-231722 and Project "IM-CLeVeR—Intrinsically Motivated Cumulative Learning Versatile Robots".

References

Agyemang, M., Barker, K., Alhajj, R.: A comprehensive survey of numeric and symbolic outlier mining techniques. Intell. Data Anal. **10**(6), 521–538 (2006)

Artac, M., Jogan, M., Leonardis, A.: Incremental pca for on-line visual learning and recognition. In: Proceedings of the of the 16th International Conference on Pattern Recognition (ICPR'02), vol. 3, pp. 781–784. IEEE Computer Society, Quebec City, QC, Canada. (2002)

Bakar, Z., Mohemad, R., Ahmad, A., Deris, M.: A comparative study for outlier detection techniques in data mining. In: 2006 IEEE Conference on Cybernetics and Intelligent Systems, pp. 1–6. IEEE (2006)

Baldassare, G.: What are intrinsic motivations? a biological perspective. In: Proceedings of the International Conference on Development and Learning and Epigenetic Robotics (ICDL-EpiRob-2011), pp. E1–E8 (2011)

Baranes, A., Oudeyer, P.-Y.: R-iac: Robust intrinsically motivated exploration and active learning. IEEE Trans. Auton. Mental Dev. **1**, 155–169 (2009)

Barto, A., Singh, S., Chentanez, N.: Intrinsically motivated learning of hierarchical collections of skills. In: Proceedings of the of the 3rd International Conference on Developmental Learning (ICDL'04), pp. 112–119 (2004)

Berlyne, D.: Conflict, Arousal and Curiosity, 1st edn. McGraw-Hill, New York (1960)

Bogacz, R., Brown, M.W., Giraud-Carrier, C.: High capacity neural networks for familiarity discrimination. Proceedings of the International Conference on Artificial Neural Networks (ICANN"99), pp. 773–778 (1999)
Chandola, V., Banerjee, A., Kumar, V.: Outlier detection: A survey. Technical report, University of Minnesota (2007)
Chandola, V., Banerjee, A., Kumar, V.: Anomaly detection: A survey. ACM Comput. Surv. **41**(3), 1–58 (2009)
Colombo, J., Mitchell, D.: Infant visual habituation. Neurobiol. Learn. Mem. **92**, 225–234 (2009)
Crook, P.A., Marsland, S., Hayes, G., Nehmzow, U.: A tale of two filters—on-line novelty detection. In: Proceedings of the of the 2002 IEEE International Conference on Robotics and Automation, ICRA 2002, pp. 3894–3899. IEEE, Washington (2002)
De Charms, R.: Personal Causation: The Internal Affective Determinants of Behaviour. Academic, New York (1968)
Deci, E., Ryan, R.: Intrinsic Motivation and Self-Determination in Human Behavior. Plenum, New York (1985)
Festinger, L.: A Theory of Cognitive Dissonance. Stanford University Press, Stanford (1957)
Fritzke, B.: Growing cell structures a self-organizing network for unsupervised and supervised learning. Neural Netw. **7**(9), 1441–1460 (1994)
Fritzke, B.: A growing neural gas network learns topologies. In: Tesauro, G., Touretzky, D.S., Leen, T.K. (eds.) Advances in Neural Information Processing Systems 7, pp. 625–632. MIT, Cambridge (1995)
Grubbs, F.E.: Procedures for detecting outlying observations in samples. Technometrics **11**, 1–21 (1969)
Gurney, K., Prescott, T., Redgrave, P.: A computational model of action selection in the basal ganglia i: A new functional anatomy. Biol. Cybern. **84**, 411–423 (2001a)
Gurney, K., Prescott, T., Redgrave, P.: A computational model of action selection in the basal ganglia ii: Analysis and simulation of behaviour. Biol. Cybern. **84**, 401–410 (2001b)
Harlow, H.: Learning and satiation of response in intrinsically motivated complex puzzle performance by monkeys. J. Comp. Physiol. Psychol. **43**, 289–294 (1950)
Hart, S., Grupen, R.: Learning generalizable control programs. IEEE Trans. Auton. Mental Dev. **3**, 216–231 (2011)
Helali, R.G.M.: Data mining based network intrusion detection system: A survey. In: Sobh, T., Elleithy, K., Mahmood, A. (eds.) Novel Algorithms and Techniques in Telecommunications and Networking, pp. 501–505. Springer, Dordrecht (2010) (Chapter 86)
Hodge, V., Austin, J.: A survey of outlier detection methodologies. Artif. Intell. Rev. **22**(2), 85–126 (2004)
Hunt, J.: Intrinsic motivation and its role in psychological development. Nebraska Symp. Motiv. **13**, 189–282 (1965)
Itti, L., Koch, C., Niebur, E.: A model of saliency-based visual attention for rapid scene analysis. IEEE Trans. Pattern Anal. Mach. Intell. **20**(11), 1254–1259 (1998)
Kaplan, F., Oudeyer, P.-Y.: Intrinsically motivated machines. In: Lungarella, M., Iida, F., Bongard, J., Pfeifer, R., (Eds.) 50 Years of Artificial Intelligence, pp. 303–314. Springer, Dordrecht (2007)
Lee, R., Walker, R., Meeden, L., Marshall, J.: Category-based intrinsic motivation. In: Proceedings of the of the Ninth International Conference on Epigenetic Robotics, pp. 81–88 (2009)
Lindeberg, T.: Feature detection with automatic scale selection. Int. J. Comput. Vis. **30**(2), 79–116 (1998)
Lisman, J., Grace, A.: The hippocampal-vta loop: Controlling the entry of information into long-term memory. Neuron **5**, 703–713 (2005)
Markou, M., Singh, S.: Novelty detection: A review. Part 1: Statistical approaches. Signal Process. **83**(12), 2481–2497 (2003a)
Markou, M., Singh, S.: Novelty detection: A review. Part 2: Neural network based approaches. Signal Process. **83**(12), 2499–2521 (2003b)

Marshall, J., Blank, D., Meeden, L.: An emergent framework for self-motivation in developmental robotics. In: Proceedings of the of the Third Int. Conference on Development and Learning (ICDL2004), pp. 104–111 (2004)

Marsland, S.: Novelty detection in learning systems. Neural Comput. Surv. **3**, 157–195 (2003)

Marsland, S., Nehmzow, U., Shapiro, J.: A real-time novelty detector for a mobile robot. In: Proceedings of the of the EUREL Conference on Advanced Robotics Systems, vol. 2, pp. 8–15 (2000)

Marsland, S., Nehmzow, U., Shapiro, J.: Vision-based environmental novelty detection on a mobile robot. In: Proceedings of the of the International Conference on Neural Information Processing (ICONIP'01), vol. 1, pp. 69–76 (2001)

Marsland, S., Nehmzow, U., Shapiro, J.: Environment-specific novelty detection. In: ICSAB: Proceedings of the Seventh International Conference on Simulation of Adaptive Behavior on From Animals to Animats, pp. 36–45. MIT, Cambridge (2002a)

Marsland, S., Nehmzow, U., Shapiro, J.: On-line novelty detection for autonomous mobile robots. Robot. Auton. Syst. **51**(2–3), 191–206 (2005)

Marsland, S., Shapiro, J., Nehmzow, U.: A self-organising network that grows when required. Neural Netw. **15**(8–9), 1041–1058 (2002b)

Martinetz, T.M., Schulten, K.J.: A neural-gas network learns topologies. In: Kohonen, T., Makisara, K., Simula, O., Kangas, J. (eds.) Artificial Neural Networks, pp. 397–402. Elsevier, Amsterdam (1991)

Merrick, K.: Self-motivated agents: Towards combined motivation models and integrated learning architectures. In: Mirolli, M., Baldassare, G. (eds.) Intrinsically Motivated Learning Systems, pp. 257–276. Springer, Berlin (2011)

Merrick, K., Maher, M.: Motivated learning from interesting events: Adaptive, multitask learning agents for complex environments. Adap. Behav. **17**(1), 7–27 (2009)

Mirolli, M., Baldassare, G.: Functions and mechanisms of intrinsic motivations. In: Mirolli, M., Baldassare, G. (eds.) Intrinsically Motivated Learning Systems, pp. 42–66. Springer, Berlin (2011)

Nehmzow, U., Neto, H.V.: Novelty-based visual inspection using mobile robots. In: Proceedings of the Towards Autonomous Robotic Systems (TAROS'04) (2004)

Nehmzow, U., Neto, H.V.: Visual attention and novelty detection: Experiments with automatic scale selection. In: Proceedings of the Towards Autonomous Robotic Systems (TAROS'06), pp. 139–146 (2006)

Neto, H.V., Nehmzow, U.: Visual novelty detection for inspection tasks using mobile robots. In: Proceedings of the of the 8th Brazilian Symposium on Neural Networks (SBRN'04) (2004)

Neto, H.V., Nehmzow, U.: Automated exploration and inspection: Comparing two visual novelty detectors. Int. J. Adv. Robot. Syst. **2**(4), 355–362 (2005a)

Neto, H.V., Nehmzow, U.: Incremental PCA: An alternative approach for novelty detection. In: Proceedings of the Towards Autonomous Robotic Systems (TAROS'05), pp. 227–233 (2005b)

Neto, H.V., Nehmzow, U.: Real-time automated visual inspection using mobile robots. J. Intell. Robot. Syst. **49**(3), 293–307 (2007a)

Neto, H.V., Nehmzow, U.: Visual novelty detection with automatic scale selection. Robot. Auton. Syst. **55**(9), 693–701 (2007b)

Otmakhova, N., Duzel, E., Deutch, A., Lisman, J.: The hippocampal-vta loop: The role of novelty and motivation in controlling the entry of information in long-term memory. In: Mirolli, M., Baldassare, G. (eds.) Intrinsically Motivated Learning Systems, pp. 277–293. Springer, Berlin (2011)

Oudeyer, P.-Y., Kaplan, F.: What is intrinsic motivation? A typology of computational approaches. Front. Neurobot. **1**(6), 1–14 (1999)

Oudeyer, P.-Y., Kaplan, F., Hafner, V.: Intrinsic motivation systems for autonomous mental development. IEEE Trans. Evol. Comput. **11**(2), 265–286 (1999)

Patcha, A., Park, J.: An overview of anomaly detection techniques: Existing solutions and latest technological trends. Comput. Netw. **51**(12), 3448–3470 (2007)

Rankin, C.: Introduction to special issue of neurobiology of learning and memory on habituation. Neurobiol. Learn. Mem. **92**, 125–126 (2009a)

Rankin, C.: Habituation revisited: An updated and revised description of the behavioral characteristics of habituation. Neurobiol. Learn. Mem. **92**, 135–138 (2009b)

Redgrave, P., Gurney, K.: The short-latency dopamine signal: A role in discovering novel actions? Nat. Rev. Neurosci. **7**, 967–975 (2006)

Ryan, R., Deci, E.: Intrinsic and extrinsic motivations: Classic definitions and new directions. Contemp. Educ. Psychol. **25**, 54–67 (2000)

Saunders, R., Gero, J.: Curious agents and situated design evaluations. In: Gero, J., Brazier, F. (eds.) Agents in Design 2002, pp. 133–149. University of Sydney, Sydney (2002)

Saunders, R., Gero, J.S.: The importance of being emergent. In: Proceedings of the of the Conference on Artificial Intelligence in Design (2000)

Schembri, M., Mirolli, M., Baldassare, G.: Evolving internal reinforcers for an intrinsically motivated reinforcement-learning robot. In: Proceedings of the of the 6th International Conference on Development and Learning (ICDL'2007), pp. 282–287 (2007)

Schmidhuber, J.: Curious model-building control systems. In: Proceedings of the of the International Joint Conference on Neural Networks, vol. 2, pp. 1458–1463, Singapore (1991a)

Schmidhuber, J.: A possibility for implementing curiosity and boredom in model-building neural controllers. In: Proceedings of the of the International Conference on Simulation of Adaptive Behavior: From Animals to Animats, pp. 222–227 (1991b)

Schmidhuber, J.: Formal theory of creativity, fun, and intrinsic motivation. IEEE Trans. Auton. Mental Dev. **2**, 230–247 (2010)

Schmidhuber, J.: Formal theory of creativity & intrinsic motivation (1990–2010): In: Mirolli, M., Baldassare, G. (eds.) Intrinsically Motivated Learning Systems, pp. 149–190. Springer, Berlin (2011)

Shahar, Y.: Dynamic temporal interpretation contexts for temporal abstraction. Ann. Math. Artif. Intell. **22**(1–2), 159–192 (1996)

Shahar, Y., Cheng, C.: Model-based visualization of temporal abstractions. Comput. Intell. **16**(2), 279–306 (2000)

Storck, J., Hochreiter, S., Schmidhuber, J.: Reinforcement-driven information acquisition in non-deterministic environments. In: Proceedings of the of the International Conference on Artificial Neural Networks (ICANN'95), vol. 2, pp. 159–164, Paris (1995)

Thompson, D.R.: Domain-guided novelty detection for autonomous exploration. In: IJCAI"09: Proceedings of the 21st International Jont Conference on Artifical Intelligence, pp. 1864–1869. Morgan Kaufmann, San Francisco (2009a)

Thompson, R.: Habituation: A history. Neurobiol. Learn. Mem. **92**, 127–134 (2009b)

Thompson, R.F., Spencer, W.A.: Habituation: A model phenomenon for the study of neuronal substrates of behaviour. Psychol. Rev. **73**(1), 16–43 (1966)

Wehmeier, S. (ed.): Oxford Advanced Learner's Dictionary, 7th edn. Oxford University Press, Oxford (2005)

White, R.: Motivation reconsidered: The concept of competence. Psychol. Rev. **66**, 297–333 (1959)

Zhang, Y., Meratnia, N., Havinga, P.J.M.: Outlier detection techniques for wireless sensor networks: A survey. IEEE Commun. Surv Tutorials, pp. 159–170 (2010)

Novelty and Beyond: Towards Combined Motivation Models and Integrated Learning Architectures

Kathryn E. Merrick

Abstract For future intrinsically motivated agents to combine multiple intrinsic motivation or behavioural components, there is a need to identify fundamental units of motivation models that can be reused and combined to produce more complex agents. This chapter reviews three existing models of intrinsic motivation, novelty, interest and competence-seeking motivation, that are based on the neural network framework of a real-time novelty detector. Four architectures are discussed that combine basic units of the intrinsic motivation functions in different ways. This chapter concludes with a discussion of future directions for combined motivation models and integrated learning architectures.

1 Introduction

The study of motivation in natural systems has a long history, including work by Aristotle, Jean Piaget and Sigmund Freud. Over the years, a broad spectrum of different motivation theories has been proposed for natural systems (Heckhausen and Heckhausen 2008). A subset of motivation theories that form the focus of this book are intrinsic motivations (Baldassarre 2011; Deci and Ryan 1985; Kaplan and Oudeyer 2007; Oudeyer and Kaplan 2007). Intrinsic motivations fall in the category of cognitive motivation theories, which includes theories of the mind that tend to be abstracted from the biological system of the behaving organism. Examples include novelty-seeking behaviour and curiosity (Berlyne 1960),

K.E. Merrick (✉)
School of Engineering and Information Technology, University of New South Wales, Australian Defence Force Academy, Northcott Drive, Canberra, ACT, Australia
e-mail: k.merrick@adfa.edu.au

G. Baldassarre and M. Mirolli (eds.), *Intrinsically Motivated Learning in Natural and Artificial Systems*, DOI 10.1007/978-3-642-32375-1_9,

competence-seeking motivation (White 1959), achievement, affiliation and power motivation (Heckhausen and Heckhausen 2008).

Artificial intelligence researchers seek to achieve a scientific understanding of the mechanisms underlying thought and intelligent behaviour in order to embody them in machines. This embodiment is achieved through abstract computational structures such as states, goals, and actions that form the fundamental units of computational models of cognition and motivation. Various different kinds of artificial models have been proposed for intrinsic motivation. Oudeyer and Kaplan (2007) provide a typology of different approaches and mechanisms from psychological and computational perspectives. Likewise, this book considers the broad classes of prediction-based (Schmidhuber 1991, 2010) models in Part II, novelty-based models (Marsland et al. 2000; Merrick and Maher 2009; Saunders 2001) in Part III and competence-based models (Barto et al. 2004; Schembri et al. 2007) in Part IV. Alternatively, the functions and mechanisms of intrinsic motivation can also be distinguished according to knowledge-based (including prediction and novelty-based) views and competence-based views as in Mirolli and Baldassarre (2012).

As our understanding of natural systems improves, new computational models will be possible that capture increasingly more of the capabilities of natural systems. For intrinsically motivated agents, this may mean incorporating multiple different kinds of intrinsic motivation with multiple different behavioural components. To achieve this, there is a need to identify fundamental units of intrinsically motivated agents and intrinsic motivation models that can be reused and combined to build more complex agents.

This chapter studies a subset of existing novelty-based models and one competence-based model of intrinsic motivation to identify fundamental units that can be combined and integrated in different agent architectures. In particular, Sect. 2 describes three models of intrinsic motivation based on the neural network framework of a real-time novelty detector: novelty, interest and competence-seeking motivation. Following this, in Sects. 3 and 4, agent architectures are presented that can use these motivation models in different ways. Section 3 describes agent models that conceptualise the fundamental units of intrinsic motivation as motivation functions that can be combined with different behavioural components. Section 4 describes agent models that conceptualise the fundamental units of intrinsic motivation as neurons in a network and integrate motivation and behaviour through shared memory. Applications of each model are discussed in Sects. 3 and 4, as well as a comparative study of the characteristics of the different motivation functions. This chapter concludes in Sect. 5 with a discussion of future directions for combined motivation models and integrated learning architectures.

2 Novelty-Based Models of Intrinsic Motivation

Psychological models of arousal, novelty and habituation (Berlyne 1960, 1966) have informed the development of computational models of novelty and curiosity. Nehmzow et al. (2012) provides a comprehensive overview of computational

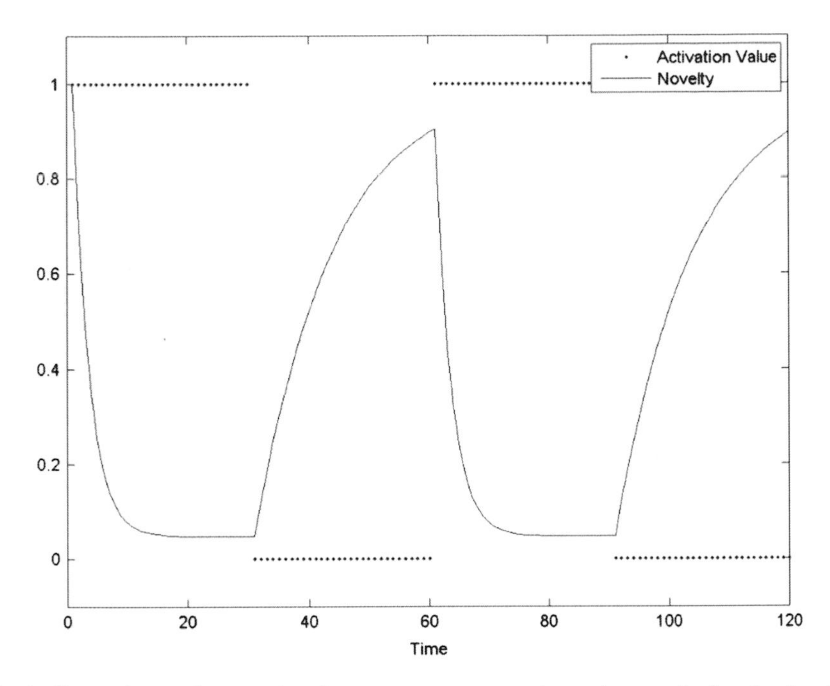

Fig. 1 Change in novelty over time in response to presentation and removal of a stimulus. The stimulus results in an activation value of 1 on presentation and 0 on removal

models of novelty for use in developmental robotics and cumulative learning applications. This chapter focuses on Stanley's model (Stanley 1976), which has formed the basis of several subsequent real-time novelty detectors, as well as models of interest, curiosity and creativity (Marsland et al. 2000; Merrick and Maher 2009; Saunders 2001). This chapter discusses how the fundamental units of a real-time novelty detector can be reused and integrated with different behavioural components to create different kinds of intrinsically motivated agents.

2.1 Modelling Novelty

In Stanley's (1976) model, the novelty N_t^k of a stimulus W^k decreases with presentation of the stimulus and increases with removal of the stimulus as shown in Fig. 1. Formally,

$$\tau \frac{\mathrm{d}N_t^k}{\mathrm{d}t} = \beta[N_0^k - N_t^k] - \varsigma_t(W^k) \tag{1}$$

$N_0^k = 1$ is the initial novelty value of a stimulus W^k at time $t = 0$, τ is a constant governing the rate of habituation and recovery of novelty and β is a constant regulating the minimum possible novelty value. $\varsigma_t(W^k)$ is a scalar activation value that is higher at times t when W^k is observed and lower when W^k is not observed.

Stanley's model has been used to implement real-time novelty detectors in a number of applications. A real-time novelty detector uses a clustering data structure such as k-means clustering (MacQueen 1967), adaptive resonance theory (ART) networks (Baraldi and Alpaydin 1998), growing neural gases (GNGs) (Fritzke 1995) or self-organising maps (SOMs) (Kohonen 1993) to generalise over attribute-based sensory data of the form $S_t = (s_t^1, s_t^2, s_t^3 \ldots s_t^J)$. Each time data is sensed, each attribute s_t^j where $j \in \{1 \ldots J\}$ is mapped to an input (sensory) neuron S^j. Sensory neurons are connected to clustering neurons by weights that are progressively adjusted according to the values of s_t^j.

As a concrete example, Marsland et al. (2000) used a SOM to create a real-time novelty detector for mobile robots. A SOM comprises a matrix $\mathbf{W}$ of K clustering neurons W^k. Each time data S^t is sensed, the closest (winning) neuron W_t^* is identified according to

$$W_t^* = \text{argmin}_{k \in \{1..K\}}(d(S_t, W^k)) \tag{2}$$

where $(d(S_t, W^k))$ is the Euclidean distance:

$$d(S_t, W^k) = \sqrt{\sum_{j=1}^{J} (S^j - w(S^j, W^k))^2} \tag{3}$$

$w(S^j, W^k)$ is a weight connecting the jth sensory neuron (associated with the jth attribute s_t^j of S_t) to the kth clustering neuron. The weights from all neurons in the topological neighbourhood of the winning clustering neuron (including the winning neuron) are then updated to reflect the new sensory data according to

$$w_{t+1}(S^j, W^k) = w_t(S^j, W^k) + \Theta_t(W^k, W_t^*)\eta_t[S^j - w_t(S^j, W^k)] \tag{4}$$

$0 \leq \eta_t \leq 1$ is the learning rate of the SOM. η_t is generally kept constant in a real-time novelty detector so that the detector is always learning.$0 \leq \Theta_t(W^k, W_t^*) \leq 1$ represents the influence on learning of a neuron's topological distance from the winning neuron. Various approaches are possible for computing $\Theta_t(.)$. As an example, Marsland et al. (2000) fix $\Theta_t(\cdot) = 1$ for the (up to) eight neurons adjacent to W_t^* in the matrix W.

Each neuron in the SOM is connected to an associated habituating neuron that holds a scalar novelty value N^k that changes according to Stanley's model in Eq. (1). Marsland et al. (2000) use $\tau = \tau_1$ for habituating neurons connected to winning SOM neurons and $\tau = \tau_2$ for all other habituating neurons. τ_1 and τ_2 are constants chosen such that $\tau_1 < \tau_2$ so habituation is faster than recovery. The activation values $\sigma_t(W^k)$ that transfer information from SOM neurons to connected habituating neurons can be computed in a number of ways. For example, Marsland et al. (2000) use

$$\varsigma_t(W^k) = \begin{cases} d(S_t, W^k) & \text{if } W^k = W_t^* \text{(i.e. if } W^k \text{ is a winning neuron at time } t) \\ 0 & \text{otherwise} \end{cases} \quad (5)$$

Using this activation function, the activation value of a given neuron decays over time. Merrick (2010a) proposes an alternative activation function that converts continuous-valued raw sensor data into a series of binary action potentials that do not decay over time:

$$\varsigma_t(W^k) = \begin{cases} 1 & \text{if } W^k = W_t^* \\ 0 & \text{otherwise} \end{cases} \quad (6)$$

The remainder of this section discusses how the underlying neural network framework of a real-time novelty detector can be adapted to create other models of intrinsic motivation. Sections 3 and 4 discuss ways that these models can be integrated with different behavioural components.

2.2 *Novelty and Interest*

Psychological literature suggests that there is an inverted U-shape relationship between novelty and interest (Heckhausen and Heckhausen 2008; Wundt 1910). That is, the most interesting experiences are often those that are moderately novel. Saunders (2001) modelled interest I_t by first using a real-time novelty detector to compute the novelty N_t^* of a stimulus W_t^*, then applying the Wundt curve:

$$\begin{aligned} I_t &= F^+(N_t^*) - F(N_t^*) \\ &= \frac{F_{\text{max}}^+ - F_{\text{avn}}^+ e^{-\rho^+(N_t^* - F_{\text{min}}^+)}}{1 + e^{-\rho^+(N_t^* - F_{\text{min}}^+)}} - \frac{F_{\text{max}}^- - F_{\text{avn}}^- e^{-\rho^-(N_t^* - F_{\text{min}}^-)}}{1 + e^{-\rho^-(N_t^* - F^- min)}} \end{aligned} \quad (7)$$

The Wundt curve in Eq. (7) is the difference of two sigmoid feedback functions $F^+(N_t^*)$ and $F^-(N_t^*)$. $F^+(N_t^+)$ provides positive feedback for the discovery of novel stimuli, while $F^-(N_t^*)$ provides negative feedback for highly novel stimuli. F_{max}^+ is a constant defining the maximum positive feedback, F_{max}^- defines the maximum negative feedback, ρ^+ and ρ^- are the slopes of the positive and negative feedback sigmoid functions, F_{min}^+ is the minimum novelty to receive positive feedback and F_{min}^- is the minimum novelty to receive negative feedback. The Wundt curve has a maximum value for moderate values of novelty. This can be seen in Fig. 2a which plots interest against novelty assuming no difference in aversion to either low or high novelty (that is $F_{\text{avn}}^+ = F_{\text{avn}}^- = 0$).

Aversion is negative, exponential feedback that modifies the positive and negative sigmoid feedback functions. The terms containing F_{avn}^+ and F_{avn}^- control the level of aversion to low and high novelty, respectively. This permits a distinction to be computed in terms of relative "negative interest" between very high or very

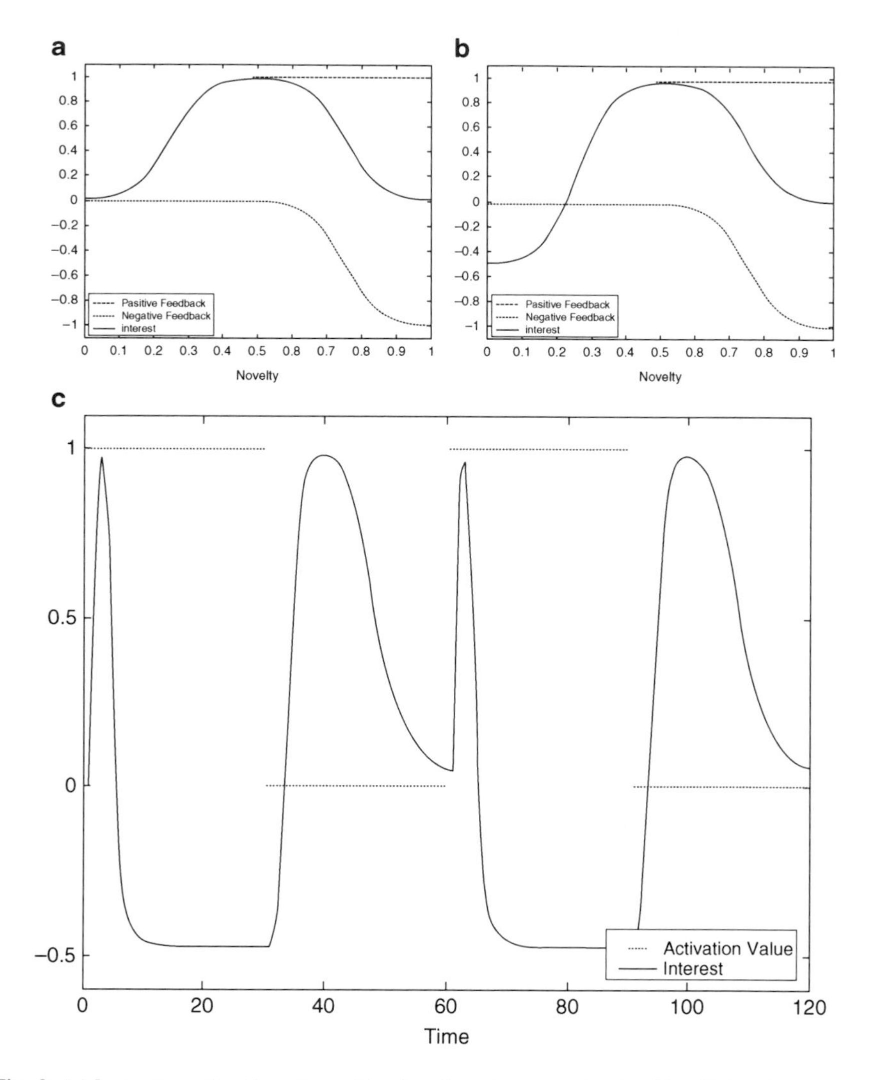

Fig. 2 (**a**) Interest as a function of novelty when there is no aversion to either high or low novelty. (**b**) Interest as a function of novelty when there is aversion to low novelty. (**c**) Change in interest over time in response to presentation and removal of a stimulus, when there is aversion to low novelty

low novelty. Figure 2b shows an interest function with aversion to low novelty. Figure 2c plots this interest function against time for an intermittent stimulus.

While other computational models of interest have also been proposed (Lenat 1976; Oudeyer and Kaplan 2004; Oudeyer et al. 2007; Schmidhuber 1991), Saunders' (2001) model is an example that builds a new model of intrinsic motivation (interest) by reusing the fundamental units of another model (novelty). The next section describes another such model for competence motivation.

2.3 Competence

Competence-based mechanisms for intrinsic motivation are characterised by the ability to measure how well a sensory-motor system is capable of achieving a certain desired goal, state or change. Competence-based motivation is important for permitting a machine to make decisions based on how well it can do something. This differs to novelty-based systems that generally make decisions based on the ability to recognise how familiar something is. In humans, these motivations work together. To achieve this synthesis in artificial systems, it is desirable to identify fundamental units of novelty and competence-based models that can permit them to work as a single intrinsic motivation system. We have already seen some of the underlying neural network components and mathematical models for novelty and interest. This section considers how components of a competence-based model can be incorporated within this framework.

Competence-based mechanisms for intrinsic motivation incorporate some form of secondary learning component (in addition to the primary clustering data structure) that maps a stimulus W^k to a response (action) A^l. Each stimulus–response mapping generally has some sort of weight or utility $U(W^k, A^l)$. A preference for a certain stimulus–response pair is learned by strengthening (increasing) $U(W^k, A^l)$. A stimulus–response mapping is forgotten by decreasing $U(W^k, A^l)$. Learned utility values $U(W^k, A^l)$ or the learning error $\Delta U(W^k, A^l)$ can thus be used as indicators of competence in this setting (Merrick 2008, 2010b).

To place this in the context of a real-time novelty detector, suppose a SOM is used to generalise over sensory data as described in Sect. 2.1. W_t^* defined by Eq. (2) is the observed stimulus at time t. The competence C_t of an agent performing action A^l when observing W_t^* can then be defined in terms of $U_t(W_t^*, A^l)$ and/or $\Delta U_t(W_t^*, A^l)$. One simple example is

$$C_t = U_t(W_t^*, A^l) \tag{8}$$

Using Eq. (8), competence is defined as the amount of accumulated (learned) utility for performing an action in a given state. This model is useful for deciding when to act. For example, an agent may be programmed to act only when competence motivation is above a given threshold. This model is less useful as an approach to lifelong attention focus because it implies that once a stimulus–response pair is learned, it will always be highly motivating, even if there are other stimulus–response pairs that have not been explored. An alternative competence motivation function that is more useful for lifelong learning is

$$C_t = \begin{cases} 1 & \text{if } \exists T \text{ such that } W_t^* = W_{t-T}^* \text{ and} \\ & (\Delta U_t(W_t^*, A_t) > \varepsilon \text{ or } 0 > \Delta U_t(W_t^*, A_t) > -\varepsilon) \\ -1 & \text{otherwise} \end{cases} \tag{9}$$

where $U_0(W_t^*, A^l) = 0$ and $\Delta U_0(W_t^*, A^l) = 0$. This motivation function rewards stimuli that are repeatable (i.e. $\exists T$ such that $W_t^* = W_{t-T}^*$) and either cause learning

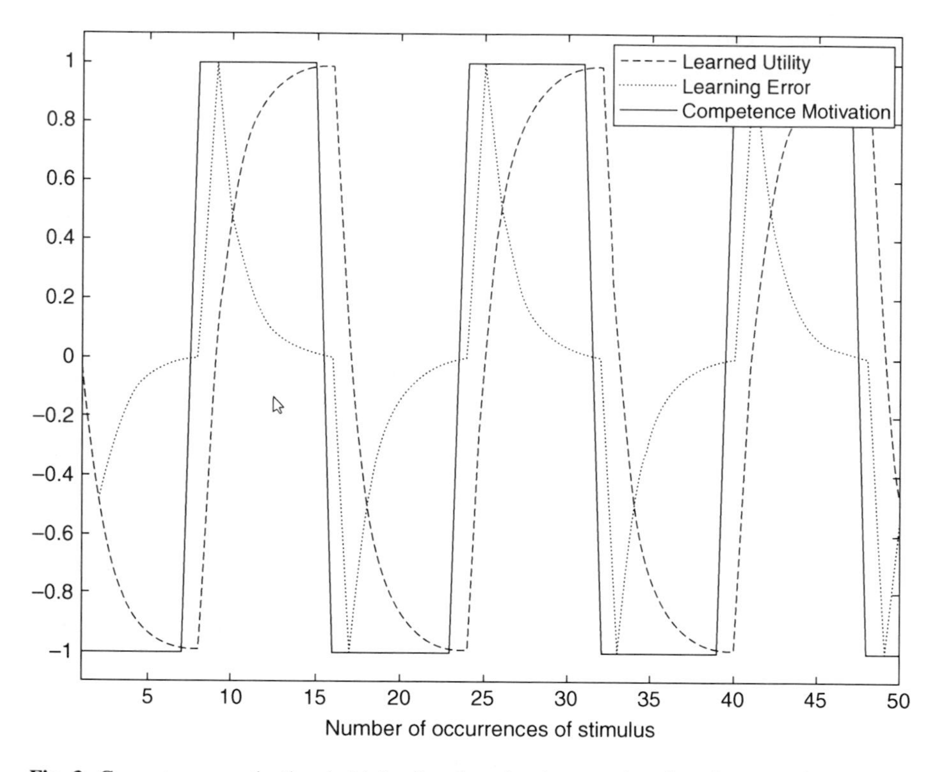

Fig. 3 Competence motivation is high when learning is occurring (learning error is large and positive) or when forgetting is complete (learning error is small and negative)

or have the potential to cause learning. Learning is represented as a "large enough" increase in U (i.e. $\Delta U > \varepsilon$), while learning potential is identified when there is a "small enough" decrease in U (i.e. $0 > \Delta U > -\varepsilon$). This latter case can be interpreted as the agent being "sure of its own incompetence". Figure 3 illustrates this competence-based motivation signal in a setting where utility $U(W_t^*, A_t)$ is updated using a reward-based learning approach that uses the competence motivation value as an immediate reward signal:

$$U_{t+1}(W_t^*, A_t) = U_t(W_t^*.A_t) + \Delta U_{t+1}(W_t^*, A_t) \tag{10}$$
$$\text{where } \Delta U_{t+1}(W_t^*, A_t) = \alpha[C_t - U_t(W_t^*, A_t)]$$

Learned utility, learning error and the corresponding competence motivation value are plotted against the number of times $W_t^* = W^k$ for some fixed k. Motivation is high when learning error is high. In other words, motivation is high while the agent is learning about the stimulus. This learning causes the learning error to drop. This eventually results in low motivation to continue learning about the stimulus. This cycle is repeated over time.

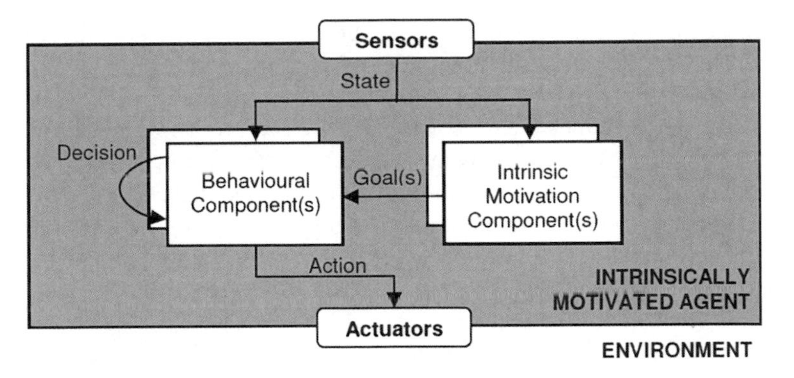

Fig. 4 Agent model for a generic intrinsically motivated agent. The behavioural component(s) connect sensors and actuators and are modulated by the intrinsic motivation component(s)

3 Intrinsically Motivated Agent Models Characterised as Motivation and Behavioural Components

This section uses the motivation functions described in Sect. 2 in a number of different intrinsically motivated agent models. For the purpose of the discussion in this chapter, an agent is defined as a software entity that can monitor its environment using sensors, reason about sensor data using some characteristic reasoning process and act to change its environment using actuators. Conceptually, two higher level fundamental units of intrinsically motivated agents are thus the motivation and behavioural components of reasoning. Motivation components signal the occurrence of certain kinds of important stimuli and trigger the agent to formulate goals, either explicitly or by rewarding certain actions. These goals are then acted on by one or more behavioural components. A generic intrinsically motivated agent is shown in Fig. 4. Sensors generate a sensed state at each time-step. One or more motivation components generate goals that are passed to one or more behavioural components. The behavioural component(s) make decisions that change the agent's internal state, or generate actions that trigger a corresponding actuator to change the state of the external environment. Three variations on this general model are discussed in the remainder of this section that combine different motivation and behavioural components. Motivations include the novelty, interest and competence models from Sect. 2. Behavioural components include reflexes, supervised learning and reinforcement learning. Applications of each model are also described.

3.1 Motivated Reflex Agents: Novelty-Seeking Agents for Computer Network Security

Reflexive behaviour is a preprogrammed response to the state of the environment (Maher and Gero 2002). Traditional reflex agents use mechanisms such as rulebases and fuzzy logic to define how the agent should respond to certain, recognised sensed states. Only recognised sensed states of the environment produce a response from the agent. In motivated reflex (MR) agents, recognised motivational states produce a response, rather than recognised sensed states. The agent can interact with complex, unknown environments without needing a preprogrammed set of recognised sensed states, because a simpler set of motivational states can be known in advance. For example, a novelty-seeking agent can be programmed to respond differently to motivational states of high or low novelty, without needing to know in advance which environmental stimuli will trigger these motivational states. This idea can be used, for example, to create novelty-seeking anomaly detection agents to detect malicious intrusions in computer networks, without knowing in advance what those intrusions might look like. An example of such a system is described in the following paragraphs.

Anomaly detection is a process that models the normal behaviour of a computer network and flags deviations from normal as intrusions (Chandola et al. 2009). Techniques include statistical models, probabilistic models, classification models and time- and frequency-based models that distinguish normal and abnormal behaviour. Anomaly detection is currently less widely used in practice than other forms of intrusion detection system (IDS) because of the difficulty of detecting zero-day attacks and their high false alarm rate. However, the potential of anomaly detection systems to adapt models of normal and abnormal activity is appealing because it removes the need for preprogrammed rules. Cumulative learning approaches to novelty detection pioneered in developmental robotics (see Nehmzow et al. 2012 for details) are a promising approach for network intrusion detection because they are online, single-pass, unsupervised learning approaches that analyse the similarity, frequency and recentness of network data. As such, they combine a number of different techniques into an approach with potential for real-time, adaptive network analysis and intrusion detection.

Shafi and Merrick (Merrick and Shafi 2009; Shafi and Merrick 2011) experimented with two novelty-seeking MR agents that differ in the way that sensor data is input to the clustering part of the novelty detector. In both algorithms, sensors read simulated network data from a comma-separated value file of 800,000 records from the KDD Cup dataset (Hettich and Bay 1999). The KDD Cup dataset is a raw traffic dump collected from simulated network traffic and converted into unique connection records. Each connection record is a vector $S_t = (s_t^1, s_t^2, s_t^3, \ldots, s_t^j)$ comprising $J = 41$ attributes (Lee and Stolfo 2001). There are thirty-nine intrusion types in the dataset.

At each time-step, the sensed state S_t comprises one connection record from the dataset. No preprocessing of the data is done aside from enumerating textual fields and standard vector normalisation of the state vector. This means that no assumptions are made about the range of values in each data field. The next step is different for the two different types of agent.

The first agent seeks novel observations using online k-means clustering of sensed states S_t.. k-Means clustering is a topology-free clustering layer with a fixed size set of neurons (called centroids). Online k-means clustering is similar to a SOM, with some notable differences described here. In k-means clustering, a winning centroid W_t^* W is selected from a list $\mathbf{W}$ of $K = 100$ centroids using Eq. (2). Weights connecting the winning centroid to each attribute of the sensed data are then updated in a similar manner to Eq. (4), but omitting the $\Theta_t(\cdot)$ term associated with the matrix topology of a SOM:

$$w_{t+1}(S^j, W^k) = w_t(S^j, W^k) + \eta_t[S^j - w_t(S^j, W^k)] \tag{11}$$

$\eta_t = 0.1$ is kept constant for all t so the clustering layer is always learning.

The second agent seeks novel events using k-means clustering of the difference vector $E_t = S_t - S_{t-1}$ between successive sensed states. A winning centroid W_t^* is selected from a list $\mathbf{W}$ of $K = 100$ centroids using a modified version of Eq. (2) as follows:

$$W_t^* = \text{argmin}_{k \in \{1 \ldots K\}} \left(\sqrt{\sum_{j=1}^{J} (E_t^j - w(S^j, W^k))^2} \right)$$

Sensory neurons S^j in this case are associated with difference in attributes $s_t^j - s_{t-1}^j$ rather than attributes themselves. Weights connecting the winning centroid to each input neuron are updated using Eq. (11).

The novelty associated with each centroid $W^k \in \mathbf{W}$ is computed using a stepwise approximation of Eq. (1). The derivative of novelty is first computed with respect to time:

$$\frac{\mathrm{d}N_{t-1}^k}{\mathrm{d}t} = \frac{\beta[N_0^k - N_{t-1}^k] - \varsigma_{t-1}(W^k)}{\tau} \tag{12}$$

where $\varsigma_{t-1}(W^k)$ is defined as in Eq. (6). The new novelty value is then computed and stored in each habituating neuron:

$$N_t^k = N_{t-1}^k + \frac{\mathrm{d}N_{t-1}^k}{\mathrm{d}t} \tag{13}$$

This concludes the intrinsic motivation component of these agents. A reflexive, behavioural component the same for both kinds of agent then distinguishes two different motivational states: high and low motivation. States of high motivation occur when the winning neuron W_t^* has high-associated novelty value, that is, $N_t^* > \Psi$. This indicates that a potentially harmful anomaly has been detected. In a real-world IDS, the agent might raise an alarm in this motivational state. In this experimental system, the agent simply writes the novelty value to a file for analysis.

Merrick and Shafi (2009, 2011) used two approaches to evaluate the performance of the agents. The first approach measured the number of first attack packets correctly recognised as such by the agent (the true positive rate). Correct recognition means that the motivated agent should assign a high novelty value to such instances. This implies that an alarm should be raised only once for the network administrator in an attack sequence. The second approach measured the number of normal data packets incorrectly identified as intrusions (the false positive rate). An optimal intrusion detection agent should never identify normal data as highly motivating. That is, it should assign low novelty values to normal data.

Using parameters, $\eta = 0.1, \beta = 1.05, \tau_1 = 3.3, \tau_2 = 14.3, N_t^k = 1 \forall k$ and $\psi = 0.4$, Merrick and Shafi (2009, 2011) found that agents seeking novel states (that is, $S^j = s_t^j$) had the higher true positive detection rate of the two agents in all four categories, but they did not adapt well to new attack types. In contrast, agents seeking novel changes (that is $S^j = S_t^j - s_{t-1}^j$) had a lower true positive detection rate, but adapted well to the new attack types in the test set. However, these agents also had a higher false positive detection rate for normal data. In general, Merrick and Shafi (2009, 2011) concluded that the false positive rate for both types of MR agent is high compared to other specialised IDSs. However, the true positive detection rate for rare attack types is also high, which suggests that with some tuning, or fusion with other IDSs, this approach may show promise as the basis for an adaptive, online, single-pass IDS.

3.2 *Motivated Supervised Learning Agents: Interest and Competence-Seeking Agents for Intelligent Environments*

Supervised learning agents learn behaviour by mimicking examples of correct behaviour from other agents, either human or artificial. In traditional supervised learning, examples tend to be hand-picked by the system designer and oriented towards a specific task or goal. In motivated supervised learning (MSL) (Merrick 2008), the learning agent uses a computational model of motivation to focus attention on a subset of examples from which to learn. One application of such agents is an intelligent environment. Intelligent environments have embedded computational and robotic devices to monitor and respond to human activities. The aim is to support and enhance human activities with adaptive computational intelligence. Adaptability has long been recognised as a key concern when developing intelligent environments (Weiser 1991). Traditional approaches support resource management, communication between devices, dynamic reconfiguration using real-time interaction models, modification of a running system, presence services and ad hoc networking. These approaches provide operating systems that can shrink and grow automatically in response to changes in the presence of devices in an intelligent room. However, they are limited in their ability to determine how the intelligent room should respond and adapt to those changes through behaviour that interacts with humans. MSL agents can permit more open-ended adaptability in such a setting. Merrick and colleagues (Merrick 2008; Merrick and Shafi 2009) conducted a number of experiments with MSL in intelligent environments, including an intelligent virtual home (Fig. 5a) and intelligent classroom (Fig. 5b) in *Second Life* (www.secondlife.com). This permits experimentation with the MSL agent model without requiring the physical infrastructure of a real building. The virtual home

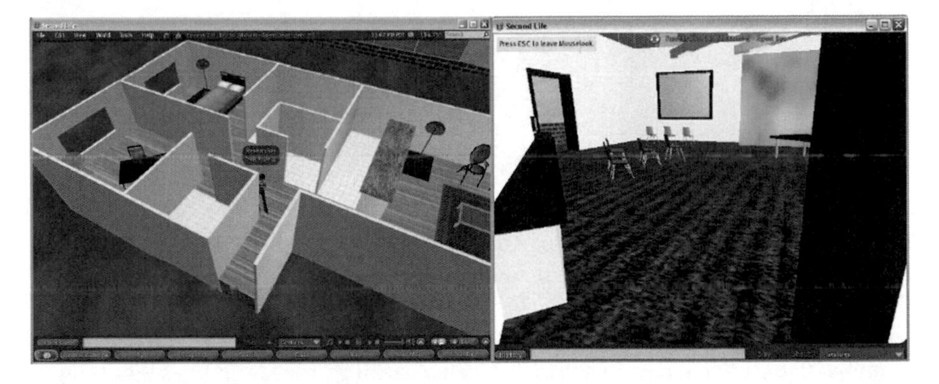

Fig. 5 (**a**) A virtual "intelligent home"; (**b**) an "intelligent classroom" (*right*) in Second Life. Images from Merrick (2008) and Merrick and Shafi (2009))

is modelled on a real-world, two-bedroom apartment. The virtual classroom is modelled on a real-world university classroom. A number of virtual devices were programmed for the virtual rooms using *Second Life's Linden Scripting Language* (LSL) including lighting, floor sensors to detect avatar presence, a television and "smart" chairs that can sense when someone is sitting on them. The middleware or "adaptive operating system" layer was implemented as a virtual ad hoc network based on the idea of a *BlipNet* (BLIPSystems 2007). A *BlipNet* consists of two main components: a *BlipServer* and BlipNodes. BlipServer software configures, monitors and controls *BlipNodes*. *BlipNodes* are hardware components that can detect, monitor and communicate with Bluetooth-enabled devices. A programming API makes it possible to create custom applications, such as MSL agents, that can monitor and control devices on the *BlipNet*. The next paragraphs describe such an agent.

At each time-step t, a MSL agent monitors the *BlipServer* to obtain the state S_t of their environment. This state comprises a list of *Second Life* object identifiers for virtual devices detected by the virtual *BlipServer*. The agent also receives a list $\mathbf{A}$ of possible actions that can be performed on these devices and, if any, an example action X_t performed by a human-controlled avatar at the current time-step. This agent model uses two motivation components and two behavioural components. An interest motivation component moderates a learning behavioural component, while a competence motivation component moderates an action-selection behavioural component. If the MSL agent senses an example action, an interest value is computed for the current sensed state S_t. Since this application is implemented in a relatively simple, noise-free virtual world, no clustering layer is used to compute interest. Instead, a list $\mathbf{W}$ is created incrementally that contains one entry corresponding to each state sensed during the agent's lifetime. At each time-step, t the agent adds a new element $W = S_t$ to $\mathbf{W}$ if there is no such element already there. Each $W^k \in \mathbf{W}$ has an associated habituating neuron that holds a scalar novelty value. All neurons in the habituating layer are updated using Eqs. (12) and (13) and the activation function:

$$\varsigma_t(W^k) = \begin{cases} 1 \text{ if } W^k = S_t \\ 0 \text{ otherwise} \end{cases}$$

Interest I_t is computed using Eq. (7) with the novelty value N_t^* associated with for $W_t^* = S_t$ as input. This completes the interest motivation component. The interest motivation component moderates a supervised learning component that uses table-based learning of associations (Steels 1996) between stimuli and examples. This behavioural component is triggered if an example X_t is sensed and W_t^* is "interesting enough" (that is, $I_t > \Phi_1$). Each element of **W** has a corresponding set of utility values of the form $U(W^k, X)$ for associations between W^k and any example X sensed in the presence of W^k. The learning process updates the strength U of the associations between W_t^* and all X in a manner similar to that proposed in Eq. (10):

$$U_{t+1}(W_t^*, X) = U_t(W_t^*, X) + \alpha[R_t - U_t(W_t^*, X)]$$

In this supervised learning model, $R_t = 1$ if $X = X_t$ or $R_t = 0$ otherwise. The parameters α govern the rate of learning. This completes the learning behavioural component. The action-selection behavioural component is triggered when no example of human behaviour is sensed, and the agent calculates that it could act on behalf of the human with high competence ($C_t > \Phi_2$). Competence is calculated using an approach based on Eq. (8) as the highest utility of any example associated with W_t^*:

$$C_t = \max_X U(W_t^*, X)$$

The actionA_t is selected as:

$$A - t = \text{argmax}_X U(W_t^*, X)$$

The experimental parameters for novelty are the same as those used in Section 3.1. Other parameters and values are $\alpha = 0.5$, $\Phi_1 = 0.7$, $\Phi_2 = 0.8$, $F^+_{\text{max}} = F^-_{\text{max}} = 1$, $\rho^+ = \rho^- = 20$, $F^+_{\text{avn}} = F^-_{\text{avn}} = 0$, $F^+_{\text{min}} = 0.25$ and $F^-_{\text{min}} = 0.75$. In a range of experiments and case studies, (Merrick and Shafi 2009; Maher et al. 2008) demonstrated the ability of MSL agents to adapt to human activities in simple, virtual, intelligent environments. The MSL agents learned behaviours such as:

- Turning on lights when an avatar entered the room.
- Turning on the TV and dimming lights when an avatar sits on the couch.
- Turning on the projector and dimming lights when avatars enter the classroom

Around six repetitions of an action or action sequence were required for the MSL agent to learn a response. This could be decreased (or increased) by modifying the values of the learning rate α or threshold parameters Φ_1 and Φ_2.

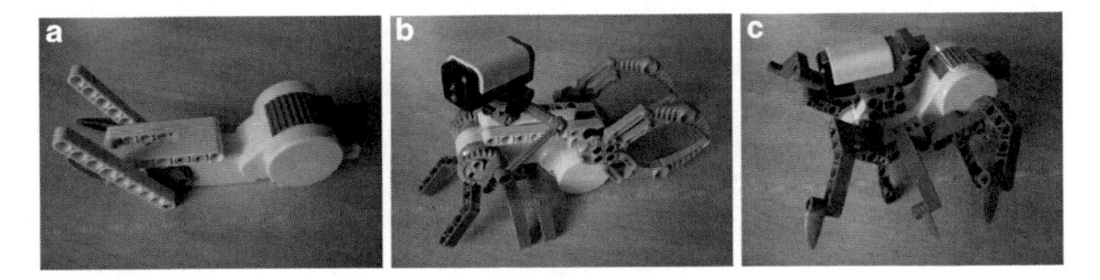

Fig. 6 Three *Lego Mindstorms* NXT robots (**a**) a snail with a single motor; (**b**) a bee with a motor and colour sensor; (**c**) an ant with a motor and accelerometer. Images from Merrick and Shafi (2009)

3.3 Motivated Reinforcement Learning Agents: Competence-Seeking Reconfigurable Robots

Reinforcement learning (RL) agents (Sutton and Barto 2000) use systematic trial and error to learn behaviours that maximise the long-term value of a reward signal. In traditional RL agents, the reward signal tends to define a specific task or goal to be achieved. In contrast, in motivated reinforcement learning (MRL), the reward signal is modelled as a motivation value defining task-independent concepts such as novelty, interest or competence. This permits MRL agents to adapt their behaviour to address tasks that are not known in advance of learning. One such example is a reconfigurable robot toy.

Reconfigurable robots such as *Lego* (http://www.lego.com) and *Meccano* (http://www.meccano.com) are technologies that support creative play. They encourage creative thinking and creative design by providing sets of basic components and connector modules that can be built into different structures. The incorporation of components for embedded automation such as motors, remote controls and programmable bricks has opened the way for traditional building packages such as *Lego* and *Meccano* to become platforms for playful learning of concepts in electronics and computer programming. Addition of components for embedded intelligence extends the capacity of such toys to encourage creative design thinking through creative play (Merrick 2008). Reconfigurable robots with embedded MRL can evolve structured behaviour adapted to their individual physical forms and thus provide the designer with feedback on the relationship between the form they are constructing and its potential behaviour.

Merrick and Scully (2009) experimented with three *Lego Mindstorms NXT* robots with different physical structures shown in Fig. 6. Each robot has a motor that can be rotated. Two of the robots also have sensors as shown in Fig. 6. At each time-step t, the agent senses the current state S_t of the robot. The sensed state is a vector of attributes describing the position of the motor and readings from any sensor present.

The current sensed state is clustered using a simplified adaptive resonance theory (SART) network (Baraldi and Alpaydin 1998). A SART network is a topology-free clustering layer that is initialised with an empty set W of neurons and grows this set of neurons when "very different" states are sensed. "Very different" in this case is defined by a validation constraint $d(S_t, W^k) < \mu$.

Each time a state S_t is sensed, the closest existing neuron that satisfies the validation constraint is sought using Eqs. (2) and (3). If such a neuron (denoted W_t^*) exists, its weights are updated according to Eq. (11). If no such neuron exists, a new neuron W_t^* is added to **W** and the weights $w(S^j, W_t^*)$ initialised with the corresponding s_t^j.

Each neuron also has an associated set of utility values of the form $U(W^k, A^l)$. In this application, every state encountered by each robot affords possible three actions: A^1 move the motor forward at a fixed speed; A^2 move the motor backwards at a fixed speed; and A^3 stop the motor. New neurons are initialised with utility values of $U_0(W^k, A^l) = 0$ for each of these actions. An associated value $\Delta U(W^k, A^l)$ is also stored, where $\Delta U_0(W^k, A^l) = 0$.

Finally, a competence motivation value C_t is computed for W_t^* using the function in Eq. (9). This completes the motivation component. In the behavioural component, the competence motivation value becomes a reward signal for learning utility values using Q-learning (Watkins and Dayan 1992):

$$U_t + 1(W_{t-1}^*, A_{t-1}) = U_t(W_{t-1}^*, A_{t-1}) + \Delta U_{t+1}(W_{t-1}^*, A_{t-1})$$

$$\text{where } \Delta U_{t+1}(W_{t-1}^*, A_{t-1}) = \alpha[C_t + \gamma \max_l U_t(W_t^*, A^l) - U_t(W_{t-1}^*, A_{t-1})]$$

The Q-learning update is computed as a function of past, present and future expected reward. γ is the discount factor for future expected reward. $\alpha = \alpha_L$ governs the rate of learning when $C > 0$ and $\alpha = \alpha_F$ governs the rate of forgetting when $C_t \leq 0$. Differentiating between learning and forgetting allows the agent to trade-off between exploration and exploitation. For example, if $\alpha_L > \alpha_F$, the robot can continue to exploit learned behaviour while exploring to discover new behaviour.

This agent was run for 1,200 time-steps (six minutes) on each robot. Parameter values were $\epsilon = 0.001$, $\alpha_L = 0.9$, $\alpha_F = 0.1$, $\gamma = 0.9$, $\mu = 0.2$ and $\eta = 0.1$. Merrick and Scully (2009) evaluated the behaviour of the robots using point-cloud matrices to visualise when actions or sequences of actions are repeated. Point-cloud matrices use colour intensity on a tXt' grid to visualise the similarity of states encountered at every pair of time-steps. The similarity of two states is computed as Euclidean distance:

$$d(s_p s_{t'}) = \sqrt{\sum_{j=1}^{J} (s_t^j - s_{t'}^j)^2}$$

The darker the pixel at position (*t,t'*) on the point-cloud matrix, the greater the similarity in the states S_t and $S_{t'}$.

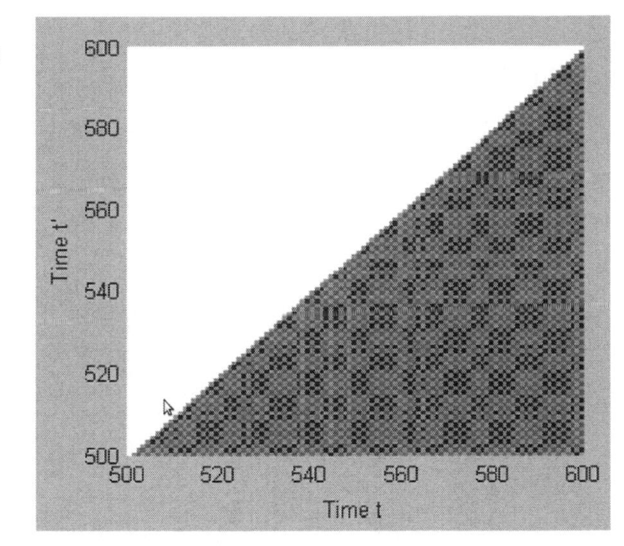

Fig. 7 A segment of a point-cloud matrix visualising the ant's walk

Merrick and Scully (2009) found that all the robots were able to learn structured behaviour cycles of between two and ten actions in length. Some of these cycles were repeated 20–30 times. The snail, for example, learned to raise and lower its antennae and the bee learned to move its head from left to right between two colour panels. The ant was perhaps the most interesting of the insect-bots as it was able to learn to "walk" motivated only by the competence-based intrinsic motivation function. The walk was somewhat jerky, with the ant learning to combine a sequence of "move-forward" and "stop-motor" actions. A segment of a point-cloud diagram showing the ant walking is shown in Fig. 7.

4 Intrinsically Motivated Agent Models Characterised as Networks of Neurons

The agent models in Sect. 3 are conceptualised as combinations of motivation and behavioural components. This permits different reflexive and learning behaviours to be combined with motivation. However, it also implies that different representations of the environment may result within each process. As an alternative, this section conceptualises the fundamental units of intrinsic motivation as neurons in a network. Motivation and behaviour are integrated through shared memory. The focus of this section is on motivated reinforcement learning (MRL) models that use a common data structure for the motivation and behavioural (reinforcement learning) components (Merrick 2010a; Merrick and Scully 2009). A comparative study is discussed of the characteristics of three motivation functions when used within this framework.

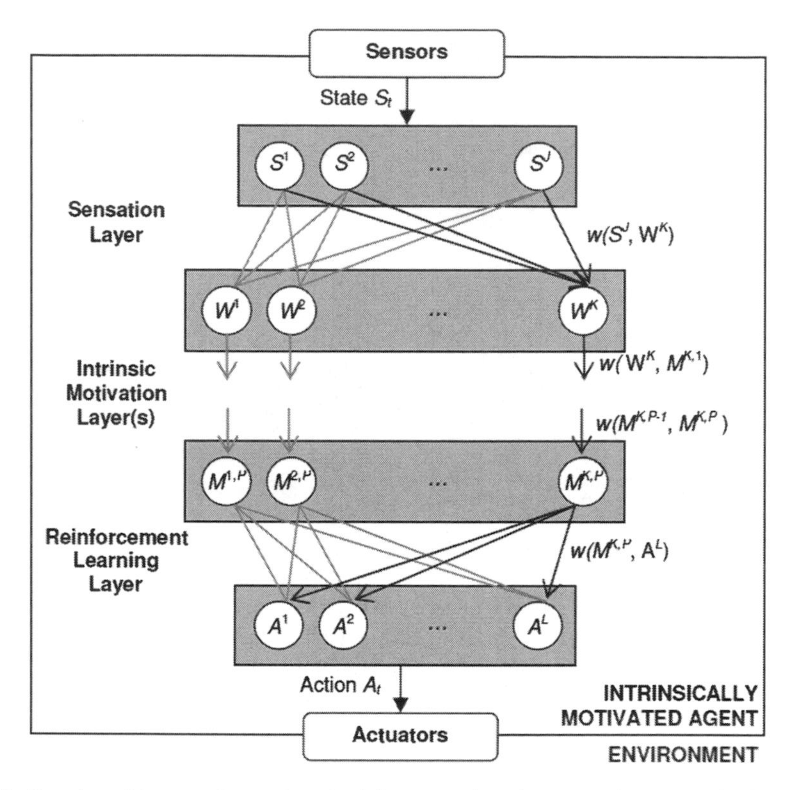

Fig. 8 Generic architecture for motivated reinforcement learning agents in a network of neurons

4.1 *Motivated Reinforcement Learning in a Network of Neurons*

This integrated MRL architecture generalises the neural network approach of a real-time novelty detector to create a multilayer neural network with a generic structure shown in Fig. 8. The fundamental units in this approach are neurons and layers of weights connecting neurons. There are four main types of neurons:

- Sensory neurons (input neurons)
- Clustering neurons (hidden neurons)
- Motivation neurons (hidden neurons)
- Action neurons (output neurons)

In each layer, one or more neurons perform the following processes:

- Get values from connected neurons in the previous layer
- Update weights connected to neurons in the previous layer
- Compute an activation value and send it to one or more neurons in the next layer

Sensory neurons S^j are responsible for inputting raw to the network. There is one sensory neuron S^j for each piece of sensor data s_t^j generated at a given time. The first layer of weights in the network is the sensation layer that generalises over the space of states (or changes in states) encountered by the agent. This layer clusters raw sensor data at a given time t to a winning clustering neuron W_t^* that best represents the data. As discussed previously in the chapter, this layer can incorporate common clustering algorithms such as k-means clustering, SOMs, SART networks or GNGs. Depending on the clustering algorithm used, there may be any number of clustering neurons and, additionally, this number can be fixed or variable. Clustering neurons can be unrelated or have a topological relationship. The winning clustering neuron is identified and updated according to the rules of the clustering algorithm, several of which have been discussed throughout this chapter [e.g. see Eqs. (2)–(4) or (11)]. An activation value is calculated and a signal sent to trigger activity in other parts of the network, starting with the first motivation layer. Various activation functions for the sensation layer have also been discussed earlier in the chapter [e.g. see Eqs. (5)–(6)].

The motivation layers have one neuron for every clustering neuron, as shown in Fig. 8. As such, they may also have a fixed or variable number of neurons, depending on the structure of the sensation layer. There may be $p = 1 \ldots P$ layers of motivation neurons, depending on the number and complexity of the motivation function(s) used. These layers may be organised in series or in parallel to permit multiple motivation functions to cooperate or compete to control learning. Weights connecting motivation neurons to clustering neurons or other motivation neurons are updated using a computational model of motivation as the update function. Various such functions have been discussed in this chapter [e.g. see Eqs. (1) and (7)–(9)]. Neurons in the pth motivation layer, output activation values $\varsigma_t(M_t^{k,p})$ to the $(p+1)$th layer or to the RL layer if $p+1 = P \cdot \varsigma_t(M_t^{k,p})$, may be defined in terms of a single weight or an aggregate such as a sum or average over several weights. In the former case, $\varsigma_t(M_t^{k,p})$ represents the influence of a single motivation. In the latter case, $\varsigma_t(M_t^{k,p})$ may represent the influence of several cooperating or competing motivations. The activation value of the Pth layer motivation neuron connected (directly or indirectly) to the winning clustering neuron at time t is denoted $\varsigma_t(M_t^*)$. Weights in the RL layer are updated to reinforce connections between stimuli and actions that are highly motivating, according to the activities of the motivation layer(s). For example, if a Q-learning approach (Watkins and Dayan 1992) is used, the weight connecting M_{t-1}^* to A_{t-1} is updated as follows:

$$w_{t+1}(M_{t-1}^*, A_{t-1}) = w_t(M_{t-1}^*, A_{t-1}) + \Delta w_{t+1}(M_{t-1}^*, A_{t-1}) \quad (14)$$

$$\Delta w_{t+1}(M_{t-1}^*, A_{t-1}) = \alpha[\varsigma_t(M_t^*) + \gamma \max_l w_t(M_t^*, A^l) - w_t(M_{t-1}^*, A_{t-1})] \quad (15)$$

α is the learning rate and γ is the discount factor for future expected motivation.

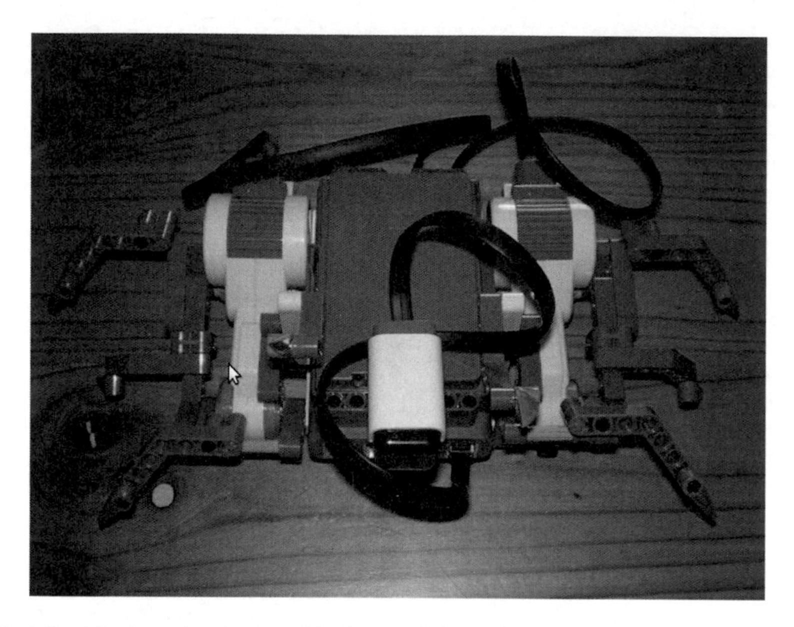

Fig. 9 A "crab" robot using the *Lego Mindstorms NXT* platform. Image from Merrick (2010a)

Neurons A^l in the action layer compute activation values $\varsigma_t(A^l) = w_t(M_t^*, A^l)$. The neuron with the highest activation value is selected to trigger its corresponding actuator:

$$A_t = \text{argmax}_l \varsigma_t(A * l) \tag{16}$$

This function greedily selects the action with the highest weight. All exploration and exploitation are assumed to be controlled by the motivation function embedded in the motivation layer.

4.2 A Comparative Study of Different Intrinsic Motivations

The applications in Sect. 3 considered intrinsic motivation functions in the presence of different behavioural components. However, when the integrated approach from Sect. 4.1 is used, it becomes possible to compare a range of motivation models in a single framework. Merrick (2010a) used such an approach to conduct a series of experiments comparing different intrinsic motivation functions on a *Lego Mindstorms NXT* "crab" robot shown in Fig. 9. The robot has two servo motors controlling the left and right sets of legs. It can move each motor forwards or backwards or stop a motor. The robot can sense whether the motors are moving or not, their rotation and direction of movement. It can also sense its acceleration and tilt in three dimensions. While this robot is relatively simple, it provides the

Table 1 Parameters values used to compare the performance different motivation models

Parameter	Description	Value
η	SART learning rate	0.1
μ	SART validation threshold	0.2
α_L	Q-learning rate	0.9
α_F	Q-forgetting rate	0.1
γ	Q-learning discount factor	0.9
β	Minimum novelty moderator	1.05
τ_1	Novelty habituation rate	3.3
τ_2	Novelty recovery rate	14.3
F^+_{min}	Minimum novelty to receive positive interest	0.5
F^-_{min}	Minimum novelty to receive negative interest	1.5
F^+_{max}, F^-max	Maximum positive/negative interest feedback	1
ρ^+, ρ^-	Gradient of approach/avoidance of novelty	10
F^+_{avn}	Aversion to low novelty	0.33
F^-_{avn}	Aversion to high novelty	0
ϵ	Competence motivation switch threshold	0.01

basic structure for a robot that can potentially learn to walk: motors to control the action of the legs and an accelerometer to monitor the movement of the body.

Three versions of the agent model in Sect. 4.1 were compared that differed in the motivation functions used. The sensation layer in all three agents used SART clustering to generalise over data from the robot's sensors as described in Sect. 3.3. The first agent had one motivation layer with the weights $w(W^k, Mk, 1)$ updated using the novelty updates in Eqs. (12) and (13). The second agent had two motivation layers. The weights $w(W^k, Mk, 1)$ were updated using the novelty updates in Eqs. (12) and (13). The weights $(M^{k,1}, M^{k,2})$ were updated using the interest function in Eq. (7). The third agent had one motivation layer with the weights $w(W^k, Mk, 1)$ updated using the competence updates in Eq. (9) with ΔU defined by Δw in Eq. (15). The RL layer for all agents is updated according to Eq. (14). An action is selected according to Eq. (16).

To permit a fair comparison of agents using the three motivation functions, common parameters use the same values. All parameters and their values are summarised in Table 1. Each agent was run five times on the robot for 4,000 time-steps (30 min). Merrick (2010a) reported a number of key results:

- The robots using all three of the motivation functions (novelty, interest and competence) show behaviour that is significantly more structured than that exhibited by a robot using random exploration.
- All motivation functions motivate exploration more than 50 % of the time on average, in preference to motivating exploitation of learned behaviours.
- Exploitation is distributed differently through robots' lifetimes depending on the motivation function used. Robots using novelty and interest-based motivation tend to exploit learned behaviour for short periods and return to the same

behaviours several times during their life. Robots using competence-based motivation exploit learned behaviours for fewer, but longer, periods.
- The robots learn only very simple behaviours including lifting and lowering their legs. The emergence of simple structured behaviours is important, but indicates that the limits of these motivation functions and basic MRL is being reached, even on this relatively simple robot structure.
- Interest-motivated agents tended to learn the longest sequences of actions.

The overall similarity in performance of the novelty and interest-based approaches was noteworthy because interest-based approaches are often favoured over novelty-seeking approaches for noisy applications such as robots. This is because novelty-based approaches are believed to be weaker than interest-based approaches in the presence of noise. Random stimuli such as sensor noise, from which little can be learned, tend to be unfamiliar and thus generate high novelty values. In practice, however, it would appear that this weakness is not apparent in a MRL setting because random stimuli by nature do not appear consistently enough to be reinforced. In other words, the frequency of stimuli is as important as their familiarity for determining novelty-based reward.

The emergence of structured behaviour cycles in this work is encouraging because it shows that structure can be generated using generic motivation functions. However, unlike the experiments in Sect. 3.3, none of the algorithms was able to motivate the crab robot to learn to walk. It is likely that alternative behaviour components that can remember and combine multiple learned policies, or policy hierarchies, will be an advantage in this area in future.

5 Towards the Future

As humans use machines to perform increasingly larger arrays of tasks, in future it is likely that intrinsic motivations will be components of more complex motivation systems that combine biological, cognitive and social motivations within a single integrated framework. Biological models of motivation will permit artificial systems to synchronise their behaviour autonomously with salient internal variables, such as battery level, heat, oil or other fluids, or with salient environmental variables. There is also a possibility for robots to synchronise their behaviour with that of humans sharing their environment. This would permit them to anticipate, predict and support those behaviours, providing a new approach to human-machine interaction. Potential applications for robots with these capabilities include home assistants and industrial robots. Cognitive models of motivation, including intrinsic motivation models, will support the development of artificial systems with the capacity for experimentation and creativity. For example, they provide a basis for building systems that are themselves capable of creative design, that can identify and use objects creatively as tools and that can discover novel problems to solve, not necessarily envisaged by the system's designers. Application areas include the

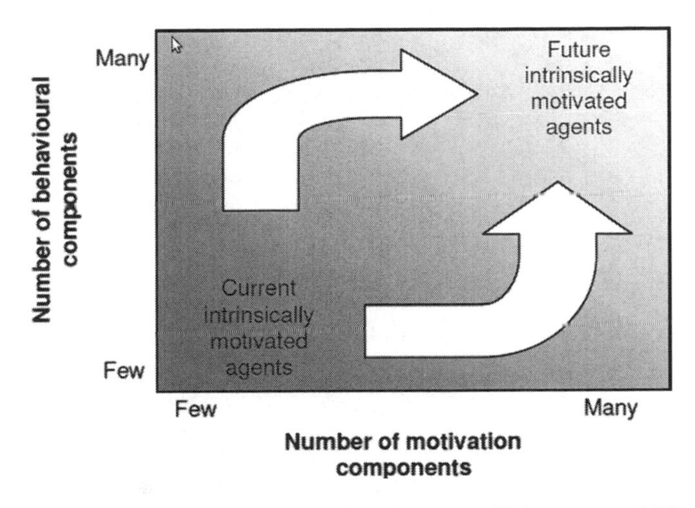

Fig. 10 Towards the future: intrinsically motivated agents will integrate multiple motivation components to select goals and multiple different behavioural components to solve to goals

architecture, engineering and construction (AEC) industry where systems that can mimic the creative role traditionally played only by humans are a long-term research goal (Gero 1992). Scientific research can also benefit from systems capable of conducting creative research and experimentation (King et al. 2009). Cognitive models of motivation such as achievement, affiliation and power motivation contribute to agent-based simulations of human decision-making (Merrick and Shafi 2011). Social models of motivation will support future artificial systems with the potential for social evolution and self-advancement. This is relevant given the current drive towards nano-technologies and robot swarms for tasks such as search and rescue in disaster zones and medical treatments (Hill et al. 2008). Figure 10 summarises the possible future trends of research in intrinsically motivated agent models. Current work combines small numbers of motivation and behavioural components. In future, artificial agents may embed multiple motivation and behavioural alternatives, based on fundamental units such as reasoning models, neurons in a network or others. This is a long-term goal towards which intrinsically motivated systems research can aspire to achieve truly autonomous artificial agents and robots capable of a wide range of complex applications.

References

Baldassarre, G.: What are intrinsic motivations? a biological perspective. In: proceedings of International Conference on Developmental Learning and Epigenetic Robotics, pp. 1–8. IEEE, New York (2011)

Baraldi, A., Alpaydin, E.: Simplified art: A new class of art algorithms. Technical report, International Computer Science Institute, Berkley (1998)

Barto, A., Singh, S., Chentanez, N.: Intrinsically motivated learning of hierarchical collections of skills. In: International Conference on Developmental Learning (2004)
Berlyne, D.: Conflict, Arousal and Curiosity. McGraw-Hill, New York (1960)
Berlyne, D.: Exploration and curiosity. Science **153**, 25–33 (1966)
BLIPSystems: Blipnet technical white paper. BLIP Systems A/S, Aalborg (2007)
Chandola, V., Banerjee, A, Kumar, V.: Anomaly detection: A survey. ACM Comput. Surv. **41**(3), 1–58 (2009)
Deci, E., Ryan, R.: Intrinsic Motivation and Self-determination in Human Behaviour. Plenum, New York (1985)
Fritzke, B.: Incremental learning of local linear mappings. In: The International Conference on Artificial Neural Networks, pp. 217–222 (1995)
Gero, J.: Creativity, emergence and evolution in design. In: Second International Roundtable Conference on Computational Models of Creative Design, pp. 1–28, Sydney (1992)
Heckhausen, J., Heckhausen, H.: Motivation and Action. Cambridge University Press, New York (2008)
Hettich, S., Bay, S.: The uci kdd archive (1999). http://kdd.ics.uci.edu/databases/kddcup99/kddcup99 (Accessed March 2009)
Hill, C., Amodeo, A., Joseph, J., Patel, H.: Nano- and microrobotics: How far is the reality. Expert Rev. **8**(12), 1891–1897 (2008)
Kaplan, F., Oudeyer, P.-Y.: Intrinsically motivated machines. In: Lungarella, M., Iida, F.J.B., Pfeifer, R. (eds.) Fifty Years of Artificial Intelligence, pp. 304–315. Springer, Berlin (2007)
King, R., et al.: The automation of science. Science **324**(5923), 85–89 (2009)
Kohonen, T.: Self-organisation and Associative Memory. Springer, Berlin (1993)
Lee, W., Stolfo, S.: A framework for constructing features and models for intrusion detection systems. ACM Trans. Inform. Syst. Security **3**(4), 227–261 (2001)
Lenat, D.: AM: An artificial intelligence approach to discovery in mathematics. Ph.D. Thesis, Stanford University (1976)
MacQueen, J.: Some methods for classification and analysis of multivariate observations. In: The Fifth Berkeley Symposium on Mathematical Statistics and Probability, pp. 281–297. University of California Press (1967)
Maher, M., Gero, J.: Agent models of 3d virtual worlds. In: ACADIA 2002: Thresholds, pp. 127–138. California State Polytechnic University (2002)
Maher, M.L., Merrick, K., Saunders, R.: Achieving Creative Behaviour Using Curious Learning Agents, AAAI Spring Symposium on Creative Intelligent Systems, March 26–28, Stanford University, pp. 40–46 (2008).
Marsland, S., Nehmzow, U., Shapiro, J.: A real-time novelty detector for a mobile robot. In: EUREL European Advanced Robotics Systems Masterclass and Conference (2000)
Merrick, K.: Designing toys that come alive: Curious robots for creative play. In: Seventh International Conference on Entertainment Computing (ICEC 2008), pp. 149–154. Carnegie Mellon University, Springer (2008)
Merrick, K.: A comparative study of value systems for self-motivated exploration and learning by robots. IEEE Trans. Auton. Mental Dev. **2**(2), 119–131 (2010a). Special Issue on Active Learning and Intrinsically Motivated Exploration in Robots
Merrick, K.: Modeling behavior cycles as a value system for developmental robots. Adap. Behav. **18**(3–4), 237–257 (2010b)
Merrick, K., Maher, M.: Motivated Reinforcement Learning: Curious Characters for Multiuser Games. Springer, Berlin (2009)
Merrick, K., Scully, T.: Modelling affordances for the control and evaluation of intrinsically motivated robots. In: Australian Conference on Robotics and Automation, CD. Sydney (2009)
Merrick, K., Shafi, K.: Agent models for self-motivated home-assistant bots. In: International Symposium on Computational Models for Life Sciences, pp. 131–150. AIP (2009)
Merrick, K., Shafi, K.: Achievement, affiliation and power: Motive profiles for artificial agents. Adap. Behav. **9**(1), 40–62 (2011)

Mirolli, M., Baldassarre, G.: Functions and mechanisms of intrinsic motivations: The knowledge versus competence distinction. In: Baldassarre, G., Mirolli, M. (eds.) Intrinsically Motivated Learning in Natural and Artificial Systems, pp. 49–72. Springer, Berlin (2012)

Nehmzow, U., Gatsoulis, Y., Kerr, E., Condell, J., Siddique, N.H., McGinnity, M.T.: Novelty detection as an intrinsic motivation for cumulative learning robots. In: Baldassarre, G., Mirolli, M. (eds.) Intrinsically Motivated Learning in Natural and Artificial Systems, pp. 185–207. Springer, Berlin (2012)

Oudeyer, P.-Y., Kaplan, F.: Intelligent adaptive curiosity: A source of self-development. In: Fourth International Workshop on Epigenetic Robotics, pp. 127–130. Lund University, Lund (2004)

Oudeyer, P.-Y., Kaplan, F.: What is intrinsic motivation? a typology of computational approaches. Front. Neurorobot. **1**(6) (2007) (online, openaccess)

Oudeyer, P.-Y., Kaplan, F., Hafner, V.: Intrinsic motivation systems for autonomous mental development. IEEE Trans. Evol. Comput. **11**(2), 265–286 (2007)

Saunders, R.: Curious design agents and artificial creativity. Ph.D. Thesis, University of Sydney, Sydney (2001)

Schembri, M., Mirolli, M., Baldassarre, G.: Evolution and learning in an intrinsically motivated reinforcement learning robot. In: Advances in Artificial Life. Proceedings of the 9th European Conference on Artificial Life (ECAL2007), Lecture Notes in Artificial Intelligence, vol. 4648, pp. 294–333. Springer, Berlin (2007)

Schmidhuber, J.: Curious model building control systems. In: International Joint Conference on Artificial Neural Networks, pp. 1458–1463. IEEE, Singapore (1991)

Schmidhuber, J.: Formal theory of creativity, fun and intrinsic motivation (1990-2010): IEEE Trans. Auton. Mental Dev. **2**(3), 230–247 (2010)

Shafi, K., Merrick, K.: A curious agent for network anomaly detection. In: The Tenth International Conference on Autonomous Agents and Multiagent Systems, pp. 1075–1076 (2011)

Stanley, J.: Computer simulation of a model of habituation. Nature **261**, 146–148 (1976)

Steels, L.: Self-organising vocabularies. Vrije Universiteit, Artificial Intelligence Laboratory, Brussels (1996)

Sutton, R., Barto, A.: Reinforcement Learning: An Introduction. MIT, Cambridge (2000)

Watkins, C., Dayan, P.: Q-learning. Mach. Learn. **8**(3), 279–292 (1992)

Weiser, M.: The computer for the 21st century. Sci. Am. **265**(3), 94–104 (1991)

White, R.: Motivation reconsidered: The concept of competence. Psychol. Rev. **66**, 297–333 (1959)

Wundt, W.: Principles of Physiological Psychology. Macmillan, New York (1910)

The Hippocampal-VTA Loop: The Role of Novelty and Motivation in Controlling the Entry of Information into Long-Term Memory

Nonna Otmakhova, Emrah Duzel, Ariel Y. Deutch, and John Lisman

Abstract The role of dopamine has been strongly implicated in reward processes, but recent work shows an additional role as a signal that promotes the stable incorporation of novel information into long-term hippocampal memory. Indeed, dopamine neurons, in addition to being activated by reward, can be activated by novelty in the absence of reward. The computation of novelty is thought to occur in the hippocampus and is carried to the dopamine cells of the VTA through a polysynaptic pathway. Although a picture of novelty-dependent processes in the VTA and hippocampus is beginning to emerge, many aspects of the process remain unclear. Here, we will consider several issues: (1) What is relationship of novelty signals coming to the VTA from the superior colliculus, as compared to those that come from the hippocampus? (2) Can dopamine released by a reward enhance the learning of novel information? (3) Is there an interaction between motivational signals and hippocampal novelty signals? (4) What are the properties of the axons that generate dopamine release in the hippocampus? We close with a discussion of some of the outstanding open issues in this field.

N. Otmakhova · J. Lisman (✉)
Biology Department, Brandeis University, 415 South Street MS 008, Waltham, MA 02454-9110, USA

E. Duzel
Institute of Cognitive Neuroscience, University College London, 17 Queen Street, London WC1N 3AR, UK

Institute of Cognitive Neurology and Dementia Research, Otto-von-Guericke Universität Magdeburg, Leipziger Str 44, 39120 Magdeburg, Germany

German Centre for Neurodegenerative Diseases (DZNE), Standort Magdeburg, Germany

A.Y. Deutch
Departments of Psychiatry and Pharmacology, Vanderbilt University Medical Center, Nashville, TN 37212, USA
e-mail: Lisman@brandeis.edu

G. Baldassarre and M. Mirolli (eds.), *Intrinsically Motivated Learning in Natural and Artificial Systems*, DOI 10.1007/978-3-642-32375-1_10,

1 Introduction

Long-term potentiation (LTP) and long-term depression (LTD) are activity-dependent changes in the strength of synapses. LTP-like changes have been observed during actual learning (Whitlock et al. 2006); furthermore, genetic alteration of proteins vital for LTP strongly affect memory (Giese et al. 1998). There is thus little doubt that LTP is one of the mechanisms that contributes to learning and memory. The field of synaptic plasticity has undergone a change from viewing LTP-mediated memory storage as a purely local process to a view that incorporates large-scale networks, including those responsible for motivation. According to the older view, which is encapsulated in Hebb's rule, memory is stored by processes that change the strength of synaptic connections and do so according to Hebb's postulate, which states that a synapse is strengthened if it has both presynaptic input and strong postsynaptic activity. The requirement for strong postsynaptic depolarization generally means that many excitatory inputs to the cell are active and that inhibitory inputs are relatively weak, a requirement that makes synaptic strengthening associative. In this sense, the Hebbian computation depends on the local synaptic events in the neuron and not on events in other brain regions. There is now strong evidence that the Hebb rule is not strictly correct because long-term synaptic modification does depend on what is happening in other brain regions. What actually occurs can, however, be appropriately called neo- Hebbian (Lisman et al. 2011) because rather than throwing out the Hebbian postulate altogether, the new rule simply adds an additional condition. Specifically, in the CA1 hippocampal system, the primary model system for studying synaptic plasticity, it was found that LTP is induced if the Hebbian condition is met but the LTP is relatively short-lasting (1–2 h), a process termed early LTP. For LTP to persist into the late phase, the cell must receive an additional signal, namely, an elevation of the neuromodulator dopamine (DA) (Frey and Morris 1998; Redondo and Morris 2011).

This raises the question of what conditions produce dopamine release. The activation of the dopaminergic system has been found to depend on several factors (Schultz 2007a,b), most notably reward. However, dopamine cells can also respond to novel stimuli in the absence of reward (Ljungberg et al. 1992). It now appears that the dopamine novelty signal can be initiated by information coming from the hippocampus itself via a polysynaptic pathway (Legault and Wise 2001); reviewed in (Lisman and Grace 2005). Because the DA signal depends on a network computation, the overall process involved in late LTP is fundamentally different from the cell-autonomous computation of the classic Hebb rule. The circuitry that underlies this neo-Hebbian computation has been termed the hippocampal-VTA loop (Lisman and Grace 2005) (Fig. 1).

The computation of novelty and its effects on memory relate importantly to the themes of this book, notably to the concept of intrinsic motivation (see Mirolli and Baldassarre 2012). It seems possible that novelty-dependent dopamine release may shape behavior just as reward-dependent dopamine release can. Thus, the neural circuitry in Fig. 1 may be relevant to the overall process of intrinsic motivation.

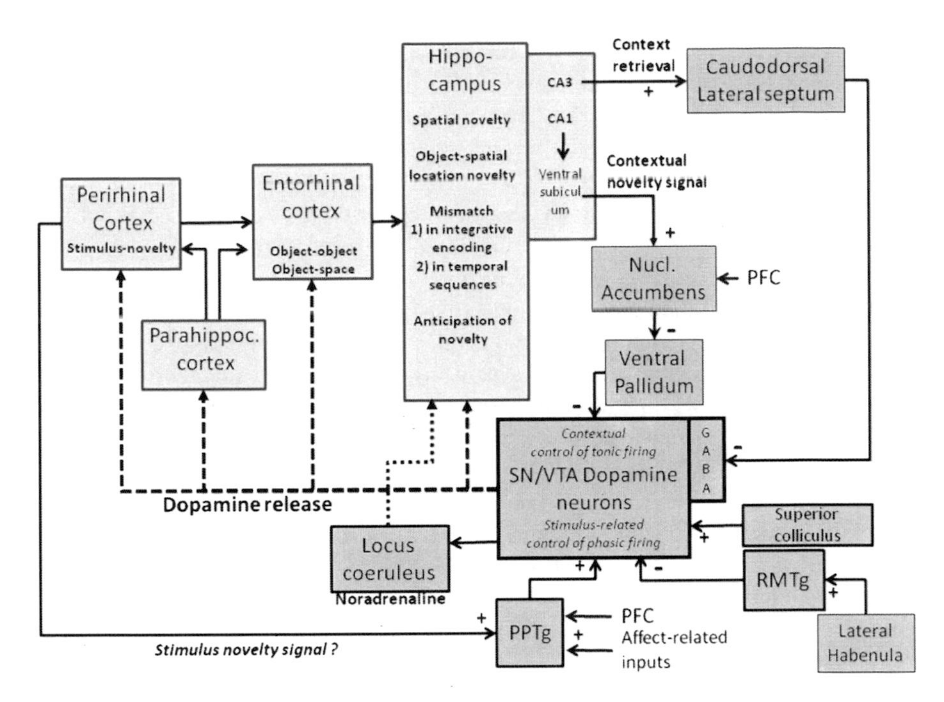

Fig. 1 Connectivity within the medial temporal lobe (MTL) and the hippocampus-ventral tegmental area (VTA) loop. *PFC* prefrontal cortex, *RMTg* rostromedial tegmental nucleus, *PPTg*, pedunculopontine tegmental nucleus

Various brain regions may contribute to this process as follows. Information about objects and their spatial location converges in the entorhinal cortex via the perirhinal and parahippocampal cortices. These inputs can be integrated in the hippocampus toward an "object-in-context" representation. Representations in the hippocampus may also include the temporal sequence of occurrence and anticipatory states associated with current goals and expectations. Hippocampal contextual novelty signals generated on the basis of such representations can increase the pool of tonically active dopamine neurons in the substantia nigra (SN)/VTA. This could allow perirhinal cortical information about stimulus novelty to generate phasic dopamine responses (italics in the figure indicate that this possibility needs experimental testing). The loop is completed by ascending dopaminergic fibers that innervate the hippocampus and other MTL structures. The dopamine released in the hippocampus functions as a permissive signal for late LTP, the enduring form of synaptic modification that underlies a form of long-term memory. Another pathway (Luo et al. 2011) originates in the CA3 region of the hippocampus and modulates the activity of GABAergic neurons in the VTA via the caudodorsal septal nucleus. This pathway may play a role in controlling dopamine release in response to the retrieval of context information. Dopaminergic neurons can also be activated by a direct input from the superior colliculus (Redgrave and Gurney 2006), and this may play a role in triggering DA release in response to perceptually salient events. Aversive events and negative prediction errors can regulate the activity of DA neurons through the lateral habenula. Finally, DA neurons can also affect the activity of locus coeruleus (LC) neurons, and activity of LC neurons can release noradrenaline and, under specific circumstances, possibly also dopamine in the hippocampus.

The goal of this chapter is to answer questions that have been raised about this loop and to discuss new areas of research that relate to loop function. The first question deals with the origin of the rapid novelty signals measured in the VTA. The role of both the superior colliculus and hippocampus is discussed. The second question examines a curious prediction: if DA enhances long-term memory, then rewards that cause DA release should enhance memory even if the rewards are not directly related to the material being learned. A third question concerns a speculation about the reason for the polysynaptic pathway from the hippocampus to the VTA. It was suggested (Lisman and Grace 2005) that this synaptic complexity might allow the interaction of novelty signals from the hippocampus and motivational signals from the PFC. Evidence relevant to this idea will be discussed. A final set of issues concerns the location of DA fibers and the nature of the dopamine signal itself. There are many technical issues involved, including issues about how a dopamine fiber can be identified. Understanding the exact mechanisms by which DA is released and taken up is necessary in order to understand the function of the system. For instance, details about the time constant of DA in the extracellular space, a time constant that will be determined both by the properties of release and the properties of uptake, bear on the interesting question of whether the DA released by one event can affect the encoding of an event that occurred at a later time. This section of this chapter is long and detailed; readers not interested in these issues may wish to jump to the final section, where we outline important remaining questions and speculate about possible answers.

2 Novelty Inputs to the VTA from both the Hippocampus and Superior Colliculus

Short-latency (phasic) novelty signals in dopamine cells were originally recorded by Schultz in monkey (Schultz et al. 1993). Some of the novelty signals seen in the VTA may originate from the superior colliculus rather than the hippocampus (Redgrave and Gurney 2006). The specific stimulus that triggered the novelty response was the opening of the door to the animals cage. Recent work shows that such visual events trigger a response in the superior colliculus, a brain region that receives direct retinal input. Ablation of the colliculus abolishes the short-latency response in the VTA, strongly arguing that colliculus generates the trigger.

There is also a short-latency response to novelty in the hippocampus, which was taken by Lisman and Grace (Lisman and Grace 2005) to be the origin of the novelty signal in the VTA. This, however, may now have to be qualified—perhaps only certain types of VTA novelty responses are of hippocampal origin.

One property of the novelty responses in the colliculus is that they strongly habituate. That is to say, a stimulus that initially evokes a large response, with repetition, rapidly comes to evoke only a small response. However, the initial stimulus presentation may well not be novel in the true sense; it may have been presented hours or days before and still evoke a maximal response. In contrast, the hippocampus, because it has access to long-term memory stores, is able to compute a true novelty response (i.e., determine whether an object was ever seen before). Habituation is thus not an appropriate term for describing the hippocampal system. Learning, in some types of experiments in which novelty has been examined in the hippocampus, can occur over days as an animal comes to "know" a new environment. For instance, one recent study showed that hippocampal CA1 firing rates were initially high in a novel environment and declined by about 50 % over several days of testing (Karlsson and Frank 2008). Interestingly, these time-dependent changes were seen only in CA1, but not CA3. In one study (Fyhn et al. 2002), firing occurred when the hidden platform in a water maze was suddenly moved. Upon finding this platform in an unexpected place, many hippocampal cells fire for about 30 s. In another experimental design in which rats explore a novel environment, it was found that CA1 pyramidal cells, but not DG cells, have an overall firing rate that is higher than in a familiar environment (Csicsvari et al. 2007; Nitz and McNaughton 2004). The firing in novel environments also shows enhanced temporal correlations, underscoring the potential complexity of the neural coding (Cheng and Frank 2008).

Other protocols used primarily in primates allow measurements of the latency of novelty responses and the responses are very fast. For instance, neurons in the rhinal cortex of monkeys, a major input structure of the hippocampus, respond to novelty within 60–90 ms (Brown et al. 2009), and electromagnetic studies in humans have confirmed that comparable novelty responses can emerge within 100 ms (Bunzeck et al. 2009). The rhinal novelty computation depends on whether the item is known or not and cannot be described as habituation. Responses in the hippocampus have yet another type of organization; they may depend on the relationship of the item to context or on changes in the sequence of items. Given the differences between the rhinal and hippocampal novelty signals, it would make sense for them to have separate pathways leading to the VTA. Consistent with this, studies in rodents have revealed a projection from the perirhinal cortex to the pedunculopontine tegmental nucleus (PPTg) (P.Burwell, personal communication; see Fig. 1), which is a major input structure for the SN/VTA. Contextual novelty signals originating in the hippocampus and stimulus novelty signals originating in the perirhinal cortex can, in principle, converge in the VTA.

Another perspective on the novelty response comes from a measure of overall activity by the activation of the immediate early gene, c-Fos. This activation is increased by novel environments (VanElzakker et al. 2008). This study further found that c-Fos expression in CA1 (but not DG or CA3) increased in proportion to the number of novel elements introduced. Such gradation has not been reported in the colliculus. Taken together, these results point to several ways in which the hippocampus and colliculus differ. Complicating the picture further, the temporal lobe region has several structures that themselves differ in the type of novelty response. Finally, recent work shows that different parts of the dopamine system (the VTA and substantia nigra) can also differ in the properties of their novelty and reward signals (Martig and Mizumori 2011). The network mechanisms that compute novelty are far from clear. Given that even an object may have a different projection on the retina depending on the objects position, distance or rotation, it might seem that virtually every input would be novel. Thus, special mechanisms must exist that compute invariance (see, e.g., Sountsov et al. 2011) and thus recognize retinal images that differ only due to changes in position, rotation, or scale as not novel. Nehmzow et al. (2012) provide an overview of models describing how novelty detection might be achieved.

3 Reward Enhances Long-Term Memory Formation

DA cell firing has been demonstrated to have a strong linkage to unpredicted reward (Schultz 2007a,b; Schultz et al. 1993). The pathways responsible for this form of dopaminergic firing have not yet been identified but are not thought to involve the hippocampus. The hippocampus is, however, likely to receive reward-related dopaminergic input, and this would be expected to enhance learning. In rodent studies, this is evident, for instance, in tasks requiring the animal to learn the location of a reward (Bethus et al. 2010). If the reward is large, the animal can form a long-term reward-location memory after a single trial, and this long-term memory can be blocked with the application of a D1 receptor antagonist into the hippocampus at the time of encoding (Bethus et al. 2010). However, if the reward is small, reward-location memory after a single exposure decays within minutes to hours (Bethus et al. 2010). A similar reward-related enhancement of hippocampus-dependent long-term memory has been observed in humans (Wittmann et al. 2005). A single exposure to a trial unique picture was enhanced when pictures were followed by monetary reward, as compared to unrewarded pictures. The results show that the long-term memory for pictures was enhanced by rewards presented at the time of encoding.

A similar type of interaction has been demonstrated for LTP itself and relates to the "synaptic tag" hypothesis (Frey and Morris 1998). This hypothesis is built on observations of CA1 LTP; notably, a weak stimulus will induce only early LTP but will persist into the late phase if given fairly contiguously with a strong stimulation of a different input. It is thought that the role of the strong stimulation is to stimulate the release of DA required to enable the protein synthesis that underlies late LTP. The strong stimulus can be given after the weak but selectively affects the weakly stimulated synapses (not unstimulated ones) because the weak synapses are "tagged."

Following this framework, Ballarini et al. (2009) found that the persistence of a memory induced by weak training could be enhanced by concurrent strong training in another task. Exactly how this interaction occurs remains to be tested. According to the synaptic tag hypothesis, it is the DA and protein synthesis produced by the strong stimulus that enhance the encoding of the weak, i.e., this is a purely biochemical process. However, an alternative (and not mutually exclusive possibility) is that DA induces a consolidation process that involves active replay of the weak events (Rossato et al. 2009)

4 Does the Motivation to Learn Affect the Hippocampal-VTA Loop?

Although many aspects of the hippocampal-VTA loop have received considerable attention, one important aspect remains relatively unexplored: the possible role of motivation in modulating the loop. Such modulation was postulated as a way of explaining the complexity of the downward part of the loop connecting the hippocampus to the VTA. The fact that this pathway is polysynaptic (through the accumbens and ventral pallidum) requires explanation. Lisman and Grace (2005) speculated that since the accumbens is also a target for prefrontal cortex input, the accumbens might be a site where motivational signals from the PFC might combine with novelty signals from the hippocampus. Perhaps then, motivation to learn might be as important as novelty in stimulating the accumbens. Synergistic activity of this kind could, by increasing DA release, enhance memory storage when the individual was motivated to learn. In a brief report, Wolosin et al. (2009) provide support for this prediction. They found that if subjects were motivated by an indication that success in the memory test would lead to high reward, then hippocampal activation, VTA activation, and memory performance were better than if subjects were promised only a modest reward.

Evidence is beginning to be published that the loop, in addition to being regulated by motivation, can affect motivational aspects of memory formation (e.g., Duzel et al. 2010). Functional MRI data show that the loop is activated by the anticipation of novelty and that memory is improved following novelty anticipation (Wittmann et al. 2007). These data converge well with suggestions from computational modeling that DA responses to novel events could act as an exploration bonus for rewards. That is, novel stimuli could motivate exploratory behavior by increasing the anticipation of possible rewards in an environment (Kakade and Dayan 2002). Compatible with this suggestion, humans show increased striatal responses to rewards if these are presented in the context of unrelated novel stimuli (Guitart-Masip et al. 2010). These suggestions and data also converge nicely with the aforementioned possibility that low levels of dopamine transporter (DAT) expression in the hippocampus may lead to prolonged effects of DA and thereby affect neural responses to events in the temporal vicinity of the novel stimuli. In fact, compared to a context in which there is only familiar information, humans show elevated medial temporal lobe responsiveness to familiar stimuli if there is novelty in the same context, and this elevation is accompanied by an overall improvement of memory (Bunzeck and Duzel 2006).

4.1 Dopaminergic Innervation of the CA1 Region

A key building block of the hippocampal-VTA loop concept (Lisman and Grace 2005) is that the hippocampus receives dopaminergic input. Evidence for dopaminergic innervations of the hippocampus is often met with skepticism because the density of dopaminergic fibers in the hippocampus is very low compared to "dopaminergic areas" such as the striatum. There are also a host of technical issues regarding the detection of a dopaminergic innervation. In this section, we review the evidence regarding DA innervation of the hippocampus, with particular attention to the localization of this innervation in the CA1 hippocampal region. This analysis is important because there is little information about the general problem of how to understand dopaminergic modulation in brain areas where the dopaminergic innervation is low but where the existence of dopaminergic receptors and dopaminergic effects of cell targets makes it clear that dopamine is functional.

The CA1 region contains a cell body region with two dendritic regions on either side, the stratum oriens and the stratum radiatum. The stratum radiatum is where the physiological evidence for a role of DA in long-term potentiation (LTP) is now clear (Frey et al. 1991; Frey and Morris 1998; Huang and Kandel 1995; Lemon and Manahan-Vaughan 2006; Li et al. 2003; Lisman and Grace 2005; Navakkode et al. 2007; Otmakhova and Lisman 1996; Swant and Wagner 2006). However, most experiments on dopamine and LTP involve the addition of exogenous dopamine or dopamine agonists/antagonists. To know whether dopamine actually modulates this region during neural activity, it is crucial to demonstrate that dopamine-containing axons from the VTA/SN innervate this region and release DA. The number of dopaminergic VTA axons in the CA1 region is certainly low. This raises the question of what is necessary for effective modulation: is low density sufficient? Alternatively, perhaps dopamine diffuses from nearby regions where dopamine innervation is higher. Still another possibility is that the dopamine contained in noradrenergic axons can account for dopamine release. In what follows, we will review the complex literature on dopamine in the hippocampus. This will entail a discussion of technical issues related to how dopamine axons from the VTA are identified and to the mechanisms by which DA is released and taken up. We close this section with a new working model for VTA-dependent dopamine release in CA1.

We begin our review by describing measurements of dopamine (DA) in the hippocampus using biochemical methods. There is a relatively rich noradrenergic innervation of the hippocampus (Swanson and Hartman 1975) in which DA is present as a precursor to norepinephrine (NE). Dopamine is synthesized by the enzyme tyrosine hydroxylase and then, in noradrenergic cells, converted into noradrenaline by the enzyme dopamine beta hydroxylase. Typically, the DA precursor pool is about 15–20 % of the concentration of NE; however, this depends on basal firing rate of NE neurons and other factors. As the reader will see, there are technical difficulties in distinguishing the DA contained in DA cells from that contained in NE cells. Early experiments sought to determine whether the DA measured in hippocampal samples was present simply as a precursor to NE. Scatton et al. (1980) analyzed NE and DA concentrations in the anterior and posterior hippocampus of control rats and animals in which the NE innervation of the hippocampus had been lesioned. In the control animals, the concentration of NE (~250 ng/g) was much greater than the DA concentration (~10 ng/g). Noradrenergic lesioning resulted in a ~100-fold decrease in hippocampal NE (to ~3 ng/g) but decreased DA by only ~30 %. However, if the sources of dopaminergic axons (ventral tegmental area, VTA and substantia nigra, SN) were also removed, then the DA content in the hippocampus dropped dramatically. This drop was observed in the anterior and posterior hippocampus. The authors further determined that DA from these midbrain DA structures comes mostly via the fimbria/fornix because undercutting this pathway depleted ~70 % of hippocampal DA. The DA content in rat hippocampus was confirmed later (Ishikawa et al. 1982), though in this work, a 10-times-higher DA content was found in a specific dorsomedial region of the hippocampus. It was also shown that in human brain, DA content in the hippocampus (~13 ng/g) is comparable to NE content (~12 ng/g) or DA content in the cortex (3–7 ng/g) (Scatton et al. 1983, 1982). The ratio of DA metabolites to DA was higher in hippocampus and cortex (as compared to striatum), suggesting a higher metabolic rate of DA (and probably its functional impact) in cortico-limbic structures. Finally, in untreated Parkinsons disease, DA content in the hippocampus was depleted by more than 75 % (Scatton et al. 1983, 1982).

A history of early attempts to visualize the dopaminergic innervation of the hippocampal formation is given by Swanson et al. (1987) and Oades and Halliday (1987). With the Falck-Hillarp histofluorescence method, it became possible to see monoamine-containing cells and their axons. Different monoamines (serotonin, DA, NE, and adrenaline) can be distinguished by their exact emission spectra, although this is difficult. To differentiate NE from DA with certainty, some studies (Fuxe et al. 1974; Hokfelt et al. 1974a) examined residual monoamine fluorescence in rats after monoamine depletion with reserpine (Fuxe et al. 1974; Hokfelt et al. 1974a) or loading with L-DOPA (a precursor of DA) while inhibiting DA beta hydroxylase (DBH) (Hokfelt et al. 1974b). Using the glyoxylic acid modification of the Falck-Hillarp approach, Hokfelt et al. (1974a) were able to detect DA axons in the hippocampal region. In a separate paper in the same year, Hokfelt et al. (1974b) commented that DA fluorescent axons were seen "only in the most ventral part of the hippocampal formation," without further specification (the hippocampal formation includes the subiculum). Swanson and Hartman (1975), subsequently analyzing the adrenergic system in rats using immunohistochemistry, noted that there were no DBH-immunoreactive axons in the fimbria, suggesting that the reported catecholamine fluorescence in the fimbria may be due to DA coming from midbrain sources and not due to NE.

The distribution of dopaminergic fibers in the rat hippocampus was investigated in more detail by Verney et al. (1985) using two methods. First, they used tyrosine hydroxylase (TH) immunohistochemistry to mark catecholamine axons. This was done after perinatal toxin injections to lesion the forebrain NE innervation. In a second method, they examined histofluorescence after loading slices of the hippocampus with DA while blocking NE and serotonin transporters so that DA may be only taken up into dopaminergic fibers, but not into NE or serotonergic axons. Although they did not observe DA axons in the dorsal hippocampus, in the ventral hippocampus, a sparse DA innervation of the stratum oriens of the CA1 field was observed, with DA axons also seen traversing the alveus. The ventral hippocampal formation received the largest DA innervation, particularly the presubiculum, but even in this region, the DA innervation was modest. Among hippocampal fields, the subiculum had the strongest innervation, followed by CA1 and the hilus of the dentate gyrus (DG). In CA1, the DA fibers were mostly observed in the alveus, stratum oriens, and stratum pyramidale. The authors claim no fibers in stratum radiatum or stratum lacunosum-moleculare, though in some figures, SR markings are evident (e.g., their Fig. 3a). It should be noted that there were no means of assessing incidental damage to DA axons by the neurotoxins used to lesion the noradrenergic innervation of the hippocampus, and thus, it is possible that the DA innervation of the hippocampus was underestimated.

In a search for possible sources of DA axons in the hippocampus of the rat, retrograde tract tracing methods were used. The retrograde markers such as horseradish peroxidase (Simon et al. 1979; Wyss et al. 1979) or wheat agglutinin (Schwab et al. 1978) were deposited into the hippocampal formation, taken up by the axons, and diffused to the cells of origin of these axons. Such retrograde-marker-labeled cells were seen in the VTA and SN. However, because both the VTA and SN contain GABAergic as well as DA neurons, no conclusion could be reached concerning the transmitter identity of the retrograde labeled cells. Swanson (1982) specifically investigated projections of the VTA and SN DA neurons by combining retrograde tract tracing with immunohistochemical detection of TH to mark DA neurons in rats. He reported a sparse projection from both the VTA and SN to the dorsal hippocampus but also reported that some of the cells projecting into the hippocampus (about 6 %) were indeed dopaminergic.

Subsequent studies analyzed dopaminergic inputs to the hippocampus in rats in more detail (Gasbarri et al. 1991, 1994a, 1996, 1997, 1994b). The authors used a few different approaches to clarify the picture. First, they used the Fink-Heimer method to stain anterogradely degenerating axons after lesions of the VTA either electrolytically (nonspecific damage) or by using DA-specific toxin, 6-hydroxydopamine (6-OH-DA). They found degenerating fibers of VTA origin in the ventral hippocampus (including the subiculum), adjacent CA1 (stratum oriens, stratum pyramidale, suprapyramidal layer, and stratum lacunosum-moleculare), CA3 (stratum oriens), and the hilus of the DG. In dorsal hippocampus, the terminal fields were sparser, being mostly in subiculum and stratum oriens of CA1 (Gasbarri et al. 1991, 1994a).

As a second approach, they added retrograde labeling techniques using markers such as Fast Blue, Nuclear Yellow, and Fluoro-Gold injected into the hippocampus. After a period of diffusion, retrogradely labeled cells were detected in the majority of midbrain dopaminergic nuclei: VTA (including the rostral linear, central linear, interfascicular, paranigral, and parabrachial pigmented nuclei) (Gasbarri et al. 1991, 1994a), SN (Gasbarri et al. 1994a), and retrorubral field (Gasbarri et al. 1996). This showed that hippocampus received input not only from the VTA but also from other midbrain DA sources. Finally, they used TH immunoreactivity to label DA-containing cells in these structures. They concluded that some retrogradely labeled cells (15–18 %) displayed TH immunoreactivity and therefore were dopaminergic (Gasbarri et al. 1994a, 1997). The combination of these approaches led to the convincing conclusion that there really are direct dopaminergic inputs to the hippocampus, though these are rather sparse. Recently, dopaminergic fibers in the CA1 region were confirmed by double immunofluorescence (Kwon et al. 2008). The DA fibers were distinguished as having enzyme TH (DA synthesis), but not DBH (synthesis of NE). The NE fibers in the same sections had both enzymes present. As the reader will note, the studies reviewed above did find evidence for DA axons in the CA1 stratum oriens but scant evidence for any in the stratum radiatum, where most physiological studies of DA have been conducted. The same is true of the recent study of Kwon et al. (2008).

Another approach is to visualize dopaminergic axons and somata using an antibody that recognizes DA itself. Using DA conjugated to glutaraldehyde as an immunogen, Geffard and colleagues were able to produce antibodies that recognize the dopamine-glutaraldehyde conjugate but are not cross-reactive with DA precursor L-DOPA or NE produced from DA (Geffard et al. 1984a,b,c). This method has been used extensively in the study of many brain areas (Arsenault et al. 1988; Goldman-Rakic et al. 1989; Onteniente et al. 1984; Van Eden et al. 1987), but not the hippocampus. Recently, one of us (AYD, unpublished) examined the distribution of DA-immunoreactive axons in the rat hippocampus. It was found that, in the entorhinal cortex, there is a moderate density of DA-immunoreactive axons. In the hippocampal formation, DA-immunoreactive axons are much less abundant. Rare long, varicose DA-immunoreactive axons of very fine caliber can be seen in the subiculum and especially the presubiculum but do not penetrate into the adjacent CA1 pyramidal cell layer. However, there is a plexus of DA-immunoreactive axons that runs along the alveus until it reaches the transition between the CA1 and CA2 fields. These DA-immunoreactive axons only very rarely emit processes that extend into the CA1 region; those medially directed axons that do emerge from the bundle along the alveus are quite short (<4 μm in length), extending into only part of the stratum oriens. These data using immunohistochemical detection of DA correspond well with the earlier data showing minimal DA axons in stratum radiatum.

How then does DA get to the DA receptors in the stratum radiatum, where most of the dopaminergic effects have been studied (Frey et al. 1991, 1990; Lemon and Manahan-Vaughan 2006; Li et al. 2003; Otmakhova and Lisman 1996)? Furthermore, stimulation of the radiatum causes DA release, as measured by radioactivity and confirmed by HPLC (Frey et al. 1990). Furthermore, in vivo microdialysis (Neugebauer et al. 2009) shows increased DA release in CA1 and dentate gyrus of the rat hippocampus due to electrical tetanic stimulation of the medial perforant path, the general cortical pathway to all hippocampal subfields.

We see three possible ways of resolving this issue:

1. There are indeed dopaminergic axons in the radiatum, but these are not labeled or detectable by current methods, perhaps because they are very small.
2. If DA axons are not present in the radiatum, perhaps DA diffuses into the radiatum from the varicosities in the plexus of dopaminergic axons that run along the alveus (and possibly stratums oriens). However, the distance from the oriens/alveus to the radiatum is up to 300 μm, longer than typical for paracrine actions of DA (Cragg et al. 2001). In evaluating whether diffusion to the radiatum is feasible, it is important to recall that, although the dopamine transporter (DAT) that takes up DA in other tissues appears to be absent in the hippocampus, as judged by immunochemistry (Coulter et al. 1995; Kwon et al. 2008; Schott et al. 2006), DA would be taken up the noradrenergic axons found in this region (Schroeter et al. 2000; Swanson and Hartman 1975); indeed, the norepinephrine transporter has a higher affinity for DA than it does for NE (Pacholczyk et al. 1991). Also relevant to the possibility of long-range DA diffusions is that DA lifetime might be further limited by oxidation. Nevertheless, even with this limitation, there are examples of long-distance (mm) DA diffusion (sometimes aided by fluid flow), as reviewed in Zoli et al. (1998). In summary, perhaps diffusion brings DA from the alveus and oriens to the radiatum, a diffusion that can occur because uptake is very weak.

   One objection to the absence of DAT must be noted. Although DAT immunoreactivity is not seen, there is pharmacological evidence for DAT: an inhibitor of DAT enhanced the effects of DA release (Swant and Wagner 2006). If the DA were entirely handled by the NE system (released and taken up by NE terminals), DAT inhibitors should have no effect. However, there is a problem with this study: the DAT inhibitor used has a high affinity for DA (<3 nM) but was used at 100 nM, a concentration where it could have had side effects. Furthermore, other experiments have directly demonstrated the role of the NE transporter rather than DAT in uptake of DA in the hippocampus (Borgkvist et al. 2011).
3. Another possibility is that the primary mechanism of DA release is from NE fibers (Curet et al. 1985; Devoto et al. 2001; Quintin et al. 1986; Scatton et al. 1984). For example, stimulation of the locus coeruleus elicits release of both NE and DA in the prefrontal cortex (Devoto et al. 2005). Apparently, although TH is the rate-limiting step in catecholamine synthesis under basal conditions, when NE neurons increase their firing rate, the NE synthetic enzyme DBH becomes rate limiting. DBH is located in the synaptic vesicle. Thus, in noradrenergic terminals, when the precursor DA is taken up into the vesicle, it is rapidly and efficiently converted to NE. However, if DBH is saturated, as is seen in response to repetitive firing of NE neurons, not all of the DA in the vesicle is metabolized to NE and the molar ratio DA:NE in the vesicle increases. Thus, when the

noradrenergic neuron is depolarized, it releases DA as well as NE. This would explain why, under basal conditions, one does not visualize DA immunoreactivity in the CA1 stratum radiatum; during high-frequency stimulation, DA would be synthesized and then released. Very recent findings provide support for the view that DA release in the hippocampus is mediated by noradrenergic axons (Smith and Greene 2012). Specifically it was shown that block of DA synthesis in noradrenergic cells blocks the DA-mediated effects of hippocampal CA1 cells produced by amphetamine.

It might seem that hypothesis 3 argues against the possibility that the VTA can influence late LTP in the CA1 region, a process that is a cornerstone of the hippocampal-VTA loop model. However, if the NE fibers that release dopamine in CA1 radiatum were themselves excited by the VTA, then VTA activity would lead to dopamine release, as posited by the model. It is therefore important that experiments have shown that the VTA synapses onto the dendrites of the NE cells and that this synaptic connection is excitatory, as evidenced by the release of dopamine in target tissues (Deutch et al. 1986). Thus, the release of dopamine by NE fibers in the radiatum is our current working hypothesis for how the VTA triggers the DA release that promotes memory encoding in the hippocampus. One interesting functional implication is that only VTA activity long enough to cause DA accumulation in NE terminal vesicle would be sufficient to trigger DA release. Thus, according to this view, target structures receiving direct input from DA axons would be affected by brief bursts of DA cell firing. In contrast, regions dependent on DA release from NE fibers might require much longer bursts because of the activity requirement for DA release.

4.2 Conclusions and Outstanding Questions

We hope the reader has come to appreciate that understanding the DA system can provide insight into learning and the interaction of motivation with learning. This is a new field that has progressed rapidly in the last few years, but many questions remain. Figure 1 summarizes some of the anatomical regions that we have discussed in this chapter, but it is important to understand that our knowledge of the connections between regions is still evolving. Indeed, Fig. 1 incorporates a new pathway that was just reported, a completely unexpected second link between the hippocampal region and the VTA (Luo et al. 2011).

The reader will no doubt have many questions regarding the timing and duration of dopamine signals that may influence memory formation and behavior. Unfortunately, most of these cannot be answered on the basis of published data. This is because measuring dopamine release has technical difficulties and has been mostly applied to the striatum. This structure has very extensive dopamine innervations and has therefore attracted the most experimental investigation.

We have emphasized various uncertainties about the nature of dopamine signaling in the hippocampus and hope this will stimulate further research. Although the nature of the axon terminals that release dopamine in the hippocampus is unclear, there is no disagreement about the fact that the dopamine transporter, DAT, is very low or absent. This strongly implies that the rate of DA uptake (perhaps into NE fibers) will be slow, and this may have interesting functional consequences. In the striatum, the role of DA is to act as a reinforcement signal that strengthens the selection process for the action just taken. The logic of this reinforcement process requires temporal precision: reinforcement should act on the particular behavior evaluated and not on behaviors that occurred several seconds previously. Thus, the pulse of DA must have duration in the seconds range. In contrast, a much longer DA pulse in the hippocampus would not have serious negative consequences; if there are events that surround a novel event and their transition into long-term memory is also enhanced, this is not problematic (indeed, there is evidence for such loose association; see below). These considerations emphasize the need for experiments that directly measure the kinetics of dopamine release in the hippocampus.

Although we have focused on the CA1 hippocampal because this is where most of the relevant experiments have been done, it is noteworthy that two other regions receive quite strong dopaminergic innervations, the entorhinal cortex and the subiculum. Experiments done during a working memory task provide a possible function for dopamine in the subiculum. It was found that units in subiculum, but not CA1, fire persistently during the delay period of the task (Deadwyler and Hampson 2004). Given the extensive work in prefrontal cortex indicating that delay period activity requires dopaminergic modulation (Sawaguchi and Goldman-Rakic 1994), the relatively high dopaminergic innervation of the subiculum makes sense. It would be useful to specifically test the role of dopamine in the dopamine-rich areas of the hippocampal region.

Functional imaging studies in humans using fMRI provide converging evidence for a hippocampal-VTA (in humans, better referred to as hippocampus-SN/VTA) loop. There is evidence for the expected co-activation of the SN/VTA and the hippocampus during encoding into long-term memory (Wittmann et al. 2005) and novelty processing (Bunzeck and Duzel 2006; Krebs et al. 2009). But in addition, activation in both structures strongly correlates in a number of novelty-related (Bunzeck et al. 2007; Krebs et al. 2011; Shohamy and Wagner 2008; Wittmann et al. 2007) and reward-related (Adcock et al. 2006) tasks. Recent developments in functional imaging will make it possible to identify and functionally image the locus coeruleus (LC), the origin of noradrenergic projections in the hippocampus. Hence, human fMRI studies can potentially provide new insights into a network-level interaction of dopaminergic and noradrenergic midbrain structures in memory consolidation (Fig. 1) (for a discussion and review, see Duzel et al. (2012).

It may seem evident that a general purpose system enabling memory consolidation in episodic memory should not be limited to novel or rewarding events but should extend also to events associated with aversive outcomes. Surprisingly, there is very little work comparing the consolidation of rewarding and aversive events (e.g., losses) in humans (although there is extensive work on the consolidation of emotionally negative stimuli). However, the observation that there are dopaminergic responses to aversive events (Bromberg-Martin et al. 2010a,b,c) suggests that dopaminergic consolidation mechanisms similar to those seen with novelty and reward may occur in the hippocampus.

Understanding the role of dopamine in memory may lead to methods that can be used to improve learning and teaching methods. First, exposure to novel or salient information could be used to improve the long-term persistence of other information given in temporal proximity. Notably, novelty-related dopamine release can induce protein synthesis that can stabilize and maintain Hebbian plasticity enacted either before or after novelty exposure (Wang et al. 2010). Initial studies in humans suggest that similar forms of novelty-related contextual memory enhancement can also be observed in humans (Fenker et al. 2008). Second, strategies based on the availability of external reward or reward anticipation to release dopamine might prove to be useful in increasing the retention of learned material.

Although the implications of novelty-related dopaminergic neurotransmission for teaching and learning are interesting, there are still many open questions. One question is which aspect of novelty drives activation of dopaminergic circuitry. According to the exploration bonus framework (Kakade and Dayan 2002), novel events carry with them a potential for reward that familiar unrewarded items have lost. Another possibility is that dopaminergic novelty signals relate to action biases rather than valence (e.g., Guitart-Masip et al. 2011). According to this view, dopaminergic neurons promote actions to approach/reap rewards or to actively avoid punishments, and they are therefore not primarily valence driven. Hence, dopaminergic responses to novel items may signal an action bias to approach and explore. The presence of such an action bias could vary with personality traits such as novelty seeking (e.g., Krebs et al. 2009). The determination of the intrinsic factors that best capture the motivational effects of novelty has the potential for providing a deep and biologically constrained understanding of motivation.

Acknowledgements John Lisman gratefully acknowledges the support of NIH Grant N.2 P50 MH060450. Emrah Duzel has been supported by the Wellcome Trust (Project Grant to ED) and the DFG (KFO 163, SFB 776 TP A7).

References

Adcock, R., Thangavel, A., Whitfield-Gabrieli, S., Knutson, B., Gabrieli, J.: Reward-motivated learning: Mesolimbic activation precedes memory formation. Neuron **50**, 507–517 (2006)

Arsenault, M., Parent, A., Seguela, P., Descarries, L.: Distribution and morphological characteristics of dopamine-immunoreactive neurons in the midbrain of the squirrel monkey (saimiri sciureus). J. Comp. Neurol. **267**(4), 489–506 (1988)

Ballarini, F., Moncada, D., Martinez, M., Alen, N., Viola, H.: Behavioral tagging is a general mechanism of long-term memory formation. Proc. Natl. Acad. Sci. U. S. A. **106**(34), 14599–604 (2009)

Bethus, I., Tse, D., Morris, R.: Dopamine and memory: Modulation of the persistence of memory for novel hippocampal nmda receptor-dependent paired associates. J. Neurosci. **30**(5), 1610–1618 (2010)

Borgkvist, A., Malmlof, T., Feltmann, K., Lindskog, M., Schilstrom, B.: Dopamine in the hippocampus is cleared by the norepinephrine transporter. Int. J. Neuropsychopharmacol. 1–10 (2011)

Bromberg-Martin, E., Matsumoto, M., Hikosaka, O.: Distinct tonic and phasic anticipatory activity in lateral habenula and dopamine neurons. Neuron **67**(1), 144–155 (2010a)

Bromberg-Martin, E., Matsumoto, M., Hikosaka, O.: Dopamine in motivational control: Rewarding, aversive, and alerting. Neuron **68**(5), 815–834 (2010b)

Bromberg-Martin, E., Matsumoto, M., Nakahara, H., Hikosaka, O.: Multiple timescales of memory in lateral habenula and dopamine neurons. Neuron **67**(3), 499–510 (2010c)

Brown, M., Henny, P., Bolam, J., Magill, P.: Activity of neurochemically heterogeneous dopaminergic neurons in the substantia nigra during spontaneous and driven changes in brain state. J. Neurosci. **29**(9), 2915–2925 (2009)

Bunzeck, N., Doeller, C., Fuentemilla, L., Dolan, R., Duzel, E.: Reward motivation accelerates the onset of neural novelty signals in humans to 85 milliseconds. Curr. Biol. **19**(15), 1294–1300 (2009)

Bunzeck, N., Duzel, E.: Absolute coding of stimulus novelty in the human substantia nigra/vta. Neuron **51**(3), 369–379 (2006)

Bunzeck, N., Schutze, H., Stallforth, S., Kaufmann, J., Duzel, S., Heinze, H., Duzel, E.: Mesolimbic novelty processing in older adults. Cereb. Cortex **17**(12), 2940–2948 (2007)

Cheng, S., Frank, L.: New experiences enhance coordinated neural activity in the hippocampus. Neuron **57**(2), 303–313 (2008)

Coulter, C., Happe, H., Bergman, D., Murrin, L.C.: Localization and quantification of the dopamine transporter: Comparison of [3h]win 35,428 and [125i]rti-55. Brain Res. **690**(2), 217–224 (1995)

Cragg, S., Nicholson, C., Kume-Kick, J., Tao, L., Rice, M.: Dopamine-mediated volume transmission in midbrain is regulated by distinct extracellular geometry and uptake. J. Neurophysiol. **85**(4), 1761–1771 (2001)

Csicsvari, J., O'Neill, J., Allen, K., Senior, T.: Place-selective firing contributes to the reverse-order reactivation of ca1 pyramidal cells during sharp waves in open-field exploration. Eur. J. Neurosci. **26**(3), 704–716 (2007)

Curet, O., Dennis, T., Scatton, B.: The formation of deaminated metabolites of dopamine in the locus coeruleus depends upon noradrenergic neuronal activity. Brain Res. **335**(2), 297–301 (1985)

Deadwyler, S., Hampson, R.: Differential but complementary mnemonic functions of the hippocampus and subiculum. Neuron **42**(3), 465–476 (2004)

Deutch, A., Goldstein, M., Roth, R.: Activation of the locus coeruleus induced by selective stimulation of the ventral tegmental area. Brain Res. **363**(2), 307–314 (1986)

Devoto, P., Flore, G., Pani, L., Gessa, G.: Evidence for co-release of noradrenaline and dopamine from noradrenergic neurons in the cerebral cortex. Mol. Psychiatry **6**(6), 657–664 (2001)

Devoto, P., Flore, G., Saba, P., Fa, M., Gessa, G.: Co-release of noradrenaline and dopamine in the cerebral cortex elicited by single train and repeated train stimulation of the locus coeruleus. BMC Neurosci. **6**(31) (2005)

Duzel, E., Bunzeck, N., Guitart-Masip, M., Duzel, S.: Novelty-related motivation of anticipation and exploration by dopamine (nomad): Implications for healthy aging. Neurosci. Biobehav. Rev. **34**(5), 660–669 (2010)

Duzel, E., Guitart-Masip, M., Weiskopf, N., Kanowski, M.: The fMRI Book, chapter Midbrain fMRI: Applications, Limitations and Challenges (2012, in revision)

Fenker, D., Frey, J., Schuetze, H., Heipertz, D., Heinze, H., Duzel, E.: Novel scenes improve recollection and recall of words. J. Cogn. Neurosci. **20**(7), 1250–1265 (2008)

Frey, U., Matthies, H., Reymann, K.: The effect of dopaminergic d1 receptor blockade during tetanization on the expression of long-term potentiation in the rat ca1 region in vitro. Neurosci. Lett. **129**(1), 111–114 (1991)

Frey, U., Morris, R.: Synaptic tagging: Implications for late maintenance of hippocampal long-term potentiation. Trends Neurosci. **21**(5), 181–188 (1998)
Frey, U., Schroeder, H., Matthies, H.: Dopaminergic antagonists prevent long-term maintenance of posttetanic ltp in the ca1 region of rat hippocampal slices. Brain Res. **522**(1), 69–75 (1990)
Fuxe, K., Hokfelt, T., Johansson, O., Jonsson, G., Lidbrink, P., Ljungdahl, A.: The origin of the dopamine nerve terminals in limbic and frontal cortex. evidence for meso-cortico dopamine neurons. Brain Res. **82**(2), 349–355 (1974)
Fyhn, M., Molden, S., Hollup, S., Moser, M., Moser, E.: Hippocampal neurons responding to first-time dislocation of a target object. Neuron **35**(3), 555–566 (2002)
Gasbarri, A., Campana, E., Pacitti, C., Hajdu, F., Tombol, T.: Organization of the projections from the ventral tegmental area of tsai to the hippocampal formation in the rat. J. Hirnforsch. **32**(4), 429–437 (1991)
Gasbarri, A., M.G., P., Campana, E., Pacitti, C.: Anterograde and retrograde tracing of projections from the ventral tegmental area to the hippocampal formation in the rat. Brain Res. Bull. **33**(4), 445–452 (1994a)
Gasbarri, A., Packard, M., Sulli, A., Pacitti, C., Innocenzi, R., Perciavalle, V.: The projections of the retrorubral field a8 to the hippocampal formation in the rat. Exp. Brain Res. **112**(2), 244–252 (1996)
Gasbarri, A., Sulli, A., Packard, M.: The dopaminergic mesencephalic projections to the hippocampal formation in the rat. Prog. Neuropsychopharmacol. Biol. Psychiatry **21**(1), 1–22 (1997)
Gasbarri, A., Verney, C., Innocenzi, R., Campana, E., Pacitti, C.: Mesolimbic dopaminergic neurons innervating the hippocampal formation in the rat: A combined retrograde tracing and immunohistochemical study. Brain Res. **668**(1–2), 71–79 (1994b)
Geffard, M., Buijs, R., Seguela, P., Pool, C., Le Moal, M.: First demonstration of highly specific and sensitive antibodies against dopamine. Brain Res. **294**(1), 161–165 (1984a)
Geffard, M., Kah, O., Onteniente, B., Seguela, P., Le Moal, M., Delaage, M.: Antibodies to dopamine: Radioimmunological study of specificity in relation to immunocytochemistry. J. Neurochem. **42**(6), 1593–1599 (1984b)
Geffard, M., Seguela, P., Heinrich-Rock, A.: Antisera against catecholamines: Specificity studies and physicochemical data for anti-dopamine and anti-p-tyramine antibodies. Mol. Immunol. **21**(6), 515–522 (1984c)
Giese, K., Fedorov, N., Filipkowski, R., Silva, A.: Autophosphorylation at thr286 of the alpha calcium-calmodulin kinase ii in ltp and learning. Science **279**(5352), 870–873 (1998)
Goldman-Rakic, P., Leranth, C., Williams, S., Mons, N., Geffard, M.: Dopamine synaptic complex with pyramidal neurons in primate cerebral cortex. Proc. Natl. Acad. Sci. U. S. A. **86**(22), 9015–9019 (1989)
Guitart-Masip, M., Bunzeck, N., Stephan, K., Dolan, R., Duzel, E.: Contextual novelty changes reward representations in the striatum. J. Neurosci. **30**(5), 1721–1726 (2010)
Guitart-Masip, M., Fuentemilla, L., Bach, D., Huys, Q., Dayan, P., Dolan, R., Duzel, E.: Action dominates valence in anticipatory representations in the human striatum and dopaminergic midbrain. J. Neurosci. **31**(21), 7867–7875 (2011)
Hokfelt, T., Fuxe, K., Johansson, O., Ljungdahl, A.: Pharmaco-histochemical evidence of the existence of dopamine nerve terminals in the limbic cortex. Eur. J. Pharmacol. **25**(1), 108–112 (1974a)
Hokfelt, T., Ljungdahl, A., Fuxe, K., Johansson, O.: Dopamine nerve terminals in the rat limbic cortex: Aspects of the dopamine hypothesis of schizophrenia. Science **184**(133), 177–179 (1974b)
Huang, Y., Kandel, E.: D1/d5 receptor agonists induce a protein synthesis-dependent late potentiation in the ca1 region of the hippocampus. Proc. Natl. Acad. Sci. U. S. A. **92**(7), 2446–2450 (1995)
Ishikawa, K., Ott, T., McGaugh, J.: Evidence for dopamine as a transmitter in dorsal hippocampus. Brain Res. **232**(1), 222–226 (1982)
Kakade, S., Dayan, P.: Dopamine: Generalization and bonuses. Neural Netw. **15**(4–6), 549–559 (2002)

Karlsson, M., Frank, L.: Network dynamics underlying the formation of sparse, informative representations in the hippocampus. J. Neurosci. **28**(52), 14271–14281 (2008)
Krebs, R., Heipertz, D., Schuetze, H., Duzel, E.: Novelty increases the mesolimbic functional connectivity of the substantia nigra/ventral tegmental area (sn/vta) during reward anticipation: Evidence from high-resolution fmri. NeuroImage **58**(2), 647–655 (2011)
Krebs, R., Schott, B., Duzel, E.: Personality traits are differentially associated with patterns of reward and novelty processing in the human substantia nigra/ventral tegmental area. Biol. Psychiatry **65**(2), 103–110 (2009)
Kwon, O., Paredes, D., Gonzalez, C., Neddens, J., Hernandez, L., Vullhorst, D., Buonanno, A.: Neuregulin-1 regulates ltp at ca1 hippocampal synapses through activation of dopamine d4 receptors. Proc. Natl. Acad. Sci. U. S. A. **105**(40), 15587–1592 (2008)
Legault, M., Wise, R.: Novelty-evoked elevations of nucleus accumbens dopamine: Dependence on impulse flow from the ventral subiculum and glutamatergic neurotransmission in the ventral tegmental area. Eur. J. Neurosci. **13**(4), 819–828 (2001)
Lemon, N., Manahan-Vaughan, D.: Dopamine d1/d5 receptors gate the acquisition of novel information through hippocampal long-term potentiation and long-term depression. J. Neurosci. **26**(29), 7723–7729 (2006)
Li, S., Cullen, W., Anwyl, R., Rowan, M.: Dopamine-dependent facilitation of ltp induction in hippocampal ca1 by exposure to spatial novelty. Nat. Neurosci. **6**(5), 526–531 (2003)
Lisman, J., Grace, A.: The hippocampal-vta loop: Controlling the entry of information into long-term memory. Neuron **46**(5), 703–713 (2005)
Lisman, J., Grace, A., Duzel, E.: A neohebbian framework for episodic memory; role of dopamine-dependent late ltp. Trends Neurosci. **34**(10), 536–547 (2011)
Ljungberg, T., Apicella, P., Schultz, W.: Responses of monkey dopamine neurons during learning of behavioral reactions. J. Neurophysiol. **67**(1), 145–163 (1992)
Luo, A., Tahsili-Fahadan, P., Wise, R., Lupica, C., Aston-Jones, G.: Linking context with reward: A functional circuit from hippocampal ca3 to ventral tegmental area. Science **333**(6040), 353–357 (2011)
Martig, A., Mizumori, S.: Ventral tegmental area and substantia nigra neural correlates of spatial learning. Learn. Mem. **18**(4), 260–271 (2011)
Mirolli, M., Baldassarre, G.: Functions and mechanisms of intrinsic motivations: The knowledge versus competence distinction. In: Baldassarre, G., Mirolli, M. (eds.) Intrinsically Motivated Learning in Natural and Artificial Systems, pp. 49–72. Springer, Berlin (2012)
Navakkode, S., Sajikumar, S., Frey, J.: Synergistic requirements for the induction of dopaminergic d1/d5-receptor-mediated ltp in hippocampal slices of rat ca1 in vitro. Neuropharmacology **52**(7), 1547–1554 (2007)
Nehmzow, U., Gatsoulis, Y., Kerr, E., Condell, J., Siddique, N.H., McGinnity, M.T.: Novelty detection as an intrinsic motivation for cumulative learning robots. In: Baldassarre, G., Mirolli, M. (eds.) Intrinsically Motivated Learning in Natural and Artificial Systems, pp. 185–207. Springer, Berlin (2012)
Neugebauer, F., Korz, V., Frey, J.: Modulation of extracellular monoamine transmitter concentrations in the hippocampus after weak and strong tetanization of the perforant path in freely moving rats. Brain Res. **1273**, 29–38 (2009)
Nitz, D., McNaughton, B.: Differential modulation of ca1 and dentate gyrus interneurons during exploration of novel environments. J. Neurophysiol. **91**(2), 863–872 (2004)
Oades, R., Halliday, G.: Ventral tegmental (a10) system: Neurobiology. 1. anatomy and connectivity. Brain Res. **434**(2), 117–165 (1987)
Onteniente, B., Geffard, M., Calas, A.: Ultrastructural immunocytochemical study of the dopaminergic innervation of the rat lateral septum with anti-dopamine antibodies. Neuroscience **13**(2), 385–393 (1984)
Otmakhova, N., Lisman, J.: D1/d5 dopamine receptor activation increases the magnitude of early long-term potentiation at ca1 hippocampal synapses. J. Neurosci. **16**(23), 7478–7486 (1996)
Pacholczyk, T., Blakely, R., Amara, S.: Expression cloning of a cocaine- and antidepressant-sensitive human noradrenaline transporter. Nature **350**(6316), 350–354 (1991)

Quintin, L., Hilaire, G., Pujol, J.: Variations in 3,4-dihydroxyphenylacetic acid concentration are correlated to single cell firing changes in the rat locus coeruleus. Neuroscience **18**(4), 889–899 (1986)

Redgrave, P., Gurney, K.: The short-latency dopamine signal: A role in discovering novel actions? Nat. Rev. Neurosci. **7**(12), 967–975 (2006)

Redondo, R., Morris, R.: Making memories last: The synaptic tagging and capture hypothesis. Nat. Rev. Neurosci. **12**(1), 17–30 (2011)

Rossato, J., Bevilaqua, L., Izquierdo, I., Medina, J., Cammarota, M.: Dopamine controls persistence of long-term memory storage. Science **325**(5943), 1017–1020 (2009)

Sawaguchi, T., Goldman-Rakic, P.: The role of d1-dopamine receptor in working memory: Local injections of dopamine antagonists into the prefrontal cortex of rhesus monkeys performing an oculomotor delayed-response task. J. Neurophysiol. **71**(2), 515–528 (1994)

Scatton, B., Dennis, T., Curet, O.: Increase in dopamine and dopac levels in noradrenergic terminals after electrical stimulation of the ascending noradrenergic pathways. Brain Res. **298**(1), 193–196 (1984)

Scatton, B., Javoy-Agid, F., Rouquier, L., Dubois, B., Agid, Y.: Reduction of cortical dopamine, noradrenaline, serotonin and their metabolites in parkinson's disease. Brain Res. **275**(2), 321–328 (1983)

Scatton, B., Rouquier, L., Javoy-Agid, F., Agid, Y.: Dopamine deficiency in the cerebral cortex in parkinson disease. Neurology **32**(9), 1039–1040 (1982)

Scatton, B., Simon, H., Le Moal, M., Bischoff, S.: Origin of dopaminergic innervation of the rat hippocampal formation. Neurosci. Lett. **18**(2), 125–131 (1980)

Schott, B., Seidenbecher, C., Fenker, D., Lauer, C., Bunzeck, N., Bernstein, H., Tischmeyer, W., Gundelfinger, E., Heinze, H., Duzel, E.: The dopaminergic midbrain participates in human episodic memory formation: Evidence from genetic imaging. J. Neurosci. **26**(5), 1407–1417 (2006)

Schroeter, S., Apparsundaram, S., Wiley, R., Miner, L., Sesack, S., Blakely, R.: Immunolocalization of the cocaine- and antidepressant-sensitive l-norepinephrine transporter. J. Comp. Neurol. **420**(2), 211–232 (2000)

Schultz, W.: Behavioral dopamine signals. Trends Neurosci. **30**(5), 203–210 (2007a)

Schultz, W.: Multiple dopamine functions at different time courses. Annu. Rev. Neurosci. **30**, 259–288 (2007b)

Schultz, W., Apicella, P., Ljungberg, T.: Responses of monkey dopamine neurons to reward and conditioned stimuli during successive steps of learning a delayed response task. J. Neurosci. **13**(3), 900–913 (1993)

Schwab, M., Javoy-Agid, F., Agid, Y.: Labeled wheat germ agglutinin (wga) as a new, highly sensitive retrograde tracer in the rat brain hippocampal system. Brain Res. **152**(1), 145–150 (1978)

Shohamy, D., Wagner, A.: Integrating memories in the human brain: Hippocampal-midbrain encoding of overlapping events. Neuron **60**(2), 378–389 (2008)

Simon, H., Le Moal, M., Calas, A.: Efferents and afferents of the ventral tegmental-a10 region studied after local injection of [3h]leucine and horseradish peroxidase. Brain Res. **178**(1), 17–40 (1979)

Smith, C.C, Greene, R.W.: CNS dopamine transmission mediated by noradrenergic innervation. J. Neurosci. **32**(18), 6072–6080 (2012)

Sountsov, P., Santucci, D.M., Lisman, J.: A biologically plausible transform for visual recognition that is invariant to translation, scale, and rotation. Front. Comput. Neurosci. **5**(53) (2011)

Swanson, L.: The projections of the ventral tegmental area and adjacent regions: A combined fluorescent retrograde tracer and immunofluorescence study in the rat. Brain Res. Bull. **9**(1–6), 321–53 (1982)

Swanson, L., Hartman, B.: The central adrenergic system. an immunofluorescence study of the location of cell bodies and their efferent connections in the rat utilizing dopamine-beta-hydroxylase as a marker. J. Comp. Neurol. **163**(4), 467–505 (1975)

Swanson, L., Kohler, C., Bjorklund, A.: The limbic region. I: The septohippocampal system. In: Bjorklund A, Hokfelt T.S.L. (eds.) Integrated Systems of the CNS, pp. 125–269. Elsevier, Amsterdam (1987)

Swant, J., Wagner, J.: Dopamine transporter blockade increases ltp in the ca1 region of the rat hippocampus via activation of the d3 dopamine receptor. Learn. Mem. **13**(2), 161–167 (2006)

Van Eden, C., Hoorneman, E., Buijs, R., Matthijssen, M., Geffard, M., Uylings, H.: Immunocytochemical localization of dopamine in the prefrontal cortex of the rat at the light and electron microscopical level. Neuroscience **22**(3), 849–862 (1987)

VanElzakker, M., Fevurly, R., Breindel, T., Spencer, R.: Environmental novelty is associated with a selective increase in fos expression in the output elements of the hippocampal formation and the perirhinal cortex. Learn. Mem. **15**(12), 899–908 (2008)

Verney, C., Baulac, M., Berger, B., Alvarez, C., Vigny, A., Helle, K.: Morphological evidence for a dopaminergic terminal field in the hippocampal formation of young and adult rat. Neuroscience **14**(4), 1039–1052 (1985)

Wang, S., Redondo, R., Morris, R.: Relevance of synaptic tagging and capture to the persistence of long-term potentiation and everyday spatial memory. Proc. Natl. Acad. Sci. U. S. A. **107**, 19537–19542 (2010)

Whitlock, J., Heynen, A., Shuler, M., Bear, M.: Learning induces long-term potentiation in the hippocampus. Science **313**(5790), 1093–1097 (2006)

Wittmann, B., Bunzeck, N., Dolan, R., Duzel, E.: Anticipation of novelty recruits reward system and hippocampus while promoting recollection. Neuroimage **38**(1), 194–202 (2007)

Wittmann, B., Schott, B., Guderian, S., Frey, J., Heinze, H., Duzel, E.: Reward-related fmri activation of dopaminergic midbrain is associated with enhanced hippocampus-dependent long-term memory formation. Neuron **45**(3), 459–467 (2005)

Wolosin, S., Liang, J., Zeithamova, D., Schmandt, N., Preston, A.: Reward modulation of hippocampal subregions during motivated associative encoding. Soc. Neurosci. (2009)

Wyss, J., Swanson, L., Cowan, W.: A study of subcortical afferents to the hippocampal formation in the rat. Neuroscience **4**(4), 463–476 (1979)

Zoli, M., Torri, C., Ferrari, R., Jansson, A., Zini, I., Fuxe, K., Agnati, L.: The emergence of the volume transmission concept. Brain Res. Brain Res. Rev. **26**(2–3), 136–47 (1998)

Part IV
Competence-Based Intrinsic Motivation Mechanisms

Deciding Which Skill to Learn When: Temporal-Difference Competence-Based Intrinsic Motivation (TD-CB-IM)

Gianluca Baldassarre and Marco Mirolli

Abstract Intrinsic motivations can be defined by contrasting them to extrinsic motivations. Extrinsic motivations are directed to drive the learning of behavior directed to satisfy basic needs related to the organisms' survival and reproduction. Intrinsic motivations, instead, are motivations that serve the evolutionary function of acquiring knowledge (e.g., the capacity to predict) and competence (i.e., the capacity to do) in the absence of extrinsic motivations: this knowledge and competence can be later exploited for producing behaviors that enhance biological fitness. Knowledge-based intrinsic motivation mechanisms (KB-IM), usable for guiding learning on the basis of the level or change of knowledge, have been widely modeled and studied. Instead, competence-based intrinsic motivation mechanisms (CB-IM), usable for guiding learning on the basis of the level or improvement of competence, have been much less investigated. The goal of this chapter is twofold. First, it aims to clarify the nature and possible roles of CB-IM mechanisms for learning, in particular in relation to the cumulative acquisition of a repertoire of skills. Second, it aims to review a specific CB-IM mechanism, the *Temporal-Difference Competence-Based Intrinsic Motivation* (TD-CB-IM). TD-CB-IM measures the improvement rate of skill acquisition on the basis of the Temporal-Difference learning signal (TD error) that is used in several reinforcement learning (RL) models. The effectiveness of the mechanism is supported by reviewing and discussing in depth the results of experiments in which the TD-CB-IM mechanism is successfully exploited by a hierarchical RL model controlling a simulated navigating robot to decide when to train different skills in different environmental conditions.

G. Baldassarre (✉) · M. Mirolli
Laboratory of Computational Embodied Neuroscience, Istituto di Scienze e Tecnologie della Cognizione, Consiglio Nazionale delle Ricerche, Rome, Italy
e-mail: gianluca.baldassarre@istc.cnr.it; marco.mirolli@istc.cnr.it

G. Baldassarre and M. Mirolli (eds.), *Intrinsically Motivated Learning in Natural and Artificial Systems*, DOI 10.1007/978-3-642-32375-1_11,

1 Introduction

Intrinsic motivations (IM) are receiving increasing attention for their potential to allow organisms and robots to acquire knowledge and skills cumulatively and in full autonomy (Baldassarre and Mirolli 2010; Barto et al. 2004; Deci et al. 2001; Oudeyer and Kaplan 2007; Schmidhuber 2010).

As further explained in Sect. 2.1, intrinsic motivations allow organisms and robots to learn skills and knowledge in the absence of a guidance from extrinsic motivations, that is, motivations related to homeostatic drives such as hunger and thirst (Baldassarre 2011) or, in the case of robots, related to the tasks dictated by the user. An important class of IM, called "Competence-Based IM" (CB-IM), is related to measurements of the capacity to solve given tasks (Sect. 2.2). CB-IM can play various subfunctions within a cognitive system. Here we focus on a specific important computational challenge which can be briefly described as *deciding what to learn when* (Sect. 2.3). This challenge stems from the fact that an agent has to learn multiple skills so as to be capable of accomplishing several different goals, as is often the case in animals and as is becoming increasingly requested in robots. Specifically, the challenge resides in the fact that when an agent has to learn several different skills, it has to decide at each moment to which skill to dedicate its learning resources.

Here we review a specific CB-IM mechanism, called *Temporal-Difference Competence-Based Intrinsic Motivation* (TD-CB-IM), that can solve this problem. The key idea is to focus learning on those skills that exhibit the maximum learning rate of competence. In particular, TD-CB-IM is based on the idea of using the TD-error learning signal that is at the heart of several reinforcement learning (RL) models (Sutton and Barto 1998) as a reward signal for a higher-level RL component within a hierarchical system.[1]

The goal of the chapter is twofold. First, it aims to clarify a specific computational problem, "deciding when to learn what," that CB-IM can solve within autonomous learning agents. To this purpose, the chapter will briefly review the overall function played by IM (Sect. 2.1), will present an analysis that contributes to clarify the difference existing between CB-IM and Knowledge-Based IM (KB-IM) (Sect. 2.2), and will illustrate the nature and importance of the deciding-when-to-learn-what problem. Second, it aims to review the TD-CB-IM. This algorithm was first presented and exploited in Schembri et al. (2007a,b,c). With respect to these papers, here we will only review the basic results of the tests of TD-CB-IM (Sect. 4), and we

[1] Reinforcement learning models mimic the trial-and-error learning processes of animals directed to achieve an extrinsic reward, in particular those studied by behaviorist psychology with instrumental learning paradigms (Lieberman 1993) (but the models are also used to capture some mechanisms of Pavlovian learning). One of the most biologically plausible RL models, the actor-critic RL model (Houk et al. 1995; Sutton and Barto 1998), is formed by (a) an *actor*, which progressively learns to select actions so to maximize rewards, and (b) a *critic*, which progressively learns to assign an evaluation (an estimate of future rewards) to each state on the basis of the received rewards (the actor is trained to act so as to move the agent toward states with higher evaluations).

will instead present a deeper analysis of the nature and properties of the algorithm (Sects. 4 and 5).

2 Competence-Based Intrinsic Motivations

2.1 *Functions of Intrinsic Motivations*

Intrinsic motivations are usually defined by contrasting them to extrinsic motivations. Extrinsic motivations (EM) refer to homeostatic drives and other mechanisms that lead organisms to engage in an activity because it will eventually lead to a valuable outcome, such as food or water. Instead, intrinsic motivations (IM), an expression first used in psychology (Harlow 1950; Ryan and Deci 2000; White 1959), refer to actions performed "for their own sake" rather than as a means to obtain a useful outcome.

From an evolutionary/adaptive perspective, extrinsic and intrinsic motivations have been proposed to have different functions (Baldassarre 2011; note that in this chapter we will focus only on the capacity of IM to produce learning signals and not on their capacity to trigger/energize behavior). EM drive the performance and learning of behaviors directed to aid homeostatic regulations and hence to improve the chances of survival and reproduction (i.e., improve biological fitness). Instead, IM have the function of leading organisms to learn complex behaviors, for example based on long chains of actions, that would never be acquired on the basis of extrinsic rewards alone. More precisely, IM generate learning signals (and motivate the execution of behaviors) that drive the learning of new knowledge and skills that *only later* are exploited to get extrinsic rewards, that is, to improve biological fitness (cf. also Singh et al. 2010). The paradigmatic example of this is represented by children at play. Children spend their first years of life acquiring in a cumulative fashion a flexible repertoire of skills, and a wide knowledge of the world, mostly guided by intrinsic motivations (von Hofsten 2007). Only later, in adult life, such skills are reused to readily assemble complex behaviors directed to increase fitness. The importance of IM for children development is also manifested by the fact that most experiments of developmental psychology successfully leverage on IM to drive the behaviors they study as it is not possible to give direct instructions to young children and babies or it is not possible (for ethical reasons) to motivate them with EM.

2.2 *Knowledge-Based and Competence-Based Intrinsic Motivation Mechanisms*

In terms of mechanisms, IM learning signals are generated on the basis of "measurements" of the level of increase of knowledge and skills done directly in the brain (Baldassarre 2011) or in the controller in the case of robots. Due to their function, the mechanisms producing IM learning signals usually cease to produce them once the knowledge or skill to which they related have been acquired (Mirolli et al. 2012; Santucci et al. 2010). This is different from EM learning signals that come back again and again with the homeostatic needs they are directed to satisfy.

Two main types of IM mechanisms can be identified: knowledge-based intrinsic motivations (KB-IM) and competence-based intrinsic motivations (CB-IM) (Oudeyer and Kaplan 2007, see also Mirolli and Baldassarre 2012). Here with *knowledge* we will intend the "capacity to predict" (i.e., in the terminology of control theory, the capacity of *forward models* to anticipate future states based on current states and planned actions; note that in reality, knowledge also includes other capabilities, for example to abstract and classify perceived stimuli, but we will not consider this here). With *competence* we will intend here the "capacity to do", that is, to change the world in a certain way when the agent intends to do so (i.e., in the terminology of control theory, the capacity of *controllers* or *inverse models* to produce suitable actions on the basis of the pursued goal state and the current state). Importantly, competence is dependent on *goals*: these are states, among all possible states, that the agent might consider as *desired states* and hence pursue with its actions. Knowledge-based IM mechanisms (here "KB-IM" for short) generate learning signals on the basis of measures of the level, or improvement, of the agent's capacity to predict. Instead, competence-based IM mechanisms (here "CB-IM" for short) generate learning signals based on measures of the level, or improvement, of the agent's capacity to achieve its goal states.

Most computational research on IM has focused on KB-IM. In a pioneering work, Schmidhuber (1991b) (see also Schmidhuber 2012, for a review) proposed an agent endowed with a predictor, learning to predict the next state based on the current state and planned action, and a reinforcement learning (RL) component, learning to produce actions based on a reward equal to the (absolute) value of the predictor's prediction error. The agent was capable of selecting actions that led the agent to explore new regions of the problem space and that led to a high error of the predictor, so fostering the improvement of the capability of prediction of the predictor itself. This system, however, was limited by the problem of getting stuck in regions of space and in activities that led to a high prediction error that could not be decreased due to the limitations of the predictor or the world intrinsic noise. To solve this problem, Schmidhuber (1991a) proposed another system that used a learning signal measuring the *improvement* of the prediction error to train the RL component. With various developments, in particular to make it applicable to real robots (e.g., Oudeyer et al. 2007; Oudeyer et al. 2012), this approach has become the IM system most used within the autonomous learning literature.

CB-IM has received much less attention than KB-IM. A possible reason is that, as we shall see, CB-IM seems to require complex hierarchical systems to be suitably investigated; this makes the investigations more challenging. Another possible reason is that measuring the improvement of competence is not easy; this is one of the main problems targeted in this chapter, and the TD-CB-IM is a possible solution to it.

To our knowledge, Barto's group (Barto et al. 2004; Singh et al. 2005) has been the first to propose a model involving CB-IM. This model was based on the RL *option framework* (Sutton et al. 1999) and grid-world tests where the learning of the policy to achieve an extrinsic reward was supported by IM learning signals. In the model, the IM learning signals are generated as follows: (a) The system is assigned different "salient states" to accomplish, and it creates a new skill (option) for each of them. (b) When pursuing one of these salient states, the system generates a reward in proportion to the probability of not achieving the target salient state from a state from which it was possible to achieve it. Although interesting, this approach suffers of a limitation analogous to the one of the KB-IM system of Schmidhuber (1991b) mentioned above: since the learning signal depends on the *level* of the skill, (probability of achieving the goal) rather than on its *improvement*, it can possibly lead the system to focus learning resources on goals that cannot be accomplished (but see Sect. 5 for a discussion of the possible conditions where this approach might work well).

2.3 Deciding When to Learn What

Within the overall function of IM (guiding the acquisition of knowledge and skills in the absence of EM), CB-IM can play a specific important subfunction within systems that have a hierarchical architecture. Before looking closely to this subfunction, we want to stress the importance of hierarchical architectures for natural and artificial intelligent systems.

The key insight is that both animals and intelligent machines and robots can benefit of an organization of their behavior based on hierarchical architectures, which are usually either structurally or functionally modular. This is particularly important when they have to learn a multiple set of skills, as it is always the case in animals and in some cases for machines/robots.[2] The importance of hierarchical modularity is due to at least three reasons. First, the acquisition of multiple skills requires data structures and storing mechanisms that avoid the problem of catastrophic forgetting (McCloskey and Cohen 1989). Catastrophic forgetting is relevant here as the acquisition of new skills can interfere and cause the forgetting of already acquired skills. Second, hierarchical modular architectures allow transferring skills and knowledge from one task to another when this is possible, thus enhancing the learning speed of new skills (see Taylor and Stone 2009, for a review). Last,

[2]By "hierarchical" we mean that some components of the system, usually processing information at a more abstract level, exert an influence on other components, usually processing information at more detailed level. By "modular" we mean that different chunks of behavior are encoded in different portions of the system. Modularity can be either "structural," that is, related to strong connections within groups of neurons and looser connections between groups, or "functional," for example leading to encode different chunks of behavior within different portions of a rather homogeneous system on the basis of specific self-organizing mechanisms.

hierarchical modular architectures facilitate the reuse of the repertoire of previously acquired skills in the exploitation phase guided by extrinsic motivations, as they facilitate the composition of such skills to produce the needed action sequences (e.g., Hart and Grupen 2011, 2012; Barto and Mahadevan 2003, for a review; see also the example presented here).

For these reasons, hierarchy and modularity represent fundamental organizational principles of animal brains (see Meunier et al. 2010 for a review), and they are exploited with success in several computational models (e.g., Baldassarre 2001, 2002b; Caligiore et al. 2010; Hart and Grupen 2011; Jacobs et al. 1991; Yao 1999; see Barto and Mahadevan 2003 for a review).

The development of hierarchical modular systems learning multiple skills presents at least three important challenges. The first challenge, discussed in Sect. 5 but not further expanded here, is related to the development of hierarchical modular architectures actually capable of storing multiple skills. The second challenge concerns the autonomous identification of tasks (goals) by the agent, again expanded in Sect. 5.

The third and last challenge, on which we focus in this chapter, is related to the agent's decision on which task, among those autonomously identified, it should allocate its attention and learning resources in each period of its life. The idea proposed here is that *the agent should train the skills that have the highest rate of improvement*. There are at least two reasons for this. First, the agent should not continue to focus learning processes on already acquired skills as this would lead it to waste time and learning resources. Second, learning of new skills can require the execution of previously acquired skills in order to create the conditions of the success of the new skills (e.g., a child has first to learn to look and reach/grasp a single toy block before having the possibility of learning to build towers formed by several toy blocks). This means that the agent should not focus on acquiring skills that, to be successful, require the execution of skills that have not yet been acquired. Behaviorally, an agent that follows these principles appears to focus learning resources on the *zone of proximal development* (Vygotsky 1978) that lays between skills already acquired and skills too difficult to be acquired. The skills in the zone of proximal development are marked by a high acquisition rate which is instead low for skills that have been already acquired or that are too difficult to be acquired.

3 Mechanisms: Measuring Competence Improvement Based on the TD-Error Learning Signal

This section explains the TD-CB-IM mechanism, which allows measuring the competence improvement of a RL agent. The mechanism (presented for the first time in Schembri et al. 2007a,b,c) is based on the exploitation of the TD error of a reinforcement learning component to infer the *rate of improvement* of the

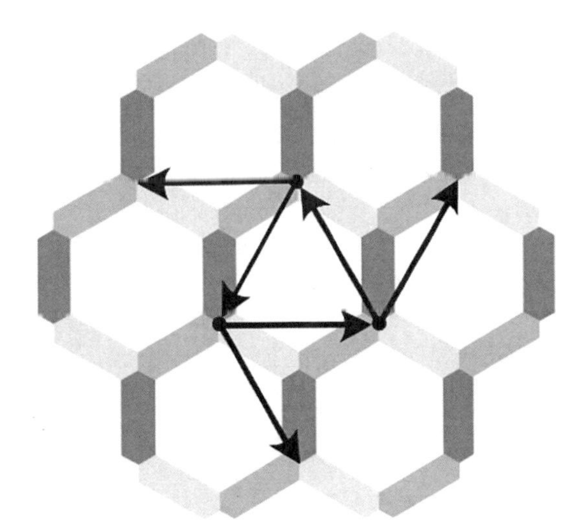

Fig. 1 The walled arena used to test the robot. The sides of the hexagons were colored with *blue* (*dark gray* in the figure), *red* (*gray*), and *green* (*light gray*). The *arrows* represent the six subtasks: for each task, the tail and the head of the arrow indicate the start and the target positions, respectively. Reprinted with permission from Schembri et al. (2007c)

skills of the component. TD-CB-IM is explained here on the basis of a hierarchical architecture, guiding a simulated robot, which exploits such mechanism to decide which skill to train among a set of skills to be acquired.

Figure 1 shows the environment used for the task that the robot has to solve. The environment is a closed arena with a colored red/green/blue pattern on the floor. The robot is a two-wheel simulated kinematic robot. The controller of the robot has to decide the translation speed and the rotation speed at each simulation step. The robot is endowed with a simplified RGB camera looking down toward the floor pattern, and the input to the controller is formed by 2×6 abstract pixels for each RGB color (in a real robot, each of these 12 abstract pixels would be the average of the activation of a portion of the camera image pixels divided in 2×6 regular parts).

The task that the robot has to solve captures a typical situation that can be faced with IM. The life of the robot is composed of two phases called "childhood" and "adulthood." The robot performance is evaluated on the basis of how fast it learns to solve a given task during adulthood. The adulthood task is composed by six subtasks, and the robot's overall performance is an average of the performance in these subtasks (see Fig. 1). In each subtask, the robot is set in a specific initial location of the arena and has to reach a specific target location (both the start and target locations are on a nonblack portion of the environment). The robot has to learn a solution to each subtask by suitably composing the skills acquired during childhood (see below). The robot gets an *extrinsic reward* of 1 when it reaches the target location of the pursued subtask and 0 otherwise.

During childhood, the robot is not informed on the final task, but it can freely explore the environment to acquire skills that can be used during adulthood to solve the final task. In particular, during childhood the robot has to acquire a repertoire of navigation skills (e.g., following a red or blue color, or turning at a certain color junction) based on (a) the guidance of *reinforcers* components and (b) the TD-CB-IM mechanism explained below.

The reinforcers that guide learning during childhood are a set of two-layer feed-forward neural networks taking as input the input of the robot camera and giving as output a reward signal ranging in $[-1, +1]$. Importantly, the connection weights of the reinforcers are evolved with a genetic algorithm (GA) that uses the robot performance in the final task as fitness function. The genetic algorithm generating the reinforcers mimics natural evolution, which generates the brain machinery of organisms that lead them to autonomously set goals. The overall (circular) evolutionary and learning cycle involving the system can hence be summarized as follows:

$$\text{Evolution} : \text{GA} \rightarrow \text{Reinforcers}$$

$$\text{Childhood} : \text{Reinforcers} + \text{TD-CB-IM} \rightarrow \text{Skill learning}$$

$$\text{Adulthood} : \text{Extrinsic rewards} \rightarrow \text{Skill composition} \rightarrow \text{Fitness} \rightarrow \text{GA}$$

Figure 2 shows the architecture of the model. The architecture is here described at a qualitative level, presenting only the critical formulas needed to explain TD-CB-IM (see Schembri et al. 2007b for other computational details on the model). The model is a two-level hierarchical reinforcement learning architecture. The higher level of the architecture is formed by a *selector* that learns to select the *experts* (3 in the experiments reported below) that form the lower level of the architecture. Each expert can control the behavior of the robot and learns though reinforcement learning. During both adulthood and childhood, at each simulation cycle, the selector selects one expert and the expert decides the robot's action. During childhood the selected expert also learns on the basis of the reinforcement signal produced by its reinforcer. During adulthood the experts do not learn but are only exploited by the selector. The selector, instead, learns in both phases of life: during adulthood it learns on the basis of the extrinsic reward related to the accomplishment of the final subtasks, whereas during childhood it learns on the basis of the TD-CB-IM mechanism. Now these processes are explained in more detail.

The selector and the experts are each formed by an actor-critic reinforcement learning model (Sutton and Barto 1998), whose actor and critic are implemented as linear approximators (two-layer feed-forward neural networks). In addition each expert has also a reinforcer associated with it. The actor of each expert is a two-layer neural network that gets the camera image as input and has two sigmoidal output units with which it controls the rotation and translation speed of the robot (each output unit sets the center of a Gaussian function on the basis of which the actual command is randomly drawn to ensure exploration).

The critic of each expert is a two-layer neural network that gets the camera image as input and has one linear output unit with which it encodes the state evaluation depending on the expert's policy. During childhood (during adulthood the experts do not learn), two successive evaluations of the expert critic, together with the expert reinforcer's reward, are used to compute the *Temporal-Difference error (TD error)* of the expert, as in the standard RL actor-critic model (Sutton and Barto 1998):

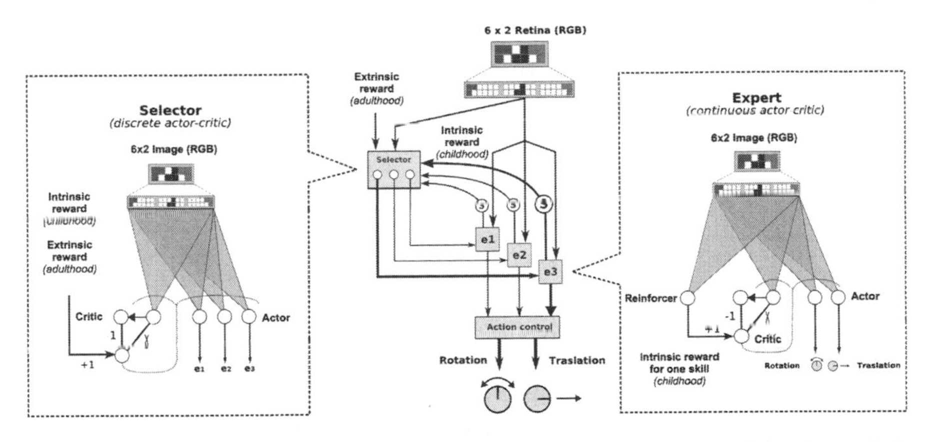

Fig. 2 The architecture of the model (*center*) with a zoom on the components of the selector (*left*) and of one expert (*right*). Reprinted with permission from Schembri et al. (2007c)

$$\mathrm{TD}_t^{\mathrm{e}} = (r_t^{\mathrm{e}} + \gamma v_t^{\mathrm{e}}) - v_{t-1}^{\mathrm{e}} \tag{1}$$

where $\mathrm{TD}_t^{\mathrm{e}}$ is the TD error, v_{t-1}^{e} and v_t^{e} are the two successive expert critic's evaluations, and r_t^{e} is the expert reinforcer's reward. The selected expert uses the learning signal TD^{e} to train its own critic component on the basis of the standard TD learning algorithm (Sutton and Barto 1998). Moreover, the selected expert trains its actor with a delta rule that moves the output units activation toward values corresponding to the executed action (which includes exploratory noise) when $\mathrm{TD}_t^{\mathrm{e}} > 0$ and away from it when $\mathrm{TD}_t^{\mathrm{e}} < 0$ (the change is done in proportion to $|\mathrm{TD}_t^{\mathrm{e}}|$).

The selector actor is a two-layer neural network that gets the camera image as input and has a number of sigmoidal output units equal to the number of experts. At each time-step, the activations of the output units are normalized so to sum to one and are used as probabilities to select, with a winner-take-all competition, the expert that controls the motor system.

Also the selector critic is a two-layer neural network. The selector critic uses two different reinforcement signals during the agent's life to compute its TD error. During adulthood, it computes the TD error, TD_t^k, on the basis of the *extrinsic reward* r^k related to the pursued subtask, k, and two succeeding evaluations related to it, v_{t-1}^k and v_t^k:

$$\mathrm{TD}_t^k = (r_t^k + \gamma v_t^k) - v_{t-1}^k \tag{2}$$

This signal is then used to train the critic's selector with the standard TD learning rule, to train the actor's selector with a delta rule, and to increase the probability of selecting the expert that in turn selects actions producing the highest TD_t^k at each state. In adulthood, at the beginning of each subtask, the selectors of the actor and the critic are reset to random weights as the policy and evaluation gradients they learn are different for each subtask and for childhood.

Most importantly, during childhood, the critic's selector uses the TD-CB-IM mechanism to compute its TD error, TD_t, and to learn. This mechanism is based on the use of the *TD error of the selected expert*, namely, $\mathrm{TD}^{\mathrm{e}}_t$, *as a reinforcement*:

$$\mathrm{TD}_t = (\mathrm{TD}^{\mathrm{e}}_t + \gamma v_t) - v_{t-1} \tag{3}$$

The fact that during childhood the selector receives the TD error of the selected expert as its reinforcement makes the critic's selector learn, for each state, to *give control to the expert which has the maximum expected learning rate in such a state.* The reason of this is that the TD error of an expert in a given state gives a measure of how much such expert learns in such a state. In fact, a positive TD error means that the expert executed an action that is on average better than the actions previously performed in such state (vice versa if the TD error is negative). If various experts are selected in a given state in successive experiences, the selector learns to produce an estimate of the average TD error that can be obtained from that state on the basis of that selection: as in standard RL, this allows it to learn to improve its decision policy, in this case with respect to the selection of the experts that have to act (and learn) in the world.

An important feature of TD-CB-IM shows that it is indeed based on a measure of competence and not of knowledge. The expert's TD error used as reward to train the selector [Eq. (3)] is *not* used in absolute value ($|\mathrm{TD}^{\mathrm{e}}_t|$) as it is done in the case of the prediction errors used by KB-IM (see Schmidhuber 2012). Indeed, even if TD-CB-IM is based on (the expert critics') prediction errors, it radically departs from KB-IM for two key reasons: (a) The prediction (of the expert critic) is about the *reward* (produced by the *reward function*), not about *world states* (produced by the *transition function*); hence, the reward is related to the success of the expert in achieving a specific goal state, not to any state that the agent might experience. (b) The *sign* of the prediction error signal (the TD error) indicates if and how much the *competence of the actor's expert* in achieving the goal is actually increasing (indeed, only if the TD error is positive there is an improvement). Instead, in the case of KB-IM (e.g., Schmidhuber 2012): (a) The prediction (of the predictor) is not about the rewards but about world states, which are neutral with respect to the skills to be acquired. (b) The sign of the prediction is not relevant as both positive and negative error signals indicate that the predictor has made an error, meaning that the *knowledge stored in such predictor* can improve.

The TD-CB-IM mechanism has other two important properties related to the fact that a second TD learning process, the one used by the selector, is used to estimate the TD error of the experts. First, this implies that the TD-CB-IM is *prospective*. Indeed, the selector critic, for the properties of TD learning, learns to produce an estimation of the true evaluations, denoted here as v^{sa}_t, that is equal to the expected sum of the future discounted TD^{e} signals that can be obtained from the current state by following the expert selection policy of the (current) selector actor (sa):

$$v^{\mathrm{sa}}_t = E\left[\mathrm{TD}^{\mathrm{e}}_t + \gamma \mathrm{TD}^{\mathrm{e}}_{t+1} + \gamma^2 \mathrm{TD}^{\mathrm{e}}_{t+2} + \ldots\right] \tag{4}$$

where $E[\cdot]$ is the expectation function. This implies that the selector learns to select an expert that not only has a high expected learning rate in the current state but that also leads to states where such expert, or other experts, can learn the most.

The second implication of the fact that the critic's selector uses a TD learning process to predict the expert TD error is that the TD-CB-IM captures the idea of focusing learning within the zone of proximal development of the agent, that is, on the experts that can learn the most in a certain developmental phase. Indeed, as the critic's selector tends to learn the v_t associated to a given state in an incremental fashion, it tends to build up an estimation of the actual v^{sa} which averages out the strong noise usually affecting TD^e, and to capture its trend value for the visited states: this value is close to zero if the expert does not learn in such state, it tends to be positive if the expert is improving its competence, and it gets again close to zero when the expert has fully acquired the skill.

4 Results

This section reviews the basic results obtained in previous work (Schembri et al. 2007a,b,c), so to show how the system behaves.

In the experiments, the genetic algorithm rapidly reaches a high performance (Fig. 3a). In this respect, the system showed to have a high degree of evolvability compared to other systems where other aspects of the architecture different from the reinforcers were evolved. For example, the architecture considered here took about 5 generations of the genetic algorithm to achieve high performance during adulthood, whereas a system where the genetic algorithm directly searched the connection weights of the actors instead of the reinforcers took about 40 generations to achieve a comparable performance, and systems where both the actors and the selector were evolved took about 80 generations (Fig. 3a). This result is likely due to the fact that it is easier to evolve the criteria (reinforcers) for guiding learning of the behavior needed to accomplish a certain task rather than directly evolving this behavior (see Schembri et al. 2007a for further details).

Figure 4a, b shows the behavior of the robot during childhood in a typical evolutionary run. At the beginning of childhood (Fig. 4a), the robot moves randomly in the arena as the selector selects random experts and the selected experts select random actions. With the progression of learning (Fig. 4b), the robot acquires a very structured exploratory behavior. Indeed, the robot explores the environment following a regular pattern that allows it to experience states that are important for accomplishing the adulthood subtasks. In particular different experts specialize and acquire different skills. With different repetitions of the simulation with different random seeds, the behaviors produced by the experts can differ, although they are all very effective in adulthood. For example, some experts make the robot follow a particular color, while others make the robot follow two colors and to avoid the third one.

Most notably, an important fact apparent from Fig. 4b is that during childhood, thanks to the TD-CB-IM, the selector has learned to select different experts for

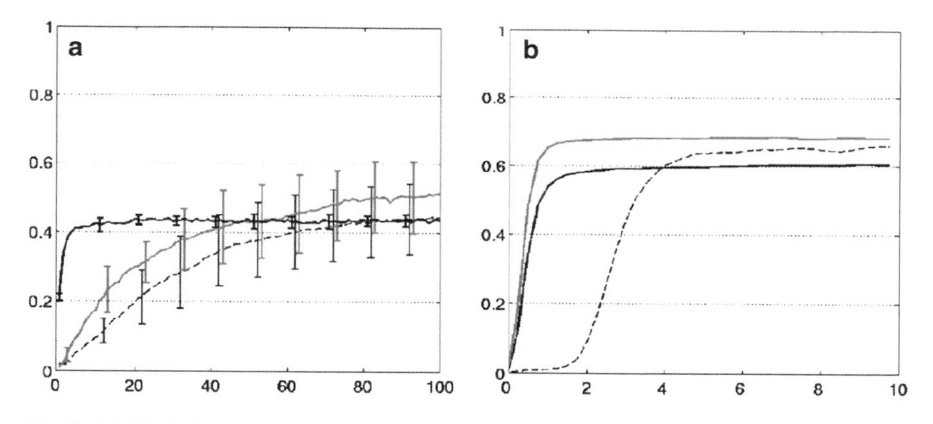

Fig. 3 (**a**) Evolution of the fitness of the best individuals (averaged over 10 runs) along 100 generations, for three conditions involving these versions of the system: evolved reinforcers, learning experts, and learning selector (*bold line*); evolved experts and learning selector (*gray line*); and evolved experts and evolved selector (*dashed line*). The graph also reports standard deviations. (**b**) Average performance during learning tests lasting 1,000,000 cycles for three conditions: evolved reinforcers, learning experts, and learning selector (*bold line*); evolved experts and learning selector (*gray line*); and simple learning expert reset before each adulthood task (*dashed line*). *Curves* refer to the average performance (normalized number of received rewards) over the ten best individuals of ten replications measured in ten tests for each of the six tasks (i.e., average of $10 \times 10 \times 6$ tests). Reprinted with permission from Schembri et al. (2007a)

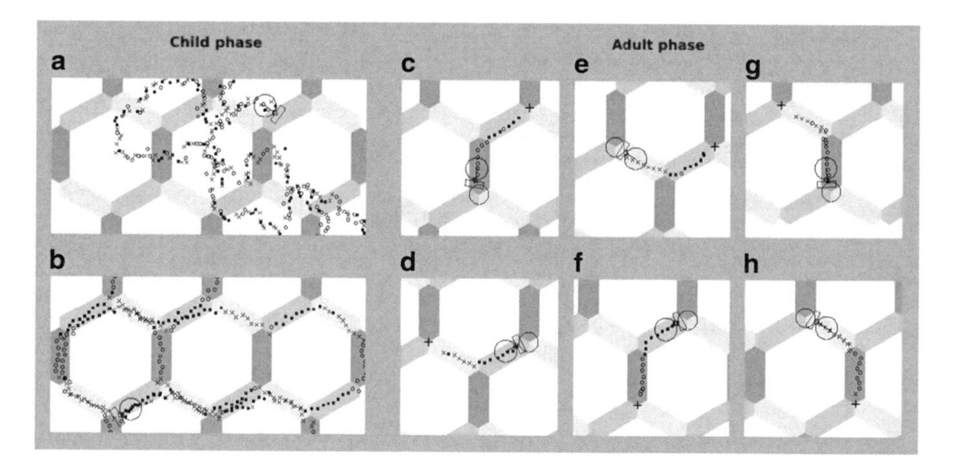

Fig. 4 Behavior of the robot: in all graphs *crosses*, *empty circles*, and *full circles* indicate the expert selected in that state (the marks are drawn every ten steps). (**a**) Childhood: behavior exhibited by the robot at the beginning of development. (**b**) Childhood: behavior exhibited by the robot after the childhood learning. (**c**–**h**) Adulthood: behavior of the robot exhibited after learning the six adulthood tasks. Reprinted with permission from Schembri et al. (2007c)

different colors of the track. The selector acquires this capability as its reward is the TD-error signal of the experts, and this leads it to select, at each state, the expert that has the highest positive TD-error signal; that is, the expert that has the highest learning rate of the competence that allows it to accomplish the skill established by its reinforcer. Following this strategy, the selector allows the different experts to acquire different skills.

A second interesting fact apparent from Fig. 4b is that the sequence with which the selector selects the experts creates a repetitive behavior based on the cyclic recall of sequences of skills. This is important as the agent is not artificially reset during childhood, so it has to procure the necessary experiences to learn. This behavior might be either the result of the structure of the environment that favors cyclic behaviors or the effect of an intended policy of the selector. In this respect, the prospective nature of the RL selector discussed in Sect. 2.1, for which the selector aims to maximize not only the next expert's TD error but rather the sum of all future TD errors (suitably discounted), might play an important role in the acquisition of such capability. Although further research is needed to understand if and how TD-CB-IM can lead to find policies that solve the "problem of the reset" autonomously, this problem is clearly an important one to be solved to obtain a fully autonomous acquisition of skills.

The childhood learning process allows the robot to acquire a repertoire of skills suitable to solve the adulthood subtasks. Fig. 4c–h shows an example of the behavior of the robot involved in solving the six adulthood subtasks. During adulthood the selector learns quite rapidly to solve each of the six subtasks by assembling the skills acquired in childhood under the guidance of TD-CB-IM. If compared to a RL system that has to learn an adulthood task from scratch, the hierarchical system takes on average four times less (compare the bold and dashed lines of Fig. 3b; for further details, see Schembri et al. 2007a). Indeed, based on the subtask external reward, during adulthood the robot needs only to learn to select the suitable expert(s) for each color and change it at color junctions. Importantly, different subtasks can be learned by composing different sequences of skills: these skills represent readily available building blocks that do not need to be acquired from scratch. In other evolutionary runs, the specialization of the experts and their selection is more fuzzy/difficult to be described than the one shown in Fig. 4, but the learning speed remains comparable.

5 Discussion and Open Challenges

5.1 *Relevance of TD-CB-IM*

This chapter has first introduced the concept of intrinsic motivations (IM), and then it has focused on a particular class of them, namely, competence-based IM (CB-IM). A first contribution of this chapter has been the analysis of the relation existing between CB-IM and the problem of the cumulative acquisition of a repertoire of skills, in particular in relation to hierarchical architectures. A fundamental function that CB-IM can play in this context is to support the *autonomous* decision about which skill to train at each moment.

The second contribution of this chapter has been to clarify the nature and functioning of a specific CB-IM mechanism, called "TD-CB-IM," and initially proposed in Schembri et al. (2007c), Schembri et al. (2007a) and Schembri et al. (2007b). TD-CB-IM exploits the TD-error learning signal used in most reinforcement learning (RL) models to measure the competence improvement of a RL agent (a mechanism similar to the one presented here, but based on the RL option framework and tested in a grid world, has been recently proposed by Stout and Barto 2010). The effectiveness of TD-CB-IM has been shown by reviewing the core aspects of a hierarchical RL model where a higher-level RL selector has to learn to give control to a number of lower-level experts, themselves based on RL models, engaged in learning different tasks. Within this architecture, the key idea of the TD-CB-IM mechanism involves the use of the experts' TD error as an index of the improvement of their competence. In particular, the TD error of experts is used as an intrinsic reinforcement for the selector. This leads the selector to learn to select, at each state, the expert with the highest competence acquisition rate. Note that this mechanism of attribution of responsibility (i.e., control and learning) is rather different from what done in other hierarchical RL models, for example in Doya et al. (2002), where the responsibility used to train RL expert modules is based on the capacity of the predictors of each module to predict the dynamics of the experienced portion of environment.

An important feature of the architecture made the mechanism prospective in the selection of experts. Indeed, as the TD error of experts is given as reward to the selector which is itself a RL model, the selector learns to select experts so as to maximize not only the immediate competence acquisition rate but also the future acquisition rate. For this reason, the selector learns to select the experts by taking in due consideration not only their (expected) learning rate but also the possibilities of learning in the states that will be visited after their actions are executed. This gives a prospective nature to the selection of the experts and leads to select sequences of skills that maximize the overall competence acquisition of the system.

The experiments reviewed here, related to a simulated robot endowed with a simplified camera, have shown how a hierarchical RL autonomous system, if endowed with a suitably system for self-identification of tasks (in this case a genetic algorithm), can benefit of the TD-CB-IM mechanism to acquire skills without the guidance of EM (i.e., in the case of robots, in complete autonomy from human intervention). Later the acquired skills can be readily composed to accomplish extrinsic tasks that would have required a long training to be accomplished or that would have never been discovered (Vigorito and Barto 2010). Although the test of the model presented here goes beyond the simple grid words usually used in RL, it is nevertheless simplified: future investigations should aim to ascertain if and how TD-CB-IM scales up to scenarios involving robots endowed with more complex sensory and motor systems.

5.2 *Intrinsic Motivations Based on Competence Improvement Versus Competence Level*

An important issue concerns the advantages and disadvantage of CB-IM mechanisms based on measures of *levels of competence*, as the one proposed by Barto et al. (2004) and Singh et al. (2005), and those based on *competence improvement*, as the TD-CB-IM presented here. In Sect. 2.2 we have said that the former is potentially affected by the problem of focusing on tasks that cannot be learned because too difficult for the system or completely unsolvable. CB-IM mechanisms based on competence improvement such as TD-CB-IM allow overcoming this problem as they focus on a task only if the system can have a competence improvement on it: if there is no improvement due to the task difficulty or the limited potentiality of the learner, the engagement with the task ceases.

However, the learning signal used by TD-CB-IM, namely, the TD error of experts, is considerably affected by noise. The reason is that when the system has not fully acquired the capability of achieving its goals, its stochastic policy continuously selects actions that can be either better or worse than the average, so the TD error continuously shifts between positive and negative values. Hence, the actual improvement of the competence of the system has to be captured as positive *average* TD error. This fact might make the CB-IM mechanisms based on competence level preferable to those based on competence improvement in case the conditions for applying them are favorable, that is, when: (a) The maximum level of achievable competence is known a priori (this is needed to compute how far the actual competence is from the maximum one). (b) We are certain that the system has the necessary capability of acquiring a full competence in the task (otherwise the system would get stuck in trying to learn tasks too difficult for it).

5.3 *Intrinsic and Extrinsic Motivations*

The model captures some essential features of the evolutionary relation between IM and EM expanded at a theoretical level in Baldassarre (2011) and only briefly tackled in the original papers where TD-CBIM was initially proposed (Schembri et al. 2007a,b,c). In particular, the model reviewed here has clearly highlighted two issues important for IM: (a) The relation existing between extrinsic motivations (EM) and IM. (b) Their adaptive function for the survival and reproduction of organisms. In this respect, the model, by dividing the life of the agent in two distinct periods involving respectively IM and EM, has stressed how the primary adaptive function of IM is to guide the acquisition of skills and knowledge in the absence of EM learning signals. These skills and knowledge can then be exploited in succeeding phases of life to rapidly assemble behaviors that contribute to adaptation under the direct guidance of EM. Beyond the organisms' life, the success of this adaptation then guides the evolutionary process to improve the IM machinery that leads to acquire certain skills instead of others (e.g., specific reinforcers in the model) and that implements the TD-CB-IM (here hardwired). Another work (Singh et al. 2010) has presented an analysis and a model on these issues. This work agrees on the function of EM and IM discussed here (e.g., the model uses two distinct IM/EM learning phases to show the potential function of IM), but argues for a continuity existing between the two from evolutionary and computational perspectives.

Linked to the latter issue, we observe that the two distinct IM/EM phases of the model reviewed here are important for theoretical analysis, but in organisms, IM and EM work at the same time (e.g., children are driven by both EM, such as those related to hunger and thirst, and IM, such as those related to curiosity and play). So, future work will have to investigate how the learning signals generated by EM and IM can be usefully arbitrated in situations where they tend to drive behavior in different directions (see Kakade and Dayan 2002 for a discussion about if and how novelty-related reinforcement signals might work together with long-term EM rewards). For example, how does a hungry child engaged in playing decide if continuing to play or looking for food?

The latter issues are relevant not only for the study of organisms but also for robotics and machine learning. Indeed, also *autonomous* robots and machines have mechanisms equivalent to the EM mechanisms of organisms. In particular, in robots EM are first related to “survival”, that is, to physical integrity, energy maintenance, etc., which are an essential precondition for the robot correct functioning. Moreover, and most importantly, in both robots and machines EM are also related to the user's requirements. Indeed, the “reproduction” of the robot/machine in several copies (eventually with variants) depends on the success of the robot/machine in accomplishing the users' requests. For this reason, the reward given to a RL robot by a user on the basis of a task useful for him/her can be considered as related to the EM of the robot. In this context, IM can be used as means in acquiring knowledge and skills before the user provides indications (i.e., EM learning signals). These previously acquired knowledge and skills allow the machine/robot to learn to solve the users' tasks much faster (e.g., see Luciw et al. 2011).

5.4 Possible Biological Correspondents of TD-CB-IM

Another important problem, not mentioned so far, concerns the investigation of the possible biological correspondents of the TD-CB-IM. The investigation of the biological mechanisms possibly underlying IM is new but growing. A first proposal comes from Kakade and Dayan (2002). The authors propose that dopamine, one of the main neuromodulators used by brain for driving trial-and-error learning, encodes information not only about primary rewards but also about *exploration bonuses*. These bonuses are quantities added to rewards or values to ensure appropriate exploration in new or changing environments. Another hypothesis is presented by Kaplan and Oudeyer (2007), who propose that the KB-IM signals generated by their model (e.g., Oudeyer et al. 2007) might correspond to tonic dopamine.

An elaborated theory on IM has been proposed within the neuroscientific literature by Redgrave and Gurney (2006) (see also Redgrave et al. 2012). The idea is that bursts of dopamine signal the detection of sudden unexpected events, for example, the unexpected onset of a light caused by the accidental pressure of a lever. These bursts of dopamine (DA), produced by the substantia nigra pars compacta (SNpc), are caused by the capacity of the superior colliculus (SC) to respond to unexpected luminance changes and, on this basis, to activate SNpc. In turn, the DA signal leads to increase the probability of execution of the actions that caused the event (putatively on the basis of trial-and-error learning processes implemented by the sensorimotor basal ganglia-cortical loops): this leads the agent to learn the experienced action-outcome contingencies and, on this basis, to later recall an action if the corresponding outcome becomes desirable (goal-based action recall; see Baldassarre et al. (2012) for a model of these processes).

A central aspect of this theory is that the dopaminergic burst is caused by apparently neutral events such as the light onset. A second important aspect is that the DA signal tends to disappear after a prolonged experience, putatively under the effect of a predictor of the phasic event that learns to progressively inhibits the sensory response (not to be confused with the inhibition inherent to the TD-error learning rule, Mirolli et al. 2012). These two aspects characterize the signal as an intrinsic rather than as an extrinsic signal. This theory has been proposed by contrasting it with the standard theories on phasic dopamine that claim that this signal corresponds to a *reward prediction error* equivalent to the TD error of RL algorithms (e.g., Schultz 2002). However, the two positions are not necessarily in contrast, as suggested by Mirolli et al. (2012) on the basis of a computational model: dopaminergic signals might indeed correspond to TD-error signals that depend on both extrinsic rewards and (intrinsic) reinforcements triggered by unexpected events and thus might have the function of driving both reward maximization and action discovery and acquisition.

Paralleling the fact that they have been less investigated with computational models, we still lack a hypothesis on the possible brain correspondents of CB-IM. Based on its features, however, we can here try to speculate a possible biological implementation of the TD-CB-IM and propose an hypothesis that builds on the theory of Redgrave and Gurney (2006) reviewed above (cf. also Mirolli and Baldassarre 2012). In this respect, an appealing feature of TD-CB-IM is that it relies upon the standard TD-error signal used by most RL models which, as mentioned above, putatively corresponds to phasic dopamine signals in brain (encoding the TD error related to either a primary reward or to a sensory prediction error). This paves the way to search a higher-level RL system in the brain that: (a) Has the capacity to select lower-level actor-critic components capable of implementing actions. (b) Receives the TD error from such lower-level actor-critic components and uses it in place of the primary reward. We put forward the hypothesis that such two components of the system might be implemented respectively by: (a) The loops formed by medial and ventral BG (mvBG) and dorsolateral prefrontal cortex (dlPFC) which have been proposed to implement higher-level RL processes captured by hierarchical RL models (Baldassarre 2002a; Botvinick et al. 2008).

(b) The striosomes of ventral BG (svBG) and their connections to the ventral tegmental area (VAT), which form a second important dopaminergic system beyond SNpc. The idea would be that mvBG-dlPFC implement the actor of the selector of the model presented here: this would play the function of learning to select large chunks of behavior (experts) implemented at a lower level within the sensorimotor BG-cortical loops. Instead, the svBG-VTA system, reached directly or indirectly by the DA caused by the lower-level sensorimotor loops, would implement the critic of the selector: this would play the function of learning to predict the learning rate of the lower-level experts as in the model presented here.

5.5 Open Problems Related to CB-IM

We see at least three open problems related to the use of CB-IM. The first is the importance of developing more powerful *hierarchical RL models* capable of storing multiple skills while avoiding catastrophic forgetting, exploiting information transfer between different tasks, and composing skills to build more complex behaviors. Various proposals already exist to face this problem: see Barto and Mahadevan (2003), for a review on hierarchical RL systems; Taylor and Stone (2009), for a review on the issue of transfer of information between tasks; Vigorito and Barto (2010), Hart and Grupen (2011), and Schembri et al. (2007a,b,c) for examples of models involving hierarchical/modular architectures and IM; and Elfwing et al. (2007) for a model that has some resemblance to the one presented here and that uses evolutionary techniques to search a hierarchy that minimizes the number of primitive subtasks that are needed for each type of problem. However, further advancements in this field are required to further develop CB-IM mechanisms.

The second open problem is related to the *autonomous identification of tasks/goals*, an important prerequisite for the functioning of the TD-CB-IM mechanism. The idea here is that a skill aims to accomplish a given *task*, that is, to accomplish a given final state (*goal*) in the environment or in the body-environment relation (e.g., "reach and get the hand in contact with a visible object" or "grasp and carry the visible object from point A to point B in space"). When tasks and goals cannot be derived from EM, they must be found autonomously through IM. CB-IM mechanisms can play the subfunction of "deciding when to learn what" only if there are several different "whats" to be learned. The pioneering work of Singh et al. (2005) circumvented the problem: the tasks were hardwired by defining a limited subset of "salient states," among all states that the agent could experience, that defined the termination states of the options to be created. The work of Schembri et al. (2007c) reviewed here solved the problem by having a genetic algorithm find reinforcers that defined the skills to be acquired by the experts on the basis of the performance of the system in the tasks of adulthood. Another solution to the problem is based on the identification of critical states having a high frequency of visits during the solution of several different tasks (e.g., the door passage connecting two environments; McGovern and Barto 2001; Pickett and Barto 2002; Thrun and Schwartz 1995). Yet another possible solution, which has however never been applied to autonomous skills discovery, might be based on the idea that relevant states are those where the agent is maximally "empowered," that is, states where their actions can lead to explore the maximum number of future states (Jung et al. 2011; Klyubin et al. 2005).

An important aspect of this problem is the relation between the need to seek the tasks to learn and the capacity of the agent to understand what it can learn and what is beyond its learning possibilities. For this reason, we think that mechanisms such as the TD-CB-IM might play an important role in the solution of the problem related to the autonomous search of tasks. Even KB-IM might play an important role in the autonomous finding of goals, as they allow the isolation of states of the world that are interesting and potentially relevant for the agent. In any case, the autonomous definition of useful goal states remains one of the most important open problems for designing systems that are capable of undergoing a prolonged autonomous accumulation of competence with the guidance of IM.

A last problem related to TD-CB-IM is the issue of scalability. Here the mechanism was tested with only a few experts/goals (e.g., three). In reality, organisms have to learn a large number of tasks. A similar condition might be encountered by future robots. The open problem is hence as follows: would the TD-CB-IM work if used to learn a large number of tasks/goals? The TD-CB-IM mechanism might have problems as its decision on when to learn what is based on a sampling of the competence improvement for each task: it does not seem efficient to continuously sample all tasks before knowing in which task the learning rate is highest. However, consider that *any* CB-IM or KB-IM mechanism used to acquire several skills would encounter this problem. This suggests to look at more general solutions. This problem is closely related to the problem regarding the autonomous identification of goals. Indeed, these two problems might actually be the same: what is the goal the system should try to learn to accomplish at each moment? In this respect, a possible solution might be that only *new goals discovered by chance*, for example, while performing previously acquired skills in new conditions, are considered for learning: this would greatly restrict the attention to goals which are new but that are within the agent's capabilities. In this condition, CB-IM mechanisms such as TD-CB-IM might be used *to continue* to engage with the discovered goal if the competence acquisition rate is above a certain level, rather than to *select* goals among the (possibly numerous) ones that are given externally as happens in the artificial conditions considered here.

Acknowledgements This research has received funds from the European Commission 7th Framework Programme (FP7/2007-2013), "Challenge 2 - Cognitive Systems, Interaction, Robotics," Grant Agreement No. ICT-IP-231722, Project "IM-CLeVeR - Intrinsically Motivated Cumulative Learning Versatile Robots."

References

Baldassarre, G.: A modular neural-network model of the basal ganglia's role in learning and selecting motor behaviours. In: Altmann, E.M., Cleermans, A., Schunn, C.D, Gray, W.D. (eds.) Proceedings of the Fourth International Conference on Cognitive Modeling (ICCM2001), pp. 37–42. Fairfax, Virgina, USA, 26–29 July 2001. Lawrence Erlbaum, Mahwah (2001)

Baldassarre, G.: A modular neural-network model of the basal ganglia's role in learning and selecting motor behaviours. J. Cogn. Syst. Res. **3**(2), 5–13. Special Issue Dynamic and Recurrent Neural Networks (2002a)

Baldassarre, G.: Planning with neural networks and reinforcement learning. Ph.D. Thesis, Computer Science Department, University of Essex, Colchester, UK (2002b)

Baldassarre, G.: What are intrinsic motivations? a biological perspective. In: Cangelosi, A., Triesch, J., Fasel, I., Rohlfing, K., Nori, F., Oudeyer, P.-Y., Schlesinger, M, Nagai, Y. (eds.) Proceedings of the International Conference on Development and Learning and Epigenetic Robotics (ICDL-EpiRob-2011), pp. E1–E8. Frankfurt, Germany, 24–27 August, 2011. IEEE, Piscataway (2011)

Baldassarre, G., Mannella, F., Fiore, V.G., Redgrave, P., Gurney, K., Mirolli, M.: Intrinsically motivated action-outcome learning and goal-based action recall: A system-level bio-constrained computational model. Neural Netw. (2012, in press)

Baldassarre, G., Mirolli, M.: What are the key open challenges for understanding the autonomous cumulative learning of skills? The Newslett. Auton. Mental Dev. Techn. Comm. (IEEE CIS AMD Newslett.) **7**(1), 11 (2010)

Barto, A., Singh, S., Chentanez, N.: Intrinsically motivated learning of hierarchical collections of skills. In: International Conference on Developmental Learning (ICDL2004). La Jolla, CA, 20–22 October, 2004. IEEE, Piscataway (2004)

Barto, A.G., Mahadevan, S.: Recent advances in hierarchical reinforcement learning. Discr. Event Dyn. Syst. **13**(4), 341–379 (2003)

Botvinick, M.M., Niv, Y., Barto, A.: Hierarchically organized behavior and its neural foundations: A reinforcement-learning perspective. Cognition **113**(3), 262–280 (2008)

Caligiore, D., Mirolli, M., Parisi, D., Baldassarre, G.: A bio-inspired hierarchical reinforcement learning architecture for modeling learning of multiple skills with continuous state and actions. In: Kuipers, B., Shultz, T., Stoytchev, A., Yu, C. (eds.) IEEE International Conference on Development and Learning (ICDL2010). Ann Arbor, MI, USA, 18–21 August, 2010 IEEE, Piscataway (2010)

Deci, E., Koestner, R., Ryan, R.: Extrinsic rewards and intrinsic motivation in education: Reconsidered once again. Rev. Educ. Res. **71**(1), 1–27 (2001)

Doya, K., Samejima, K., Katagiri, K.-I, Kawato, M.: Multiple model-based reinforcement learning. Neural Comput. **14**(6), 1347–1369 (2002)

Elfwing, S., Uchibe, E., Doya, K., Christensen, H.: Evolutionary development of hierarchical learning structures. IEEE Trans. Evol. Comput. **11**(2), 249–264 (2007)

Harlow, H.F.: Learning and satiation of response in intrinsically motivated complex puzzle performance by monkeys. J. Comp. Physiol. Psychol. **43**, 289–294 (1950)

Hart, S., Grupen, R.: Learning generalizable control programs. IEEE Trans. Auton. Mental Dev. **3**(1), 216–231 (2011)

Hart, S., Grupen, R.: Intrinsically motivated affordance discovery and modeling. In: Baldassarre, G., Mirolli, M. (eds.) Intrinsically Motivated Learning in Natural and Artificial Systems. Springer, Berlin (2012, this volume)

Houk, J.C., Adams, J.L., Barto, A.G.: A model of how the basal ganglia generate and use neural signals that predict reinforcement. In: Houk, J.C., Davids, J.L., Beiser, D.G. (eds.) Models of Information Processing in the Basal Ganglia, pp. 249–270. The MIT Press, Cambridge (1995)

Jacobs, R., Jordan, M., Nowlan, S., Hinton, G.: Adaptive mixtures of local experts. Neural Comput. **3**(1), 79–87 (1991)

Jung, T., Polani, D., Stone, P.: Empowerment for continuous agent-environment systems. Adap. Behav. **19**(1), 16–39 (2011)

Kakade, S., Dayan, P.: Dopamine: Generalization and bonuses. Neural Netw. **15**(4–6), 549–559 (2002)

Kaplan, F., Oudeyer, P.-Y.: In: Search of the neural circuits of intrinsic motivation. Front. Neurosci. **1**, 225–236 (2007)

Klyubin, A., Polani, D., Nehaniv, C.: Empowerment: A universal agent-centric measure of control. In: The 2005 IEEE Congress on Evolutionary Computation, vol. 1, pp. 128–135. Edinburg UK, 2–4 September, (2005)

Lieberman, D.A.: Learning, Behaviour and Cognition. Pacific Grove, CA: Brooks/Cole (1993)

Luciw, M., Graziano, V., Ring, M., Schmidhuber, J.: Artificial curiosity with planning for autonomous perceptual and cognitive development. In: Cangelosi, A., Triesch, J., Fasel, I., Rohlfing, K., Nori, F., Oudeyer, P.-Y., Schlesinger, M., Nagai, Y. (eds.) IEEE International Conference on Development and Learning (ICDL2011), pp. E1–8. IEEE, Frankfurt, Germany, 24–27 August, 2011. Piscataway (2011)

McCloskey, M., Cohen, N.: Catastrophic interference in connectionist networks: The sequential learning problem. In: Bower, G.H. (ed.) The Psychology of Learning and Motivation, vol. 24, pp. 109–165. Academic Press, San Diego (1989)

McGovern, A., Barto, A.: Automatic discovery of subgoals in reinforcement learning using diverse density. Technical report of the faculty publication series, University of Massachusetts – Amherst, Computer Science Department (2001)

Meunier, D., Lambiotte, R., Bullmore, E.T.: Modular and hierarchically modular organization of brain networks. Front. Neurosci. **4**, 200 (2010)

Mirolli, M., Baldassarre, G.: Functions and mechanisms of intrinsic motivations: The knowledge versus competence distinction. In: Baldassarre, G., Mirolli, M. (eds.) Intrinsically Motivated Learning in Natural and Artificial Systems. Springer, Berlin (2012, this volume)

Mirolli, M., Santucci, V.G., Baldassarre, G.: Phasic dopamine as a prediction error of intrinsic and extrinsic reinforcement driving both action acquisition and reward maximization: A simulated robotic study. Neural Netw. (2012, submitted)

Oudeyer, P.-Y., Banares, A., Frédéric, K.: Intrinsically motivated learning of real world sensorimotor skills with developmental constraints. In: Baldassarre, G., Mirolli, M. (eds.) Intrinsically Motivated Learning in Natural and Artificial Systems. Springer, Berlin (2012, this volume)

Oudeyer, P.-Y., Kaplan, F.: What is intrinsic motivation? a typology of computational approaches. Front. Neurorobot. **1**, 6 (2007)

Oudeyer, P.-Y., Kaplan, F., Hafner, V.V.: Intrinsic motivation systems for autonomous mental development. IEEE Trans. Evol. Comput. **11**(2), 265–286 (2007)

Pickett, M., Barto, A.: Policyblocks: An algorithm for creating useful macro-actions in reinforcement learning. In: Sammut, C., Hoffmann, A.G. (eds.) Proceedings of the Nineteenth International Conference on Machine Learning, pp. 506–513. Sydney, Australia, 8–12 July 2002. Morgan Kaufmann, San Francisco (2002)

Redgrave, P., Gurney, K.: The short-latency dopamine signal: A role in discovering novel actions? Nat. Rev. Neurosci. **7**(12), 967–975 (2006)

Redgrave, P., Gurney, K., Stafford, T., Thirkettle, M., Lewis, J.: The role of the basal ganglia in discovering novel actions. In: Baldassarre, G., Mirolli, M. (eds.) Intrinsically Motivated Learning in Natural and Artificial Systems. Springer, Berlin (2012, this volume)

Ryan, R., Deci, E.: Intrinsic and extrinsic motivations: Classic definitions and new directions. Contemp. Educ. Psychol. **25**, 54–67 (2000)

Santucci, V.G., Baldassarre, G., Mirolli, M.: Biological cumulative learning through intrinsic motivations: A simulated robotic study on development of visually-guided reaching. In: Johansson, B., Sahin, E., Balkenius, C. (eds.) Proceedings of the Tenth International Conference on Epigenetic Robotics (EpiRob2010), pp. 121–128. Lund, Sweden. Lund: Lund University Cognitive Studies vol.149 (2010)

Schembri, M., Mirolli, M., Baldassarre, G.: Evolution and learning in an intrinsically motivated reinforcement learning robot. In: Almeida e Costa Fernando, Rocha, L.M., Costa, E., Harvey, I., Coutinho, A. (eds.) Advances in Artificial Life. Proceedings of the 9th European Conference on Artificial Life (ECAL2007), Lisbon, Portugal, 10–14 September 2007. Lecture Notes in Artificial Intelligence, vol. 4648, pp. 294–333. Springer, Berlin (2007a)

Schembri, M., Mirolli, M., Baldassarre, G.: Evolving childhood's length and learning parameters in an intrinsically motivated reinforcement learning robot. In: Berthouze, L., Dhristiopher, P.G., Littman, M., Kozima, H., Balkenius, C. (eds.) Proceedings of the Seventh International Conference on Epigenetic Robotics, vol. 134, pp. 141–148. Lund, Sweden. Lund: Lund University Cognitive Studies vol. 149 (2007b)

Schembri, M., Mirolli, M., Baldassarre, G.: Evolving internal reinforcers for an intrinsically motivated reinforcement-learning robot. In: Demiris, Y., Mareschal, D., Scassellati, B., Weng, J. (eds.) Proceedings of the 6th International Conference on Development and Learning, pp. E1–6. London, UK, 11–13 July 2007. IEEE, Piscataway (2007c)

Schmidhuber, J.: Curious model-building control systems. In: Proceedings of the International Joint Conference on Neural Networks, vol. 2, pp. 1458–1463 Singapore, 18–21 November (1991a)

Schmidhuber, J.: A possibility for implementing curiosity and boredom in model-building neural controllers. In: Meyer, J.-A., Wilson, S. (eds.) From Animals to Animats: Proceedings of the First International Conference on Simulation of Adaptive Behavior, Paris, France, December, 1990 pp. 222–227, MIT, Cambridge (1991b)

Schmidhuber, J.: Formal theory of creativity, fun, and intrinsic motivation (1990–2010): IEEE Trans. Auton. Mental Dev. **2**(3), 230–247 (2010)

Schmidhuber, J.: Maximizing fun by creating data with easily reducible subjective complexity. In: Baldassarre, G., Mirolli, M. (eds.) Intrinsically Motivated Learning in Natural and Artificial Systems. Springer, Berlin (2012, this volume)

Schultz, W.: Getting formal with dopamine and reward. Neuron **36**(2), 241–263 (2002)

Singh, S., Barto, A., Chentanez, N.: Intrinsically motivated reinforcement learning. In: Saul, L.K., Weiss, Y., Bottou, L. (eds.). Advances in Neural Information Processing Systems 17: Proceedings of the 2004 Conference. Vancouver, British Columbia, Canada, 13–18 December 2004. MIT, Cambridge (2005)

Singh, S., Lewis, R., Barto, A., Sorg, J.: Intrinsically motivated reinforcement learning: An evolutionary perspective. IEEE Trans. Auton. Mental Dev. **2**(2), 70–82 (2010)

Stout, A., Barto, A.G.: Competence progress intrinsic motivation. In: Kuipers, B., Shultz, T., Stoytchev, A., Yu, C. (eds.) IEEE International Conference on Development and Learning (ICDL2010). Ann Arbor, MI, USA, 18–21 August, 2010. IEEE, Piscataway (2010)

Sutton, R., Precup, D., Singh, S.: Between MDPs and semi-MDPs: A framework for temporal abstraction in reinforcement learning. Artif. Intell. **112**, 181–211 (1999)

Sutton, R.S., Barto, A.G.: Reinforcement Learning: An Introduction. MIT, Cambridge (1998)

Taylor, M., Stone, P.: Transfer learning for reinforcement learning domains: A survey. J. Mach. Learn. Res. **10**, 1633–1685 (2009)

Thrun, S., Schwartz, A.: Finding structure in reinforcement learning. In: Tesauro, G., Touretzky, D, Leen, T. (eds.) Advances in Neural Information Processing Systems 7 (NIPS1994), Denver, Colorado, USA, pp. 385–392. MIT, Cambridge (1995)

Vigorito, C., Barto, A.: Intrinsically motivated hierarchical skill learning in structured environments. IEEE Trans. Auton. Mental Dev. **2**(2), 132–143 (2010)

von Hofsten, C.: Action in development. Dev. Sci. **10**(1), 54–60 (2007)

Vygotsky, L.S.: Mind in society: The development of higher psychological processes. Cambridge, MA: Harvard University Press (1978)

White, R.W.: Motivation reconsidered: The concept of competence. Psychol. Rev. **66**, 297–333 (1959)

Yao, X.: Evolving artificial neural networks. In: Proceedings of the IEEE, vol. 87, pp. 1423–1447. (1999)

Intrinsically Motivated Affordance Discovery and Modeling

Stephen Hart and Roderic Grupen

Abstract In this chapter, we argue that a single intrinsic motivation function for affordance discovery can guide long-term learning in robot systems. To these ends, we provide a novel definition of "affordance" as the latent potential for the closed-loop control of environmental stimuli perceived by sensors. Specifically, the proposed intrinsic motivation function rewards the discovery of such control affordances. We will demonstrate how this function has been used by a humanoid robot to learn a number of general purpose control skills that address many different tasks. These skills, for example, include strategies for finding, grasping, and placing simple objects. We further show how this same intrinsic reward function is used to direct the robot to build stable models of when the environment affords these skills.

1 Introduction

Computational approaches for accumulating long-term control knowledge have eluded psychologists and roboticists since the beginning of research in artificial intelligence. In order for an agent to learn over a lifetime, it must figure out how to take actions that have some measurable effect on the world and be motivated to exercise such actions to understand their consequences. In this chapter, we examine a single fixed *intrinsic reward function* that addresses these issues in a unified framework.

S. Hart (✉)
Manufacturing Systems Research Laboratory, General Motors R&D, 30500 Mound Road, Warren, MI 48090, USA
e-mail: stephen.hart@gm.com

R. Grupen
Department of Computer Science, University of Massachusetts Amherst, 140 Governors Drive, Amherst, MA 01003, USA
e-mail: grupen@cs.umass.edu

G. Baldassarre and M. Mirolli (eds.), *Intrinsically Motivated Learning in Natural and Artificial Systems*, DOI 10.1007/978-3-642-32375-1_12,

Intrinsically motivated learning is an area of research that has recently provided new tools for autonomous systems to learn over the long term. It alleviates the intractability of more traditional adaptive control learning approaches in which human programmers are required to supply specific (extrinsic) reward criteria for every task. However, much of the existing work in the intrinsic motivation literature has focused on how an agent can explore its environment to gather as much information as possible (cf., Oudeyer et al. 2007). In contrast, we propose a framework in which the robot is intrinsically motivated to control interactions with the environment—learning new control programs and learning how to predict their outcomes in a large variety of run-time situations.

The intrinsic motivator we propose was previously introduced in work by the authors (Hart 2009b; Hart and Grupen 2011; Hart et al. 2008a,b) in which we demonstrated how to use this motivator to learn generalizable control strategies for uncovering environmental affordances. In this chapter, we will review this work and extend it by showing how the same motivator can create probabilistic models concerning the conditions in which the environment affords these strategies. We call these models "control affordance models" as they provide direct perception of the functional attributes of objects. Functional representations provide a convenient way of organizing cognitive structures in agents by providing direct measures of the completeness of background knowledge. Moreover, they provide a simple means of experimental verification. To verify whether a test object affords grasping, for example, the agent need only take the requisite action and observe the result.

This chapter is organized as follows. In Sect. 2, we discuss relevant work on affordance learning and intrinsic motivation in both the machine learning and psychology literature. In Sect. 3 we provide an overview of the foundational framework we use called the *control basis*. Section 4 formally defines control affordances and introduces an intrinsic reward function for control affordance discovery and modeling. Section 5 demonstrates how this reward function can guide a robot to learn generalizable control strategies for uncovering control affordances and then use these strategies to model the environmental contexts in which they occur. We conclude with a discussion of future work.

2 Related Work

2.1 Affordance Learning

Gibson initially proposed the "theory of affordances," suggesting that organisms perceive their environment in terms of their ability to interact with it (Gibson 1977). Thus, it is a natural area of study for embodied learning agents such as robots. Chemero defined affordances as a relationship between an agent and an object in terms of the potential for action (Chemero 2003). Applying these theories to robotics, researchers have examined how a robot can learn probabilistic models of affordances for pushing and grasping objects (Fitzpatrick et al. 2003), tool use (Stoytchev 2005), and navigation (Modayil and Kupiers 2007).

The multi-sensory autonomous cognitive systems (MACS) group proposed a general model of affordances in terms *entities*, *behaviors*, and *effects* (Şahin et al. 2007). In this work, machine learning algorithms are used to predict the perceptual effects of taking actions that involve objects (or entities). The MACS formulation has been explored on a mobile robot platform to learn affordances for traversability, pushability, and liftability (by means of a magnetic gripper), as well as to ground planning operators for extended tasks (Uğur et al. 2009).

A number of researchers have provided a formalism of affordances called "object-action complexes" (or OACs), also grounded in the robot's sensory data, but ultimately used for higher-level planning tasks (Krüger et al. 2011, 2009). The OACs framework has been used in various situations, such as to predict grasp affordances from the visual appearance of an object for a robot gripper (Detry et al. 2009; Kraft et al. 2008).

In this work, robot actions are typically simple preprogrammed activities that require no sensory feedback to measure "success," as usually defined by the programmer, or are not goal directed. As a result, these activities do not ground behavioral objectives in the robot's closed-loop interaction dynamics. In contrast, this chapter will examine a formulation of affordances that arises from a robot's dynamic interactions with its environment.

2.2 Intrinsic Motivation

Intrinsic motivators for behavior have been extensively studied in psychology. Hull introduced the concept of "drives" such as hunger, pain, sex, or escape, defined in terms of deficits that the organism wishes to reduce to achieve homeostatic equilibrium (Hull 1943). Later researchers extended the Hullian theory by introducing drives for manipulation (Harlow 1950) and for exploration (Montgomery 1954). Festinger suggested that there is a drive to reduce the cognitive dissonance between internal knowledge structures and the current perception of the organism's world (Festinger 1957). Primary motivators to reduce the discrepancy between cognitive structures and experience were introduced by Kagan (1972). Hunt suggested that children, in fact, seek to reduce such incongruity (Hunt 1965). The motivator discussed in this chapter provides a unique perspective as it attempts to link together the drive for manipulation with the drive for building cognitive models.

In the computational literature, Schmidhuber examined how intrinsic motivation techniques can be used to shape reward in reinforcement learning systems (Schmidhuber 1991). Barto et al. demonstrated how to intrinsically motivate a reinforcement learning agent to learn a reusable set of skills (called *options* in the RL literature) that can be applied in different but possibly related tasks (Barto et al. 2004). The behavioral skills learned in our proposed framework are similar to options except that they automatically generate their own state/action spaces as necessary to achieve new behavior.

Oudeyer et al. (2007) make two useful distinctions in statistical models of intrinsic motivation: those that predict the consequences of an agent's action (Huang and Weng 2002) and those that predict the errors in those predictions (a meta-predictor) (Herrmann et al. 2000). The former approach, the authors argue, results in systems that will focus on challenging situations that may be too complex to ever get a handle on. The latter approach remedies this issue by using the meta-predictor to recognize that certain situations are too complex, or unlearnable. This meta-predictor looks at both learning rate and the contextual similarity between learning contexts to capture such situations. This work is important to the framework presented in this document because it introduces the idea of a *memory* to the computational intrinsic motivation literature and is consistent with the theories of Festinger, Kagan, and Hunt.

Oudeyer and Kaplan also provide a taxonomy of intrinsic reward functions that distinguishes between *knowledge-based* and *competence-based* motivators (Oudeyer and Kaplan 2007). Knowledge-based approaches are based on measures of modeling or prediction error. Competence-based approaches are based on measures of changing levels of mastery in terms of what an agent can accomplish. The intrinsic reward function for control affordance discovery and modeling introduced in this chapter is both knowledge-based and competence-based. In order to define this function, however, we first need to introduce the representational framework necessary called the *control basis*.

3 The Control Basis Framework

The *control basis* framework (Huber and Grupen 1996; Huber et al. 1996) provides a formal structure for constructing hierarchical and multi-objective closed-loop programs from discrete combinations of sensory and motor resources. We briefly summarize the main components of this framework that are relevant to the proposed intrinsic reward function and definition of control affordance. The interested reader is invited to follow the provided references for more examples and details.

3.1 The Combinatorics of Control Actions

Actions in the control basis are constructed by using a robot's controllable degrees of freedom to suppress observable errors by gradient descent of potential functions. Formally, the control basis is defined by three discrete sets $\langle \Phi, \Sigma, \mathcal{T} \rangle$ as follows.

Perceptual Entities Σ: Signals are continuous streams of data that are provided by sensor devices (cameras, strain gauges, microphones, motor encoders, etc.). There may be several signals derived from a single physical sensor. For example, a contact load cell on the fingertip of a robot hand may produce multidimensional force signals from which Cartesian contact positions and normals can be computed. "Perceptual entities" $\sigma \subseteq \Sigma$ represent real-valued features derived from these signals. Each σ could be a single feature from a single signal, such as a contact position, or it could be a collection of such features, such as the collection of joint angles describing the kinematic structure. Additionally, it could be derived from a robot's internal knowledge structures like an occupancy map, or a distribution of positions where interesting objects tend to be located in the world.

Motor Variables $\mathcal{T}$*:* Motor units in $\mathcal{T}$ are "low-level" embedded controllers corresponding to independently actuatable degrees of freedom in the robot. Controllers in the control basis submit "higher-level" reference inputs $\mathbf{u}_\iota$ to groups of motor units $\tau \subseteq \mathcal{T}$ to move collections of motor units concurrently.

Potential Functions Φ*:* Potential functions $\phi \in \Phi$ map the values of perceptual entities to real-valued scalar potentials such that $\phi : \sigma \to \mathbb{R}$. A scalar potential can be viewed as a measure of the strain in the system between an observed situation and a goal specified by percepts in Σ. The gradient, therefore, acts as a virtual force that decreases the distance between a set of observable features and a reference condition. Rimon and Koditschek enumerated the conditions for a class of *navigation functions* that can formally be used as control functions (Koditschek and Rimon 1990; Rimon and Koditschek 1992). If these conditions are met, then the gradient of these functions will lead asymptotically to equilibrium set points. Examples of potential functions that have been used successfully in the control basis include fields that describe kinodynamic conditioning (Hart and Grupen 2007), harmonic function path planners (Connolly and Grupen 1994), and force closure functions for grasping and manipulation (Platt et al. 2010).

The control basis provides a comprehensive way of combining sensory, motor, and computational resources into equilibrium set-point controllers where $\nabla_\tau \phi(\sigma) = 0$. In particular, primitive closed-loop controllers are combinations $\langle \phi \in \Phi, \sigma \subseteq \Sigma, \tau \subseteq \mathcal{T} \rangle$. We designate a primitive controller $c = \langle \phi, \sigma, \tau \rangle$ with the special notation $\phi|_\tau^\sigma$. Controllers compute displacements to motor units using the gradient of potential functions computed from sensory signals. The instantaneous gradient of a potential function $\phi(\sigma)$ with respect to a collection of motor units τ is defined by the control Jacobian:

$$\mathbf{J} = \frac{\partial \phi(\sigma)}{\partial \mathbf{u}_\tau}. \tag{1}$$

Controller displacements are computed by the following linear approximation:

$$\Delta \mathbf{u}_\tau = \mathbf{J}^\# \Delta \phi(\sigma) \kappa \tag{2}$$

where κ is a small positive gain and $\mathbf{J}^\#$ is the Moore-Penrose pseudo-inverse of $\mathbf{J}$. When $\min_\sigma \phi(\sigma) = 0$, as is often the case, Eq. (2) can be written in the simplified form:

$$\Delta \mathbf{u}_\tau = -\mathbf{J}^\# \phi(\sigma) \kappa. \tag{3}$$

Multi-objective control actions are constructed by combining control primitives in a prioritized fashion such that they can be executed in parallel to provide co-articulated behavior. Consider two control actions, a higher priority controller c_1 and a lower priority controller c_2. To ensure that the lower priority controller does not destructively interfere with the progress of the higher priority controller, they are combined using null-space projection (Nakamura 1991). For a twofold control relationship that controls the same set of motor variables $\tau \subseteq \mathcal{T}$, the prioritized composite control law is defined as

$$\Delta \mathbf{u}_\tau = \mathbf{J}_1^\# \Delta\phi_1(\sigma_1)\kappa_1 + \mathbf{N}_1 \left(\mathbf{J}_2^\# \Delta\phi_2(\sigma_2)\kappa_2\right), \tag{4}$$

where $\mathbf{N}_1$ is the null-space matrix of the higher priority controller such that $\mathbf{N}_1 = (\mathbf{I} - \mathbf{J}_1^\# \mathbf{J}_1)$. Equation (4) can be extended to control laws of n-fold concurrency relationships. The control expression $c_2 \triangleleft c_1$—read, "c_2 *subject-to* c_1"—provides a useful shorthand notation for such relationships.

3.1.1 Example: Kinematically Conditioned Reaching

A simple example of a multi-objective control law concerns moving the Cartesian end-effector location of a 7-DOF serial-chain manipulator toward a target position while simultaneously keeping the arm's joints away from range of motion constraints. For the sake of discussion (and to keep the control composition simple), we will assume that there are no obstacles as these would require a more complex control composition.

The position of the arm and the target position will be designated $\mathbf{x}_{\text{arm}} \in \mathbb{R}^3$ and $\mathbf{x}_{\text{target}} \in \mathbb{R}^3$, respectively. Additionally, let $\mathbf{q} = [q_1 \ldots q_n]$ be the seven-dimensional vector of joint angles for the manipulator with range of motion centers $\tilde{\mathbf{q}}$. The manipulator arm is controlled by the collection of motor units τ_q that accepts reference control inputs $\mathbf{u}_q$.

In this example, the sensor and motor "resources" for constructing closed-loop controllers are the sets $\Sigma = \{\mathbf{x}_{\text{arm}}, \mathbf{x}_{\text{target}}, \mathbf{q}, \tilde{\mathbf{q}}\}$ and $\mathcal{T} = \{\tau_q\}$. The set of potential functions Φ in this example will consist of simple quadratic potentials on the position error of the end-effector and on the error between the current manipulator configuration and the nominal (midrange) configuration.

Motion Control: The first control primitive, c_1, constructed from sets $\langle \Phi, \Sigma, \mathcal{T} \rangle$ implements Cartesian position control for the end effector by sending commands to the motor units τ_q. It uses the perceptual entities $\sigma_x = \{\mathbf{x}_{\text{arm}}, \mathbf{x}_{\text{target}}\}$ and the potential function:

$$\phi_1(\sigma_x) = \frac{1}{2}(\mathbf{x}_{\text{target}} - \mathbf{x}_{\text{arm}})^T (\mathbf{x}_{\text{target}} - \mathbf{x}_{\text{arm}}). \tag{5}$$

Joint displacements are computed according to the control expression:

$$\Delta \mathbf{u}_1 = -\mathbf{J}_1^{\#} \phi_1(\sigma_x) \kappa_1 \tag{6}$$

$$= -\left(\frac{\partial \phi_1(\sigma_x)}{\partial \mathbf{u}_q} \right)^{\#} \phi_1(\sigma_x) \kappa_1 \tag{7}$$

$$= -\left(\frac{\partial \phi_1(\sigma_x)}{\partial \mathbf{x}_{\text{arm}}} \frac{\partial \mathbf{x}_{\text{arm}}}{\partial \mathbf{u}_q} \right)^{\#} \phi_1(\sigma_x) \kappa_1 \tag{8}$$

$$= -\left(\mathbf{J}_{\phi_1} \mathbf{J}_m \right)^{\#} \phi_1(\sigma_x) \kappa_1 \tag{9}$$

$$= \mathbf{J}_m^{\#} \left(\mathbf{x}_{\text{target}} - \mathbf{x}_{\text{arm}} \right) \kappa_1 \tag{10}$$

where $\mathbf{J}_{\phi_1} = \partial \phi_1(\sigma_x) / \partial \mathbf{x}_{\text{arm}}$ and $\mathbf{J}_m = \partial \mathbf{x}_{\text{arm}} / \partial \mathbf{u}_q$ is the manipulator Jacobian.

Kinematic Conditioning: The second control primitive, c_2, is constructed to kinematically condition the manipulator toward the middle of its range of motion, $\tilde{\mathbf{q}}$. It uses the perceptual entities $\sigma_q = \{\mathbf{q}, \tilde{\mathbf{q}}\}$ and the potential function

$$\phi_2(\sigma_q) = \frac{1}{2} (\tilde{\mathbf{q}} - \mathbf{q})^T (\tilde{\mathbf{q}} - \mathbf{q}) \tag{11}$$

and computes joint displacements according to the control equation:

$$\Delta \mathbf{u}_2 = -\mathbf{J}_2^{\#} \phi_2(\sigma_q) \kappa_2 \tag{12}$$

$$= -\left(\frac{\partial \phi_2(\sigma_q)}{\partial \mathbf{u}_q} \right)^{\#} \phi_2(\sigma_q) \kappa_2 \tag{13}$$

$$= (\tilde{\mathbf{q}} - \mathbf{q}) \kappa_2. \tag{14}$$

The multi-objective control law $c_2 \triangleleft c_1$ moves the end effector toward the desired Cartesian goal while conditioning its joints in the null space:

$$\Delta \mathbf{u}_q = \Delta \mathbf{u}_1 \kappa_1 + \mathbf{N}_1 \Delta \mathbf{u}_2 \kappa_2. \tag{15}$$

3.2 State Estimation

The dynamics observed when a controller interacts with the environment supports a natural discrete abstraction of the underlying continuous state space. One simple discrete state definition based on *quiescence* events and controller relevance was proposed in Hart et al. (2008b). Quiescence events occur when a controller reaches the neighborhood of a fixed point where the gradient vanishes (and the goal of the action is achieved). Specifically, the state of controller c_i at time k is represented by the classifier p_i^k such that

$$p_i^k = \begin{cases} X & : \quad c_i \text{ not activated,} \\ - & : \quad \text{features in } \sigma \text{ are not observed,} \\ 0 & : \quad |\dot{\phi}| > \epsilon_i, \\ 1 & : \quad |\dot{\phi}| \leq \epsilon_i, \text{quiescence,} \end{cases} \tag{16}$$

where ϵ_i is a small, positive constant.

Given a collection of n distinct primitive controllers, a discrete state space $\mathcal{S}$ can be formed where the state vector at time k is defined as $\mathbf{s}^k = [p_1^k \dots p_n^k]$ and $\mathbf{s}^k \in \mathcal{S}$. Using this representation, policies π (possibly stochastic) can be specified to map states in $\mathcal{S}$ to actions in $\mathcal{A}$ (where the actions may be either the n primitive controllers or multi-objective control laws assembled from their combination). We call the collection of states, actions, and policy a *control basis program*. For convenience, controllers and control programs are given names (written in capital letters) that intuitively reflect their nominal function under certain conditions—for example, GRASP or STEP.

3.2.1 Example: Finding and Tracking Visual Features

Consider a control basis program called SEARCHTRACK that has the action set $\mathcal{A}_{\text{st}} = \{\text{SEARCH, TRACK}\}$. The TRACK controller moves a 2-DOF pan/tilt camera to track highly saturated visual "blobs." Specifically, it uses a quadratic potential function to track the centroid coordinates of such blobs, $\boldsymbol{\gamma}^{\text{sat}}$, using the motor units of the camera τ_{pt}. The SEARCH controller produces references for τ_{pt} sampled from a probability distribution of configurations where the saturated blob features have led to TRACK quiescence in the past, $Pr(\mathbf{u}_{\text{pt}}|p_{\text{track}} = 1)$. This distribution is encoded in the form of a multidimensional Gaussian that is estimated from experience.

These controllers define a state vector $\mathbf{s} = [p_{\text{search}}\ p_{\text{track}}]$ (with the time indexes dropped for notational simplicity). A policy in this state and action space for finding and tracking highly saturated blobs that only uses primitive control actions at each step is shown in Fig. 1. The program begins in state [XX] and executes the TRACK controller. If a highly saturated blob is present, the program enters state [X0] where the policy suggests continuing with this controller until it quiesces in state [X1]. If such a blob is not initially present, a transition to state [X−] occurs and the policy switches to the SEARCH controller—moving the pan/tilt camera to a new configuration sampled from the search distribution—and trying the TRACK controller again once it finishes (repeating this process if necessary).

3.3 Hierarchy in the Control Basis

In conjunction with a reward function that assigns value to each state (or state/action pair), reinforcement learning (RL) techniques such as Q-learning can be used

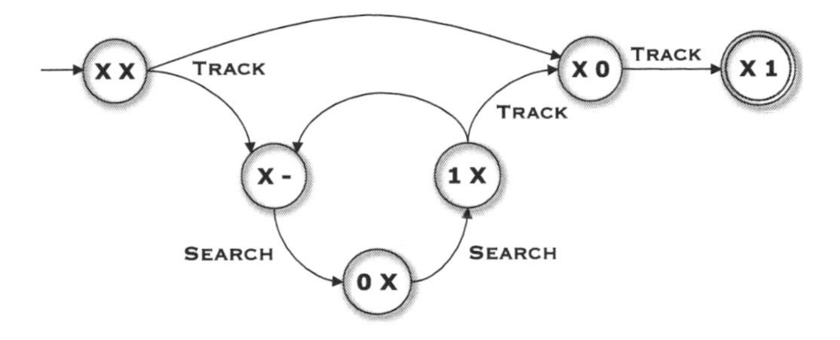

Fig. 1 The policy for a control basis program called SEARCHTRACK

to estimate state-action value functions that satisfy the Bellman optimality equation (Sutton and Barto 1998). These value functions are directly analogous to potential functions for discrete state/action spaces. The control basis takes advantage of this observation by allowing an abstraction of sensorimotor programs—with all the internal state they require—in terms of the single, four-predicate state logic of Eq. (16). Although a program can have a significant amount of internal structure, a hierarchical learning agent can view this program as a single, temporally extended action a_i whose state is represented by a single predicate p_i in the same way that it views all other control basis actions. In the next section, we consider a special reward function—particular to the control basis—for affordance discovery.

4 Intrinsically Motivated Affordance Modeling and Discovery

Reinforcement learning algorithms allow a learning agent to acquire policies for selecting actions in states in order to maximize expected cumulative return—defined by a reward function specified a priori—over time. In the control basis, they provide a mechanism for a robot to learn how to sequence controllers into policies, such as the one shown in Fig. 1, that lead to desired attractor states. In this section we define an intrinsic reward function (Sect. 2.2) designed to allow a robot to learn *multiple* control programs for interacting with its environment along with the situations in which they are likely to apply. More specifically, this intrinsic motivator rewards a robot for discovering and modeling the *control affordances* in its environment.

4.1 Control Affordances

The control basis framework provides the representational foundations for computationally encoding control affordances. When a control action is able to effectively track an environmental stimulus—closing the loop between the dynamics of the environmental source and the dynamics of the robot's motor systems—it signifies that the environment affords that control action.

Environmental tracking controllers are defined in terms of the special subset of perceptual entities, $\sigma_{\text{env}} \subseteq \Sigma$, that represent signals that originate in the robot's environment. The set σ_{env} includes, for example, visual features observed on a robot's camera images and force contact features observed on a robot's fingertip load cells.

Definition 1 (Environmental Tracking Controller). The controller c_i is an environmental tracking controller if it uses features from $\sigma_{\text{env}} \subseteq \Sigma$ to evaluate the potential function $\phi \in \Phi$. The set of environmental tracking controllers is defined as $\mathcal{C}_t$.

The TRACK controller introduced in Sect. 3.2.1 is an example of an environmental tracking controller. A controller that maintains a constant pressure on an object with a finger or collection of fingers would also be an environmental tracking controller.

Control affordances are captured in the control basis framework through the ability to execute environmental tracking controllers until quiescence.

Definition 2 (Control Affordance). The environment affords controller c_i at time k if (1) c_i is an environmental tracking controller and (2) the status of that controller (16) $p_i^k = 1$.

Control affordances are thus measured not only in terms of perceptual stimuli but also in terms of the robot's ability to engage these stimuli with its motor resources in stable control configurations. If a robot can use its cameras to keep an object in the center of its field of view over an extended period of time, the environment affords the tracking of that object. If a robot can maintain a constant contact force with its fingertips to keep an object in its hand, the environment affords holding that object. The onset of a control affordance is defined by the Boolean variable

$$b_i^k = \left((p_i^{k-1} \neq 1) \wedge (p_i^k = 1)\right) \tag{17}$$

capturing the "discovery" event, at time k, that the current context affords controller c_i.

4.2 Control Affordance Modeling

Gibson's concept of affordance relies not only on the ability of an organism to perform a particular action but also on the ability for that organism to recognize the contexts in which that action is possible (Gibson 1977). We define the environmental context $\mathbf{f} \in \mathcal{F}$ as the vector of information observed through a robot's perceptual entities σ_{env}. The likelihood of context $\mathbf{f}$ affording controller c_i is defined as a probability distribution we call a *control affordance model*.

Definition 3 (Control Affordance Model). A control affordance model for environmental tracking controller $c_i \in \mathcal{C}_t$ is defined as the probability distribution $Pr(p_i = 1|\mathbf{f})$ where $\mathbf{f}$ is the environmental context.

Put simply, these models capture the likely environmental conditions in which controllers are expected to converge. As such, control affordance models can be thought of as representing the *initiation set* of admissible environmental states in which c_i is afforded.

In practice, control affordance models can be represented by a variety of means. For simplicity, we define this distribution as a multivariate normal distribution with the same dimension as the variable $\mathbf{f}$ such that $Pr(p_i = 1|\mathbf{f}) \sim \mathcal{N}_i(\boldsymbol{\mu}_i, \boldsymbol{\Sigma}_i)$. As this distribution must be estimated from experience, we define the parameter estimates for this distribution at time k as $\hat{\boldsymbol{\mu}}_i^k$ and $\hat{\boldsymbol{\Sigma}}_i^k$. As experience is gathered, one possibility of measuring the "completeness" of this model can be captured by examining how the covariance estimate changes over time. As the model grows more stable, new information should provide little change to this estimate. We define this change in terms of a "habituation" variable

$$h_i^k = ||\hat{\boldsymbol{\Sigma}}_i^k - \hat{\boldsymbol{\Sigma}}_i^{k-1}||_1, \tag{18}$$

where $||\cdot||_1$ is the entry-wise norm. Because h_i^k captures a measure of "learning progress" with respect to a given control affordance, it can be used to direct a robot to take actions that provide the most new information.

4.3 Intrinsic Reward

Given the above definitions, we can now introduce the main contribution of this chapter: an intrinsic reward function that rewards the discovery and modeling of control affordances.

Definition 4 (Intrinsic Control Affordance Discovery Reward). The intrinsic reward for control affordance discovery is defined as

$$r^k = \sum_i \left(h_i^k r_i^k - \rho_i\right), \tag{19}$$

where

$$r_i^k = \begin{cases} 1 & : \quad (b_i^k \wedge (c_i \in \mathcal{C}_t)) \\ 0 & : \quad \text{otherwise} \end{cases}, \tag{20}$$

ρ_i is a small, positive cost for running controller c_i, and h_i^k is the habituation variable that modulates the level of reward based on modeling progress [Eq. (18)].

Equation (19) provides an aggregate reward value based on all controllers that quiesce at a given time. In the remainder of this chapter, we will briefly overview how this intrinsic reward function can guide a robot to learn generalizable control skills—called *schema*—and then use these schema to estimate affordance models that capture the contexts in which they apply.

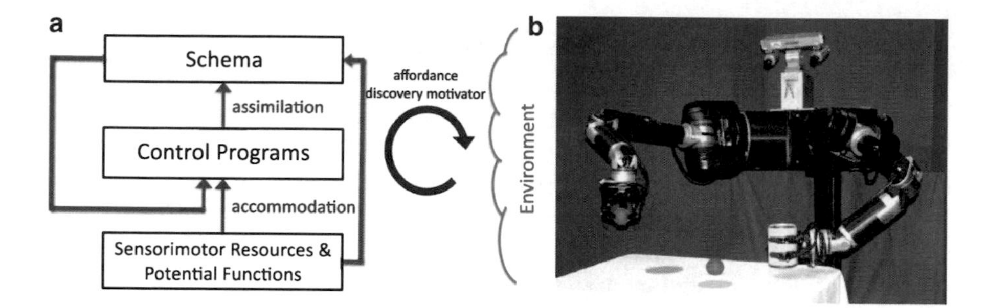

Fig. 2 (**a**) The process of schema learning. (**b**) The bimanual robot "Dexter"

5 Intrinsically Motivated Control Knowledge

Generalizable skills in the control basis are assembled from the bottom-up as the robot finds policies for discovering new affordances and generalized from the top-down as the robot learns how these policies apply in different contexts. This approach is consistent with Piaget's notions of *accommodation*, in which an organism finds new ways to "mold" itself to its environment as new situations present themselves, and *assimilation*, in which resulting knowledge structures are fit to new situations with robust contingency plans (Piaget 1952). Following Piaget, we call a generalized skill in the proposed framework, a *schema*.

Figure 2a shows an overview of the schema learning procedure. Through a process of accommodation, a robot acquires control basis programs that lead to the control of environmental signals. Through a process of assimilation, the robot discovers how to re-parameterize these programs with different sensory or motor resources to be able to apply them to different contexts. The resulting generalized control programs—or schema—can be reused hierarchically in new phases of accommodation to support cumulative skill acquisition. Both the accommodation and the assimilation processes are governed by the robot's intrinsic drive for affordance discovery introduced in Sect. 4.

5.1 Skill Accommodation

In each phase of accommodation, a robot uses intrinsically motivated reinforcement learning to acquire new programs for controlling environmental stimuli [via Eq. (19)]. As robot programmers, we have the ability to control the particular context in which these programs are learned, or instead to allow the robot to explore options through stochastic sampling processes in more open-ended situations. If we choose to control the context, we can structure the environment to teach the robot about particular control affordances that we believe are important (e.g., graspability, stackability). This structure might arise from presenting certain objects in the robot's workspace or by limiting the control combinations $\langle \phi \in \Phi, \sigma \subseteq \Sigma, \tau \subseteq T \rangle$ we allow the robot to explore at any given time.

5.1.1 Example Programs Acquired by Accommodation

A number of control programs were taught to Dexter (Fig. 2b) in structured phases of accommodation. Dexter has a two degree of freedom pan/tilt head equipped with two Sony color cameras and two 7-DOF whole-arm manipulators (Barrett Technologies, Cambridge, MA). Each WAM is equipped with a 3-finger Barrett Hand with a F/T load cell on each fingertip. Each hand has four degrees of freedom (one for each finger and one for the spread angle between two of these fingers).

Each program is modeled as a distinct Markov decision process (MDP) with a state and action set obtained from a set of control basis actions as described in Sect. 3. Policies in each of these MDPs were learned using the Q-Learning update rule and the intrinsic reward function in Eq. (19) in no more than 25 learning episodes each. For a more complete description of each of these programs and the contexts in which they were learned, the interested reader is directed toward (Hart 2009a).

SearchTrack is a program, similar to the example provided in Sect. 3.2.1, that uses Dexter's pan/tilt head to find and track highly saturated visual blobs using a policy of multi-objective control laws.

ReachTouch is a program Dexter learned that hierarchically combines SEARCH-TRACK with other reaching and force tracking controllers in order to assert "touchability" affordances with the robot's right hand. REACHTOUCH allows Dexter to physically engage highly saturated objects that are not physically presented to it. Because of the geometric structure of Dexter's hand, simultaneously controlling the contact forces between all three of the robot's fingertips and an object often forms a primitive robotic analog of the palmar grasp reflex in humans. In such a way, this formulation demonstrates how an embodied system's morphology can be exploited to accomplish behavior.

BimanualTouch is a program that the robot learned to get more touchability affordances from small, graspable objects. It provides a strategy for Dexter to pick up an object with one hand (using REACHTOUCH) and bring it into contact with the other hand at a location that is well conditioned kinematically. This behavior is important for bimanual grasps and actions that transfer objects between hands.

VisualInspect is a program that Dexter acquired for picking up an object and inspecting it for additional visual tracking affordances that are initially unavailable due to inadequate sensing geometry. It too uses REACHTOUCH hierarchically. Such a program is useful for close inspection of objects and can be used for purposes of high-fidelity classification.

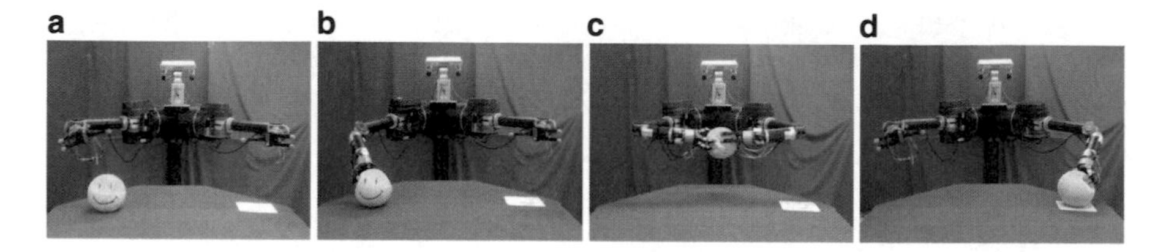

Fig. 3 Dexter executing PICKANDPLACE. In frame (**a**), the (*light-colored*) goal is placed far to the robot's left, while the object is on its right. Frames (**b**) and (**c**) show the robot using REACHTOUCH and BIMANUALTOUCH to pick up the object and pass it between its hands so that it can be brought to the distant goal location (**d**)

PickAndPlace allows Dexter to pick up one object and bring it into contact with another, regulating the resulting interaction forces that occur. It uses either REACHTOUCH or BIMANUALTOUCH as appropriate to allow the robot to transport objects to areas within its full workspace (as seen in Fig. 3).

These control programs represent a set of skills that the robot learned in successive stages of accommodation. Combinations of these control programs provide a number of strategies that Dexter can use to discover visual and tactile control affordances in its environment. Furthermore, they represent a cumulative skill set that applies to increasingly complex contexts and that can provide support for tasks such as sorting, classification, or inspection.

5.2 *Skill Assimilation*

Phases of accommodation generate new skills in restricted environmental contexts and with restricted control options. Restricting the explorable options is an appropriate way for a human teacher to bootstrap intrinsically motivated behavior.It is necessary, however, to also consider how the robot can generalize the control programs it learns in these restricted contexts to more complex situations through additional phases of assimilation. Assimilation relies on finding alternative sensor and effector resources for control programs that can be used to achieve reward in contexts that differ from the training context. Such a situation can occur when a new object is introduced that shares common salient attributes with other objects in the training context, but differs in other ways. For example, a new object can vary in color, scale, mass, position, and/or velocity in a manner that does not affect the performance of the skill if contingencies are discovered that re-parameterize the skill with appropriate sensor and/or effect or resources for this case.

Assimilation is accomplished in the control basis by factoring existing control programs into *declarative* and *procedural* components (Hart et al. 2008a). The declarative component provides an abstraction of the control policy learned in the accommodation phase so that it can be re-parameterized with alternative sensory and motor resources and thus be used in different run-time contexts. If $c = \phi|_{\tau}^{\sigma}$ is a specific controller, let $a = \phi|_{*}^{*}$ be an abstract controller that accepts alternative

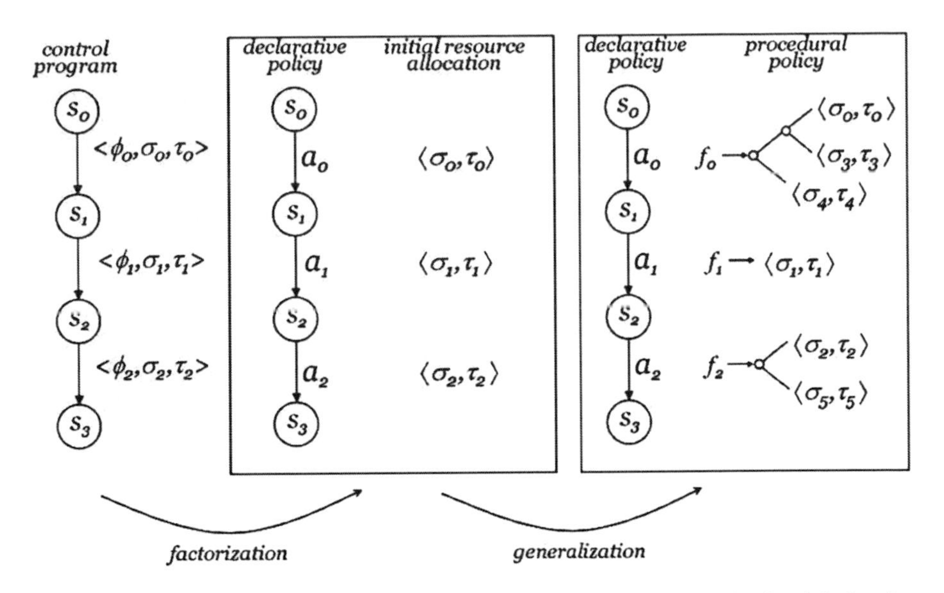

Fig. 4 Sensorimotor programs in the control basis can be factored into procedural and declarative components and generalized to new environmental contexts $\mathbf{f}_i \in \mathcal{F}$

sensorimotor resource allocations from Σ and $\mathcal{T}$ (where $*$ is the "wildcard" operator). The procedural component provides the strategy for parameterizing the entire declarative policy with particular sensory and motor resources based on the context in order to maximize the likelihood of receiving reward. The control knowledge consisting of both the declarative and procedural policies for controlling environmental stimuli in multiple contexts is what we call a control basis schema.

Figure 4 illustrates how control basis programs are generalized. Here, a policy is first learned in an accommodation phase using specific sensory and motor signals from Σ and $\mathcal{T}$ and in a particular environmental context. The policy is then factored into declarative (abstract) and procedural components. The abstract actions are then reallocated based on the run-time environmental contexts $\mathbf{f} \in \mathcal{F}$ in order to preserve the original transition structure of the learned policy (Hart et al. 2008a). For example, a re-parameterized SEARCHTRACK—a program learned to find and track highly saturated visual blobs by moving the robot's pan/tilt head—can be assimilated to find and track visual blobs of different hue, saturation, or intensity values, or to find and maintain contact with objects by moving the robot's arm, hand, and fingers (Hart 2009a).

5.2.1 Example: ReachTouch Generalization

In Sect. 5.1.1, we introduced the REACHTOUCH program Dexter acquired in an accommodation phase to grab highly saturated objects with its right hand. Following the construction of this program and its decomposition into declarative and procedural components, the robot assimilated conditions that recommend different resource allocations based on characteristics of the object attended to.

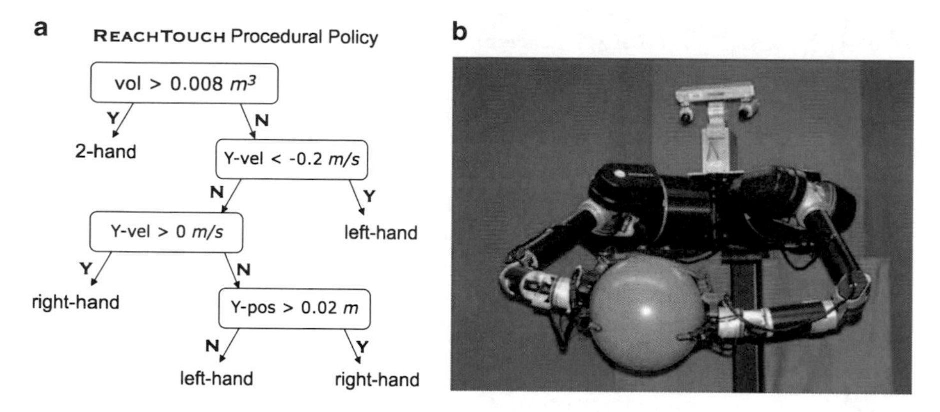

Fig. 5 The learned procedural policy (**a**) for allocating arms to reach behavior based on object volume, position, and velocity. The y-axis of the robot's coordinate frame is lateral to the robot. In frame (**b**), two arms are allocated to a grasping task based on object volume

Specifically, the robot learned a procedural policy for selecting motor synergies in $\mathcal{T}$ (i.e., the appropriate hand/arm) to use to grab objects based on their position, velocity, and size. This policy was learned using the C4.5 algorithm (Quinlan 1993) to classify the boundary regions within the feature vector $\mathbf{f} = [\mathbf{x}, \dot{\mathbf{x}}, V]$, where $\mathbf{x}$ is the Cartesian position of the object in the robot's coordinate system, $\dot{\mathbf{x}}$ is the object's velocity, and V is its observed spatial volume. Procedural policy decisions concerning which motor synergy to choose are made to preserve the state/action transition structure of ReachTouch that leads to the accumulation of intrinsic reward.

Figure 5 shows the procedural policy the robot learned after 50 learning trials. If the object has appreciable volume, a 2-handed reach is selected. In general, smaller stationary objects recommend using the hand closest to the object or that anticipates the object's movement. This policy reflects clear common sense knowledge about handedness, scale, and velocity concerning one- and two-hand ReachTouch options.

Once procedural strategies for a schema are learned, any other program that employs that schema automatically inherits this new knowledge. For example, once contingencies for handedness and locale are acquired by the ReachTouch schema, the BimanualTouch, VisualInspect, and PickAndPlace schema (which each use ReachTouch to grab objects) can exploit those contingencies as well to increase their applicability to different contexts.

5.3 *Affordance Modeling*

When learning a control policy during phases of accommodation or assimilation, it is sufficient only that *some* positive reward is achieved when a rewarding controller runs till quiescence. We now examine how the robot can exploit *how much* reward is

Algorithm 1 MODELAFFORDANCES($\mathcal{A}$)

1: initialize all initial expected returns (for each action) to zero.
2: **repeat**
3:     choose $a \in \mathcal{A}$ with highest expected reward
4:     execute a
5:     observe context $\mathbf{f}$
6:     **if** a leads to reward by Eq. (19) **then**
7:         update $Pr(p_i = 1|\mathbf{f})$, h_i for each controller $c_i \in \mathcal{C}_t$ if $p_i = 1$
8:     **end if**
9:     update expected reward for each $a \in \mathcal{A}$
10: **until** $\forall\,(c_i \in \mathcal{C}_t)\,(h_i \leq 0)$

received to focus on actions that provide the most "interesting" knowledge about the world. As discussed in Sect. 4.3, the proposed intrinsic reward function modulates the amount of reward returned based on a habituation factor h (18). This factor provides a simple measure of the expected information gain of taking actions in the current context. Therefore, in the absence of an explicit task, the robot can choose the most informative action among multiple options.

One simple formulation of this process is for a robot to use its schema to explore the visual and tactile affordances related to a visual cue it samples from its environment. For example, if Dexter observes a blue object, it will instantiate a version of SEARCHTRACK that tries to find and track blue visual cues and a version of REACHTOUCH that tries to reach out and grab that cue. With an action set $\mathcal{A}$ defined by a robot's set of schema, the n-armed bandit formalization (Berry and Fristedt 1985) can be used for selecting which of its possible n actions is probabilistically likely to lead to the most expected intrinsic reward. The choice of action will depend on the current level of habituation of the control affordances that each schema is likely to uncover.

The method for choosing actions and building affordance models is illustrated by the MODELAFFORDANCES() procedure (Algorithm 1). This procedure simply chooses which action to execute based on its likely expected reward. When running an action results in the quiescence of environmental tracking controllers $c_i \in \mathcal{C}_t$, the robot can update its corresponding control affordance models $Pr(p_i = 1|\mathbf{f})$ and habituation metrics, h_i, based on the environmental context $\mathbf{f}$. This procedure continues until all models have habituated.

5.3.1 Example: Building Control Affordance Models

We provided training episodes for Dexter to build control affordance models with respect to each of the objects seen in the top row of Fig. 6. For simplicity, we focused only on allowing the robot to learn affordances based on the hue(s), location, and shape properties of these objects.

Specifically, three learning episodes were performed in which the robot first sampled the ith color blob feature with centroid $\boldsymbol{\gamma}_i^{\text{hue},m} \in \Sigma$ from one of ten

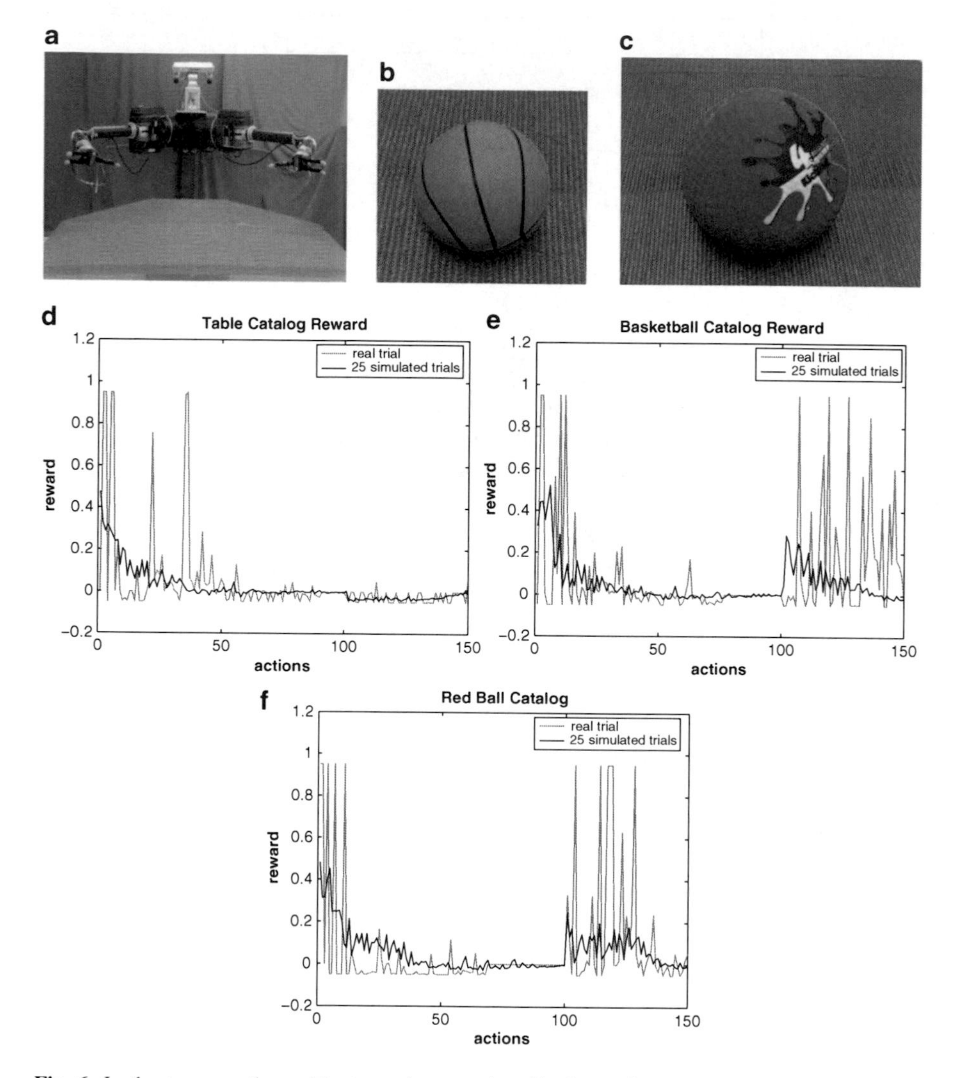

Fig. 6 In the *top row*, three objects used to test the affordance discovery algorithm with Dexter are shown: (**a**) a large green table, (**b**) a small basketball, and (**c**) a red ball with smaller colored features on it. Plots (**d**)–(**f**) show the reward per action over a sequence of 150 actions for the real and simulated trials. The addition of the PICKANDPLACE option after 100 actions shows an increase in activity for the two objects that afford that behavior

discretized channels of hue space ($m \in [1, 10]$). In each of these episodes, the sampled blob corresponded to one of three objects in Fig. 6. For the first 100 actions of each episode, the robot explored an action set $\mathcal{A}$ = {NOOP, SEARCHTRACK, REACHTOUCH, BIMANUALTOUCH, VISUALINSPECT} using the MODELAFFORDANCES($\mathcal{A}$) procedure. This action set consists of the specified schema parameterized by the sampled hue feature and a zero-cost NOOP action that does nothing. All other controllers executed by a schema were set to have a fixed cost of $\rho = 0.05$. As the robot performs each episode and gathers information about the contexts that lead to the discovery of control affordances, corresponding control affordance models were constructed based on the location and the scale of the visual cue (both on the image plane or in Cartesian space).

After 100 actions were performed, a PICKANDPLACE schema was added to the action set, where the sampled visual feature was designated as the PICK goal. The robot explored this augmented action set for an additional 50 actions. This "late addition" of a new action choice demonstrates how new skills, as they are acquired, provide new possibilities for intrinsic reward in areas of the environment (i.e., objects) that had previously habituated. After a single trial of 150 training actions for each of these episodes, 25 additional simulated trials were performed using the transition dynamics and estimated affordance models learned on the robot to generate simulated samples.

Figure 6d–f shows the reward plots for each of the three objects during both the real robot trials (shown in gray) and the simulated trials (shown in black). These plots quantitatively illustrate the robot's growing competency in modeling the affordances in its environment. For all three objects, the trial on the real robot shows a number of large spikes in reward during the early part of the first stage of learning where all of the affordances are "interesting." These spikes correspond to situations in which the robot chooses to run schemas that result in significant new information. All three objects afford a number of visual and tactile affordances discoverable through the robot's set of schema. In all cases, however, the reward tends toward 0 as the control affordance models habituate, resulting in only a negligible amount after about 50 actions. After the introduction of the PICKANDPLACE schema at action 100, however, additional activity can be observed for the orange and red balls (but not for the table, as the robot cannot pick that object up and deliver it to another location). The plots that average the reward received per action over 25 (simulated) trials show this habituation more clearly.

As a robot explores its environment, it can start collecting likely co-occurring collections of affordances together into structures called *catalogs*. For example, the affordances pertaining to the green table in the previous example indicate that the table affords TRACK and TOUCH, but not PLACE. The basketball, however, also affords PLACE because it is small enough to be picked up by the robot. A full discussion concerning catalogs is beyond the scope of this chapter as it is ongoing research (cf., Hart 2009a), but it provides an area of interesting future consideration as the robot uses the proposed intrinsic reward function to learn new skills and build new models.

6 Discussion

In this chapter we have demonstrated how a single, fixed intrinsic reward function for control affordance discovery can guide a robot to acquire generalizable control programs (called *schema*) that it can then use to intelligently model the conditions in which these schema apply. Our approach contributes to the intrinsic motivation literature by providing a mechanism to guide both autonomous skill development and the acquisition of knowledge about the world. The proposed reward function, according to the taxonomy of Oudeyer and Kaplan (2007), is both competence-based—in that it can guide a robot to learn new skills and generalizations of those skills—and knowledge based—in that it can guide a robot to focus on the affordances that provide the most expected information gain when explored.

There are many areas of consideration to pursue in future work both concerning the control basis framework itself and the intrinsic reward function:

- The control basis is designed to provide a combinatoric means of creating and exploring control programs. We have not examined, however, how it can improve the dynamic performance of those control programs as they interact with the world. Future work concerns methods for optimizing the dynamics of interactions by refining control basis policies.
- In this chapter we examined three situations in which the proposed intrinsic reward function can build knowledge: skill acquisition, skill generalization, and world modeling. In the examples, each of these phases of learning was performed independently to illustrate the power of the proposed function. It would be interesting, however, to examine how these three phases could occur simultaneously in an integrated framework that relies less on the human programmer to structure the run-time context and more on open-ended autonomous exploration.
- Many of the illustrative examples in this chapter relied on modeling the environmental context $\mathbf{f} \in \mathcal{F}$ in order to make salient information conspicuous to the robot. In these examples, this vector was chosen by the human programmer. In general, however, this will not be feasible and will require autonomous methods for feature selection and dimensionality reduction. Methods for reducing the set of possible sensory signals to those that are relevant for the task at hand are an interesting area of consideration.
- Finally, the formulation of affordance models as multivariate Gaussian distributions was a choice made for simplicity, not generality. In situations where the variation in the modeled data is not Gaussian, this choice would be insufficient. A more general representation for modeling these distributions is currently under investigation.

References

Barto, A., Singh, S, Chentanez, N.: Intrinsically motivated learning of hierarchical collections of skills. In: Proceedings of the International Conference on Development and Learning (ICDL), La Jolla, CA, USA October (2004)

Berry, D.A., Fristedt, B.: Bandit problems: Sequential allocation of experiments. In: Monographs on Statistics and Applied Probability, vol. viii+275. Chapman & Hall, London (1985)

Chemero, A.: An outline of a theory of affordances. Ecol. Psychol. **15**(3), 181–195 (2003)

Connolly, C., Grupen, R.: Nonholonomic path planning using harmonic functions. Technical Report 94-50, University of Massachusetts, Amherst (1994)

Detry, R., Popovic, M., Touati, Y., Baseski, E., Krüger, N, Piater, J.: Autonomous learning of object-specific grasp affordance densities. In: ICRA 2009 Workshop Approaches to Sensorimotor Learning on Humanoid Robots, Kobe, Japan (2009)

Festinger, L.: A Theory of Cognitive Dissonance. Evanston, Row, Peterson (1957)

Fitzpatrick, P., Metta, G., Natale, L., Rao, S., Sandini, G.: Learning about objects through action: Initial steps towards artificial cognition. In: IEEE International Conference on Robotics and Automation, Taipei, Taiwan (2003)

Gibson, J.J.: The theory of affordances. In: Perceiving, Acting and Knowing: Toward an Ecological Psychology, pp. 67–82. Lawrence Erlbaum Associates, Hillsdale (1977)

Harlow, H.: Learning and satiation of response in intrinsically motivated complex puzzle performances by monkeys. J. Comp. Psychol. Psychol. **43**, 289–294 (1950)

Hart, S.: The Development of Hierarchical Knowledge in Robot Systems. Ph.D. Thesis, Department of Computer Science, University of Massachusetts, Amherst (2009a)

Hart, S.: An intrinsic reward for affordance exploration. In: Proceedings of the 8th IEEE International Conference on Development and Learning (ICDL), Shanghai, China (2009b)

Hart, S., Grupen, R.: Natural task decomposition with intrinsic potential fields. In: Proceedings of the 2007 International Conference on Intelligent Robots and Systems (IROS), San Diego, CA (2007)

Hart, S., Grupen, R.: Learning generalizable control programs. IEEE Trans. Auton. Mental Dev. **3**(3), 216–231 (2011)

Hart, S., Sen, S., Grupen, R.: Generalization and transfer in robot control. In: 8th International Conference on Epigenetic Robotics (Epirob08), University of Sussex, Brighton, UK (2008a)

Hart, S., Sen, S., Grupen, R.: Intrinsically motivated hierarchical manipulation. In: Proceedings of the 2008 IEEE Conference on Robots and Automation (ICRA), Pasadena, CA (2008b)

Herrmann, J., Pawelzik, K., Geisel, T.: Learning predictive representations. Neurocomputing **32–33**, 785–791 (2000)

Huang, X., Weng, J.: Novelty and reinforcement learning in the value system of developmental robots. In: Proceedings of the 2nd International Workshop on Epigenetic Robotics: Modeling Cognitive Development in Robotic Systems. Edinburgh, Scotland (2002)

Huber, M., Grupen, R.: A hybrid discrete dynamic systems approach to robot control. Technical Report 96-43, Department of Computer Science, University of Massachusetts Amherst, Amherst (1996)

Huber, M., MacDonald, W, Grupen, R.: A control basis for multilegged walking. In: Proceedings of the Conference on Robotics and Automation. IEEE, Minneapolis, MN, USA (1996)

Hull, C.: Principles of Behavior: An Introduction to Behavior Theory. Appleton-Century-Croft, New York (1943)

Hunt, H.: Intrinsic motivation and its role in psychological development. Nebraska Symp. Motiv. **13**, 189–282 (1965)

Kagan, J.: Motives and development. J. Pers. Soc. Psychol. **22**, 51–66 (1972)

Koditschek, D., Rimon, E.: Robot navigation functions on manifolds with boundary. Adv. Appl. Math. **11**(4), 412–442 (1990)

Kraft, D., Pugeault, N., Baseski, E., Popović, M., Kragic, D., Kalkan, S., Wörgötter, F, Krüger, N.: Birth of the object: Detection of objectness and extraction of shape through object action complexes. In: Proceedings of the 2008 International Conference on Cognitive Systems, Karlsruhe, DE (2008)

Krüger, N., Geib, C., Piater, J., Petrick, R., Steedman, M., Wörgötter, F., Ude, A., Asfour, T., Kraft, D., Omrcen, D., Agostini, A, Dillmann, R.: Object-action complexes: Grounded abstractions of sensori-motor processes. Robot. Auton. Syst. **59**(10), 740–757 (2011)

Krüger, N., Piater, J., Wörgötter, F., Geib, C., Petrick, R., Steedman, M., Ude, A., Asfour, T., Kraft, D., Omrcen, D., Hommel, B., Agostino, A., Kragic, D., Eklundh, J., Kruger, V, Dillmann, R.: A formal definition of object action complexes and examples at different levels of the process hierarchy. http://www.paco-plus.org (2009)

Modayil, J., Kupiers, B.: Autonomous development of a grounded object ontology by a learning robot. In: Proceedings of the Twenty-Second Conference on Artificial Intelligence (AAAI-07), Vancouver, British Columbia (2007)
Montgomery, K.: The role of exploratory drive in learning. J. Comp. Psychol. Psychol. **47**, 60–64 (1954)
Nakamura, Y.: Advanced Robotics: Redundancy and Optimization. Addison-Wesley, Reading (1991)
Oudeyer, P., Kaplan, F.: What is intrinsic motivation? a typology of computational approaches. Front. Neurorobot. **1**(2) (2007)
Oudeyer, P., Kaplan, F, Hafner, V.V.: Intrinsic motivation systems for autonomous mental development. IEEE Trans. Evol. Comput. **11**, 265–286 (2007)
Piaget, J.: The Origins of Intelligence in Childhood. International Universities Press, New York (1952)
Platt, R., Fagg, A.H, Grupen, R.A.: Null space grasp control: Theory and experiments. IEEE Trans. Robot. Autom. **26**, 282–295 (2010)
Quinlan, J.: C4.5: Programs for Machine Learning. Morgan Kaufmann, San Mateo (1993)
Rimon, E., Koditschek, D.: Exact robot navigation using artificial potential functions. IEEE Trans. Robot. Autom. **8**(5), 501–518 (1992)
Şahin, E., Çakmak, M., Doğar, M., Uğur, E, Üçoluk, G.: To afford or not to afford: A formalization of affordances toward affordance-based robot control. Adap. Behav. **4**(15), 447–472 (2007)
Schmidhuber, J.: Adaptive curiosity and adaptive confidence. Technical Report FKI-149-91, Institut fur Informatik, Technische Universitat Munchen (1991)
Stoytchev, A.: Toward learning the binding affordances of objects: A behavior-grounded approach. In: Proceedings of the AAAI Spring Symposium on Developmental Robotics. Stanford University, Stanford, CA (2005)
Sutton, R., Barto, A.: Reinforcement Learning. MIT, Cambridge (1998)
Uğur, E., Oztop, E, Şahin, E.: Learning object affordances for planning. In: ICRA 2009 Workshop Approaches to Sensorimotor Learning on Humanoid Robots, Kobe, Japan (2009)

Part V
Mechanisms Complementary to Intrinsic Motivations

Intrinsically Motivated Learning of Real-World Sensorimotor Skills with Developmental Constraints

Pierre-Yves Oudeyer, Adrien Baranes, and Frédéric Kaplan

Abstract Open-ended exploration and learning in the real world is a major challenge of developmental robotics. Three properties of real-world sensorimotor spaces provide important conceptual and technical challenges: unlearnability, high dimensionality, and unboundedness. In this chapter, we argue that exploration in such spaces needs to be constrained and guided by several combined developmental mechanisms. While intrinsic motivation, that is, curiosity-driven learning, is a key mechanism to address this challenge, it has to be complemented and integrated with other developmental constraints, in particular: sensorimotor primitives and embodiment, task space representations, maturational processes (i.e., adaptive changes of the embodied sensorimotor apparatus), and social guidance. We illustrate and discuss the potential of such an integration of developmental mechanisms in several robot learning experiments.

A central aim of developmental robotics is to study the developmental mechanisms that allow lifelong and open-ended learning of new skills and new knowledge in robots and animals (Asada et al. 2009; Lungarella et al. 2003; Weng et al. 2001). Strongly rooted in theories of human and animal development, embodied computational models are built both to explore how one could build more versatile and adaptive robots, as in the work presented in this chapter, and to explore new understandings of biological development (Oudeyer 2010).

P.-Y. Oudeyer (✉) · A. Baranes
INRIA Bordeaux, France
e-mail: pierre-yves.oudeyer@inria.fr

F. Kaplan
EPFL-CRAFT, Lausanne, Switzerland

G. Baldassarre and M. Mirolli (eds.), *Intrinsically Motivated Learning in Natural and Artificial Systems*, DOI 10.1007/978-3-642-32375-1_13,

Building machines capable of open-ended learning in the real world poses many difficult challenges. One of them is exploration, which is the central topic of this chapter. In order to be able to learn cumulatively an open-ended repertoire of skills, developmental robots, like animal babies and human infants, shall be equipped with task-independent mechanisms which push them to explore new activities and new situations. However, a major problem is that the continuous sensorimotor space of a typical robot, including its own body as well as all the potential interactions with the open-ended surrounding physical and social environment, is extremely large and high dimensional. The set of skills that can potentially be learnt is actually infinite. Yet, within a lifetime, only a small subset of them can be practiced and learnt. Thus, the central question: How to explore and what to learn? And with this question comes an equally important question: What *not* to explore and what *not* to learn? Clearly, exploring randomly and/or trying to learn all possible sensorimotor skills will fail. Exploration strategies, mechanisms, and constraints are needed and appear in two broad interacting families in animals and humans: internally guided exploration and socially guided exploration. Within the large diversity of associated mechanisms, as we will illustrate in this chapter, intrinsic motivation, a peculiar example of internal mechanism for guiding exploration, has drawn a lot of attention in the recent years, especially when related to the issue of open-ended cumulative learning of skills as shown by other chapters in this book (Barto 2012; Dayan 2012; Mirolli and Baldassarre 2012; Redgrave et al. 2012; Schlesinger 2012; Schmidhuber 2012).

Intrinsic motivation was identified in humans and animals as the set of processes which push organisms to spontaneously explore their environment even when their basic needs such as food or water are satisfied (Berlyne 1960; Deci and Ryan 1985; White 1959). It is related to curiosity-driven learning and exploration, but is actually broader since it applies, for example, to the processes that push us to persist in trying to solve puzzles or improve our sport skills when not driven by extrinsic motivations such as the search for social status or money. A very large body of theories of intrinsic motivation, and its interaction with extrinsic motivation, has flourished in psychology and educational sciences at least since the middle of the twentieth century (Ryan and Deci 2000). Many of them have consisted in trying to understand which features of given activities could make them intrinsically motivating or "interesting" for a particular person at a particular moment of time. In this context, "interestingness" was proposed to be understood as related to concepts such as novelty (Hull 1943; Montgomery 1954), reduction of cognitive dissonances (Festinger 1957; Kagan 1972), optimal incongruity (Berlyne 1960; Hunt 1965), effectance and personal causation (De Charms 1968; White 1959), or optimal challenge (Csikszentmihalyi 1996).

Following those ideas, either a priori or a posteriori, many computational systems were built to formalize, implement, and evaluate intrinsically motivated exploration and learning, also referred as curiosity-driven machine learning or active learning (Lopes and Oudeyer 2010). These models came from various fields such as statistics and "optimal experiment design" (e.g., Fedorov 1972), active learning (e.g., Angluin 1988; Castro and Novak 2008; Chaloner and Verdinelli

1995; Cohn et al. 1994; Thrun 1992, reinforcement learning (e.g., Barto et al. 2004; Brafman and Tennenholtz 2001; Schmidhuber 1991; Sutton 1990; Szita and Lorincz 2008), computational neuroscience (e.g., Dayan and Belleine 2002; Doya 2002), and developmental robotics (e.g., Baldassarre and Mirolli 2012; Baranes and Oudeyer 2009; Blank et al. 2002; Hart and Grupen 2008; Huang and Weng 2002; Merrick 2012; Oudeyer and Kaplan 2007; Oudeyer et al. 2007, Schembri et al. 2007a; Schmidhuber 2006, 2010). Correspondingly, many formal measures of "interestingness," either heuristics or optimal regarding some criteria—and associated algorithms to compute them—were devised, including principles such as the maximization of prediction error (Meyer and Wilson 1991; Thrun 1992), the local density of already queried/sampled points (Whitehead 1991), the maximization of the decrease of the global model variance (Cohn et al. 1996), or maximal uncertainty of the model (Thrun and Moller 1992), among others. Those principles and algorithms were then integrated in various framings, a particularly interesting one being intrinsically motivated reinforcement learning, allowing to approach sequential decision problems in a unified approach (e.g., Barto et al. 2004; Mirolli and Baldassarre 2012; Schmidhuber 1991) and see (Dayan 2012; Kakade and Dayan 2002; Sutton 1990) for a related approach using exploration bonuses.

In spite of this diversity of techniques, many of these computational approaches where not designed initially for developmental learning and make assumptions that are incompatible with their use for learning in real developmental robots. Indeed, a combination of the following assumptions, which do not hold for a developmental robot, is often made for active exploration models:

- **Assumption 1.** It is possible to learn a model of the complete world/space within the lifetime of the learning agent.
- **Assumption 2.** The world is learnable everywhere.
- **Assumption 3.** The noise is homogeneous.

These assumptions are very useful and relevant when the goal is to have a machine learn a predictive or control model of a whole bounded relatively small domain (e.g., sensorimotor space) and when it is yet very expensive to make one single measure/experiment. Examples include the control of automatic biological or chemical experiments (Faller et al. 2003; Kumar et al. 2010) or learning to visually recognize a finite set of visual categories (Tong and Chang 2001). The associated techniques, for example, those based on principles such as "search for maximal novelty or uncertainty," allow the learner to efficiently minimize the number of necessary experiments to perform in order to acquire a certain level of knowledge or a certain level of competence for controlling the given domain.

Furthermore, the models designed explicitly in a developmental learning framing were often elaborated and experimented in simple simulated worlds, even sometimes in discrete grid worlds, which allowed researchers to perform easily systematic experiments but introduced a bias on the properties of sensorimotor spaces. As a consequence, many of these models consisted in mechanisms that either also implicitly made the assumptions described in the previous paragraph or could not (or were not shown in practice) to scale to real-world high-dimensional robot spaces.

Yet, the challenges of exploration and developmental learning become very different as soon as one uses real high-dimensional redundant bodies, with continuous sensorimotor channels, and an open-ended unbounded environment. Real sensorimotor spaces introduce three fundamental properties to which exploration and learning mechanisms should be robust:

- *Unlearnability*: There are very large regions of sensorimotor spaces for which predictive or control models cannot be learnt. Some of these regions of the sensorimotor space are definitively unlearnable, such as, the relations between body movement and cloud movements (one cannot learn to control the displacement of clouds with one's own body actions) or the relation between the color of a cat and the color of the next car passing in the road (a developmental robot shall not be "spoon fed" with the adequate causal groupings of variables he may observe but rather shall discover by itself which are the sensible groupings). Some other regions of the sensorimotor space are unlearnable at a given moment of time/development, but may become learnable later on. For example, trying to play tennis is unlearnable for a baby who did not even learn to grasp objects yet, but it becomes learnable once he is a bit older and has acquired a variety of basic skills that he can reuse for learning tennis.
- *High dimensionality*: A human child has hundreds of muscles and hundreds of thousands of sensors, as well as a brain able to generate new representational spaces based on those primitive sensorimotor channels, that are used by the organism to interact with novel objects, activities, situations, or persons. Given this apparatus, even single specific skills such as hand–eye coordination or locomotion involve continuous sensorimotor spaces of very high low-level dimensions. Furthermore, action and perception consist in manipulating dynamic sequences within those high-dimensional spaces, generating a combinatorial explosion for exploration. As explained below, this raises the well-known problem of the curse-of-dimensionality (Bishop 1995), which needs to be addressed even for single specific skill learning involving the learning of forward and inverse models given a control space and a task space (Nguyen-Tuong and Peters 2011; Sigaud et al. 2011);
- *Unboundedness*: Even if the learning organism would have a sort of "oracle" saying what is learnable and what is not at a given moment of time, real sensorimotor spaces would still have the property of unboundedness: The set of learnable predictive models and/or skills is infinite and thus much larger than what can be practiced and learnt within a lifetime. Just imagine a one-year-old baby who is trying to explore and learn how to crawl, touch, grasp, and observe objects from various manners. First of all, with a given object in a given room, say, for example, a book, there is a very large amount of both knowledge and skills, of approximately equal interest for any measure of interestingness, to be learnt, for example, learning to throw the book in various boxes in the room, at various lengths, with a various number of flips, with a final position

on various sides, and using various parts of the body (hands, shoulders, head, legs, ...); learning to predict the sequence of letters and drawings in it; learning to see what kind of noise it makes when torn up at various places with various strengths, hit on various objects; learning how it tastes; learning how it can fly out of the window; and learning how individual pages fly when folded in various manners, ... Now, imagine what the same child may learn with all the other toys and objects in the room, then with all the toys in the house and in the one of neighbors. As it can walk, of course the child could learn to discover the map of his garden and of all the places he could crawl to. Even with no increase of complexity, the child could basically always find something to learn. Actually, this would even apply if there would be no objects, no house, and no gardens around the child: The set of skills he could learn to do with its sole own body, conceptualized as an "object/tool" to be discovered and learnt, is already unbounded in many respects. And even if obviously there are some cognitive and physical bounds on what he can learn (e.g., bounds on the possible speeds one can run at), those bounds are initially unknown to the learner (e.g., the child initially does not know that it is impossible to run over a certain speed; thus, he will need mechanisms to discover this and avoid spending its life trying to reach speeds that are not physically possible), and this is part of what is here called the challenge of unboundedness.

Considering some particular aspects of those challenging properties, in particular, related to unlearnability, some specific computational models of "interestingness" and intrinsically motivated exploration were elaborated. In particular, measures of interestingness based on the *derivative* of the evolution of performances of acquired knowledge or skills, such as maximal increase in prediction errors, also called "learning progress" (Oudeyer et al. 2007; Schmidhuber 1991), maximal compression progress (Schmidhuber 2006), or competence progress (Bakker and Schmidhuber 2004; Baranes and Oudeyer 2010a; Modayil et al. 2010; Stout and Barto 2010), were proposed. These measures resonate with some models in active learning, such as related to the principle of maximal decrease of model uncertainty (e.g., Cohn et al. 1996) but were sometimes transformed into heuristics which make them computationally reasonable in robotic applications (e.g., Oudeyer et al. 2007; Schmidhuber 1991), which is not necessarily the case for various theoretically optimal measures. These measures also resonate with psychological theories of intrinsic motivation based on the concept of "optimal level" (e.g., Berlyne 1960; Csikszentmihalyi 1996; White 1959; Wundt 1874), which state that the most interesting activities are those that are neither too easy nor too difficult, that is, are of the "right intermediate complexity." Yet, if modeled directly, "optimal level" approaches introduce the problem of what is "intermediate," that is, what is/are the corresponding threshold(s). Introducing the *derivative* of knowledge or competences, such as in prediction progress or competence progress-based intrinsic motivations, allows us to transform the problem into a maximization problem where no thresholds have to be defined and yet allowing learning agents to focus in practice on activities of intermediate complexity (e.g., Oudeyer et al. 2007).

A central property of the "interestingness" measures based on the increase of knowledge or competences is that they can allow a learning agent to discover which activities or predictive relations are unlearnable (and even rank the levels of learnability) and thus allow it to avoid spending too much time exploring these activities when coupled with an action-selection system such as in traditional reinforcement learning architectures and where the reward is directly encoded as the derivative of the performances of the learnt predictive models of the agent (Schmidhuber 1991). This has been demonstrated in various computational experiments (Baranes and Oudeyer 2009; Oudeyer and Kaplan 2006; Schmidhuber 1991, 2006). An interesting side effect of these measures, used in an intrinsic motivation system and in dynamical interaction with other brain modules as well as the body and the environment, is also the fact that it allows the self-organization of developmental stages of increasing complexity, sharing many similarities with both the structural and statistical properties of developmental trajectories in human infants (Oudeyer et al. 2007). Some models even suggest that the formation of higher-level skills such as language and imitation bootstrapping could self-organize through intrinsically motivated exploration of the sensorimotor space and with no language-specific biases (Oudeyer and Kaplan 2006).

Yet, those approaches to intrinsically motivated exploration and learning address only partially the challenge of unlearnability and leave largely unaddressed the challenges of high dimensionality and unboundedness in real robots. First of all, while efforts have been made to make these approaches work robustly in continuous sensorimotor spaces, computing meaningful associated measures of interest still requires a level of sampling density which makes those approaches become more and more inefficient as dimensionality grows. Even in bounded spaces, the processes for establishing measures of interestingness can be cast into a form of nonstationary regression problem, which as most regression problems in high dimension faces the curse-of-dimensionality (Bishop 2007). Thus, without additional mechanisms, like the ones we will describe in this chapter, the identification of unlearnable zones where no knowledge or competence progress happens is a process that becomes inefficient in high dimensions. The second limit of those approaches if used alone relates to unboundedness. Actually, whatever the measure of "interestingness," if it is only based in a way or another on the evaluation of performances of predictive models or of skills, one is faced with the following circular problem:

- Those measures were initially designed to efficiently guide exploration.
- Those measures need to be "measured/evaluated."
- By definition, they cannot be known in advance, and the "measure of interestingness" of a given sensorimotor subspace can only be obtained if at least explored/sampled a little bit.
- In order to obtain meaningful measures, those subspaces cannot be too large and are ideally quite local.
- In unbounded spaces, by definition, all localities (even at the maximal granularity allowing to obtain meaningful measures, which is anyway initially unknown to the learner) cannot be explored/sampled within a lifetime.

– Thus, one has to decide which subspaces to sample to evaluate their interestingness, that is, one has to find an efficient meta-exploration strategy, and we are basically back to our initial problem with an equivalent meta-problem. This meta-problem for evaluating interestingness requires a less dense local sampling of subspaces than the problem of actually learning mappings and skills within those subspaces, but as the space is unbounded and thus infinite, this theoretical decrease in required sampling density does not make the meta-problem more tractable from a computational complexity point of view.

As a matter of fact, this argument can also be made directly starting from the framing of intrinsically motivated exploration and learning within the reinforcement learning framework, that is, intrinsically motivated reinforcement learning. Indeed, in this framework, one reuses exactly the same machinery and architectures than in more traditional reinforcement learning, but instead of using a reward function which is specific to a given practical problem, one uses a measure of interestingness such as the ones discussed above (e.g., a reward is provided to the system when high prediction errors or high improvement of skills/options are observed). In such a way, the system can be made to learn how to achieve sequences of actions that will maximize the sum of future discounted rewards, for example, the sum of future discounted prediction errors or competence progress. But essentially, this defines a reinforcement learning problem which has the same structure as traditional reinforcement learning problems and especially similar to *difficult* traditional reinforcement learning problems given that the reward function will typically be highly nonstationary (indeed, prediction errors or competences and their evolution are both locally and globally nonstationary because of learning and of the external coupling of action selection and the reward function itself). Most importantly, as all reinforcement learning problems applied to unbounded/infinite state-spaces, exploration is a very hard problem (Sutton and Barto 1998): Even if the world would be discrete but with an unbounded/infinite number of states and associated number of options, how should exploration proceed? This problem is especially acute since when a "niche" of prediction or competence progress/errors has been well explored and learnt, it provides no more rewards and new sources of intrinsic rewards must permanently be found. And as intrinsically motivated reinforcement learning was formulated as a way to explore efficiently the world to acquire potentially general skills that may be reused later on for solving specific problems, we can indeed recast the meta-problem we just described as a meta-exploration problem.

Existing approaches of intrinsically motivated exploration can provide efficient mechanisms which allow a robot to decide whether it is interesting to *continue* or *stop* to explore a given sensorimotor subspace (or a local predictive model or a skill/option or simply a subset of states) which it has *already* began to explore a little bit. But due to unboundedness, strategies for exploration that may allow efficient organized acquisition of knowledge and skills need also mechanisms for answering to the question: What should *not* be explored *at all*?

The main argument that is put forward in this chapter is that complementary developmental mechanisms should be introduced in order to constrain

the growth of the size, dimensionality, and complexity of practically explorable spaces. Those mechanisms, that we call *developmental constraints* and are inspired by human development, should essentially allow the organism to automatically introduce self-boundings in the unbounded world (including their own body), such that intrinsically motivated exploration is allowed only within those bounds and then progressively releasing constraints and boundings to increase the volume of explorable sensorimotor spaces, that is, the diversity of explorable knowledge and skills.

Indeed, there is actually no mystery: Efficient unconstrained exploration, even intrinsically motivated, of unbounded infinite complex spaces, especially high-dimensional spaces, is impossible within a lifetime. Adaptive constraints and bounds have to be introduced, and ideally, these constraints should be as little ad hoc, as little hand-tuned, and as little task-specific as possible while compatible with the real world (i.e., a real body within the real physical environment).

The study of developmental constraints complementing or interacting with or even integrated within intrinsically motivated exploration and learning has been the central topic of the research outlined in this chapter. This is achieved with the long-term goal of elaborating architectures allowing a robot to acquire developmentally a repertoire of skills of increasing complexity over a significant duration (at least on the order of one month) and in large high-dimensional sensorimotor spaces in an unbounded environment (which contrasts strongly with the existing experiments with real robots lasting most often a few minutes, at best a few hours, and allowing the acquisition of a limited repertoire of skills). Most of these developmental constraints that we are investigating are strongly inspired by constraints on human infant development, from which we take the fundamental insight that *complex acquisition of novel skills in the real world necessitates to leverage sophisticated innate capabilities/constraints as well as social constraints and constraints provided by self-organization* that may unfold with time in interaction with the environment during the course of epigenesis. In the following, we will describe some of them and explain how they may facilitate, sometimes considerably, the exploration and acquisition of complex skills in real-world sensorimotor spaces, more precisely:

- *Parameterized dynamic sensori and motor primitives, also referred as muscle synergies, and their use in adequate embodiments:* Human infants do not learn to control their whole body movements "pixel by pixel." Rather, they are born with muscle synergies, that is, neurally embedded dynamical systems that generate parameterized coordinated movements, for example, CPGs. These motor primitives can considerably decrease the size of the explorable space and transform complex low-level action planning problems in higher-level low-dimensional dynamical system tuning problems. As we will show, their combination with intrinsic motivation is essential for the acquisition of dynamic motor skills in experiments like the Playground Experiment (Oudeyer and Kaplan 2006; Oudeyer et al. 2007). We will also discuss the fact that adequate body morphologies can in addition facilitate the self-organization of movement structures and thus be potentially leveraged by intrinsically motivated exploration and learning.

- *Task-level intrinsically motivated exploration:* While biological bodies are very high dimensional and redundant, motor tasks considered individually often consist in controlling effects in relatively low-dimensional task spaces. For example, while locomotion or reaching involves the coordination of a high number of muscular fibers, these activities aim at controlling only the three-dimensional trajectory of the body center of mass or of the hand. When human infants explore such sensorimotor spaces, they directly explore what they can do in the task space/space of effects (Bremner and Slater 2003; Rochat 1989) and rather spend their time exploring how to produce varieties of effects with sufficient means rather than exploring all means to achieve a single effect. Doing this, they exploit the low dimensionality of task spaces in combination with the high redundancy of their bodies. We will argue that similarly, intrinsic motivation in robots should operate directly in tasks spaces. We will illustrate the efficiency of this approach by presenting experiments using the SAGG-RIAC competence-based intrinsic motivation system, pushing the robot to actively explore and select goals in its task space.
- *Maturational constraints:* Human infants are not born with complete access to all their potential degrees of freedom. The neural system, partly through myelination, as well as the body, progressively grows, opening for control new muscle synergies and increasing the range and resolution of sensorimotor signals. We will illustrate how such maturational processes can be modeled and adaptively coupled with intrinsic motivation in the McSAGG-RIAC system (Baranes and Oudeyer 2011), allowing a robot to learn skills like reaching or omnidirectional locomotion not only faster but also with a higher asymptotic performance in generalization.
- *Social guidance:* Last but not least, social interaction should be a central companion to intrinsic motivation. The interaction between those two guiding mechanisms is at the center of educational research (Ryan and Deci 2000). We will argue that this shall probably also become the case in developmental robots and discuss the various kinds of bidirectional interaction between social guidance and intrinsic motivation that shall be useful for open-ended learning in the real world.

The choice of these families of developmental constraints on intrinsic motivation was here driven by our own investigations toward addressing the challenges of unlearnability, high dimensionality, and unboundedness and is not intended to be a comprehensive list of potentially useful mechanisms (e.g., developmental biases on representations, on mechanisms for creating abstractions, on operators for combining and re-using knowledge and skills, and on statistical inference should be equally important; see Baldassarre and Mirolli 2012; Dayan 2012; Hart and Grupen 2012; Mirolli and Baldassarre 2012). Furthermore, as already explained earlier, we are still very far away from being able to address the challenge of open-ended cumulative learning in unbounded spaces in the real world, and the approaches we present are still preliminary in this respect. Thus, our goal is mainly to draw attention to potential routes that may be pursued to address a fundamental problem of developmental robotics that has been so far largely overlooked.

1 Intrinsic Motivation and Embodied Sensorimotor Primitives

1.1 Bootstrapping Learning in the "Great Blooming, Buzzing Confusion"

The problem of discovering structure and learning skills in the "great blooming, buzzing confusion" of a high-dimensional body equipped with a wide diversity of sensors like the eyes, ears, nose, or skin, as stated by William James (James 1890), might seem a daunting task. Hopefully, animal and human babies do not learn to see the world pixel by pixel, and likewise, they do not learn to control their whole body movements "pixel by pixel." Rather, they are born with neurally embedded dynamical systems which, on the sensori side, allow them to be able to detect and track a number of higher-level structures right from the start and, on the motor side, allow them to tune motor and muscle synergies which already generate parameterized coordinated movements (d'Avella et al. 2003; Lee 1984; Ting and McKay 2007). Examples of innate sensori primitives include visual movement detection and tracking systems (Bronson 1974), basic human facial expression perception (Johnson 2001; Meltzoff and Moore 1977), or special auditory filters tuned for speech processing in humans (Sekuler and Blake 1994). Examples of motor primitives include central pattern generators such as for leg oscillations (Cazalets et al. 1995), synergies for reaching with the hand (d'Avella et al. 2006), closing the fingers in a coordinated manner such as used in grasping (Weiss and Flanders 2004), or of course skills such as breathing or swallowing (Dick et al. 1993). Of course, the existence of these primitives does not avoid the fundamental need for learning, even for the most basic skills: Those primitives are typically parameterized and thus can typically be seen as parameterized dynamical systems which semantics (affordances in particular), parameter values to be set and combination for achieving given tasks have to be learnt. For example, central pattern generators are typically neurally implemented as complex dynamical system generating oscillatory movements which can be tuned by controlling a number of high-level parameters (e.g., inputs to the neural dynamical system), and learning will consist, for example, in discovering that such a motor primitive can be used to "move" the whole body and in learning which tuning of the dynamical system produces which movement of the whole body. Yet, these sensorimotor primitives can considerably decrease the dimensionality and thus the size of the explorable sensorimotor spaces and transform complex low-level action planning problems in simpler higher-level dynamical system tuning problems.

The use of a repertoires of innate parameterized sensorimotor primitives has been key in some of the most advanced real-world intrinsically motivated robot experiments so far, such as in the Playground Experiment (Oudeyer and Kaplan 2006; Oudeyer et al. 2007) or in Hart and Grupen (2008) where primitives were based on sophisticated control-theoretic sensorimotor feedback loops. In parallel, several projects investigating the use of options in intrinsically motivated reinforcement learning can be related to this concept of motor primitives, for example, experiments such as in Barto et al. (2004); Stout and Barto (2010) assumed the existence of a number of innate temporally extended skill "templates," called "options," and corresponding to macro-actions which can be conceptualized as parameterized motor primitives. In those simulations, even if the world is discrete and finite, the system is nevertheless shown to be able to learn to achieve complex skills corresponding to long sequences of actions that are extremely difficult to learn with standard exploration procedures and only low-level actions. In other words, those simulations also provide examples of how innate motor primitives can leverage the potentialities of intrinsically motivated exploration. To give a more precise illustration of such uses of sensorimotor primitives with intrinsic motivation, we will now outline the Playground Experiment (Oudeyer and Kaplan 2006; Oudeyer et al. 2007). Other experiments such as those described in the references above would be equally relevant to illustrate this point, and the reader is referred to them for more details.

1.2 Intrinsically Motivated Acquisition of Affordances and Skills in the Playground Experiment

The Playground Experiment was introduced as an experimental setup allowing us to show how one particular kind of intrinsic reward system, called "Intelligent Adaptive Curiosity" (IAC), could allow a real-world robot with high-dimensional continuous sensorimotor channels to acquire continuously new skills of increasing complexity. As detailed in Oudeyer et al. (2007), the central idea of IAC (which was later importantly refined in R-IAC (Baranes and Oudeyer 2009) was to push the robot to explore certain dynamic motor activities in certain sensorimotor contexts where its predictions of the consequences of its actions in given contexts were improving maximally fast, similarly to what was also proposed in Schmidhuber (1991). A specificity of IAC was the introduction of algorithmic heuristics allowing us to compute prediction progress efficiently and robustly in relatively large continuous sensorimotor spaces. Such an approach based on the optimization of prediction progress belongs to the family of "knowledge-based" intrinsic motivation systems (Oudeyer and Kaplan 2008). Yet, even if driven by the acquisition of knowledge, the whole process is fundamentally active (active choice of actions or sequences of actions in given sensory contexts), and the forward models that are learnt can easily and efficiently be reused for control as soon as one uses nonparametric statistical approaches such as in memory-based approaches such as those presented in Moore (1992) and adapted in Oudeyer et al. (2007), multimap learning approaches such as in Calinon et al. (2007); Ghahramani (1993), or a mixture of nonparametric and multimap approaches (Cederborg et al. 2010). As a consequence, such active knowledge acquired through knowledge-based intrinsically motivated exploration can readily and directly be used for efficient control, as quantitatively shown in Baranes and Oudeyer (2009), and, thus, the IAC system allows the robot to learn a repertoire of *skills* of progressively increasing complexity in the Playground Experiment.

1.2.1 Parameterized Motor Primitives in the Playground Experiment

As argued in the previous paragraph, previous articles presenting the Playground Experiment largely focused on the study of IAC and its role in the obtained results. Yet, a second essential ingredient was the use of parameterized dynamic motor primitives as well as sensory primitives, on top of which exploration and learning was actually happening. Here, we try to emphasize the role of those innate (but still very plastic thanks to their parameters) structures to show two complementary points:

- These parameterized motor primitives consist in complex closed-loop dynamical policies which are actually temporally extended macro-actions (and thus could very well be described in terms of options) that include at the low-level long sequences of micro-actions but controlled at the high level only through the setting of a few parameters; thus, behind the apparently "single-step look ahead" property of the system at the higher level, the Playground Experiment shows the acquisition of skills consisting in complex *sequences* of actions.
- The use of those parameterized motor primitives allows the robot to encode those whole sequences of micro-actions into constrained compact low-dimensional static projections that permit an exploration with IAC that is made considerably easier than if all physically possible movements had been made possible and explorable "pixel by pixel."

1.2.2 Experimental Setup and Description of Primitives

The Playground Experiment setup involves a physical Sony AIBO robot which is put on a baby play mat with various toys, some of which affording learnable interactions, and an "adult robot" which is preprogrammed to imitate the vocalization of the learning robot when this later robot produces a vocalization while looking in the direction of the adult robot (see Fig. 1). The AIBO robot is equipped with four legs, each equipped with three degrees of freedom controlled by servomotors (the degrees of freedom are not controlled directly but through the many dimensions of the control architecture of the motors), with one head with four degrees of freedom

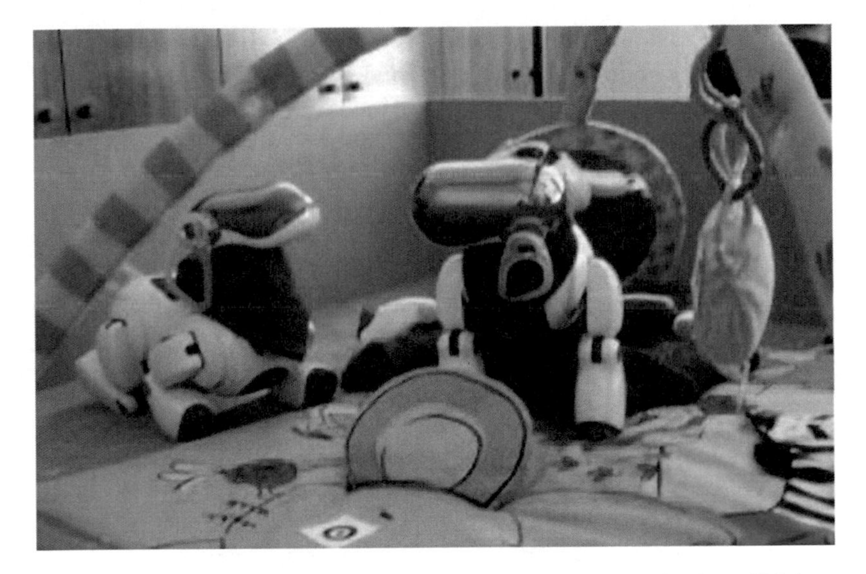

Fig. 1 The playground experiment setup involves a physical Sony AIBO robot which is put on a baby play mat with various toys, some of which affording learnable interactions, and an "adult robot" which is preprogrammed to imitate the vocalization of the learning robot when this later robot produces a vocalization while looking in the direction of the adult robot. The learning robot is equipped with a repertoire of innate parameterized sensorimotor primitives and learns driven by intrinsic motivation how to use and tune them to affect various aspects of its surrounding environment. Complex self-organized developmental trajectories emerge as a result of intrinsically motivated exploration, and the set of acquired skills and affordances increases along with time

including a mouth, with a loudspeaker, as well as with a video camera, an infrared distance sensor mounted on the chin and a microphone. Here, the back legs are blocked so that the robot is not able to locomote, similarly to young human infants in the first months of their life. Given such a rich sensorimotor apparatus in such an environment, it is clear that if action generation and exploration started at the level of millisecond-wide force commands in the motors and no further constraints on the movement profiles were added and if perception started from the level of individual camera pixels or millisecond-wide spectrogram auditory features, the sensorimotor space would be so large that learning and development would be highly inefficient if not impossible.

In order to avoid this problem, the following parameterized motor and sensory primitives are made available to the robot and can be used either alone or in combination (concurrently or in sequence in theory, but so far, the Playground Experiment was only made with the concurrency combination operator):

– *Bashing motor primitive:* This motor primitive allows the robot to produce a bashing movement with either one of its two forelegs and is parameterized by two real numbers indicating the strength and angle of the bashing movement. Based on these parameters, a lower-level control-theoretic architecture first selects the appropriate group/synergy of motors to be used (depending on the angle, motors of the right or left leg shall be used) and then starting from a template movement of the tip of the leg in its operational/task space (Khatib 1987), uses it to define a target trajectory to be followed by the tip of the leg with a certain acceleration profile (corresponding to the force parameter), which is then passed to a lower-level closed-loop action-selection mechanism which generates the appropriate motor currents/torques, in response to real-time position/speed/acceleration errors measured proprioceptively within the motor, at a frequency around 1 kHz and based on a standard PID algorithm (Chung et al. 2008). As a consequence, once the two high-level parameters of the primitive have been set, an automatic dynamical system/policy is generated and is launched to control leg movements, which thanks to the low-level PID servoing controller react and are robust to potential external perturbations. While the parameterization of these bashing movements compresses drastically the generation of movement, it still allows the robot to produce a constrained but very large number of movements that are not unlike the reaching primitives of young human infants. Also to be noted is the fact that special values $(-1, -1)$ are used for the parameters to inhibit the primitive (it is not launched), and this applies to all other motor primitives. Concurrency and combination of primitives are managed through this encoding mechanism.

- *Crouch-biting motor primitive:* This motor primitive allows the robot to crouch down while opening the mouth and then finally closing the mouth, in which an object may potentially be bitten. It is parameterized by the amplitude of the crouch movement and optionally by a parameter controlling the timing of the closing of the mouth. Furthermore, this primitive is such that it keeps the orientation of the head as it is before the primitive is launched, which basically allows to have the effect of this primitive partially controlled by the use of other concurrent motor primitives controlling the head, such as the "turn head" primitive below. Once the parameters are set, a control-theoretic low-level system very similar to the one for the bashing motor primitive is launched: Given the set of motors associated with this primitive, here those of the two legs and of the mouth, and a reference target trajectory of each of these motors (which shape is spline-like) and directly controlled by the parameters, a low-level PID-based motion tracking system is launched to control the low-level sequences of motor torque/current commands.
- *Turning the head motor primitive:* This motor primitive allows the robot to direct its head in a direction determined by two parameters controlling its head pan and tilt. Again, those parameters trigger a lower-level control loop that gets the head from the current position to the desired orientation through low-level torque control. This motor primitive is essential for the robot since the head supports the camera and the infrared sensor. Thus, this motor primitive allows the robot to direct its sensors in given directions of the environment.
- *Vocalization motor primitive:* This motor primitive allows the robot to produce vocalizations consisting of prototypical "baba"-like sounds which are parameterized by their fundamental frequency, more precisely their mean pitch value. Of course, the AIBO robot does not have a physical vocal tract, so a

speech synthesizer is used instead (which may be seen himself as a model of a vocal tract), and the dynamic sounds to be produced are constrained to be basic syllables, corresponding to "canonical babbling" [innate stereotypical coordinated actions of many muscles in the human mouth (MacNeilage 2008)], for which the robot is only authorized to modify the mean pitch.

- *Movement sensory primitive:* This sensory primitive allows the robot to assess whether something is moving, for example, oscillating, right in the direction in front of its nose where the infrared sensor is positioned. It basically consists in a filter operating on short-time windows of the past infrared sensor values, which is then saturated to provide a binary value (0 if no movement is detected and 1 if a movement is detected). This sensory primitive is not unlike the innate movement detectors of the visual system of human infants (Bronson 1974).
- *Visual object detection sensory primitive:* This sensory primitive allows the robot to assess whether an "object" is visually present in its narrow field of view, an object being defined as a group of pixels with certain saliency properties. In the Playground Experiment, those measures of saliency were short-cut by the use of visual markers directly put on objects to be perceived as "salient." This sensory primitive thus provides high-level filters upon the pixel matrix of the camera, which are functionally not unlike the facial presence and facial expression innate detectors in human infants.
- *Mouth-grabbing sensory primitive:* This sensory primitive allows the robot to assess whether he is holding something in the mouth or not and relies on the use of a filter above the proprioceptive sensors in the mouth, saturated so that the end value is also binary.
- *Auditory pitch sensor:* This sensory primitive allows the robot to measure the mean pitch of the sounds perceived in the short past, typically being a continuous value when a vocalization has been produced by the other robot and either a value 0 or a random value for noises produces during motor interaction with objects. This sensor is automatically disabled while the learning robot is producing its own vocalizations (but it could very well not be the case, which would also produce interesting behaviors).

1.2.3 What the Robot May Explore and Learn

The sensorimotor primitives described in the previous paragraph constitute a significant amount of innate structures provided to the robot. Yet, those motor and sensory motor primitives are tools which semantics, parameterization, combination, and affordances both among themselves and with the environment should be learnt. Indeed, from the point of view of the robot, each of these primitives is black boxes in which uninterpreted numbers can be sent and from which uninterpreted numbers can be read. The relations among those black boxes, especially between the motor and sensory primitives, are also totally unknown to the robot. In practice, this means that the robot does not know initially things such as the fact that using the "bashing primitive" can produce controllable values in the "movement sensory primitive" (an object oscillating after being bashed) and when applied in certain regions of its sensorimotor space (with particular parameter values in relation to the position of an object) and in coordination with the "turning head primitive" which allows to direct the sensors in the direction of the physical effect of the bashing primitive. Another example is that the robot shall not know that predictable, and, thus, controllable, auditory sensations corresponding to the adult robot's vocalization shall be triggered by vocalizing while at the same time looking in the direction of the other robot, and the robot shall not know how particular parameters of the vocalization itself can affect the imitation of the adult robot (which is by the way perceived just as other standard salient "objects"). As a result, in the Playground Experiment, the robot has to explore and learn how the use of the motor primitives, with their continuous space of parameters, as well as their concurrent combination (e.g., bashing with given parameters achieved concurrently with turning the head with given parameters), allows (or does not allow) to predict and control the values of subsets of the sensory primitives. Details are described in Oudeyer and Kaplan (2006) and Oudeyer et al. (2007).

In spite of the fact that those motor and sensory primitive considerably constrain and reduce the sensorimotor space to be explored for acquiring action knowledge and thus skills, it is still a rather large space in comparison with the physical time necessary to achieve one single sensorimotor experiment (i.e., experimenting how a vocalization with certain parameters might make a toy move—actually, the robot shall discover that this is not possible—or make one of the surrounding objects, the adult robot, produce another vocalization). Indeed, in its most simple version, the above primitives still define a six-dimensional continuous space of motor parameters and a four-dimensional space of sensory parameters, constituting a ten-dimensional sensorimotor space. Such a dimensionality shall not be daunting for sampling and modeling an abstract space in a computer simulation where individual experiments last a few milliseconds and are thus cheap in terms of time. Yet, for robots as for living animals, actions take time and a reaching, bashing, or vocalization attempt lasts at least two or three seconds. As a consequence, sampling randomly the space of sensorimotor experiments would lead to inefficient and slow acquisition of the learnable skills. This is the reason why the use of sensorimotor primitives in combination with intrinsically motivated exploration can really allow each mechanism to leverage the potentialities of each other.

1.2.4 Results of Experiments

We outline here the various results that came out of repeated experiments. For further details, the reader is referred to Oudeyer and Kaplan (2006) and Oudeyer et al. (2007). During an experiment, which lasts approximately half a day, we store all the flow of values of the sensorimotor channels, as well as a number of features that help us to characterize the dynamics of the robot's development. Indeed, we measure the evolution of the relative frequency of the use of the different actuators and motor primitives (analogous measures were also used to study the behavioral

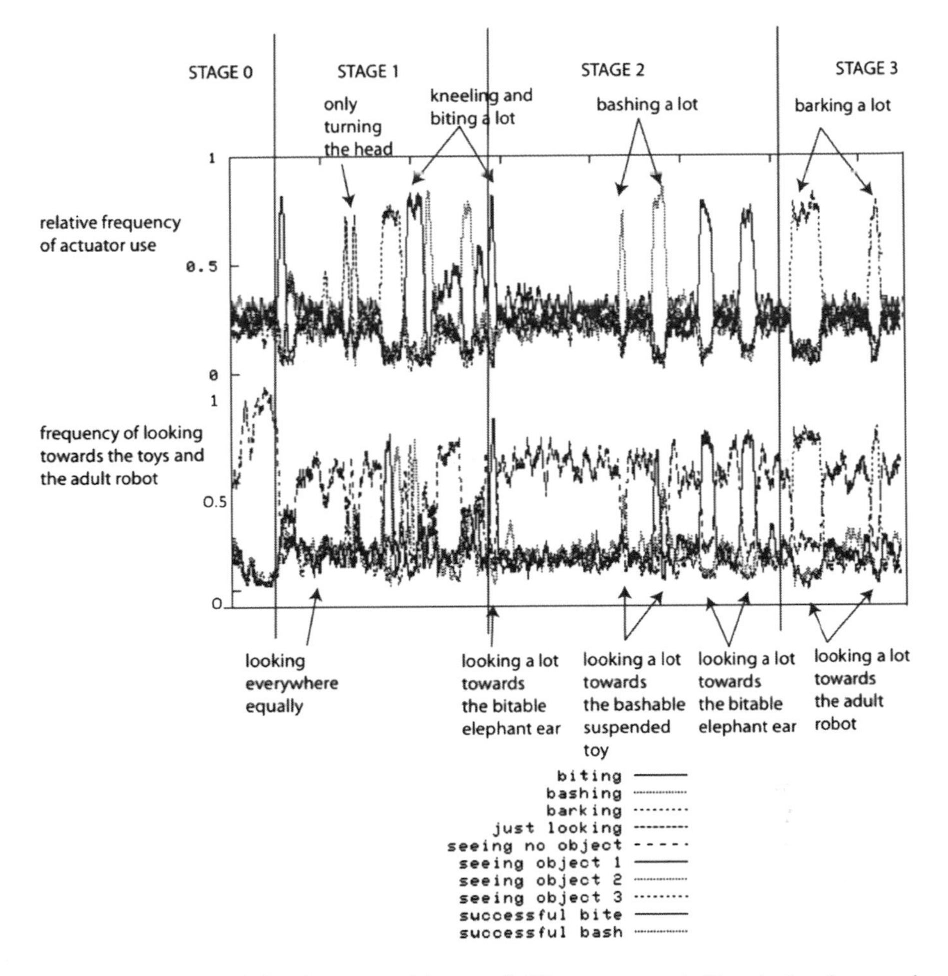

Fig. 2 *Top curves*: relative frequency of the use of different motor primitives in the playground experiment. *Bottom curves*: frequency of looking toward each object and, in particular, toward the "adult" preprogrammed robot. We can observe that the robot explores, and thus learns, progressively more complex and more affordant skills

structure of intrinsically motivated exploration in Schmidhuber 2002). In particular, we also constantly measure the direction in which the robot is turning its head. Figure 2 shows details of an example for a typical run of the experiment.

Self-Organization of Developmental Stages and Affordance Learning. From the careful study of the curves in Fig. 2, augmented with the study of the trace of all the situations that the robot encountered, we observe that (1) there is an evolution in the behavior of the robot; (2) this evolution is characterized by qualitative changes in this behavior; and (3) these changes correspond to a sequence of more than two phases of increasing behavioral complexity, that is, we observe

Table 1 Stages in the robot's developmental sequence

Description	Stage 0	Stage 1	Stage 2	Stage 3
Individuation of actions	−	+	+	+
Biting and bashing with the right affordances	−	−	+	+
Focused vocal interactions with the adult	−	−	−	+

the emergence of several successive levels of behavioral patterns. Moreover, it is possible to summarize the evolution of these behavioral patterns using the concept of stages, where a stage is here defined as a period of time during which some particular behavioral patterns occur significantly more often than random and did not occur significantly more often than random in previous stages. This definition of a stage is inspired from that of Piaget (Piaget 1952). These behavioral patterns correspond to combinations of clear deviations from the mean in the curves in Fig. 2. This means that a new stage does not imply that the organism is now only doing new things, but rather that among its activities, some are new. Here are the different stages that are visually denoted in Fig. 2 and Table 1:

- *Stage 0:* The robot has a short initial phase of random exploration and body babbling. This is because during this period, the sensorimotor space has not yet been partitioned in significantly different areas. During this stage, the robot's behavior is equivalent to the one we would obtain using random action selection: We clearly observe that in the vast majority of cases, the robot does not even look or act toward objects, and, thus, its action on the environment is quasi-absent. This is due to the fact that the sensorimotor space is vast, and, only in some small subparts, some nontrivial learnable phenomena can happen given its environment.
- *Stage 1:* Then, there is a phase during which the robot begins to focus successively on playing with individual motor primitives but without the adequate affordances: First, there is a period where it focuses on trying to bite in all directions (and stops bashing or producing sounds), then it focuses on just looking around, then it focuses on trying to bark/vocalize toward all directions (and stops biting and bashing), then to bite, and finally to bash in all directions (and stops biting and vocalizing). Sometimes, the robot not only focuses on a given actuator but also looks in a focused manner toward a particular object at the same time: Yet, there is no affordance between the actuator used and the object it is looking at. For example, the developing robot tries to bite the "adult" robot or to bark/vocalize toward the elephant ear. Basically, in this stage, the robot is learning to decompose its motor space into differentiable subparts which correspond to the use of different (combination of) motor primitives. This results from the fact that using one or two primitives at time (typically either bashing/biting/vocalizing together with turning the head in a particular direction) makes the $SM(t) \rightarrow S(t+1)$ easier to learn, and so at this stage in its development, this is what the robot judges as being the largest niche of learning progress.

– *Stage 2:* Then, the robot comes to a phase in which it discovers the precise affordances between certain motor primitives and certain particular "objects": It is now focusing either on trying to bite a biteable object (an elephant ear) and on trying to bash a bashable object (a suspended toy). Furthermore, the trace shows that it does actually manage to bite and bash successfully quite often, which shows how such capabilities can be learnt through general curiosity-driven learning since no reward specific to these specific tasks is preprogrammed. This focus on trying to do actions toward affordant objects is a result of the splitting mechanism of IAC (Oudeyer et al. 2007), which is a refinement of the categorization of the sensorimotor space that allows the robot to see that, for example, there is more learning progress to be gained when trying to bite the biteable object that when trying to bite the suspended toy or the "adult" robot (indeed, in that case, nothing happens because they are too far, and so the situation is always very predictable and does not provide a decrease in the errors in prediction).
– *Stage 3:* Finally, the robot comes to a phase in which it now focuses on vocalizing toward the "adult" robot and listens to the vocal imitations that it triggers. Again, this is a completely self-organized result of the intrinsic motivation system driving the behavior of the robot: This interest for vocal interactions was not preprogrammed and results from exactly the same mechanism which allowed the robot to discover the affordances between certain physical actions and certain objects. The fact that the interest in vocal interaction appears after the focus on biting and bashing comes from the fact that this is an activity which is a little bit more difficult to learn for the robot, given its sensorimotor space and the playground environment: Indeed, this is due to the continuous sensory dimensions which are involved in vocalizing and listening, as opposed to the binary sensory dimensions which are involved in biting and bashing.

We made several experiments, and each time, we got a similar global structure in which a self-organized developmental sequence pushed the robot toward practicing and learning activities of increasingly organized complexity, particularly toward the progressive discovery of the sensorimotor affordances as well as the discovery for vocal interactions. In particular, in the majority of developmental sequences, there was a transition from a stage where the robot acted with the wrong affordances to a stage where it explored motor primitives with the right affordances and in particular finishing by a stage where it explored and focused on vocal interactions. Nevertheless, we also observed that two developmental sequences are never exactly the same, and the number of stages sometimes changes a bit or the order of intermediary stages is sometimes different. We then conducted systematic experiments to assess statistically those properties, as described in Oudeyer et al. (2007), and we found that strong structural regularities were appearing in a statistically significant manner and, at the same time, that diversity of the details, and cases which varied importantly from the mean, appeared. This is particularly interesting since this duality between universal regularities and diversity in development pervades human infant development, as described in the developmental psychology literature (Berk 2008;

Fisher and Silvern 1985), a property which has been so far only poorly understood and for which such a computational experiment suggests original hypothesis.

Formation of Developmental Cognitive Categories. In addition to driving the exploration of the space of sensory and motor primitives and their combinations in given environmental contexts, the IAC architecture builds internal categorization structures, called "regions" (Oudeyer et al. 2007), and used to separate sensorimotor subspaces of various level of "interestingness," that is, of various level of learnability/controllability. As argued in Kaplan and Oudeyer (2007), those categories initially made at the service of the intrinsic motivation system are formed gradually, and their properties reflect important properties of fundamental general conceptual categories to be discovered by the human/robot child: In particular, it allows the learning agent to separate its own body—that is, the self (maximally controllable), from inanimate surrounding objects (moderately controllable), from other living entities (less controllable but still important niches of learning progress), and finally from the unlearnable and uncontrollable. A similar approach to the bootstrapping of these fundamental cognitive categories was also presented in Kemp and Edsinger (2006).

Skill Acquisition: From the Knowledge of Action Consequences to Direct Control. In the Playground Experiment, exploration is driven by the search of maximal improvement of the predictions of the consequences of using motor primitives upon sensory primitives in given environments. Thus, it is actively driven by the acquisition of knowledge about the consequences of actions, that is, by the acquisition of "forward models." If forward models would be encoded using parametric regression methods such as standard neural networks, then it would be complicated and highly inefficient to transform this knowledge into a competence, that is, to reuse this knowledge to achieve practical goals, and, thus, one may say that the learning agent would not have learnt skills. Hopefully, research in robot learning and stochastic control theory based on statistical inference has shown that if forward models are encoded using certain forms of nonparametric models (Bishop 2007), such as in memory-based approaches (Schaal and Atkeson 1995), then there are simple and efficient methods to directly reuse the acquired knowledge to achieve efficient control, even in high-dimensional highly redundant robot bodies (Baranes and Oudeyer 2009; Moore 1992). It has also been shown in the same literature that instead of either learning forward or inverse models with experimental data collected by a robot of the type in the Playground Experiment, one could learn both at the same time using multimap models, such as in Gaussian Mixture Regression (Calinon et al. 2007; Cederborg et al. 2010; Ghahramani 1993). In the Playground Experiment, nonparametric models similar to (Moore 1992) were used and thus allow the robot to acquire permanently new *skills* as it is exploring the world, even if driven by the acquisition of new *knowledge* about the consequences of its actions. A second collateral advantage of using nonparametric statistical approaches over parametric approaches such as standard neural networks is that it avoids catastrophic forgetting: New experiments by the robot allow it to acquire novel skills without forgetting any of the previously learnt knowledge and skills. In more recent experiments, such as experiments about a new version of IAC, called R-IAC, which is algorithmically more robust from several respects, a combination of nonparametric learning and multimap regression based on Gaussian mixtures was used, and it was quantitatively shown how it could be reused efficiently for controlling a high-dimensional redundant body (Baranes and Oudeyer 2009).

1.2.5 Embodiment and Morphological Computation

We have just seen how sensorimotor primitives, viewed as dynamical systems controlling high-dimensional bodies but tuned by low-dimensional parameters, could be considerably useful when combined with intrinsic motivation for learning complex sensorimotor skills in a real robot. Actually, the efficiency of those primitives is tightly related to the morphological properties of the body in which they are used. First, the inputs and structure of those primitives only make sense within a given body structure. Second, the outputs of those primitives do not entirely determine the movements/behavior of the robot body: Indeed, the physics of real-world robots is such that gravity and its interaction with the inertia of the robot, in combination with the compliance and other dynamical properties of materials and actuators, also impact importantly the resulting movements/behavior. Furthermore, the morphology of a robot might be more or less affordant with the environment (Gibson 1986) and thus make the control of various aspects of the environment more or less easy to learn, for example, it will be much more difficult to learn how to grasp an egg for a robot with a gripper made of two stiff metal fingers than for a robot with a multi-finger soft compliant hand. Equally, a robot with an anthropomorphic head with a wide-angle camera will more easily trigger and perceive human social cues than a robot with no head and a narrow-angle camera directed to its foot.

Thus, the impact of morphology on control and behavior is paramount. An adequately designed morphology can allow to significantly reduce the complexity of its traditional control code/system for a given set of tasks and can even be conceptualized as replacing traditional digital control computations by "physical" or "morphological computation" (Paul 2004; Pfeifer and Bongard 2006; Pfeifer et al. 2007; Pfeifer and Scheier 1999). A number of experiments exploring this principle have been presented in the literature, concerning skills such as grasping (Yokoi et al. 2004), quadruped locomotion (Iida and Pfeifer 2004), robot fish swimming (Ziegler et al. 2006), insect navigation (Franceschini et al. 1992), as well as biped humanoid locomotion or emergent physical human–robot interfaces (Ly et al. 2011; Ly and Oudeyer 2010; Oudeyer et al. 2011). The body itself, as a physical dynamical system subject to the laws of physics, should actually be considered as any other complex dynamical system, which can potentially generate spontaneously organized structures through self-organization (Ball 1999).

As a consequence, the spontaneous structures potentially generated by the body complement and interact with the structures provided by sensorimotor primitives and shall equally be leveraged for intrinsically motivated learning of sophisticated sensorimotor skills in the real world. Like when one uses a given set of innate sensorimotor primitives, a given body with given morphological properties is by definition particular. These innate constraints of course introduce biases: They will help the robot to acquire certain families of skills rather than other families of skills. But this is in no way incompatible with the goal of building machines capable of open-ended development and learning. Indeed, "open-ended learning" does not imply that the robot shall be able to learn universally *anything* but rather simply that he shall be able to learn continuously novel skills. Again, due to unboundedness in particular, efficient universal skill learning in the real world is probably impossible, and constraints at all levels need to be employed to make learning of particular *families* of skills in particular *families* of environment. This actually applies to intrinsic motivation systems themselves, for which no measure of "interestingness" might be universally useful, as argued in the evolutionary perspective presented in Singh et al. (2010). Furthermore, using particular constraints, in particular morphological constraints, for a particular family of skills and environments does not mean either that they are necessarily ad hoc. For example, the human body has very particular properties that considerably help the acquisition of a versatile and diverse repertoire of motor skills.

1.2.6 Limits and Perspectives

The Playground Experiment has shown how a high-dimensional robot could learn incrementally a repertoire of diverse and relatively complex skills and affordances through curiosity-driven exploration. We have argued above that these results could be obtained thanks to the use of innate parameterized motor and sensory primitives as much as to the use of an intrinsic motivation system. Yet, next to these promising results, many limits and avenues for improvement may be found in both the experimental setup and the algorithmic approach.

Firstly, while we have explained that knowledge-based intrinsically motivated exploration allowed to acquire skills as a side effect when using nonparametric and/or multimap models, one could wonder what could be gained by using competence-based intrinsically motivated exploration (Bakker and Schmidhuber 2004; Baranes and Oudeyer 2010a; Oudeyer and Kaplan 2008; Schembri et al. 2007b; Stout and Barto 2010), that is, an architecture *directly* driven by the acquisition of skills (see also Rolf et al. 2010 for a related approach). In principle, there may be good reasons to use competence-based approaches to mimic animal and human development given the central importance of skills for the survival of living beings and for the usefulness of robots (see Part IV of this book). In the Playground Experiment, it may be noted that the motor parameter space is much larger and more complex than the space defined by the sensory primitives, that is, the command/action space is much larger than the task/effect space. This is partly the result of having redundant motor primitives. If one is eventually interested in the skills that the robot may learn and if skills are defined in terms of what changes in the external (or internal) environment the robot can produce by its actions (e.g., making an object move, being grasped, or produce sounds), then this means that one should prefer that the robot learns one strategy to achieve all possible effects rather than many strategies to achieve only a subset of potential effects. Thus, in such redundant spaces, it would be interesting that exploration be driven directly by the evolution of performances for producing effects in task spaces, hence directly by evolution of competences. In Sect. 2, we will present an example of such competence-based intrinsic motivation system where active exploration takes place directly in the task space (i.e., realizing what is sometimes called goal babbling Rolf et al. 2010) and show quantitatively how it can improve the speed of skill acquisition in a high-dimensional highly redundant robot.

Secondly, while the use of such sensorimotor primitives in combination with intrinsic motivation is probably necessary for bootstrapping developmental learning in real sensorimotor spaces, it addresses only very partially and in a limited manner the fundamental problem of unboundedness. As shown above, the use of sensorimotor primitives can be used as a transform mapping a high-dimensional continuous problem into a much lower-dimensional continuous problem. Harnessing dimensionality is fundamental, but it is nevertheless not sufficient to address unboundedness. Indeed, low-dimensional spaces could very well be themselves infinite/unbounded, for example, one could typically have a motor or sensory primitive with parameters or values in an unbounded space, or alternatively one could very well have an infinite number of low-dimensional bounded sensorimotor primitives. In such contexts, intrinsic motivation systems face the meta-exploration problem: Evaluating "interestingness" itself becomes very difficult. As argued above, unboundedness is probably an obstacle that shall not be attacked frontally. Rather, mechanisms for introducing "artificial" bounds are necessary (in addition to the bounds created by intrinsic motivation systems once interestingness has been efficiently evaluated). This is what was done in the Playground Experiment: All parameters of motor primitives, as well as all sensory values, were bounded in a compact hypercube within R^n, and there was a small number of motor primitives.

This self-bounding approach may be a bit too drastic and problematic for allowing open-ended acquisition of novel skills upon a longer lifetime duration. A first, aspect of the limits of such an artificial bounding is related to the very introduction of fixed relatively ad hoc bounds on the values of sensorimotor primitive parameters. It might be difficult to tune those bounds manually in order to allow the spaces to be explorable and learnable, and once the robot has reached these boundaries of what can be learnt and explore, an obstacle to further development appears. Introducing bounds is essential, but clearly autonomous open-ended development needs more flexibility. One possible way of addressing this challenge is to consider the possibility of using maturational mechanisms, inspired by the progressive growth and maturation of the body and brains of living beings, which permit to control the dynamic self-tuning and self-expansion of these bounds. This includes mechanisms controlling, for example, the progressive increase of the sensitivity of sensors or of the number of degrees of freedoms and range of motor commands. Section 3 will present a system combining such maturational constraints with intrinsically motivated learning and draw some perspectives on the future challenges that this entails.

A second aspect of introducing such artificial boundings is related to the use of fixed and limited set of motor and sensory primitives. This equally limits the extent to which open-ended development may be achieved on a longer time scale. A first important direction of research in order to remove this barrier is to generalize the introduction of operators for combining primitives and make them recursive. Only a simple concurrency combination operator was available in the Playground Experiment, but many other kinds of operators could be imagined. The most obvious one is sequencing, allowing the robot to learn higher-level skills involving plans based on the motor primitives (thus, in addition to the low-level motor sequences inside the motor primitives), that may be coupled with operators allowing to encapsulate such plans/high-level skills into macros that can be reused as atomic actions. Those objectives are at the center of research combining intrinsically motivated reinforcement learning and option theory and more generally approaches to cumulative learning, and the reader is referred to the following articles for an overview of those techniques (Bakker and Schmidhuber 2004; Barto et al. 2004; Ring 1994; Sutton et al. 1999; Wiering and Schmidhuber 1997). A second equally important direction of research to go beyond a fixed set of sensorimotor primitives is social learning: Mechanisms such as learning by imitation or demonstration may be very useful to help a robot acquire novel primitives and novel combinations of those primitives. More generally, while research on intrinsically motivated skill acquisition has largely focused on pure autonomous learning for methodological reasons, human infants learn and develop through a strong interaction of intrinsically driven learning and social guidance. Likewise, this interaction should probably be key in the strategies to be employed to face the challenge of open-ended development in an unbounded world, which we will discuss in Sect. 4.

2 Intrinsically Motivated Exploration and Learning Directly in Task Spaces

As argued earlier in this chapter, robots are typically equipped with a very large sensorimotor space, in which motor policies are typically embedded in high-dimensional manifolds. Yet, many real-world tasks consist in controlling/effecting only a limited number of sensory variables based on the use of high-dimensional motor commands. For example, a hand reaching task consists in positioning the hand in a three-dimensional visual space, which contrasts with the many muscles that need to be activated to achieve this reaching. A biped locomotion task is defined in terms of the three-dimensional trajectory of the center of mass, achieved with very high-dimensional control of all the degrees of freedom of the body. Related to this high dissimilarity between the dimensionality of many tasks and the dimensionality of their associated control/joint space is the fact that human and robot motor systems are highly redundant. Goals in a task space (e.g., the position of the hand in three dimension) can typically be reached by many motor programs.

This property can importantly be exploited to design intrinsic motivation systems that drive exploration in such high-dimensional redundant spaces.[1] Knowledge-based intrinsic motivation systems and traditional active learning heuristics drive exploration by the active choice of motor commands and measure of their consequences, which allows to learn forward models that can be reused as a side effect for achieving goals/tasks: This approach is suboptimal in many cases since it explores in the high-dimensional space of motor commands and considers the achievement of tasks only indirectly. A more efficient approach consists in directly actively exploring the space of goals within task spaces, and then learn associated local coupled forward/inverse models (possibly through local goal-driven active exploration) that are useful to achieve those goals. For example, if we consider the learning of a hand reaching task, the knowledge-based approach would actively sample the set of joint motor commands and observe the resulting three-dimensional hand position. This exploration process will not consider the distribution of explored hand position and, in addition to being embedded in a high-dimensional space if the arm has many degrees of freedom, may lead to learning many joint motor commands that produce the same hand position while not necessarily learning how to reach many other hand positions. On the other hand, task-level exploration will directly and actively explore the space of goals, actively choosing three-dimensional hand configurations to be reached and then launch a lower-level process for exploration of the joint space directed to the selected goal. Here, rather than learning many motor programs allowing to reach one goal, the robot will learn to reach many goals, maybe with few motor solutions for each goal. This allows to exploit redundancy and low dimensionality of the task space. Such a task-level approach belongs the family of competence-based intrinsic motivation systems (Oudeyer and Kaplan 2008).

In the next section, we illustrate how this approach can be useful in the context of the SAGG-RIAC architecture. Actually, as it happens in SAGG-RIAC, task-level/goal exploration and control-level/joint exploration can be integrated in a single hierarchical active learning architecture. This architecture is organized in two levels: at a higher level, the robot chooses actively goals to explore (e.g., points in the visual space that may be reached by its hand), and, at a lower level, the robot actively performs local exploration to learn how to reach goals selected at the higher level. Hence, globally, the exploration is guided by motor exploration in the task space, where goals are defined as particular configurations to reach (possibly under certain constraints, e.g., a goal may be to reach a given position with the tip of the arm through a straight line or while minimizing the spent energy). Yet, in spite of having a task space which dimensionality can be considerably smaller than the control space (e.g., often below five), sophisticated exploration heuristics have to be used due to a specific novel problem that appears in goal-babbling/task-level exploration. Indeed, a human or a robot does not know initially what parts of

[1] Part of the material presented in this section is adapted from Baranes and Oudeyer (2010a, 2012).

the task space are "reachable": The robot knows neither its learning limits nor its physical limits. If we take again the example of the reaching task, initially the robot will not know which part of the three-dimensional visual space can or cannot be reached with its hand. Some goals may be impossible to reach because of physical limitation, some other goals may be too difficult to learn to reach given its inference capabilities, and some other goals may be too difficult to reach now but become reachable later on after learning basic motor programs that can be reused for these more difficult goals. Thus, efficient exploration requires that the robot identifies quickly the parts of the task space where goals are not reachable at a given point of its development and focus exploration on trying to learn goals that are actually reachable and thus learnable. This directly leads to the idea of transposing the concept of "prediction improvement"—characterizing the (non)interestingness of motor commands in knowledge-based architectures into a concept of "competence improvement" and characterizing the (non)interestingness of goals in the task space.

2.1 SAGG-RIAC: Multilevel Active Learning

In order to illustrate the interest of task-level exploration, we outline here the SAGG-RIAC active learning architecture, introduced in Baranes and Oudeyer (2010a), and present it in the context of a reaching task example (but it can be trivially adapted to other sensorimotor spaces). We also present experiments evaluating the gain compared to knowledge-based architectures such as R-IAC. SAGG-RIAC transposes some of the basic ideas of R-IAC, combined with ideas from the SSA algorithm (Schaal and Atkeson 1994), into a mutilevel active learning algorithms, called *Self-Adaptive Goal Generation R-IAC (SAGG-RIAC) algorithm*. Unlike R-IAC that was made for active learning of forward models, we show that this new algorithm allows for efficient learning of inverse models in redundant robots by leveraging the lower-level dimension of the task space. The central idea of *SAGG-RIAC* consists in pushing the robot to perform babbling in the goal/operational space, as opposed to motor babbling in the actuator space, by self-generating goals actively and adaptively in regions of the goal space which provide a maximal competence improvement for reaching those goals. Then, a lower-level active motor learning algorithm, inspired by the SSA algorithm (Schaal and Atkeson 1994), is used to allow the robot to locally explore how to reach a given self-generated goal. Hence, it follows the inspiration of both the SSA algorithm, which constrains the exploration to a tube of data targeted to a specific goal, and of "learning progress" approaches to intrinsic motivation: It explores in an open-ended manner the space of goals, focusing on those where local improvement of the competence to reach them is maximal.

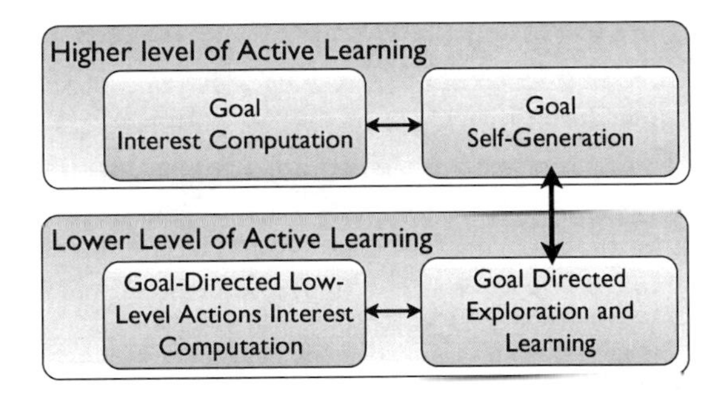

Fig. 3 Global architecture of the SAGG-RIAC algorithm. The structure is composed of two parts defining two levels of active learning: a higher level, which considers the active self-generation and self-selection of goals, and a lower level, which considers the goal-directed active choice and active exploration of lower-level actions, to reach the goals selected at the higher level

2.2 *Global Architecture*

Let us consider the definition of competence-based models outlined in Oudeyer and Kaplan (2008) and extract from it two different levels for active learning defined at different time scales (Fig. 3):

1. The higher level of active learning (higher time scale) considers the *active self-generation and self-selection of goals*, depending on a measure of interestingness based on the level of achievement of previously generated goals.
2. The lower level of active learning (lower time scale) considers the *goal-directed active choice and active exploration* of lower-level actions to be taken to reach the goals selected at the higher level and depending on another local measure of interestingness based on the evolution of the quality of learnt inverse and/or forward models.

2.2.1 Model Formalization

Let us consider a robotic system whose configurations/states are described in both an actuator space S and an operational/task space S'. For given configurations $(s_1, s'_1) \in S \times S'$, a sequence of actions $a = \{a_1, a_2, \ldots, a_n\}$ allows a transition toward the new states $(s_2, s'_2) \in S \times S'$ such that $(s_1, s'_1, a) \Rightarrow (s_2, s'_2)$. For instance, in the case of a robotic manipulator, S may represent its actuator/joint space, S' the operational space corresponding to the Cartesian position of its end-effector, and a may be velocity or torque commands in the joints.

In the frame of SAGG-RIAC, we are interested in the reaching of *goals*, from starting states. Also, we formalize starting states as configurations $(s_{\text{start}}, s'_{\text{start}}) \in S \times S'$ and goals, as a desired $s'_g \in S'$. All states are here considered as potential starting states; therefore, once a goal has been generated, the lower level of active learning always try to reach it by starting from the current state of the system.

When a given goal is set, the low-level process of goal-directed active exploration and learning to reach this goal from the starting state can be seen as exploration and learning of a motor primitive $\Pi_{(s_{\text{start}}, s'_{\text{start}}, s'_{\text{g}}, \rho, \mathbf{M})}$, parameterized by the initiation position $(s_{\text{start}}, s'_{\text{start}})$, the goal s'_{g}, constraints ρ (e.g., linked with the spent energy), and parameters of already learnt internal forward and inverse models $\mathbf{M}$.

Also, according to the self-generation and self-selection of goals at the higher level, we deduce that the whole process (higher and lower time scales) developed in SAGG-RIAC can be defined as an autonomous system that explores and learns *fields of parameterized motor primitives*.

2.2.2 Lower Time Scale: Active Goal-Directed Exploration and Learning

The goal-directed exploration and learning mechanism can be carried out in numerous ways. Its main idea is to guide the system toward the goal, by executing low-level actions, which allows it to progressively explore the world and create a model that may be reused afterward. Its conception has to respect two imperatives:

1. A model (inverse and/or forward) has to be computed during the exploration and has to be available for a later reuse, in particular, when considering other goals.
2. A learning feedback has to be added, such that the exploration is active, and the selection of new actions depends on local measures about the evolution of the quality of the learnt model.

In the experiment introduced in the following, we will use a method inspired by the SSA algorithm introduced by Schaal and Atkeson (Schaal and Atkeson 1994). Other kinds of techniques, for example, based on natural actor-critic architectures in model-based reinforcement learning (Peters and Schaal 2008), could also be used.

2.2.3 Higher Time Scale: Goal Self-generation and Self-selection

The goal self-generation and self-selection process relies on a feedback defined using a notion of competence and more precisely on the competence improvement in given subregions of the space where goals are chosen. The following part details the technical formalization of this system.

2.2.4 Measure of Competence

A reaching attempt in direction of a goal is defined as terminated according to two conditions:

1. A timeout related to a maximal number of micro-actions/time steps allowed has been exceeded.
2. The goal has effectively been reached.

We introduce a measure of competence $\gamma_{s'_g}$ for a given reaching attempt as depending on a measure of *similarity* C (i.e., typically a distance measure) between the state s'_f reached when the goal reaching attempt has terminated and the actual goal s'_g of this reaching attempt and the respect of constraints ρ. The measure of similarity C, and thus the measure of competence, is as general as the measure of prediction error could be in RIAC. As seen below, we set equations so that $\gamma_{s'_g}$ is always a negative number, such that the lower the value is, the lower the competence (one can be unboundedly bad, i.e., the distance between the reached configuration and the goal can in general be growing toward infinity), and the higher the value, the higher the competence (which becomes maximal when the goal is perfectly reached). Thus, we define $\gamma_{s'_g}$ as

$$\gamma_{s'_g} = \begin{cases} C(s'_g, s'_f, \rho) & \text{if } C(s'_g, s'_f, \rho) \leq \varepsilon_C < 0 \\ 0 & \text{otherwise} \end{cases}$$

with ε_C a tolerance factor where $C(s'_g, s'_f, \rho) > \varepsilon_C$ corresponds to a goal reached. Thus, a value $\gamma_{s'_g}$ close to 0 represents a system that is competent to reach the goal s'_g respecting constraints ρ. A typical instantiation of C, without constraints, is defined as $C(s'_g, s'_f, \emptyset) = \|s'_g - s'_f\|^2$, which is the direct transposition of prediction error in R-IAC (which here becomes goal reaching error). Yet, other equally general examples of similarity or distance measures could be used, possibly including normalizing terms such as in the experiments below.

Definition of Local Competence Progress. The active goal self-generation and self-selection relies on a feedback linked with the notion of competence introduced above and more precisely on the monitoring of the progress of local competences. We firstly define this notion of local competence: Let us consider different measures of competence $\gamma_{s'_i}$ computed for reaching attempts to different goals $s'_i \in S', i > 1$. For a subspace called a region $R \subset S'$, we can compute a measure of competence γ_R that we call a *local measure* such that

$$\gamma_R = \left(\frac{\sum_{s'_j \in R} (\gamma_{s'_j})}{|R|} \right) \tag{1}$$

with $|R|$, cardinal of R.

Let us now consider different regions R_i of S' such that $R_i \subset S'$, $\bigcup_i R_i = S'$. (initially, there is only one region that is then progressively and recursively split; see below and Fig. 4). Each R_i contains attempted goals $\{s'_{t_1}, s'_{t_2}, \ldots, s'_{t_k}\}_{R_i}$, and corresponding competences obtained $\{\gamma_{s'_{t_1}}, \gamma_{s'_{t_2}}, \ldots, \gamma_{s'_{t_k}}\}_{R_i}$, indexed by their relative time order $t_1 < t_2 < \cdots < t_k | t_{n+1} = t_n + 1$ of experimentation inside this precise subspace R_i (t_i are not the absolute time but integer indexes of relative order in the given subspace (region) being considered for goal selection). The interest value, described by Eq. (2), represents *the absolute value of the derivative of the local competence value inside R_i, hence the local competence progress, over a*

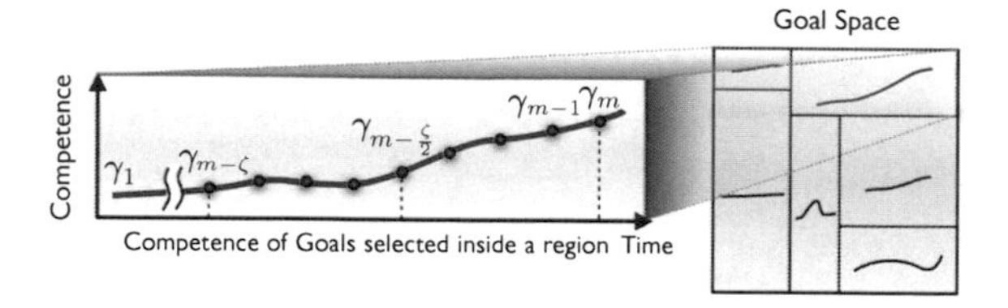

Fig. 4 Illustration of how a goal space can be split into subregions, in each of which competence progress is monitored. The action-selection system decides most of the time (typically 70 %) to explore goals with regions of highest learning progress (the probability of choosing a region is proportional to competence progress) but still for meta-exploration dedicates a part of its time (typically 30 %) to explore other randomly chosen regions

sliding time window of the ı *more recent goals attempted inside* R_i (see Baranes and Oudeyer 2011 for a justification of the absolute value):

$$\text{interest}(R_i) = \frac{\left| \left(\sum_{j=|R_i|-\zeta}^{|R_i|-\frac{\zeta}{2}} \gamma_{s'_j} \right) - \left(\sum_{j=|R_i|-\frac{\zeta}{2}}^{|R_i|} \gamma_{s'_j} \right) \right|}{\zeta} \tag{2}$$

Goal Self-Generation Using the Measure of Interest. Using the previous description of interest, the goal self-generation and self-selection mechanism has to carry out two different processes (see Fig. 4):

1. Split of the space S' where goals are chosen, into subspaces, according to heuristics that allow to maximally distinguish areas according to their levels of interest.
2. Select the subspaces where future goals will be chosen.

Such a mechanism has been described in the Robust-Intelligent Adaptive Curiosity (R-IAC) algorithm introduced in Baranes and Oudeyer (2009) but was previously applied to the actuator space S rather than to the goal/task space S' as we do in SAGG-RIAC. Here, we use the same kind of methods like a recursive split of the space, each split being triggered once a maximal number of goals $g_{\max}$ have been attempted inside. Each split is performed such that maximizes the difference of the interest measure described above; in the two resulting subspaces, this allows to easily separate areas of different interest and, thus, of different reaching difficulty.

Finally, goals are chosen according to the following heuristics that mix three modes, and once at least two regions exist after an initial random exploration of the whole space:

1. $Mode(1)$: In p_1% percent (typically $p_1 = 70\,\%$) of goal selections, the algorithm chooses a random goal inside a region chosen with a probability proportional to its interest value:

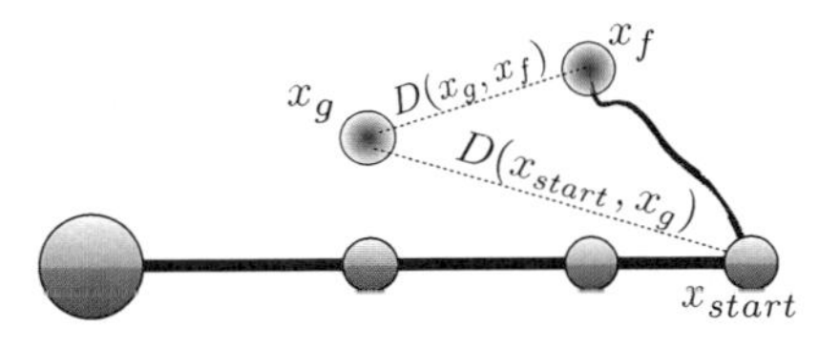

Fig. 5 Values used to compute the competence $\gamma_{s'_g}$, considering a manipulator of three degrees of freedom, in a two dimensions operational space. Here, the arm is set in a position called *rest position* $(\theta_{\text{rest}}, x_{\text{rest}})$

$$P_n = \frac{|\text{interest}_n - \mathbf{min}(\text{interest}_i)|}{\sum_{i=1}^{|R_n|} |\text{interest}_i - \mathbf{min}(\text{interest}_i)|} \tag{3}$$

where P_n is the probability of selection of the region R_n and $interest_i$ corresponds to the current *interest* of regions R_i.

2. $Mode(2)$: In p_2 % of cases (typically $p_2 = 20$ %), the algorithm selects a random goal inside the whole space.
3. $Mode(3)$: In p_3 % (typically $p_3 = 10$ %), it performs a random experiment inside the region where the mean competence level is the lowest.

Developmental Constraints for the Reduction of the Initiation Set: To improve the quality of the learnt inverse model, we add a heuristic inspired by observations of (Berthier et al. 1999) who noticed that infant's reaching attempts were often preceded by movements that either elevated their hand or moved their hand back to their side. By analogy, using such heuristics can directly allow a highly redundant robotic system to reduce the space of initiation states used to learn to reach goals and also typically prevent it from experimenting with too complex actuator configurations. Also, we add it in SAGG-RIAC, by specifying a rest position $(s_{\text{rest}}, s'_{\text{rest}})$ settable without any need of planning from the system, that is, set for each $r \in n\mathbb{Z}$ subsequent reaching attempts.

2.3 *Experimenting SAGG-RIAC on a Reaching Task*

In the following, we consider a n-dimensions manipulator controlled in position and speed (as many of today's robots), updated at discrete time values, called *time steps*. The vector $\theta \in \mathbb{R}^n = S$ represents joint angles and $x \in \mathbb{R}^m = S'$, the position of the manipulator's end-effector in m dimensions, in the Euclidian space S' (see Fig. 5 where $n = 15$ and $m = 2$). We evaluate how the SAGG-RIAC algorithm can be used by a robot to learn how to reach all reachable points in the environment S' with this arm's end-effector. Learning both the forward and inverse kinematics is here an online process that arises each time a micro-action is executed by the manipulator: By doing movements, the robot stores measures $(\theta, \Delta\theta, \Delta x)$ in its memory; these measures are then reused online to compute the Jacobian $J(\theta) = \Delta x / \Delta \theta$ locally and the associated Moore-Penrose pseudo-inverse to move the end-effector in a desired direction $\Delta x_{desired}$ fixed toward the self-generated goal. Also, in this experiment, where we suppose S' Euclidian and do not consider obstacles, the direction to a goal can be defined as following a straight line between the current end-effector's position and the goal (thus, we avoid using complex planning, which is a separate problem and thus allows us to interpret more easily the results of the experiments).

2.3.1 Evaluation of Competence

In this experiment, we do not consider constraints ρ and only focus on the reaching of goal positions x_{g}. We define the cost function C and thus the competence as linked with the Euclidian distance $D(x_{\mathrm{g}}, x_{\mathrm{f}})$, between the goal position and the final reached position x_{f}, which is normalized by the starting distance $D(x_{\mathrm{start}}, x_{\mathrm{g}})$, where x_{start} is the end-effector's starting position:

$$C(x_{\mathrm{g}}, x_{\mathrm{f}}, x_{\mathrm{start}}) = -\frac{D(x_{\mathrm{g}}, x_{\mathrm{f}})}{D(x_{\mathrm{start}}, x_{\mathrm{g}})} \tag{4}$$

where $C(x_{\mathrm{g}}, x_{\mathrm{f}}, x_{\mathrm{start}}) = min_C$ if $D(x_{\mathrm{start}}, x_{\mathrm{g}}) = 0$ and $D(x_{\mathrm{g}}, x_{\mathrm{f}}) \neq 0$.

2.3.2 Addition of Subgoals

Computing local competence progress in subspaces/regions typically requires the reaching of numerous goals. Because reaching a goal can necessitate several actions and thus time, obtaining competence measures can be long. Also, without biasing the learning process, we improve this mechanism by taking advantage of the Euclidian aspect of S': We increase the number of goals artificially, by adding subgoals on the pathway between the starting position and the goal, where competences are computed. Therefore, considering a starting state x_{start} in S' and a self-generated goal x_{g}, we define the set of l subgoals $\{x_1, x_2, \ldots, x_l\}$ where $x_i = (i/l) \times (x_{\mathrm{g}} - x_{\mathrm{start}})$, that have to be reached before attempting to reach the terminal goal x_{g}.

2.3.3 Local Exploration and Reaching

Here, we propose a method, inspired by the SSA algorithm (Schaal and Atkeson 1994), to guide the system to learn on the pathway toward the selected goal position x_{g}. The system is organized around two alternating phases: *reaching* phases, which involve a local controller to drive the system from the current position x_{c} toward the goal, and *local exploration* phases, which allow to learn the inverse model of the system in the close vicinity of the current state and are triggered when the reliability of the local controller is too low. These mechanisms are stopped once the goal has been reached or a timeout exceeded. Let us here describe the precise functioning of those phases in our experiment:

Reaching phase: The reaching phase deals with creating a pathway to the goal position x_g. This phase consists of determining, from the current position x_c, an optimal movement to guide the end-effector toward x_g. For this purpose, the system computes the needed end-effector's displacement $\Delta x_{next} = v.\frac{x_c - x_g}{\|x_c - x_g\|}$ (where v is the velocity bounded by v_{max} and $\frac{x_c - x_g}{\|x_c - x_g\|}$ a normalized vector in direction of the goal) and performs the action $\Delta\theta_{next} = J^+.\Delta x_{next}$, with J^+, pseudo-inverse of the Jacobian estimated in the close vicinity of θ and given the data collected by the robot so far. After each action Δx_{next}, we compute the error $\varepsilon = \|\widetilde{\Delta x}_{next} - \Delta x_{next}\|$ and trigger the exploration phase in cases of a too high value $\varepsilon > \varepsilon_{max} > 0$.

Exploration phase: This phase consists in performing $q \in \mathbb{N}$ small random explorative actions $\Delta\theta_i$, around the current position θ. This allows the learning system to learn the relationship $(\theta, \Delta\theta) \Rightarrow \Delta x$, in the close vicinity of θ, which is needed to compute the inverse kinematics model around θ.

2.4 Results

2.4.1 Goal-Directed Exploration and Learning

In the experiment introduced in this section, we consider the robotic system presented above with a n-DOF arm on a plane, with $n = 7$, 15, or 30 (thus, the problem has, respectively, 16, 32, and 62 continuous dimensions, if one considers the fact that the motor space is spanned by the position and speed of each joint and the task space has two dimensions) . We set the dimensions of S' as bounded in intervals $x_g \in [0; 150] \times [-150; 150]$, where 50 units are the total length of the arm, which means that the arm covers less than $1/18$ of the space S' where goals can be chosen (i.e., the majority of areas in the operational/task space are not reachable, which has to be discovered by the robot). We fix the number of subgoal per goal to 5 and the maximal number of elements inside a region before a split to 50. We also set the desired velocity $v = 0.5$ units/movement and the number of explorative actions $q = 20$. Moreover, we reset the arm to the rest position $(\theta_{rest}, x_{rest})$, where the arm is straight (position displayed in Fig. 5), every $r = 2$ reaching attempts. This allows the system to reduce the initiation set and avoid experimenting with too complex joint positions where the arm is folded and where the Jacobian is more difficult to compute.

2.4.2 Qualitative Results

Figure 6 shows histograms of the self-generated goal positions (goals without subgoals) with $n = 15$ and created regions, after the execution of 200,000 time

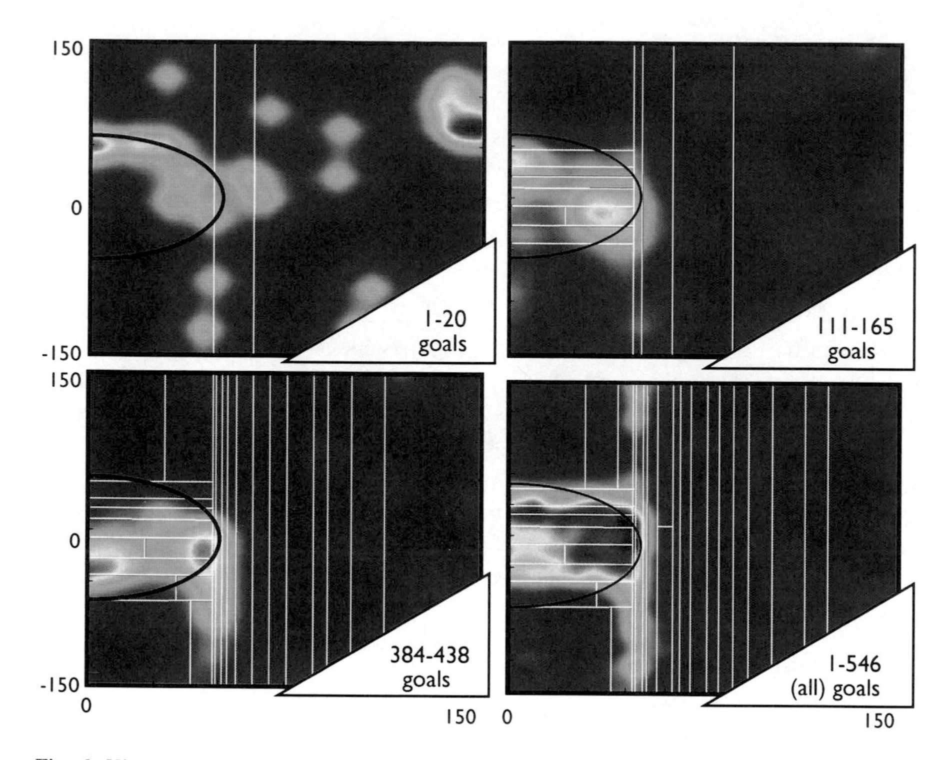

Fig. 6 Histograms of self-generated goals and regions with a 15 DOF robotic planar arm (split by white lines) displayed over time windows indexed by the number of performed goals, for an experiment of 200,000 time steps (i.e., micro-actions). The black half-circle represents the contour of the area reachable by the arm according to its length of 50 units

steps (i.e., micro-actions). Each subfigure represents data obtained during a time window indexed on the number of generated goals: The first one (upper-left) shows that in the very beginning of learning (20 goals correspond to 100 goals and subgoals), the system is already splitting the space and seems to discriminate the left third of the space, where the reachable area is (contoured by the black half-circle on each subfigure). Upper-right and lower-left subfigures show examples of areas where goals are generated over time; we can observe that the highest amount of goals that are chosen remains inside the reachable area: The system is indeed discovering that only a subpart is reachable, the interest value becoming null in totally unreachable areas where the competence typically takes small values or even reaches the threshold min_C. The last subfigure (lower-right) represents the position of all goals that have been self-generated and allows to observe that SAGG-RIAC is able to highly discriminate unreachable areas over time and to focus its goal self-generation in the whole reachable subspace. Finally, observing regions, we can globally notice that the system splits the reachable space into regions in the first quarter of goal generations (upper-right subfigure) and then continues to split the space inside unreachable regions, in order to potentially release new areas of interest.

It is also important to notice that coupling the lower level of active learning inspired by SSA with the heuristic of returning to x_{rest} every two subsequent goals creates an increasing radius of known data around x_{rest}, inside the reachable space. Indeed, the necessity to be confident in the local model of the arm to shift toward new positions makes the system progressively explore the space, and resetting it to its rest position makes it progressively explore the space by beginning close to x_{rest}. Finally, goal positions that are physically reachable but far from this radius typically present a low competence to be reached initially, before the radius spreads enough to reach them, which creates new areas of interest and explains the focalization on reachable areas far from x_{rest} (see Fig. 6). Therefore, the exploration also proceeds by going through reachable subspaces of growing complexity of reachability.

2.4.3 Quantitative Results

In the following evaluation, we consider the same robotic system as previously and design two experiments. This experiment considers a large space $S' = [0; 150] \times [-150; 150]$, where one can evaluate the capability of SAGG-RIAC to discriminate and avoid to explore unreachable areas. Here, we repeated the experiment with $n = 7, 15, 30$ dofs as well as by taking two geometries for the arm: one where all segments have equal length and one where the length is decreasing with the golden number ratio. All configurations of experiments were repeated 15 times in order to obtain proper statistics. We compare the following exploration techniques:

1. SAGG-RIAC.
2. SAGG-Random, where goals are chosen randomly (higher level of active learning (RIAC) disabled).
3. ACTUATOR-RANDOM, where small random movements $\Delta\theta$ are executed.
4. ACTUATOR-RIAC, which corresponds to the original RIAC algorithm, which uses the decrease of the prediction error $(\theta, \Delta\theta) \rightarrow \Delta x$ to compute an interest value and split the space $(\theta, \Delta\theta)$.

Also, to be comparable to SAGG-RIAC, for each other techniques, we reset the position of the arm to the *rest position* every max time steps, max being the number of time steps needed to consecutively reach the two more distant reachable positions. Figure 7 shows the evolution of the capability of the system to reach 100 test goals (independently and uniformly distributed in the reachable area) using the inverse model learnt by each technique, starting from, half the time, the rest positions. The observations of the curves show several things. First, SAGG-RIAC allows both the robot to learn faster and to reach the highest absolute level of performance in *all* cases, and an ANOVA analysis shows a level of significance of this result $p = 0.002$ at the end of the experiment for 15 dofs. Thus, like in the previous experiment, we see that SAGG-RIAC allows both larger speed and higher generalization ability. The second observation that we can make is that random exploration in the joint space (ACTUATOR-RANDOM) is the second best method for 7 dofs, then third for 15 dofs, and then last for 30 dofs, illustrating the curse of dimensionality.

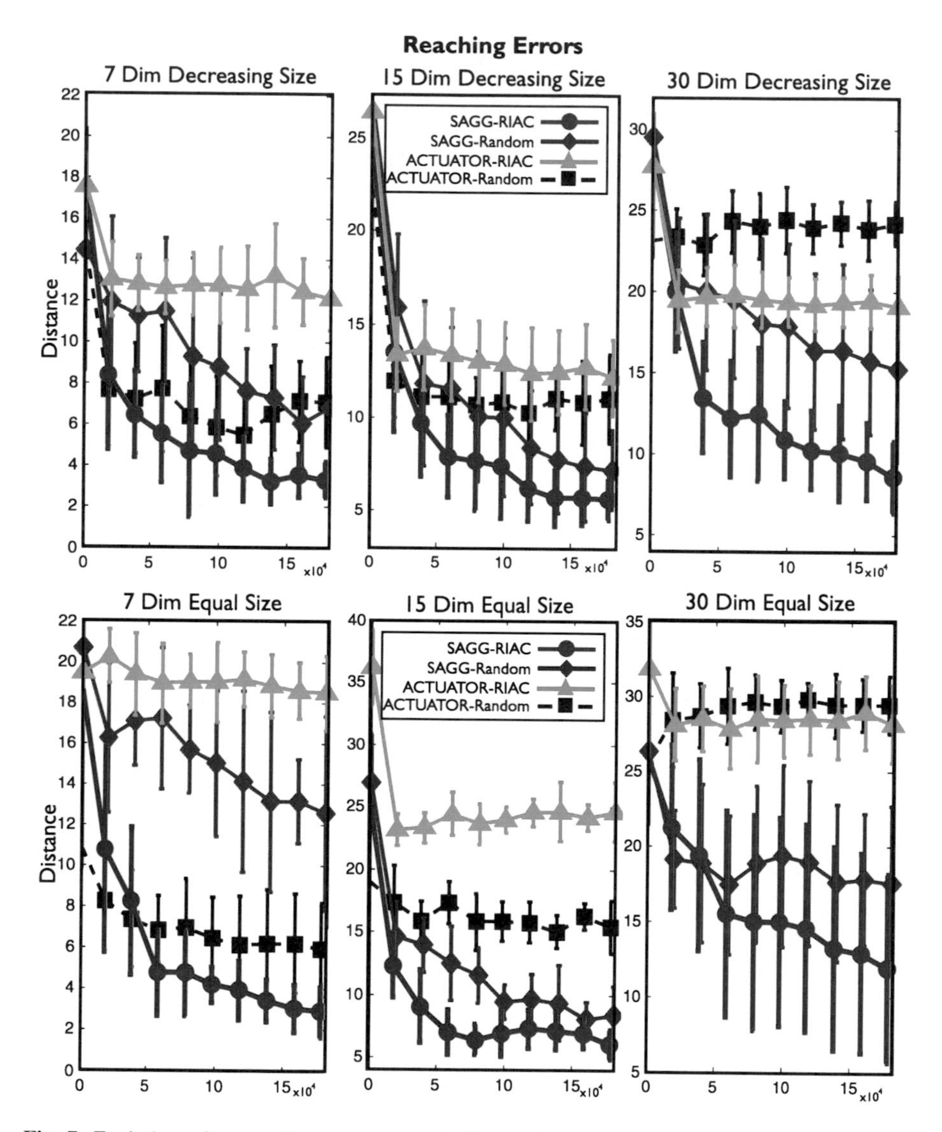

Fig. 7 Evolution of mean distances goal-end effector (reaching errors) after reaching attempts over an independently randomly generated set of test goals. Here, SAGG-RIAC and SAGG-RANDOM are only allowed to choose goals within $S' = [0; 150] \times [-150; 150]$ (i.e., the set of reachable goals is only a small subset of eligible goals)

Inversely, the evolution of performances of SAGG-RANDOM and SAGG-RIAC degrades gracefully as dimension grows, showing how exploration in the operational space allows to harness the curse-of-dimensionality by exploiting the redundancy of the robotic system and the low dimensionality of the operational space. Yet, one sees that SAGG-RIAC is consistently and significantly more efficient than

SAGG-RANDOM, which is explained by the fact that SAGG-RANDOM pushes too often the robot to try to reach unreachable goals, while SAGG-RIAC is capable of quickly focusing in reachable goals. Finally, we again see that ACTUATOR-RIAC is not robust to the increase of dimensionality in such continuous spaces.

More systematic studies should of course be done, but these results already indicate the high potential of *competence-based motor learning* in general, even using random goal self-generation.

3 Maturationally Constrained Intrinsically Motivated Exploration

Task-level exploration by competence-based intrinsic motivation architectures can considerably decrease the dimensionality of the spaces to be explored and leverage the potentially high redundancy of sensorimotor spaces for more efficient exploration and acquisition of new skills. Yet, task spaces may often be unbounded or characterized by a volume of the "interesting" regions much smaller than the overall volume of the sensorimotor space, even when there are very few dimensions, and in those cases task-level exploration and competence-based architectures become as inefficient as knowledge-based architectures. For example, the three-dimensional space around a human is unbounded, and both for reaching or locomotion tasks, the space of potential goals to be reached is thus unbounded. As said above, the human or the robot does not know its limits initially, so why shall he not try to reach with its hand the mountains five kilometers ahead in its visual field or why shall he not try to run at one hundred kilometers per hour? In the reaching experiment presented in previous section, the task space was in fact artificially and rather arbitrarily bounded: While including many parts that were not reachable, it was still severely bounded, which allowed goal exploration to succeed. As argued at the beginning of this chapter, mechanisms for self-bounding the explorable space are necessary, but they should be less ad hoc. To reach this objective, one may take inspiration from maturational mechanisms in biological organisms.[2]

The progressive biological maturation of infant's brain, motor and sensor capabilities, including changes in morphological properties of the body, introduces numerous important constraints on the learning process (Schlesinger 2008). Indeed, at birth, all the sensorimotor apparatus are neither precise enough nor fast enough to allow infants to perform complex tasks. The low visual acuity of infants (Turkewitz and Kenny 1985) and their incapacity to efficiently control distal muscles and to detect high-frequency sounds are examples of constraints reducing the complexity and limiting the access to the high-dimensional and unbounded space where

[2]Part of the material presented in this section is adapted from Baranes and Oudeyer (2011).

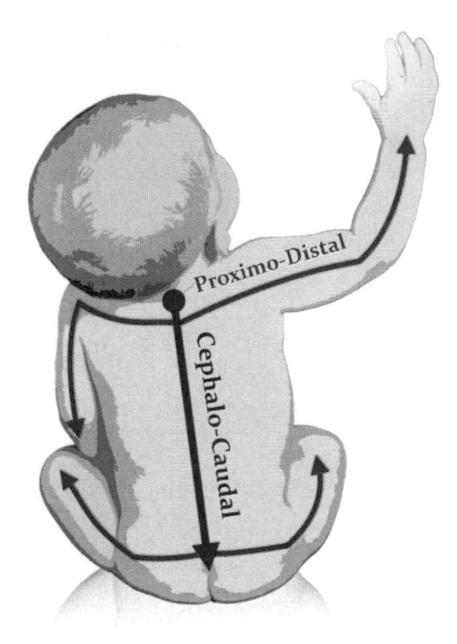

Fig. 8 The proximo-distal and cephalocaudal law: infants explore and learn in priority their torso and shoulder for reaching movements and progressively their elbow, and the same process happens in the gradual exploration and mastery of the neck-feet axis

they evolve (Bjorklund 1997). Maturational constraints play an important role in learning, by partially determining a developmental pathway. Numerous biological reasons are part of this process, like the brain maturation, the weakness of infants' muscles, or the development of the physiological sensory system. In the following, we focus on constraints induced by the brain *myelination* (Eyre 2003). Related to the evolution of a substance called myelin and usually qualified by the term white matter, the main impact of myelination is to help the information transfer in the brain by increasing the speed at which impulses propagate along axons (connections between neurons). Here, we focus on the myelination process for several reasons, this phenomenon being responsible for numerous maturational constraints, effecting the motor development but also the visual or auditory acuity, by making the number of degrees of freedom, and the resolution of sensory–motor channels increase progressively with time.

Actually, infants' brain does not come with an important quantity of white matter, myelination being predominantly a postnatal process, taking place in a large part during the first years of life. Konczak (Konczak et al. 1997) and Berthier (Berthier et al. 1999) studied mechanisms involved in reaching trials in human infants. In their researches, they expose that goal-directed reaching movements are ataxic in a first time and become more precise with time and training. Also, they show that for all infants, the improving efficiency of control follows a proximo-distal way, which means that infants use in priority their torso and shoulder for reaching movements and, progressively, their elbow (Berthier et al. 1999); see Fig. 8. This evolution of control capabilities comes from the increasing frequency of the muscular impulses, gradually, in shoulders and elbows. This phenomenon, directly related to the myelination of the motor cortex, then allows muscles to become stronger at the same time, by training, which then increases their possibility to experiment wider sets of positions. Myelin is also responsible for brain responses to high visual and sound frequencies. Therefore, like introduced in Turkewitz and Kenny (1985), children are not able to detect details in images, which is also a reason, of imprecise reaching movements.

Coupling Maturation and Intrinsic Motivation. Maturational mechanisms could easily be integrated with an intrinsic motivation system, where the space explorable with intrinsic motivation would grow as new degrees of freedom and higher resolutions or ranges are released and timed by a maturational clock. If the maturational clock is purely dependent on physical time, then maturation influences intrinsically motivated exploration. But what may be potentially even more useful is that maturation could in return be accelerated or slowed down based on how fast (or slow) new competences are acquired by the intrinsically motivated organism. This means that intrinsically motivated exploration would not only be a mechanism for deciding "what to learn" but also a self-regulating mechanism indirectly regulating the growth of the complexity of the very space in which exploration takes place. If one imagines that maturation not only releases new degrees of freedoms in sensorimotor channels but also capabilities of statistical inference mechanisms (e.g., increasing the size of the hypothesis space to search), then one would have an intrinsic motivation system which actively explores its environment and at the same time actively regulates both the bounds of this explorable space and the capabilities of the learning system that it is driving. Such an integration of maturation and intrinsic motivation is what has been explored in the McSAGG architecture, coupling SAGG-RIAC with maturational constraints (Baranes and Oudeyer 2010b). Such an approach is also supported by theories of brain and behavior development that highlight the strong interaction between maturational processes and learning processes (Johnson 2001). The following section presents an outline of the system as well as results that show how it can improve the efficiency of intrinsically motivated learning on the same reaching task than in previous section.

3.1 McSAGG: Maturationally Constrained Competence-Based Architecture

It is important to notice the multilevel aspect of maturational constraints: Maturation can apply to motor actions/commands in the joint/control space as well as to goals in task spaces; also, maturational constraints can apply to sensors, such as the capacity to discriminate objects and, so here, to declare a goal as reached. The global idea is to control all of these constraints using an evolving term $\psi(t)$, called *adaptive maturational clock*, which increase, influencing the lifting of constraints, depends on the global learning evolution and is typically nonlinear. The main problem raised is to define a measure allowing the robot learner to control the evolution of this clock. For instance, in the Lift-Constraint, Act, Saturate (LCAS) algorithm,

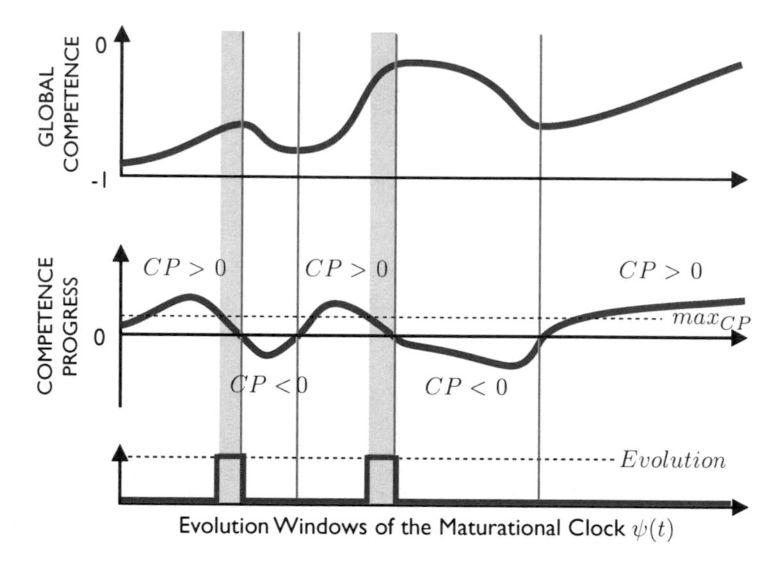

Fig. 9 Values used to compute the competence $\gamma_{s'_g}$, considering a manipulator of three degrees of freedom, in a two dimensions operational space

(Lee et al. 2007) use a simple discrete criteria based on a saturation threshold. (Lee et al. 2007) consider a robotic arm whose end-effector's position is observed in a task space. This task space is segmented into spherical regions of specified radius used as output for learning the forward kinematics of the robot. Each time, the end-effector explores inside a region, this one is activated. Once every region is activated, saturation happens, and the radius of each region decreases so that the task space becomes segmented with a higher resolution and allows a more precise learning of the kinematics. In the following section, we take inspiration from the LCAS algorithm and define a measure based on the competence progress allowing us to control a continuous and nonlinear evolution of the maturational clock.

3.1.1 Stage Transition: Maturational Evolution and Intrinsic Motivations

Often considered as a process strictly happening in the first years of life, myelin continues to be produced even in adults while learning new complex activities (Scholz et al. 2009). Also, in a developmental robotics frame, we set the maturational clock $\psi(t)$ which controls the evolution of each release of constraint, as depending on the learning activity and especially on the progress in learning by itself. Here, the main idea is to increase $\psi(t)$ (lifting constraints), *when the system is in a phase of stabilization of its global competence level, after a phase of progression* (see Fig. 9). This stabilization is shown by a low derivative of the averaged competence level computed in the whole goal space S' in a recent time window $[t_{n-\frac{\zeta}{2}}, t_n]$ and the progression, by an increase of these levels in a preceding time window $[t_{n-\zeta}, t_{n-\frac{\zeta}{2}}]$. We thus use a description analogous to the notion of competence progress used to define our measure of interest. Therefore, considering competence values estimated for the ζ last reaching attempts $\{\gamma_{s'_{n-\zeta}}, \ldots, \gamma_{s'_n}\}_{S'}$, $\psi(t)$ evolves until reaching a threshold ψ_{max} such that

$$\psi(t+1) = \psi(t) + \min\left(\max_{evol}; \frac{\lambda}{CP(\{\gamma_{s'_{n-\zeta/2}}, \ldots, \gamma_{s'_n}\})}\right)$$

$$\text{if} \begin{cases} 0 < CP(\{\gamma_{s'_{n-\zeta/2}}, \ldots, \gamma_{s'_n}\}) < \max_{CP} \textit{ and} \\ CP(\{\gamma_{s'_{n-\zeta}}, \ldots, \gamma_{s'_{n-\zeta/2}}\}) > 0 \text{ and } \psi(t) < \psi_{max} \end{cases}$$

and $\psi(t+1) = \psi(t)$ otherwise, where $\max_{evol}$ is a threshold limiting a too rapid evolution of ψ, $\max_{CP}$ a threshold defining a stable competence progress, λ a positive factor, and $CP(\{\gamma_{s'_{n-\zeta/2}}, \ldots, \gamma_{s'_n}\})$ a measure of competence progress (in the experiments presented in this section, no absolute value is used, i.e., intrinsic rewards are only provided for increases in competence). As the global interest of the whole space is typically nonstationary, the maturational clock becomes typically nonlinear and stops its progression when the global average of competence decreases, due to the lifting of previous constraints. In Fig. 9, the increase of $\psi(t)$ is denoted as evolution periods.

3.1.2 Constraints Modeling

3.1.2.1 Constraints Over the Control Space

In this model, we concentrate on three kinds of maturational constraints over the control and perceptual space, that is, constraints on motor programs explorable to reach goals and over perception used to achieve those programs or evaluate whether goals are reached or not, directly inspired by consequences of the myelination process and which are controlled by $\psi(t)$. These constraints are general and can be integrated in numerous kinds of robots.

The first constraint describes the *limitation of frequency of muscular impulses*, applied to the control of the limbs, which is responsible of the precision and complexity of control (Konczak et al. 1997). Also corresponding to the frequency of feedback updating movements to achieve a trajectory, we define the constraint $f(t)$ as increasing with the evolution of the maturational clock:

$$f(t) = \left(-\frac{(p_{max} - p_{min})}{\psi_{max}}.\psi(t) + p_{max}\right)^{-1} \quad (5)$$

where p_{max} and p_{min} represents maximal and minimal possible time periods between control impulses.

The second studied constraint relies on the sensor abilities. Here, we consider the *capacity to discriminate objects* as evolving over time, which here corresponds to an evolving value of ε_D, the tolerance factor allowing to decide of a goal as reached. We thus set ε_D as evolving and, more precisely, decreasing over the maturational clock, from $\varepsilon_{D_{max}}$ to $\varepsilon_{D_{min}}$:

$$\varepsilon_D(t) = -\frac{(\varepsilon_{D_{max}} - \varepsilon_{D_{min}})}{\psi_{max}}.\psi(t) + \varepsilon_{D_{max}} \tag{6}$$

Finally, we set another constraint, implementing a mechanism analogous to the proximo-distal law described above. Here, we consider the ranges r_i within which motor commands in the control space can be chosen, as increasing over maturational time following a proximo-distal way over the structure of the studied embodied system. This typically allows larger movements and further goals to become explorable and thus learnable:

$$r_i(t) = \min(\psi(t).k_i, r\max_i) \tag{7}$$

where k_i represents an intrinsic value determining the difference of evolution velocities between each joint. In the case of a robotic arm such as in the reaching task and if one denotes $i = 1, \ldots, l$ the joints in the control space, then the proximo-distal law can be implemented by choosing $k_1 \geq k_2 \geq \cdots \geq k_n$, where k_1. In the quantitative experiments below, we only use this later constraint.

3.1.2.2 Constraints Over the Goal Space

As explained above, evolving maturational constraints can also be set on the space of explorable goals, in which active learning algorithm such as SAGG-RIAC can learn to discover reachable and unreachable areas. A simple but powerful (as shown below) manner to model those constraints is to let the robot start from a relatively small volume goal space around one or several seeds and then have the goal space grow as a sphere which radius R_{goal} increases with the maturational clock:

$$R_{goal} = \psi(t).G_{const} \tag{8}$$

3.1.3 Experiments on Maturationally Constrained Learning of Arm Kinematics

Here, we consider a simulated robotic arm with the same reaching task than in the previous section on task-level exploration.

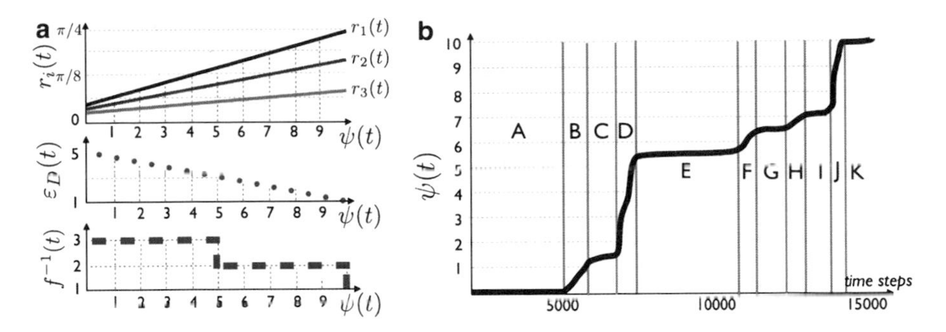

Fig. 10 (**a**) Exploration of maturational constraints over values taken by the maturational clock $\psi(t)$, for a manipulator of three-dof. (**b**) Evolution of the maturational clock over time, for a given experiment. Vertical splits are added manually, to let appear what we call *maturational stages*, which are described as periods between important changes of the evolution of $\psi(t)$ (change of the second derivative of $\psi(t)$)

In a first qualitative experiment, we consider the case of a $n = 3$ DOF arm, put in a two-dimensional environment. We set the arm with a global length of 50 units and fix the proportion of each limb as 3/5, 2/5, and 1/5 of this length and fix $\psi_{\max} = 10$. Figure 10a shows the different constraints $r_i(t)$, ε_{D}, and $f^{-1}(t)$ over values that take the maturational clock $\psi(t)$. We can firstly observe increasing ranges $r_i(t)$, defined such that $r_3(t) < r_2(t) < r_1(t)$, which respects the proximo-distal constraint meaning that joints closer to the basis of the arm have a controllable range which increase faster than further joints. Figure 10a also shows the evolutions of $\varepsilon_{\mathrm{D}}(t)$, from 5 to 1 units over $\psi(t)$, and $f^{-1}(t)$, representative of the time period between the manipulator's update control signals, from 3 to 1 time steps. The evolution of the frequency has been decided as being not continuous, to let us observe the behavior of the algorithm when a sudden change of complexity arises for a constraint. We run an experiment over 15,000 time steps, which corresponds to the selection of about 7,500 goals. During the exploration, we observe the evolution of the maturational clock $\psi(t)$ over time (black curve in Fig. 10b) which evolves nonlinearly, depending on the global progress of competence. Letters from A to K are added from an external point of view; they are described as periods between important changes of the evolution of $\psi(t)$ (evolution of the second derivative of $\psi(t)$) and represent what we call *maturational stages*. We describe two types of stages, *stationary stages* like A, C, E, G, I, K, where the maturational clock evolves slowly, which corresponds to time period (over time steps) where the global competence progress is either stable or negative, and *evolution stages*, like B, D, F, H, J, where the maturational clock is evolving with a high velocity.

We can emphasize two important maturational stages: the first one, A, which corresponds to a non-evolution of $\psi(t)$; this is due to the need of the mechanism to obtain a minimal number of competence measures, before computing the global progress to decide of a release of constraints. Also, the stable stage E, which appears

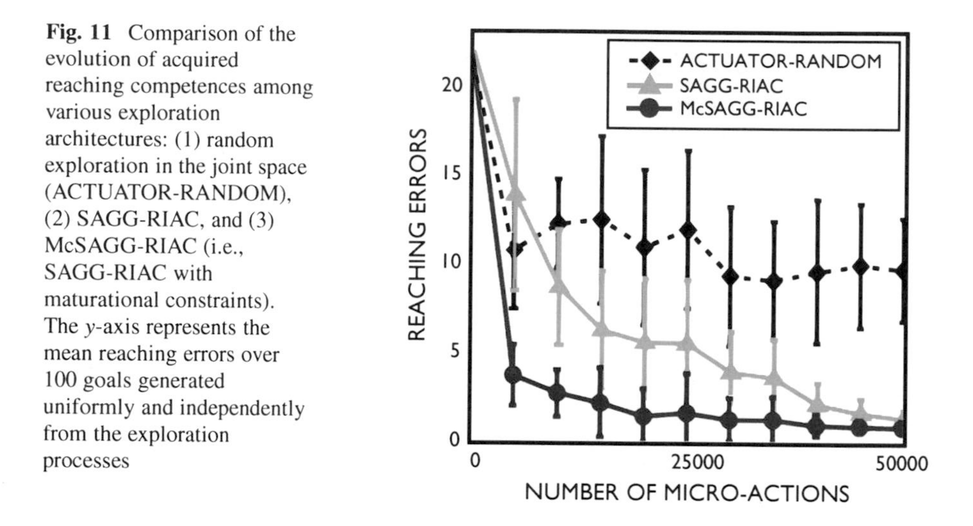

Fig. 11 Comparison of the evolution of acquired reaching competences among various exploration architectures: (1) random exploration in the joint space (ACTUATOR-RANDOM), (2) SAGG-RIAC, and (3) McSAGG-RIAC (i.e., SAGG-RIAC with maturational constraints). The *y*-axis represents the mean reaching errors over 100 goals generated uniformly and independently from the exploration processes

after that $\psi(t)$ reaches the value 5 can be explained by the sudden change of frequency $f(t)$ from $1/3$ to $1/2$ update per time step, that is produced precisely at $\psi(t) = 5$. This is an effective example that clearly shows the capability of the McSAGG algorithm to slow down the evolution of the maturational clock in cases of an important change of complexity of the accessible body and world, according to constraints.

Another experiment can be made to assess the quantitative gain that can be obtained by using maturational constraints in terms of acquired competence to reach goals spread in the reachable space. In this experiment, we use $n = 15$ degrees of freedom in the robotic arm. Figure 11 shows the evolution of competences to reach a set of goals uniformly spread over the reachable space and chosen independently from the exploration process. We observe that using maturational constraints still improves importantly SAGG-RIAC, which was itself already shown to improve other active learning strategies as explained in the previous section.

3.1.4 Maturationally Constrained Learning of Quadruped Locomotion: Coupling Maturational Constraints, Motor Synergies, and Intrinsic Motivation

The following experiment gives an example of how the combination of three families of constraints presented so far, that is, intrinsically motivated exploration in the task space, motor synergies, and maturational constraints, can leverage each other in order to allow a robot to learn a field of motor skills in a high-dimensional complex motor space: learning omnidirectional quadruped locomotion (see Fig. 12).

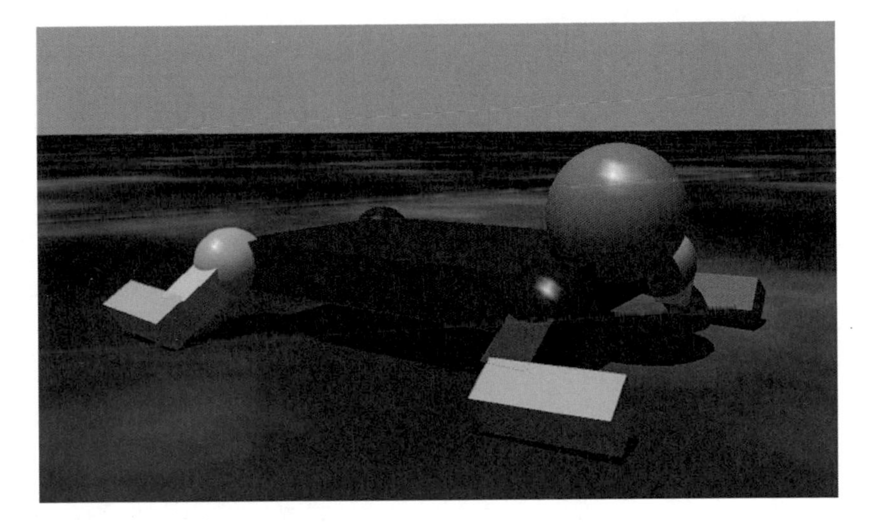

Fig. 12 The simulated quadruped. Physics is simulated using ODE and the Breve simulator (http://www.spiderland.org/)

3.1.4.1 Robotic Setup

In the following experiment, we consider a quadruped robot. Each of its leg is composed of two joints, the first one (the closest to the robot's body) is controlled by two rotational DOF and the second by one rotation (one DOF). Each leg therefore consists of 3 DOF, the robot having in its totality 12 DOF (see Fig. 12).

This robot is controlled using motor synergies Υ which directly specify the phase and amplitude of sinusoids which control the precise rotational value of each DOF trajectory over time (the synergies define target trajectories which are then dynamically tracked by a closed-loop low-level PID controller). These synergies are parameterized using a set of 24 continuous values, 12 representing the phase ph of each joint and the 12 others, the amplitude am: $\Upsilon = \{\mathrm{ph}_{1,2,\ldots,12}; \mathrm{am}_{1,2,\ldots,12}\}$. Each experimentation consists of launching a motor synergy Υ for a fixed amount of time, starting from a fixed position. After this time period, the resulting position x_{f} of the robot is extracted into three dimensions: its position (u, v) and its rotation θ. The correspondence $\Upsilon \rightarrow (u, v, \theta)$ is then kept in memory as a learning exemplar.

The three dimensions u, v, θ are used to define the goal space of the robot. Also, it is important to notice that precise areas reachable by the quadruped cannot be estimated beforehand. In the following, we set the original dimensions of the goal space to $[-45; 45] \times [-45; 45] \times [-2\pi; 2\pi]$ on axis (u, v, θ), which was a priori larger than the reachable space. Then, after having carried out numerous experimentations, it appeared that this goal space was actually more than 25 times the size of the area accessible by the robot (see red contours in Fig. 14).

The implementation of our algorithm in such a robotic setup aims to test if the SAGG-RIAC and McSAGG-RIAC driving methods allow the robot to learn to attain

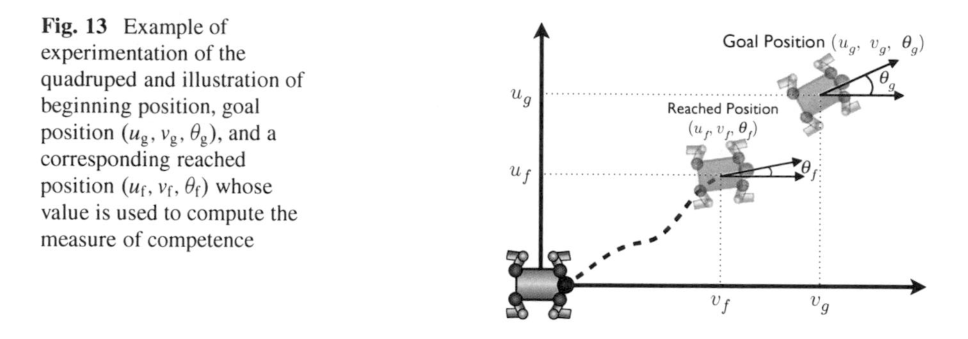

Fig. 13 Example of experimentation of the quadruped and illustration of beginning position, goal position (u_g, v_g, θ_g), and a corresponding reached position (u_f, v_f, θ_f) whose value is used to compute the measure of competence

a maximal amount of reachable positions, avoiding the selection of many goals inside regions which are unreachable or alternatively that have previously been visited.

3.1.4.2 Measure of Competence

In this experiment, we do not consider requirements ρ and only focus on reaching goal positions $x_g = (u_g, v_g, \theta_g)$. In each iteration, the robot is reset to a rest configuration, and goal positions are defined in the robot's own body referential (see Fig. 13). We define the cost function C and thus the competence as linked with the Euclidian distance $D(x_g, x_f)$ after a reaching attempt, which is normalized by the original distance between the rest position, and the goal $D(x_{origin}, x_g)$ (see Fig. 13). This allows, for instance, assigning a same competence level when considering a goal at 1 km from the origin position, which the robot approaches at 0.1 km, and a goal at 100 m, which the robot approaches at 10 m.

In this measure of competence, we consider the rotation factor θ and compute the Euclidian distance using (u, v, θ). Also, dimensions of the goal space are rescaled in [0;1]. Each dimension therefore has the same weight in the estimation of competence (an angle error of $\theta = \frac{1}{2\pi}$ is as important as an error $u = \frac{1}{90}$ or $v = \frac{1}{90}$):

$$C(x_g, x_f, x_{start}) = -\frac{D(x_g, x_f)}{||x_g||} \tag{9}$$

where $C(x_g, x_f, x_{start}) = 0$ if $||x_g|| = 0$.

3.1.4.3 Local Exploration and Reaching

Reaching a goal x_g necessitates the estimation of a motor synergy Υ_i leading to this chosen state x_g. Considering a single starting configuration (the rest configuration) for each experimentation and motor synergies Υ, the forward model which defines this system can be written as the following:

$$\Upsilon \rightarrow (u, v, \theta) \tag{10}$$

Here, we have a direct relationship which only considers the 24 parameters $\{ph_{1,2,\ldots,12}; am_{1,2,\ldots,12}\}$ as inputs of the system and a position in (u, v, θ) as output. We thus have a direct relationship and no context or possible set point, as used in the arm experiment. Also, when considering the inverse model $(u, v, \theta) \rightarrow \Upsilon$ that has to be estimated, the low level of active learning that we use cannot be directly derived from SSA. Instead, we use the following optimization mechanism that can be divided into two different phases: a reaching phase and an exploration phase.

3.1.5 Reaching Phase

The reaching phase deals with reusing the data already learned to compute an inverse model $((u, v, \theta) \rightarrow \Upsilon)_L$ in the locality L of the intended goal $x_g = (u_g, v_g, \theta_g)$. In order to create such an inverse model (numerous can exist), we extract the potentially more reliable data using the following method:

We first compute the set L of the l nearest neighbors of (u_g, v_g, θ_g) and their corresponding motor synergies using an ANN method (Muja and Lowe 2009):

$$L = \{\{u, v, \theta, \Upsilon\}_1, \{u, v, \theta, \Upsilon\}_2, \ldots, \{u, v, \theta, \Upsilon\}_l\} \tag{11}$$

Then, we consider the set M which contains l sets of m elements:

$$M = \left\{ \begin{array}{c} \{\{u, v, \theta, \Upsilon\}_1, \{u, v, \theta, \Upsilon\}_2, \ldots, \{u, v, \theta, \Upsilon\}_m\}_1 \\ \{\{u, v, \theta, \Upsilon\}_1, \{u, v, \theta, \Upsilon\}_2, \ldots, \{u, v, \theta, \Upsilon\}_m\}_2 \\ \ldots \\ \{\{u, v, \theta, \Upsilon\}_1, \{u, v, \theta, \Upsilon\}_2, \ldots, \{u, v, \theta, \Upsilon\}_m\}_l \end{array} \right\}$$

where each set $\{\{u, v, \theta, \Upsilon\}_1, \{u, v, \theta, \Upsilon\}_2, \ldots, \{u, v, \theta, \Upsilon\}_m\}_i$ corresponds to the m nearest neighbors of each Υ_i, $i \in L$ and their corresponding resulting position (u, v, θ).

For each set $\{\{u, v, \theta, \Upsilon\}_1, \{u, v, \theta, \Upsilon\}_2, \ldots, \{u, v, \theta, \Upsilon\}_m\}_i$, we estimate the standard deviation σ of their motor synergies Υ :

$$N = \cup_{i \in M} \left\{ \sigma \left(\Upsilon_j \in \{\{u, v, \theta, \Upsilon\}_{1,\ldots,m}\}_i \right) \right\} \tag{12}$$

Finally, we select the set $O = \{\{u, v, \theta, \Upsilon\}_1, \{u, v, \theta, \Upsilon\}_2, \ldots, \{u, v, \theta, \Upsilon\}_m\}$ inside M such that it minimizes the standard deviation of its synergies:

$$O = \arg\min_N M \tag{13}$$

From O, we estimate a linear inverse model $((u, v, \theta) \rightarrow \Upsilon)$ by using a pseudo-inverse as introduced in the reaching experiment and obtain the synergy Υ_g which corresponds to the desired goal (u_g, v_g, θ_g).

3.1.5.1 Exploration Phase

The system here continuously estimates the distance between the goal x_g and the closest already reached position x_c. If the reaching phase does not manage to make the system come closer to x_g, that is, $D(x_g, x_t) > D(x_g, x_c)$, with x_t as last experimented synergy in an attempt toward x_g, the exploration phase is triggered.

In this phase, the system first considers the nearest neighbor $x_c = (u_c, v_c, \theta_c)$ of the goal (u_g, v_g, θ_g) and gets the corresponding known synergy Υ_c. Then, it adds a random noise *rand*(24) to the 24 parameters $\{\text{ph}_{1,2,\ldots,12}, \text{am}_{1,2,\ldots,12}\}_c$ of this synergy Υ_c which is proportional to the Euclidian distance $D(x_g, x_c)$. The next synergy $\Upsilon_{t+1} = \{\text{ph}_{1,2,\ldots,12}, \text{am}_{1,2,\ldots,12}\}_{t+1}$ to experiment can thus be described using the following equation:

$$\Upsilon_{t+1} = \begin{pmatrix} \{\text{ph}_{1,2,\ldots,12}, \text{am}_{1,2,\ldots,12}\}_c \\ + \lambda \cdot \text{rand}(24) \cdot D(x_g, x_c) \end{pmatrix} \tag{14}$$

where rand(i) returns a vector of i random values in $[-1; 1]$, $\lambda > 0$, and $\{\text{ph}_{1,2,\ldots,12}, \text{am}_{1,2,\ldots,12}\}_c$ the motor synergy which corresponds to x_c.

3.1.5.2 Constraining the Goal Space

In the following, we constrain the goal space using the same maturational mechanism used in the maturationally constrained reaching task presented above. The goal space starts as a small sphere centered around the position $(u, v, \theta) = (0, 0, 0)$, which corresponds to the rest position where the quadruped starts every displacement. Then, according to the evolution of the maturational clock, the radius of this sphere increases, until covering the entire goal space.

3.1.5.3 Constraining the Control Space

Due to the high number of parameters controlling each motor synergy, the learning mechanism faces a highly redundant system. Also, because our framework considers important the fact of performing a maximal amount of tasks (i.e., goals in the task space), instead of different ways to perform a same task, constraints on the control space can be considered.

Let us consider the 24-dimensional space controlling phases and amplitudes as defined as $S = [-2\pi; 2\pi]^{12} \times [0; 1]^{12}$. We set the constrained subspace where possible values can be taken as $[\mu_i - 4\pi\sigma; \mu_i + 4\pi\sigma]^{12} \times [\mu_j - \sigma; \mu_j + \sigma]^{12} \in S$, where μ defines a seed, different for each dimension, around which values can be taken according to a window of size 2σ, σ being function of the maturational clock $\psi(t)$. The value of those seeds is typically an innate constraint over the maturational constraints that should be the result of a biological evolutionary process. As we did not use evolutionary optimization here, we took a short-cut by handcrafting the value of each seed according to the following mechanism: first, we run an experiment only using constraints in the goal space. Once this experiment terminated, we compute histograms of phases and amplitude experimented with during the exploration process. Then, the seed selected for each dimension corresponds to the maximum of the histogram, which represents the most used value during this experiment. Whereas different seeds could be imagined, we found that these handcrafted seeds were adequate for the learning efficiency of the robot.

3.1.5.4 Qualitative Results

Figure 14a presents representative examples of histograms of positions explored by the quadruped inside the goal space u, v, θ after 10,000 experimentations (running of motor synergies during the same fixed amount of time) and Fig. 14b shows examples of the repartitions of positions inside the goal space after 10,000 experimentations, when using the following exploration mechanisms:

ACTUATOR-RANDOM corresponds to a uniform selection of parameters controlling motor synergies (values inside the 24-dimensional space of phases and amplitude). ACTUATOR-RIAC corresponds to the original version of R-IAC (Baranes and Oudeyer 2009) that actively generates actions inside the same space of synergies as ACTUATOR-RANDOM. SAGG-RANDOM is a method where the learning is situated at the level of goals which are generated uniformly in the goal space u, v, θ. Here, the low level of active learning used is the same as in SAGG-RIAC. Then, the SAGG-RIAC method corresponds to the self-generation of goals actively inside the whole goal space, while McSAGG-RIAC also considers maturational constraints in both control and goal spaces.

Displaying both histograms and reached positions (i.e., displacement in the robot's own referential) allows observing different important qualitative aspects of the learning process: Whereas histograms efficiently show the relative quantities of positions which have been experimented in the goal space u, v, θ, they prevent the precise observation of the volume where positions have been reached. This information is then displayed by observing the repartition of visited positions (see Fig. 14b).

Comparing the two first exploration mechanisms (ACTUATOR-RANDOM and ACTUATOR-RIAC) we cannot distinguish any notable difference, the space explored appears similar, and the extent of explored space on the (u, v) axis is comprised in the interval $[-5; 5]$ for u and $[-2.5; 2.5]$ for v on both graphs. Nevertheless, these results are important when comparing histograms of exploration (Fig. 14a) and visited positions (Fig. 14b) to the size of the reachable area (red lines in Fig. 14). It indeed shows that, in the 24-dimensional space controlling motor

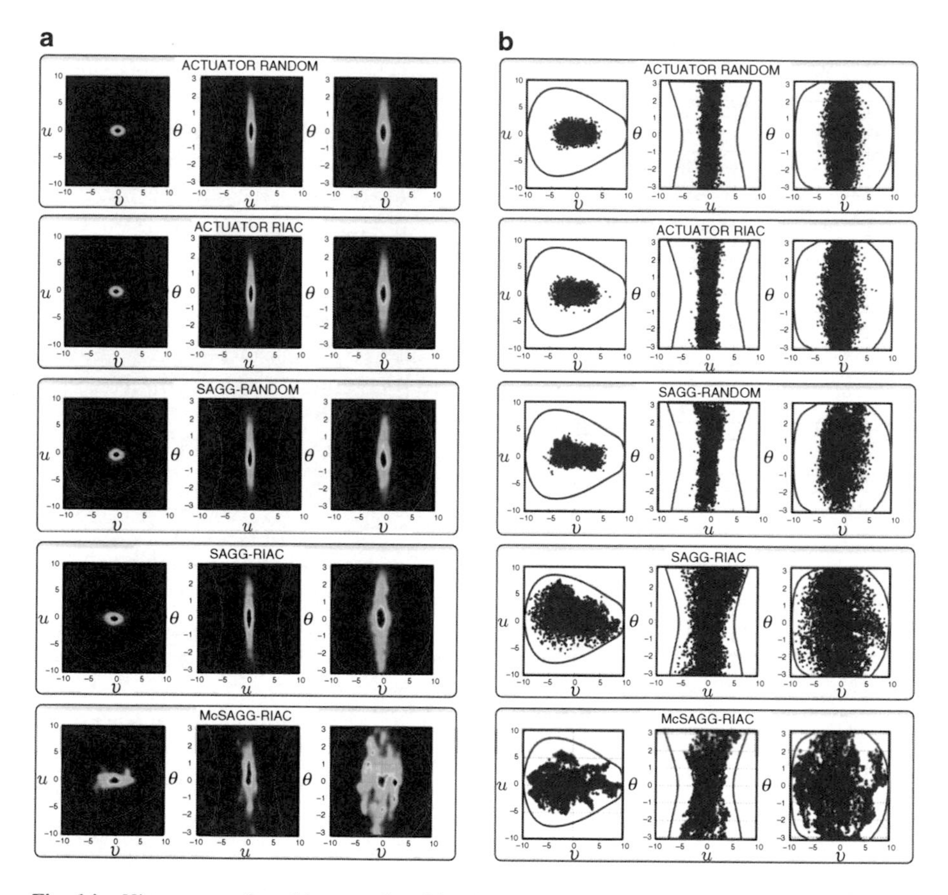

Fig. 14 Histograms of positions explored by the quadruped inside the goal space u, v, θ after 10,000 experimentations (running a motor synergy during a fixed amount of time), using different exploration mechanisms

synergies, an extremely large part of values leads to positions close to $(0, 0, 0)$ and thus does not allow the robot to perform a large displacement. It allows us to see that reaching the entire goal space is a difficult task, which could be discovered using exploration in the space of motor synergies, only after extremely long time periods. Moreover, we notice that the difference between u and v scales is due to the inherent structure of the robot, which simplifies the way to go forward and backward rather than shifting left or right.

Considering SAGG methods, it is important to note the difference between the reachable area and the goal space. In Fig. 14, red lines correspond to the estimated reachable area that is comprised of $[-10; 10] \times [-10; 10] \times [-\pi; \pi]$, whereas the goal space is much larger: $[-45; 45] \times [-45; 45] \times [-2\pi; 2\pi]$. We are also able to notice the asymmetric aspect of its repartition according to the v-axis, which is due to the decentered weight of the robot's head.

The SAGG-RANDOM method seems to slightly increase the space covered on the u- and v-axis compared to ACTUATOR methods, as shown by the higher concentration of positions explored in the interval $[-5; -3] \cup [3; 5]$ of u. However, this change does not seem very important when comparing SAGG-RANDOM to any previous algorithm.

SAGG-RIAC, contrary to SAGG-RANDOM, shows a large exploration range compared to other methods: The surface in u has almost twice as much coverage than using previous algorithms and, in v, up to three times; there is a maximum of 7.5 in v where the previous algorithms were at 2.5. These last results emphasize the capability of SAGG-RIAC to drive the learning process inside reachable areas that are not easily accessible (hardly discovered by chance). Nevertheless, when observing histograms of SAGG-RIAC, we can notice the high concentration of explored positions around $(0, 0, 0)$, the starting position where every experimentation is launched. This signifies that, even if SAGG-RIAC is able to explore a large volume of the reachable space, as shown in Fig. 14b, it still spends many iterations exploring the same areas.

According to the repartition of positions shown in Fig. 14b for the McSAGG-RIAC exploration mechanism, we can notice a volume explored comparable to the one explored by SAGG-RIAC. Nevertheless, it seems that McSAGG-RIAC visits a slightly lower part of the space, avoiding some areas, while explored area seems to be visited with a higher concentration. This higher concentration is confirmed via observation of histograms of McSAGG-RIAC: Indeed, whereas every other methods focused during a large part of their exploration time around the position $(0, 0, 0)$, McSAGG-RIAC also focuses in areas distant from this position. The higher consideration of different areas is due to constraints fixed in the goal space, which allows a fast discovery of reachable goals and ways to reach them, whereas without constraints, the system spends high amount of time attempting unreachable goals and thus performs movements which have a high probability to lead to position close to $(0, 0, 0)$. Also, small areas not visited can be explained by the high focalization of McSAGG-RIAC in others, as well as the limitation of values taken in the control space.

3.1.5.5 Quantitative Results

In this section, we aim to test the efficiency of the learned database to guide the quadruped robot to reach a set of goal positions from its rest configuration. Here, we consider a test database of 100 goals and compute the distance between each goal attempted and the reached position. Figure 15 shows performances of methods introduced previously. Also, in addition to the evaluation of the efficiency of McSAGG-RIAC with constraints in both control and goal spaces (called McSAGG-RIAC In&Out in Fig. 15), we introduce the evaluation of McSAGG-RIAC when only using constraints on the goal space (McSAGG-RIAC Out).

First of all, we can observe the higher efficiency of SAGG-RIAC compared to methods ACTUATOR-RANDOM, ACTUATOR-RIAC, and SAGG-RANDOM

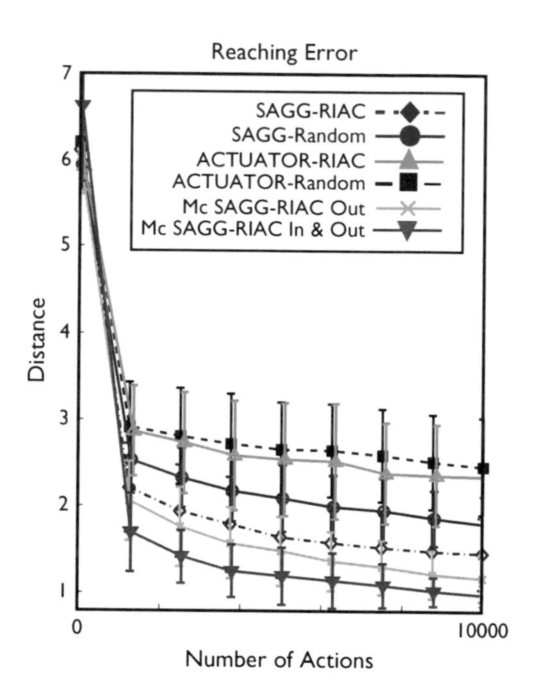

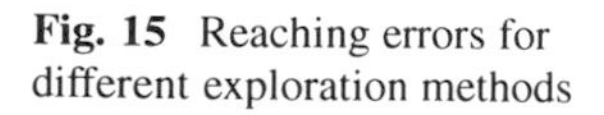

Fig. 15 Reaching errors for different exploration methods

which can be observed after only 1,000 iterations. The high decreasing velocity of the reaching error (in the number of experimentations) is due to the consideration of regions limited to a small number of elements (30 in this experiment). It allows the system to create a very high number of regions within a small interval of time, which helps the system to discover and focus on reachable regions and its surrounding area.

ACTUATOR-RIAC shows slightly more efficient performances than ACTUATOR-RANDOM. Also, even if SAGG-RANDOM is less efficient than SAGG-RIAC, we can observe its highly decreasing reaching errors compared to ACTUATOR methods, which allow it to be significantly more efficient than these method when considered at 10,000 iterations.

McSAGG-RIAC Out shows better results than SAGG-RIAC since the beginning of the evolution (1,000 iterations) and decreases with a higher velocity until the end of the experiment. This illustrates the high potential of coupling constraints situated in the goal space and SAGG-RIAC in such a complex robotic setup.

Eventually, we can observe that using both constraints in both control and goal spaces as introduced by McSAGG-RANDOM In and Out allows to obtain significantly more efficient results than SAGG-RIAC without constraints ($p = 0.0055$ at the end of the exploration process) and better than when only using constraints in the goal space with a measure of significance $p = 0.05$.

In such a highly redundant robot, coupling different types of maturational constraints with the SAGG-RIAC process thus allows to obtain significantly better performances than when using the SAGG-RIAC competence-based intrinsic motivation algorithm without maturational constraints. It is important to note that "better performances" means here not only faster learning but better asymptotic generalization, as was already shown in earlier work on active learning (Cohn et al. 1994).

3.1.5.6 Summary

These experiments exemplify the high efficiency of methods that drive the exploration at the level of goals and then show that adding up maturational constraints improves significantly the efficiency of intrinsically motivated exploration and learning. As illustrated by qualitative results, SAGG methods, and especially SAGG-RIAC and McSAGG-RIAC, allow the robot to drive efficiently to explore large spaces containing areas hardly discovered by chance, when limits of reachability are impossible to predict. In spite of using motor primitives that already drastically reduce the huge space of physically possible quadruped movements, the dimensionality of the control space is still high, and, in such spaces, the experiment showed how McSAGG-RIAC could significantly improve the performances in generalization over SAGG-RIAC for learning precise omnidirectional locomotion.

Eventually, we conclude that the bidirectional coupling of maturational constraints and intrinsic motivation shall allow the self-focalization of goals inside maturationally restrained areas, which maximizes the information needed for constraints to evolve, increasing progressively the complexity of the accessible world and thus of the acquired competences. Thus, it will be highly stimulating in the future to explore more systematically, and in various sensorimotor spaces, how the results outlined here could be reproduced and extended.

4 Integrating Intrinsic Motivation with Socially Guided Learning

Because of its very nature, intrinsic motivation has often been studied separately (as in the developmental robotics literature) and opposed [as in the psychology and educational theory literature (Ryan and Deci 2000)], to socially guided learning, many forms of which can be seen as extrinsically driven learning. Yet, in the daily life of humans, these two families of mechanisms strongly interact. Intrinsic motivation can motivate a child to follow the lessons of an interesting teacher. But reversely and most importantly for the main question approached in this chapter, social guidance can drive a learner into new intrinsically motivating spaces/activities which it may continue to explore alone and for their own sake but might not have discovered without the social guidance. For example, many people practice activities like Sudoku, tennis, painting, or sculpture driven by intrinsic motivation, but most of them discovered the very existence of those explorable activities by observing others practice it. Furthermore, while they practice activities like painting or Sudoku driven by intrinsic motivation, they may acquire new strategies for achieving those intrinsically motivated activities by observing others or by listening to their advices. Thus, social guidance is often a fundamental mechanism allowing an intrinsically motivated learner both to discover new potential explorable task spaces as well as new example of successful control strategies.

This role of social guidance shall quickly become essential and necessary for any robot built for open-ended development in high-dimensional unbounded spaces, even when equipped with advanced competence-based intrinsic motivation operating on sophisticated sensorimotor primitives and with maturational constraints. Indeed, there are at least three important potential limits to the developmental constraints on intrinsic motivation presented so far in this chapter, that we describe in the following:

How to discover isolated islands of learnable goals? While maturational constraints in a task space can allow us to harness the problem of unboundedness by growing progressively the explorable region(s), it may as a side effect make it difficult for a sole intrinsic motivation system to discover disconnected islands of learnability in the whole task space. Let us take the example of a grasping task space defined in terms of the shape properties of objects. This is an unbounded space since the space of all objects around us is infinite (especially if we include things like walls, trees, or clouds as potential objects to learn how to grasp). Using maturational constraints in a competence-based approach would amount to start from a few basic object shapes for which to explore grasp motor commands and see how they work and then progressively and continuously extend the space of explorable shapes to try to grasp. This would allow the robot to learn efficiently how to grasp a growing set of object shapes. Yet, the shape space is complicated, and there are many object shapes which the robot could learn to grasp but will never learn because either it would take too much time for the maturationally growing explorable space to reach them or because they are surrounded by unlearnable shapes that would prevent the explorable space to grow and reach them. Social guidance could be of essential help here: Instead of waiting that the explorable space grows until reaching those objects, a simple social signal drawing the attention and motivation of the learner toward new specific objects in these islands could be used to start a new local and growing region of exploration around this object. The same applies to all kinds of task spaces. Initial work toward this objective has been presented in Nguyen et al. (2011).

How to discover new explorable task spaces? All the experiments presented above, similarly to what exists in many other models of intrinsically motivated exploration in the literature, assumed a small finite set of predefined tasks spaces, that is, a small set of groups of variables describing aspects of the world that the robot may learn to manipulate through exploration. The reaching task experiment involved only one such task space, while the Playground Experiment mixed several predefined task spaces. As a consequence, the robot could potentially achieve open-ended development of skills within those task spaces but was impossible for it to learn skills outside those task spaces, for the simple reason that they had no mechanism for discovering and representing novel task spaces, that is, novel groups of variables potentially interesting to learn to manipulate. In principle, modifications of the associated intrinsic motivation architecture could be done to address this limitation. One could provide the robot with a very large set of potential task space variables, as well as with operators to build new such variables, and then use a higher level active exploration mechanisms which would generate, sample, and select the new task spaces in which lower-level intrinsically motivated exploration could provide competence progress. Yet, even if one would constrain task spaces to be composed of only limited number of dimensions/variables (e.g., below six or seven), such an approach would have to face a very hard combinatorial problem. If one would like to learn the same kind of task variety as a human infant does, then the number of variables that may be considered by the learner shall be large. And as a mechanical consequence, the number of potential subsets of these variables, defining potentially new task spaces, would grow exponentially in such a way that even active exploration would be again inefficient. Thus here again, social guidance may be essential: Either through observation or direct gestural or linguistic guidance, a learner may infer the task dimensions/variables that characterize a new task space to explore later on through intrinsic motivation. The literature on robot learning by imitation/demonstration has already developed statistical inference mechanisms allowing to infer new task constraints/dimensions (Calinon et al. 2007; Cederborg et al. 2010; Lopes et al. 2009; Ng and Russell 2000). These techniques could usefully be reused by intrinsically motivated learning architectures to expand efficiently the set of explorable task spaces. Initial work in this direction has, for example, been presented in Thomaz and Breazeal (2008).

How to discover new explorable sensorimotor primitives? Similarly to task spaces, all the experiments presented earlier and many other approaches in the literature assumed that the set of sensorimotor "tools," that is, sensorimotor variables and the primitives operating on them, were predefined and finite. Of course, using techniques like reinforcement learning can allow a robot to learn how new sequences of motor commands can allow it to achieve a given task, but the dimensions in which these elementary commands are encoded are typically finite and predefined (but yet might be high dimensional). Likewise, the set of sensorimotor primitives, providing the structure necessary to bootstrap the intrinsically motivated learning of many complicated tasks as argued earlier, is often predefined and thus limited. Just like for expanding the space of explorable task spaces, social guidance can also be an essential mechanism allowing a robot to discover new useful control dimensions, and new associated motor primitives, that it may reuse to explore a task space through intrinsic motivation. Let us take the example of the "playing tennis" space. In addition to being a space typically discovered by seeing others play tennis, observation of others is also crucial for the discovery of (1) which control variables are important, such as, the relative position of the feet to the net at the moment of striking the ball, and (2) which motor primitives based on those control dimensions shall be explored, such as, the forehand, backhand, or volley motor primitives.

Once prototypical backhand or volley primitives have been observed, the learner can explore through intrinsic motivation the space of variations of these primitives and how to tune their parameters to the real-time trajectory of the ball. But without the observation of such movements in others, learning to play tennis efficiently would be an extremely difficult challenge. Finally, at a finer grain, when prototypes and dimensions for new sensorimotor primitives have been discovered, social guidance can continue to play in concert with intrinsic motivation by continuously providing new examples of variations of those primitives that may be repeated and explored by the learner (e.g., see Nguyen et al. 2011). Again, the literature on robot learning by imitation/demonstration has elaborated many algorithms allowing the acquisition of new motor primitives (Billard et al. 2008; Calinon et al. 2007; Cederborg et al. 2010; Grollman and Jenkins 2010), and future research in developmental robotics might strongly benefit from integrating computational models of intrinsic motivation and socially guided learning.

5 Conclusion

Research on computational approaches to intrinsic motivation has allowed important conceptual advances in developmental robotics in the last decade, opening new horizons for the building of machines capable of open-ended learning and development. Many kinds of models and formalisms have been proposed and integrated in sophisticated architectures, such as in intrinsically motivated reinforcement learning, coming from a wide variety of research groups and backgrounds, ranging from machine learning, statistics, cognitive modeling to robotics. Diverse proof-of-concept experiments have also been achieved.

Yet, several important challenges are now in need to be addressed. Among them, a paramount objective is to study how it is possible to scale those conceptual and proof-of-concept initial results to the real world. How can a robot, equipped with a rich sensorimotor apparatus, develop new skills in an open high-dimensional unbounded uncontrolled environment, just as human children do? We are very far from having both conceptual and technical answer(s) to this question. Intrinsic motivation will certainly be a key element, but this chapter has shown that it can only become useful and used when other complementary mechanisms are harmoniously integrated in a single developmental architecture. Intrinsic motivation alone is indeed nearly helpless in unconstrained unbounded sensorimotor spaces. The growth of complexity should be controlled by the interaction of intrinsic motivation and other families of developmental constraints. In this chapter, we have argued that sensorimotor primitives, self-organization and embodiment, task space representations, maturational mechanisms, and social guidance should be considered as essential complements to intrinsic motivation for open-ended development in the real world. Other families of mechanisms, which we did not discuss, will be equally important, including developmental biases on representations, on mechanisms for creating abstractions, on operators for combining and reusing knowledge and skills and creating novel representations, or on statistical inference.

The challenges posed by the real world cannot be reduced to mere algorithmic complexity and/or efficiency problems. Unlearnability, high dimensionality, and unboundedness introduce new fundamental conceptual obstacles. Constraints and biases, either innate or self-organized, either static or evolving, are unavoidable for any real-world developmental learning system. And most probably, those constraints that include intrinsic motivation together with maturation or social guidance will function efficiently only when integrated together properly. How shall social guidance, in its many different forms, be integrated with computational models of intrinsically motivated learning? How shall maturation and intrinsic motivation control each other? How novel sensorimotor primitives and associated higher-level representations and abstractions can be constructed through the interaction of intrinsic motivation, maturation, and social learning? Which constraints should be pre-wired explicitly, and which one should be self-organized? Can we understand how a given body/embodiment can help the development of certain families of skills rather than others? These fundamental questions shall become an essential target of research on intrinsic motivation and developmental robotics.

Furthermore, the unavoidability of constraints and biases in the real world indicates that no general purpose machine can be made capable of learning universally and, at the same time efficiently, anything in any environment. As a consequence, a set of fundamental conceptual questions raised by trying to scale to the real world concern the very concept of open-ended and task-independent learning: We should try to understand better how this property that we observe in human children is different from omni-capable any-task learning. Related to this, we should try to understand how certain families of constraints in certain families of environment allow or disallow the development of certain families of skills.

Finally, future research shall strongly rely on larger-scale, "more real-world" experiments with high-dimensional robots in environments functionally and structurally as similar as those encountered by human infants. There were many good reasons for conducting toy-level experiments so far, but this had the consequence to short-cut much of the specific conceptual and technical difficulties posed by the real world. Confronting to the reality shall be an efficient constraint to guide research in a direction that may allow robots to acquire novel skills like human infants do. Furthermore, an associated methodological need for future research is to construct both explanations and understanding of our experiments such as to provide an appropriate emphasis on all components/constraints that allow these experiments to actually "work." Because one may be most interested by intrinsic motivation, it is sometimes tempting to emphasize the role of intrinsic motivation in the interpretation of experimental results. This is illustrated by the Playground Experiment: While often presented, including by us, under the light of the concepts of "learning progress" and intrinsic motivation, its success was actually due to the *combination* and *interaction* of "learning progress"-based intrinsic motivation with an innate parameterized repertoire of dynamic sensorimotor primitives.

As long held by the embodied and situated cognition literature, adaptive behavior as well as sensorimotor and cognitive development shall not be the result of isolated localized components but rather the results of the dynamical interactions of all the components of a complete creature—mental and body components—among themselves and with their physical and social environment. Thus, research on intrinsic motivation shall now focus on "boundaries": Establishing coordinated links between intrinsic motivation and its functional boundaries, that is, with the other constraints on exploration and learning of the complete creature, shall help robots to control better the progressive growth of the boundaries of their own knowledge and capabilities.

Acknowledgements Many of the ideas presented in this chapter benefited from discussions and joint work with our colleagues, in particular, Jérome Béchu, Fabien Benureau, Thomas Cederborg, Fabien Danieau, Haylee Fogg, David Filliat, Paul Fudal, Verena V. Hafner, Matthieu Lapeyre, Manuel Lopes, Olivier Ly, Olivier Mangin, Mai Nguyen, Luc Steels, Pierre Rouanet, and Andrew Whyte. This research was partially funded by ERC Starting Grant EXPLORER 240007.

References

Angluin, D.: Queries and concept learning. Mach. Learn. **2**, 319–342 (1988)

Asada, M., Hosoda, K., Kuniyoshi, Y., Ishiguro, H., Inui, T., Yoshikawa, Y., Ogino, M., Yoshida, C.: Cognitive developmental robotics: A survey. IEEE Trans. Auton. Mental Dev. **1**(1), 12–34 (2009)

Bakker, B., Schmidhuber, J.: Hierarchical reinforcement learning based on subgoal discovery and subpolicy specialization. In: Proceedings of the 8th Conference on Intelligent Autonomous Systems (IAS-8) (2004)

Baldassarre, G., Mirolli, M.: Temporal-difference competence-based intrinsic motivation (TD-CB-IM): A mechanism that uses the td-error as an intrinsic reinforcement for deciding which skill to learn when. In: Baldassarre, G., Mirolli, M. (eds.) Intrinsically Motivated Learning in Natural and Artificial Systems, pp. 255–276. Springer, Berlin (2012)

Ball, P.: The Self-made Tapestry-Pattern formation in nature. Oxford University Press, New York (1999)

Baranes, A., Oudeyer, P.-Y.: Riac: Robust intrinsically motivated exploration and active learning. IEEE Trans. Auton. Mental Dev. **1**(3), 155–169 (2009)

Baranes, A., Oudeyer, P.-Y.: Intrinsically motivated goal exploration for active motor learning in robots: A case study. In: Proceedings of IEEE/RSJ International Conference on Intelligent Robots and Systems (IROS 2010) (2010a)

Baranes, A., Oudeyer, P.-Y.: Maturationally constrained competence-based intrinsically motivated learning. In: Proceedings of IEEE International Conference on Development and Learning (ICDL 2010) (2010b)

Baranes, A., Oudeyer, P.-Y.: The interaction of maturational constraints and intrinsic motivations in active motor development. In: Proceedings of IEEE ICDL-Epirob 2011 (2011)

Baranes, A., Oudeyer, P-Y.: Active Learning of Inverse Models with Intrinsically Motivated Goal Exploration in Robots, Robotics and Autonomous Systems, http://dx.doi.org/10.1016/j.robot.2012.05.008, (2012)

Barto, A., Singh, S., Chenatez, N.: Intrinsically motivated learning of hierarchical collections of skills. In: Proceedings of the 3rd International Conference Development Learning, San Diego, pp. 112–119 (2004)

Barto, A.G.: Intrinsic motivation and reinforcement learning. In: Baldassarre, G., Mirolli, M. (eds.) Intrinsically Motivated Learning in Natural and Artificial Systems, pp. 17–47. Springer, Berlin (2012)
Berk, L.: Child Development. Allyn and Bacon, Boston (2008)
Berlyne, D.: Conflict, Arousal and Curiosity. McGraw-Hill, New York (1960)
Berthier, N.E., Clifton, R., McCall, D., Robin, D.: Proximodistal structure of early reaching in human infants. Exp. Brain Res. **127**(3), 259–269 (1999)
Billard, A., Calinon, S., Dillmann, R., Schaal, S.: Robot programming by demonstration. In: Handbook of Robotics. Springer, Berlin (2008)
Bishop, C.M.: Neural Networks for Pattern Recognition. Oxford University Press, Oxford (1995)
Bishop, C.M.: Pattern Recognition and Machine Learning (Information Science and Statistics). Springer, Berlin (1st ed., 2006/corr. 2nd printing edition, 2007)
Bjorklund, D.: The role of immaturity in human development. Psychol. Bull. **122**(2), 153–169 (1997)
Blank, D., Kumar, D., Meeden, L., Marshall, J.: Bringing up robot: Fundamental mechanisms for creating a self-motivated, self-organizing architecture. Cybern. Syst. **36**(2), 125–150 (2002)
Brafman, R., Tennenholtz, M.: R-max: A general polynomial time algorithm for near-optimal reinforcement learning. In: Proceedings of IJCAI'01 (2001)
Bremner, J., Slater, A. (eds.): Theories of Infant Development. Blackwell, Cambridge (2003)
Bronson, G.: The postnatal growth of visual capacity. Child. Dev. **45**(4), 873–890 (1974)
Calinon, S., Guenter, F., Billard, A.: On learning, representing and generalizing a task in a humanoid robot. IEEE Trans. Syst. Man Cybern. B, **37**(2), 286–298 (2007)
Castro, R., Novak, R.: Minimax bounds for active learning. IEEE Trans. Inform. Theory **54**, 151–156 (2008)
Cazalets, J., Borde, M., Clarac, F.: Localization and organization of the central pattern generator for hindlimb locomotion in newborn rat. J. Neurosci. **15**, 4943–4951 (1995)
Cederborg, T., Ming, L., Baranes, A., Oudeyer, P.-Y.: Incremental local online gaussian mixture regression for imitation learning of multiple tasks. In: Proceedings of IEEE/RSJ International Conference on Intelligent Robots and Systems (IROS 2010) (2010)
Chaloner, K., Verdinelli, I.: Bayesian experimental design: A review. J. Stat. Sci. **10**, 273–304 (1995)
Chung, W., Fu, L.-C., Hsu, S.-H.: Motion control. In: Handbook of Robotics, pp. 133–159. Springer, Berlin (2008)
Cohn, D., Atlas, L., Ladner, R.: Improving generalization with active learning. Mach. Learn. **15**(2), 201–221 (1994)
Cohn, D., Ghahramani, Z., Jordan, M.: Active learning with statistical models. J. Artif. Intell. Res. **4**, 129–145 (1996)
Csikszentmihalyi, M.: Creativity-Flow and the Psychology of Discovery and Invention. Harper Perennial, New York (1996)
d'Avella, A., Portone, A., Fernandez, L., Lacquaniti, F.: Control of fast-reaching movement by muscle synergies combinations. J. Neurosci. **26**(30), 7791–7810 (2006)
d'Avella, A., Saltiel, P., Bizzi, E.: Combinations of muscle synergies in the construction of a natural motor behavior. Nat. Neurosci. **6**, 300–308 (2003)
Dayan, P.: Exploration from generalisation mediated by multiple controllers. In: Baldassarre, G., Mirolli, M. (eds.) Intrinsically Motivated Learning in Natural and Artificial Systems, pp. 73–91. Springer, Berlin (2012)
Dayan, P., Belleine, W.: Reward, motivation and reinforcement learning. Neuron **36**, 285–298 (2002)
De Charms, R.: Personal Causation: The Internal Affective Determinants of Behavior. Academic, New York (1968)
Deci, E., Ryan, M.: Intrinsic Motivation and Self-determination in Human Behavior. Plenum, New York (1985)
Dick, T., Oku, Y., Romaniuk, J., Cherniack, N.: Interaction between cpgs for breathing and swallowing in the cat. J. Physiol. **465**, 715–730 (1993)

Doya, K.: Metalearning and neuromodulation. Neural Netw. **15**(4–5), 495–506 (2002)
Eyre, J.: Development and Plasticity of the Corticospinal System in Man. Neural Plast.; **10**(1–2), 93–106 (2003)
Faller, D., Klingmüller, U., Timmer, J.: Simulation methods for optimal experimental design in systems biology. Simulation **79**, 717–725 (2003)
Fedorov, V.: Theory of Optimal Experiment. Academic, New York (1972)
Festinger, L.: A Theory of Cognitive Dissonance. Row & Peterson, Evanston (1957)
Fisher, K., Silvern, L.: Stages and individual differences in cognitive development. Annu. Rev. Psychol. **36**, 613–648 (1985)
Franceschini, N., Pichon, J., Blanes, C.: From insect vision to robot vision. Phil. Trans. R. Soc. Lond. B **337**, 283–294 (1992)
Ghahramani, Z.: Solving inverse problems using an em approach to density estimation. In: Mozer, M., Smolensky, P., Toureztky, D., Elman, J., Weigend, A. (eds.) Proceedings of the 1993 Connectionist Models Summer School (1993)
Gibson, J.: The Ecological Approach to Visual Perception. Lawrence Erlbaum Associates, Hillsdale (1986)
Grollman, D.H., Jenkins, O.C.: Incremental learning of subtasks from unsegmented demonstration. In: International Conference on Intelligent Robots and Systems, Taipei (2010)
Hart, S., Grupen, R.: Intrinsically motivated hierarchical manipulation. In: Proceedings of the 2008 IEEE Conference on Robots and Automation (ICRA) (2008)
Hart, S., Grupen, R.: Intrinsically motivated affordance discovery and modeling. In: Baldassarre, G., Mirolli, M. (eds.) Intrinsically Motivated Learning in Natural and Artificial Systems, pp. 279–300. Springer, Berlin (2012)
Huang, X., Weng, J.: Novelty and reinforcement learning in the value system of developmental robots. In: Prince, C., Demiris, Y., Marom, Y., Kozima, H., Balkenius, C. (eds.) Proceedings of the 2nd International Workshop on Epigenetic Robotics : Modeling Cognitive Development in Robotic Systems, pp. 47–55. Lund University Cognitive Studies 94, Lund (2002)
Hull, C.L.: Principles of Behavior: An Introduction to Behavior Theory. Appleton-Century-Croft, New York (1943)
Hunt, J.M.: Intrinsic motivation and its role in psychological development. Nebraska Symp. Motiv. **13**, 189–282 (1965)
Iida, F., Pfeifer, R.: Cheap and rapid locomotion of a quadruped robot: Self-stabilization of bounding gait. In: Proceedings of the 8th International Conference on Intelligent Autonomous Systems (IAS-8), Amsterdam, Netherlands, Groen, F. et al. (Eds.) (2004)
James, W.: The Principles of Psychology. Harvard University Press, Cambridge (1890)
Johnson, M.: Functional brain development in humans. Nat. Rev. Neurosci. **2**(7), 475–483 (2001)
Kagan, J.: Motives and development. J. Pers. Soc. Psychol. **22**, 51–66 (1972)
Kakade, S., Dayan, P.: Dopamine: Generalization and bonuses. Neural Netw. **15**, 549–559 (2002)
Kaplan, F., Oudeyer, P.-Y.: The progress-drive hypothesis: An interpretation of early imitation. In: Nehaniv, C., Dautenhahn, K. (eds.) Models and Mechanisms of Imitation and Social Learning: Behavioural, Social and Communication Dimensions, pp. 361–377. Cambridge University Press, Cambridge (2007)
Kemp, C., Edsinger, A.: What can i control?: The development of visual categories for a robots body and the world that it influences. In: In 5th IEEE International Conference on Development and Learning (ICDL-06), Special Session on Autonomous Mental Development (2006)
Khatib, O.: A unified approach for motion and force control of robot manipulators: The operational space formulation. IEEE J. Robot. Autom. **3**(1), 43–53 (1987)
Konczak, J., Borutta, M., Dichgans, J.: The development of goal-directed reaching in infants. Learning to produce task-adequate patterns of joint torque. Exp. Brain Res. **106**(1), 156–168 (1997)
Kumar, S., Narasimhan, K., Patwardhan, S., Prasad, V.: Experiment design, identification and control in large-scale chemical processes. In: The 2010 International Conference on Modelling, Identification and Control (ICMIC), pp. 155–160 (2010)

Lee, M., Meng, Q., Chao, F.: Staged competence learning in developmental robotics. Adap. Behav. **15**(3), 241–255 (2007)
Lee, W.: Neuromotor synergies as a basis for coordinated intentional action. J. Mot. Behav. **16**, 135–170 (1984)
Lopes, M., Melo, F., Montesano, L.: Active learning for reward estimation in inverse reinforcement learning. In: Proceedings of European Conference on Machine Learning (ECML/PKDD) (2009)
Lopes, M., Oudeyer, P.-Y.: Active learning and intrinsically motivated exploration in robots: Advances and challenges (guest editorial): IEEE Trans. Auton. Mental Dev. **2**(2), 65–69 (2010)
Lungarella, M., Metta, G., Pfeifer, R., Sandini, G.: Developmental robotics: A survey. Connect. Sci. **15**(4), 151–190 (2003)
Ly, O., Lapeyre, M., Oudeyer, P.-Y.: Bio-inspired vertebral column, compliance and semi-passive dynamics in a lightweight robot. In: Proceedings of IEEE/RSJ International Conference on Intelligent Robots and Systems (IROS 2011) (2011)
Ly, O., Oudeyer, P.-Y.: Acroban the humanoid: Playful and compliant physical child-robot interaction. In: ACM Siggraph Emerging Technologies, pp. 1–1 (2010)
MacNeilage, P.: The Origin of Speech. Oxford University Press, Oxford (2008)
Meltzoff, A., Moore, M.: Imitation of facial and manual gestures by human neonates. Science **198**(4312), 75–8 (1977)
Merrick, K.E.: Novelty and beyond: Towards combined motivation models and integrated learning architectures. In: Baldassarre, G., Mirolli, M. (eds.) Intrinsically Motivated Learning in Natural and Artificial Systems, pp. 209–233. Springer, Berlin (2012)
Meyer, J.A., Wilson, S.W. (eds.): A Possibility for Implementing Curiosity and Boredom in Model-Building Neural Controllers. MIT/Bradford Books, Cambridge (1991)
Mirolli, M., Baldassarre, G.: Functions and mechanisms of intrinsic motivations: The knowledge versus competence distinction. In: Baldassarre, G., Mirolli, M. (eds.) Intrinsically Motivated Learning in Natural and Artificial Systems, pp. 47–72. Springer, Berlin (2012)
Modayil, J., Pilarski, P., White, A., Degris, T., Sutton, R.: Off-policy knowledge maintenance for robots. In: Proceedings of Robotics Science and Systems Workshop (Towards Closing the Loop: Active Learning for Robotics) (2010)
Montgomery, K.: The role of exploratory drive in learning. J. Comp. Physiol. Psychol. **47**, 60–64 (1954)
Moore, A.: Fast, robust adaptive control by learning only forward models. In: Advances in Neural Information Processing Systems, vol. 4 (1992)
Muja, M., Lowe, D.: Fast approximate nearest neighbors with automatic algorithm. In: International Conference on Computer Vision Theory and Applications (VISAPP'09) (2009)
Ng, A.Y., Russell, S.: Algorithms for inverse reinforcement learning. In: Proceedings of the 17th International Conference on Machine Learning, pp. 663–670. Morgan Kaufmann, San Francisco (2000)
Nguyen, M., Baranes, A., Oudeyer, P.-Y.: Bootstrapping intrinsically motivated learning with human demonstrations. In: Proceedings of IEEE ICDL-Epirob 2011 (2011)
Nguyen-Tuong, D., Peters, J.: Model learning in robotics: A survey. Cogn. Process. **12**(4), 319–340 (2011)
Oudeyer, P.-Y.: On the impact of robotics in behavioral and cognitive sciences: From insect navigation to human cognitive development. IEEE Trans. Auton. Mental Dev. **2**(1), 2–16 (2010)
Oudeyer, P.-Y. Kaplan, F.: The discovery of communication. Connect. Sci. **18**(2), 189–206 (2006)
Oudeyer, P.-Y. Kaplan, F.: What is intrinsic motivation? A typology of computational approaches. Front. Neurorobot. **1**, 6 (2007)
Oudeyer, P.-Y. Kaplan, F.: How can we define intrinsic motivations ? In: Proceedings of the 8th Conference on Epigenetic Robotics (2008)
Oudeyer, P.-Y., Kaplan, F., Hafner, V.: Intrinsic motivation systems for autonomous mental development. IEEE Trans. Evol. Comput. **11**(2), 265–286 (2007)
Oudeyer, P.-Y., Ly, O., Rouanet, P.: Exploring robust, intuitive and emergent physical human–robot interaction with the humanoid acroban. In: Proceedings of IEEE-RAS International Conference on Humanoid Robots (2011)

Paul, C.: Morphology and computation. In: Proceedings of the International Conference on the Simulation of Adaptive Behaviour (2004)
Peters, J., Schaal, S.: Natural actor critic. Neurocomputing **71**, 1180–1190 (2008)
Pfeifer, R., Bongard, J.C.: How the Body Shapes the Way We Think: A New View of Intelligence. MIT/Bradford Books, Cambridge (2006)
Pfeifer, R., Lungarella, M., Iida, F.: Self-organization, embodiment, and biologically inspired robotics. Science **318**, 1088–1093 (2007)
Pfeifer, R., Scheier, C.: Understanding Intelligence. MIT, Boston (1999)
Piaget, J.: The Origins of Intelligence in Childhood. International University Press, New York (1952)
Redgrave, P., Gurney, K., Stafford, T., Thirkettle, M., Lewis, J.: The role of the basal ganglia in discovering novel actions. In: Baldassarre, G., Mirolli, M. (eds.) Intrinsically Motivated Learning in Natural and Artificial Systems, pp. 129–149. Springer, Berlin (2012)
Ring, M.: Continual learning in reinforcement environments. Ph.D. Thesis, University of Texas at Austin, Austin (1994)
Rochat, P.: Object manipulation and exploration in 2- to 5-month-old infants Dev. Psychol. **25**, 871–884 (1989)
Rolf, M., Steil, J., Gienger, M.: Goal babbling permits direct learning of inverse kinematics. IEEE Trans. Auton. Mental Dev. **2**(3), 216–229 (2010)
Ryan, R.M., Deci, E.L.: Intrinsic and extrinsic motivations: Classic definitions and new directions. Contem. Educ. Psychol. **25**(1), 54–67 (2000)
Schaal, S., Atkeson, C.G.: Robot juggling: An implementation of memory-based learning. Control Syst. Mag. 57–71 (1994)
Schaal, S., Atkeson, C.G.: Robot learning by nonparametric regression, In: Proceedings of Intelligent Robots and Systems 1994 (IROS 94) pp. 137–153 (1995)
Schembri, M., Mirolli, M., Baldassare, G.: Evolving internal reinforcers for an intrinsically motivated reinforcement learning robot. In: Demiris, Y., Scassellati, B., Mareschal, D. (eds.) Proceedings of the 6th IEEE International Conference on Development and Learning (ICDL2007) (2007a)
Schembri, M., Mirolli, M., G., B.: Evolution and learning in an intrinsically motivated reinforcement learning robot. In: Springer (ed.) Advances in Artificial Life. Proceedings of the 9th European Conference on Artificial Life, Berlin, pp. 294–333 (2007b)
Schlesinger, M.: Heterochrony: It's (all) about time! In: Studies, L.U.C. (ed.) Proceedings of the Eighth International Workshop on Epigenetic Robotics: Modeling Cognitive Development in Robotic Systems, Sweden, pp. 111–117 (2008)
Schlesinger, M.: Investigating the origins of intrinsic motivations in human infants. In: Baldassarre, G., Mirolli, M. (eds.) Intrinsically Motivated Learning in Natural and Artificial Systems, pp. 367–392. Springer, Berlin (2012)
Schmidhuber, J.: Curious model-building control systems. Proc. Int. Joint Conf. Neural Netw. **2**, 1458–1463 (1991)
Schmidhuber, J.: Exploring the predictable. In: Ghosh, S., Tsutsui, S. (eds.) Advances in Evolutionary Computing: Theory and Applications, pp. 579–612. Springer, New York (2002)
Schmidhuber, J.: Optimal artificial curiosity, developmental robotics, creativity, music, and the fine arts. Connect. Sci. **18**(2), 173–187 (2006)
Schmidhuber, J.: Formal theory of creativity. IEEE Trans. Auton. Mental Dev. **2**(3), 230–247 (2010)
Schmidhuber, J.: Maximizing fun by creating data with easily reducible subjective complexity. In: Baldassarre, G., Mirolli, M. (eds.) Intrinsically Motivated Learning in Natural and Artificial Systems, pp. 95–128. Springer, Berlin (2012)
Scholz, J., Klein, M., Behrens, T., Johansen-Berg, H.: Training induces changes in white-matter architecture. Nat. Neurosci. **12**(11), 1367–1368 (2009)
Sekuler, R., Blake, R.: Perception. McGraw-Hill, New York (1994)
Sigaud, O., Salaün, C., Padois, V.: On-line regression algorithms for learning mechanical models of robots: A survey. Robot. Auton. Syst. **59**(12), 1115–1129 (2011)

Singh, S., Lewis, R., Barto, A., Sorg, J.: Intrinsically motivated reinforcement learning: An evolutionary perspective. IEEE Trans. Auton. Mental Dev. **2**(2), 70–82 (2010)
Stout, A., Barto, A.: Competence based intrinsic motivation. In: Proceedings of IEEE International Conference on Development and Learning (ICDL 2010) (2010)
Sutton, R.: Integrated architectures for learning, planning, and reacting based on approximating integrated architectures for learning, planning, and reacting based on approximating dynamic programming. In: Proceedings of the International Machine Learning Conference, pp. 212–218 (1990)
Sutton, R., Barto, A.: Reinforcement learning: An introduction. MIT, Cambridge (1998)
Sutton, R., Precup, D., Singh, S.: Between mdpss and semi-mdps: A framework for temporal abstraction in reinforcement learning. Artif. Intell. **112**, 181–211 (1999)
Szita, I., Lorincz, A.: The many faces of optimism: A unifying approach. In: Proceedings of ICML'08 (2008)
Thomaz, A., Breazeal, C.: Experiments in socially guided exploration: Lessons learned in building robots that learn with and without human teachers. Connect. Sci. **20**(2–3), 91–110 (2008)
Thrun, S.: The role of exploration in learning control. In: White, D., Sofge, D. (eds.) Handbook for Intelligent Control: Neural, Fuzzy and Adaptive Approaches. Van Nostrand Reinhold, Florence (1992)
Thrun, S., Moller, K.: Active exploration in dynamic environments. In: J. Moody, S., Hanson, R.L. (ed.) Proceedings of the Advances of Neural Information Processing Systems, vol. 4 (1992)
Ting, L., McKay, J.: Neuromechanics of muscle synergies for posture and movement. Curr. Opin. Neurobiol. **17**, 622–628 (2007)
Tong, S., Chang, E.: Support vector machine active learning for image retrieval. In: Proceedings of the Ninth ACM International Conference on Multimedia, MULTIMEDIA'01, pp. 107–118. ACM (2001)
Turkewitz, G., Kenny, P.: The role of developmental limitations of sensory input on sensory/perceptual organization. J. Dev. Behav. Pediatr. **6**(5), 302–306 (1985)
Weiss, E., Flanders, M.: Muscular and postural synergies of the human hand. J. Neurophysiol. **92**, 523–535 (2004)
Weng, J., McClelland, J., Pentland, A., Sporns, O., Stockman, I., Sur, M., Thelen, E.: Autonomous mental development by robots and animals. Science **291**, 599–600 (2001)
White, R.: Motivation reconsidered: The concept of competence. Psychol. Rev. **66**, 297–333 (1959)
Whitehead, S.: A Study of Cooperative Mechanisms for Faster Reinforcement Learning. Tr-365, University of Rochester, Rochester (1991)
Wiering, M., Schmidhuber, J.: Hq-learning. Adap. Behav. **6**, 219–246 (1997)
Wundt, W.: Grundzuge der physiologischen Psychologie. Engelmann, Leipzig (1874)
Yokoi, H., Hernandez, A., Katoh, R., Yu, W., Watanabe, I., Maruishi, M.: Mutual adaptation in a prosthetics application. In: Embodied Artificial Intelligence. LNAI, vol. 3139. Springer, Heidelberg (2004)
Ziegler, M., Iida, F., Pfeifer, R.: Cheap underwater locomotion: Roles of morphological properties and behavioural diversity. In: Proceedings of the International Conference on Climbing and Walking Robots (2006)

Investigating the Origins of Intrinsic Motivation in Human Infants

Matthew Schlesinger

Abstract One of the earliest behaviors driven by intrinsic motivation is visual exploration. In this chapter, I highlight how the development of this capacity is influenced not only by changes in the brain that take place after birth but also by the acquisition of oculomotor skill. To provide a context for interpreting these developmental changes, I then survey three theoretical perspectives that are available for explaining how and why visual exploration develops. Next, I describe work on the development of perceptual completion, which offers a case study on the development of visual exploration and the role of oculomotor skill. I conclude by discussing a number of challenges and open questions that are suggested by this work.

1 Introduction

In contrast to many other species, including gorillas, chimpanzees, and monkeys, human infants are born comparatively helpless and physically immature (Antinucci 1989; Bjorklund 1997). The fact that humans are unable to survive after birth without assistance from others has a number of important consequences. For example, humans have evolved a complex set of caretaking behaviors that promote attachment and emotional bonding between parents and offspring (Bowlby 1969). Another important consequence is that human infants spend the first several months of life relatively immobile: Reaching and grasping do not begin to emerge until age

M. Schlesinger (✉)
Department of Psychology, Southern Illinois University Carbondale, Carbondale, IL, USA
e-mail: matthews@siu.edu

G. Baldassarre and M. Mirolli (eds.), *Intrinsically Motivated Learning in Natural and Artificial Systems*, DOI 10.1007/978-3-642-32375-1_14,

3 months, while crawling develops approximately 5 months later. As a result, there is a strong developmental bias in young infants to begin learning about the physical world by exploring it visually.

The goal of this chapter is to highlight the development of visual exploration in human infants, not only as a case study in intrinsic motivation (IM) but also as part of a more general claim that visual exploration is perhaps the earliest expression of many of the essential components of IM (e.g., curiosity, novelty, and surprise). It should be stressed at the outset, however, that the current chapter focuses on a dimension of IM that is somewhat distinct from the way it is conceptualized in the rest of the volume. In particular, here I emphasize IM as a "motor" or "psychological force" that directs or causes behavior. It is a biological mechanism that "kick starts" action in an adaptive way by generating sensorimotor data that are essential for early perceptual and cognitive development. This differs from (but is also highly compatible with) the more conventional view of IM as a mechanism that generates learning signals.

Accordingly, the rest of this chapter is organized into four sections. In the first section, I briefly survey the core developmental changes that occur in visual perception during the first year of infancy, including the shift from exogenous to endogenous control of visual attention. The second section reviews some of the major concepts and theoretical approaches that are available for linking the development of visual exploration to the study of IM in infants (e.g., assimilation and accommodation). In the third section, I focus on how visual selective attention—a critical skill that underlies visual exploration—begins to emerge and develop in early infancy. In particular, this section presents recent empirical work that utilizes behavioral and computational methods as an integrated approach for studying the development of visual exploration in young infants. The fourth and final section raises a number of fundamental challenges and open questions concerning the development based on IM.

2 Developmental Components of Visual Exploration

Parents often note that when their newborn infant is in a quiet, alert state, they are remarkably "focused" or "attentive." The infant may become engrossed with a mobile hanging above the crib, the mother's face, or perhaps their own hand as it moves through the visual field. In this context, it is tempting to wonder: What does the infant see? How clear is their vision, and how do they interpret or make sense of their visual experience? In addition, what is driving or motivating this process? Are infants systematically studying and absorbing the features of their visual world, or is this behavior simply an instance of "tuning out" with their eyes open?

The question of what engages young infants' attention and what influences their visual-exploratory activity can be framed as a developmental task. Much like sucking, grasping, crawling, and other basic motor behaviors, learning to see is a sensorimotor skill that infants develop in the first year of life. From this

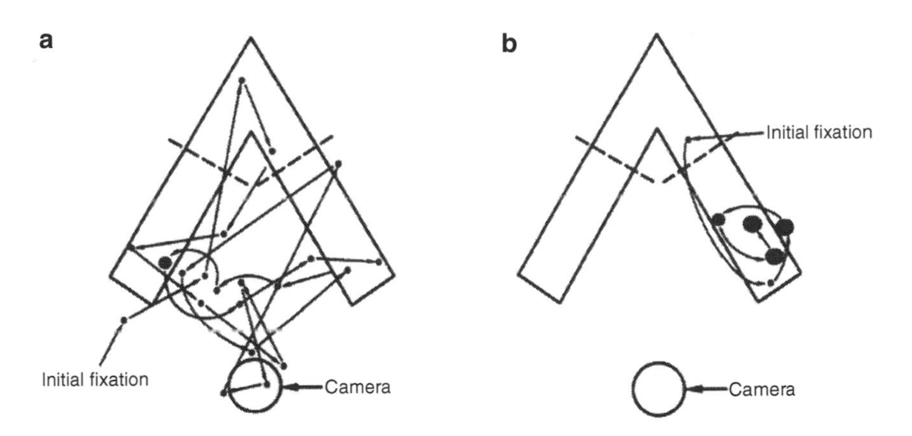

Fig. 1 Gaze patterns produced by two infants (Bronson 1991). The scan pattern on the *left* (**a**) was produced by a 12-week-old and has many brief fixations, distributed over the stimulus, while the scan pattern on the *right* (**b**) was produced by a 2-week-old and has several long fixations focused on the lower right portion of the stimulus

perspective, the sequence of changes that occur in visual perception between birth and 12 months is in many ways a process of acquiring increasingly complex and hierarchically organized or integrated behaviors. These behaviors not only improve infants' ability for information pick-up (e.g., efficient visual scanning), but they also provide essential data for the process of conceptual development (e.g., object recognition, object permanence, and perception of causality).

To help illustrate the kinds of changes that occur in visual exploration during early infancy, Fig. 1 presents two samples of gaze behavior in young infants from a study of visual encoding in 2- and 12-week-olds (Bronson 1991). During the study, infants viewed an inverted-V figure while their eye movements were recorded with a camera located beneath the figure. For each infant, the initial fixation is indicated by a small dot, and subsequent gaze shifts are indicated by the links between the dots. The size of each dot indicates the relative dwell time of the fixation, with larger dots representing longer dwell times. The sample on the left (Fig. 1a) highlights two important aspects of efficient scanning behavior that are typical of 12-week-olds: (1) Individual fixations (the small dots) are relatively well distributed, spanning most of the stimulus, and (2) dwell or fixation times are fairly brief (i.e., less than 1 s each). In contrast, 2-week-old infants tend to produce scanning patterns like those on the right (Fig. 1b), which include comparatively long fixations (i.e., 2–3 s) that only span a small portion of the stimulus.

These data indicate that a fundamental shift in oculomotor control occurs during early infancy. In this section, I highlight changes at two levels that are part of this shift and which play a critical role in the development of visual exploration during the first year: (1) maturation of the neural substrate and (2) the transition from exogenous to endogenous control of attention.

2.1 Maturation of the Neural Substrate

The neural pathway from the retina to the visual cortex is not fully functional at birth, but instead undergoes a number of important changes during the first few months of postnatal life (Banks and Bennett 1988; Johnson 1990). While the development of this pathway is largely constrained by maturational factors, visual input also plays a significant role. Greenough and Black (1999) describe the process as experience-expectant development. In particular, a basic neural pathway is biologically "hardwired" and then as a series of typical experiences occur (e.g., visual or auditory input), structures and connections within the pathway become more specifically shaped or tuned. In the case of early visual processing, synapses between neurons are initially "overproduced" and then selectively pruned as a function of input into the visual system (e.g., stimulation of the left and right eyes).

One of the most important examples of growth in the early visual system involves changes in the structure of the fovea. In this case, it is also an example that has direct impact on the development of visual exploration, because the changes that occur are associated with not only an increase in visual acuity (i.e., detail vision) but also the emergence of color perception. As Banks and Bennett (1988) highlight, there are several anatomical differences between foveal cones in the newborn infant and those in adults. For example, the outer segments of these cones (which are responsible for "capturing" photons and channeling them toward the inner segments) are significantly larger in newborn infants. As a result, neonate visual acuity is highly nearsighted (e.g., approximately 20/400). Over time, the outer segments gradually shrink, which increases the packing density of cones and leads to an improvement in visual acuity. In addition, Banks and Bennett (1988) note that color perception also improves as the likelihood of capturing photons increases.

While the previous example emphasizes anatomical changes at the sensory level, there are also several changes taking place within the cortex that support the development of visual exploration. For instance, Canfield and Kirkham (2001) highlight maturation of the prefrontal cortex (PFC) and, in particular, the frontal eye fields (FEF). In adults, FEF activity is associated with anticipatory eye movements, which typically occur prior to (or during the occlusion of) a visual target and suggest that the movement is not only voluntary but also planned or programmed on the basis of pre-target information. When does this area begin to develop in infants? The evidence available to answer this question is somewhat mixed and varies depending on the paradigm used to measure saccade planning and voluntary eye movements. However, as I note in the next section (Exogenous to Endogenous Control), a conservative estimate for evidence of FEF activity in infants is age 6 months (e.g., Johnson 1990), while a more liberal estimate is 3–4 months (e.g., Haith et al. 1993).

A third neural substrate that plays an essential role in visual exploration is the development of visual cortex and, in particular, the growth of horizontal connections in area V1. While the emergence of these connections is not well studied in humans, work with other mammals (e.g., ferrets, see Ruthazer and Stryker 1996) illustrates the *experience-expectant* developmental pattern: A broad, coarse set of horizontal connections form during late prenatal development, and these connections are subsequently pruned in the first few weeks after birth. An additional source of evidence is provided by lesion and single-cell studies with nonhuman primates, which demonstrate that these connections support the perception of contours (e.g., Albright and Stoner 2002; Hess and Field 1999).

The ability to perceive contours is a critical prerequisite for visual exploration, in at least two ways. First, as Fig. 1 highlights, efficient and systematic scanning of a visual stimulus cannot occur unless fixations are distributed over the entire stimulus. Without contour perception, the stimulus may appear as a disorganized collection of features (e.g., patches of high and low contrast), and the observer may be unable to determine whether a particular region has already been fixated or not. Second, contour perception also enables the observer to integrate surfaces of an object that are separated due to an occluding surface (e.g., an animal standing behind the trunk of a tree). In effect, horizontal connections between V1 neurons create a perceptual "fill-in" mechanism, in which objects are perceived as coherent wholes despite being partially occluded (e.g., Albright and Stoner 2002).

2.2 Exogenous to Endogenous Control

In parallel with underlying changes in neural structure and function, oculomotor activity also develops systematically during early infancy. There are numerous examples that provide support for a broad, consistent developmental trend: (1) Between 0 and 2 months, infants' visual activity is largely stimulus-driven and controlled by exogenous factors such as luminance and motion, and (2) by age 2 months, endogenous control of vision begins to emerge, enabling infants to deploy their visual attention in a more structured or systematic manner (e.g., Haith 1980). I briefly describe here a few important examples of this shift from exogenous to endogenous control of vision.

First, a key hallmark of endogenous control of vision is that it is predictive or anticipatory. For example, the visual expectation paradigm (VEP) investigates the development of predictive eye movements by presenting infants with sequences of images that appear at specific locations (e.g., Haith and Goodman 1988). The ability to learn simple sequences, such as images that alternate consecutively at two locations (e.g., A–B–A–B), does not appear to develop until age 2 months, while predictive scanning of more complex sequences (e.g., A–A–B–A–A–B) begins to develop by age 3 months (Haith et al. 1993; Wentworth and Haith 1998).

It is worth noting that while the neural circuitry underlying the capacity for predictive visual behavior in human infants has not yet been identified, single-cell recordings with mature monkeys have implicated the FEF as a critical area. In particular, activity in the FEF is not only associated with anticipatory eye movements during tracking of an occluded target, but this activity is also associated with an error signal that occurs when predictive movements are inaccurate (Barborica and Ferrera 2004; Ferrera and Barborica 2010). At the end of Sect. 4, I describe how we are using these findings to design a biologically inspired model that integrates bottom-up perceptual salience and prediction learning.

As Fig. 1a illustrates, a second important feature of endogenous vision is that it is systematic or exhaustive. For example, Maurer and Salapatek (1976) recorded the gaze patterns of 1- and 2-month-old infants as they viewed pictures of faces. The younger infants tended to spend less time looking at the faces than the older infants, and their fixations were often limited to the outer edges of the faces. In contrast, the older infants distributed their fixations more evenly over the pictures, and in particular, they spent significantly more time viewing the internal features of the faces (e.g., eyes, nose, and mouth). It is important to note not only that systematic scanning behavior is a skill that continues to develop beyond age 2 months but also that there is variability in the rate at which individual infants develop. I return to this issue later in this chapter, where I discuss the development of visual selective attention.

Finally, a third component of endogenous control of vision that develops in early infancy involves competition between multiple, salient objects, or locations in the visual field and the ability to adaptively distribute attention to these locations. Dannemiller (2000) investigated the development of this skill between ages 2 and 5 months, by presenting infants with a moving bar that was embedded within a field of stationary bars of different colors. Two major findings emerged from this work. First, Dannemiller found that detection of the moving target significantly improved with age. Thus, older infants were more sensitive to the motion of the target object and less distracted by the stationary bars. Second, Dannemiller also found that the spatial distribution of the colored, stationary bars had a stronger influence on the older infants. In particular, older infants benefited when relatively salient, stationary bars were positioned on the same side as the moving target, while the performance of younger infants was relatively unaffected by the placement of the salient, stationary bars.

3 Linking Visual Exploration and Intrinsic Motivation: A Theoretical Bridge

The review presented thus far highlights both the biological and behavioral changes that underlie the development of visual exploration. Neural growth and physiological development help make possible more efficient and adaptive modes of information pick-up, and at the same time, visual scanning strategies become progressively more complex, endogenously controlled, and sensitive to visual features in the environment. While these changes provide infants with the means to explore the world in increasingly powerful ways, however, they remain somewhat descriptive. Thus, although they are necessary components or tools of visual exploration, they do not provide direct answers to two fundamental questions. First, why do infants explore the visual world? In other words, is the exploratory process intrinsically motivated, and if so, what is the basis for this motivation? Second, how does the IM for visual exploration arise, and how is it manifested in infants' visual behavior?

In this section, I survey some of the prevailing answers that developmental researchers have proposed to address these questions. In particular, I describe three complementary theoretical approaches: (1) evolutionary theory, (2) Piagetian theory, and (3) information-processing theory. It is important to stress that these approaches are not mutually exclusive, but in fact overlap considerably. In addition, they can be viewed as complementary accounts as each focuses on a particular dimension or level of organism–environment interaction and development.

Thus, evolutionary theory emphasizes the role of adaptation and survival at the species level, including mechanisms for encoding various aspects of exploratory behavior (e.g., drives or instincts) in the genetic code. While Piaget also highlights the importance of adaptation, his account is focused at the level of the individual and, in particular, on the growth of knowledge structures (i.e., schemes) through active manipulation of the environment. Finally, information-processing theory shares many features with evolutionary (i.e., biological) and Piagetian theory. However, a unique feature of this approach is its emphasis on providing explicit mechanistic accounts for how sensory information is acquired, stored, and subsequently used to guide action.

3.1 Evolutionary Theory

According to evolutionary theory, newborn infants' gaze behavior is a product of mammalian and primate evolution. By this view, infants are born with an innate behavioral "program" that directs visual attention. This program has the implicit goal of providing optimal visual stimulation, which promotes the growth and development of the neural pathways that support vision. For example, Haith (1980) proposes the *high firing rate principle*, which includes a set of basic heuristics that guide visual activity, such as (1) when there is no visual input, move the eyes, and (2) if an edge (i.e., adjacent regions of high and low luminance) is encountered, move the eyes over the edge.

A similar approach is proposed by Sporns and Edelman (1993), who emphasize the concept of biological or intrinsic value systems. According to this view, value systems are species-specific neural circuits that evolve through the process of natural selection and become activated during sensorimotor activity. In the case of visual exploration, for example, eye movements create stimulation on the retina, which modulates neural activity throughout the visual stream (e.g., lateral geniculate nucleus and occipital cortex). These patterns of sensorimotor activity result in increased value (e.g., release of dopamine), which strengthens the neural circuits that are active during visual exploration.

Evolutionary theory provides a clear answer to the question of why infants explore their environment visually: because this behavior promotes brain development (Edelman 1987). It also provides a preliminary answer to the question of how it develops: Due to its adaptive significance, visual exploration was selected as an innate behavior in humans through the process of evolution and natural selection. However, where evolutionary theory falls short is in providing a detailed account of how visual exploration develops after birth, and in particular, how the value or motivation system interacts with specific environmental experiences over time to produce the developmental trajectory observed in human infants.

3.2 Piagetian Theory

A highly influential approach to understand the link between IM and visual exploration is offered by Piaget's theory of cognitive development (Piaget 1952). Two central concepts are assimilation and accommodation. Assimilation is the tendency to use familiar or preexisting behaviors when interacting with an object. For example, after young infants master the ability to nurse, they will often examine new objects by exploring them with their mouth. Accommodation, instead, is the modification of preexisting behaviors or schemes, or the invention of new schemes, which gradually become coordinated and integrated with previous schemes. Imagine, for example, that an infant who tends to explore objects with the mouth is given a piece of ice. At first, the ice goes in the mouth (assimilation), but it is quickly spit out. The infant subsequently discovers that the ice slides when pushed (accommodation), and so a novel scheme begins to form as the infant plays with their new toy.

It is important to note that Piaget proposed several distinct forms of assimilation. Functional assimilation, for example, is the tendency to "exercise" an existing behavior or scheme. Piaget suggested that functional assimilation plays a fundamental role in the acquisition of new skills (i.e., as the scheme is beginning to form). This view is consistent with the observation parents often make while their infants develop a new capacity, such as learning to reach or crawl, as the infant appears entirely focused on "practicing" or deliberately rehearsing the ability over and over again. Generalizing assimilation, instead, is the tendency to extend schemes that have been acquired with familiar objects toward novel or unfamiliar ones.

Taken together, functional and generalizing assimilation provide a straightforward answer to the questions of why and how visual exploration develops (Piaget 1952). First, functional assimilation means that visual exploration is the tendency to exercise the schemes associated with visual activity (e.g., fixations, saccades, and pursuit of moving objects). Given an object to look at, an infant will automatically engage their visual schemes. According to Piaget, the functioning of these schemes is analogous to the biological activity of physical organs, such as the relation between food and the digestive system or air and the respiratory system. While this view overlaps with the approach offered by evolutionary theory, an important distinction is that Piaget's account also predicts the transition from exogenous to endogenous control of vision. In particular, Piaget suggests that the "automatic" or reflexive exercising of visual activity—that is, functional assimilation—should diminish over time, as the new skill becomes mastered.

Second, generalizing assimilation also clearly defines the role of IM in the development of visual exploration. Specifically, Piaget proposes the *moderate novelty principle* as a core feature of visual exploration (Ginsburg and Opper 1988; Piaget 1952). According to this principle, as infants generalize preexisting schemes to new objects, they do not select those objects arbitrarily. Instead, infants tend to orient toward new objects which are neither too easily assimilated nor those that require entirely new schemes (i.e., completely familiar or unfamiliar objects, respectively).

By this view, infants' oculomotor activity patterns or schemes—where and how they explore the visual world—are intimately tied to their preexisting perceptual categories. Thus, Piaget proposes a dynamic and reciprocal connection between seeing and knowing: Infants' visual-exploratory skill level determines the objects they perceive and recognize, while their current perceptual categories influence how they seek out new visual features. In other words, the process of exploratory skill development leads to the discovery of new perceptual features and categories, and vice versa.

3.3 Information-Processing Theory

A third approach that relates IM and visual exploration is offered by information-processing theory, which both overlaps with and is complementary to Piaget's theory (e.g., Case 1985; Klahr and MacWhinney 1998; Siegler and Jenkins 1989). However, there are two important distinctions. First, information-processing theory uses the modern computer as a metaphor for understanding mental processes and consequently tends to focus on a relatively narrow set of phenomena, including perception, attention, and memory. Second, and more importantly, while Piaget relies on the somewhat abstract process of equilibration (i.e., the balance between assimilation and accommodation) as the primary mechanism for driving development, information-processing theory instead emphasizes maturation of the underlying neural substrate (i.e., "hardware") and the acquisition of new and more efficient or powerful strategies for gathering and using information (i.e., "software"; for related discussion, see Case 1985).

One of the most direct ways that information-processing theory links IM and visual exploration is through the concepts of curiosity, novelty, and surprise. For example, *template-matching theory* (e.g., Charlesworth 1969; Sokolov 1963) proposes that as infants view an object or event, they compare the visual input produced by that experience with a corresponding internal representation (e.g., mental image or memory). By this view, the amount of interest or curiosity an infant shows in an object—which is operationalized and measured by their looking time—is a function of how well represented the object is: Completely familiar objects have robust internal representations, and so the comparison process terminates quickly (i.e., the infant rapidly loses interest). In contrast, objects that are moderately novel have weak or incomplete internal representations and, as a result, generate a longer comparison process as the representation is updated with new sensory data (i.e., mild curiosity or interest).

In many ways, this account is comparable to Piaget's moderate novelty principle. However, an interesting difference between the theories arises in the case of a highly novel object. While Piaget might predict that a highly novel object should generate a low level of interest, there is some evidence to suggest that such objects may in fact be strongly aversive to young infants. For example, Fox et al. (1979) proposed that stranger wariness or anxiety—which emerges around age 6 months and is marked by distress, fear, and crying in the presence of unfamiliar adults—is the result of improvement in long-term memory. By this view, the fear is not in response to perceived danger but rather is a reaction to the inability to retrieve an image from memory that corresponds to the face of the stranger. In order to evaluate their hypothesis, Fox et al. (1979) conducted a longitudinal study of infants between ages 5 and 14 months and, as predicted, found that improvements in memory reliably preceded the development of stranger anxiety.

Finally, an interesting issue raised by information-processing theory is the question of whether individual differences in processing or encoding speed during infancy can accurately predict later intelligence. For example, Bronson (1991) noted considerable variability between infants at age 3 months in the strategies used to scan objects. Information-processing theorists have proposed that infants who scan visual stimuli rapidly and efficiently are thus able to create internal representations more effectively than infants who scan slowly and unsystematically (e.g., Bornstein and Sigman 1986) and that this difference between infants may be diagnostic of more general differences in intelligence or intellectual ability. Indeed, in a meta-analysis of 23 studies, McCall and Carriger (1993) found substantial support for a predictive relation between visual processing during infancy and intelligence in later childhood. In effect, infants who are faster visual processors grow up to be more intelligent children (as assessed by standard IQ tests). While these data do not provide a direct link between IM during infancy and intelligence in older children, they do suggest that early forms of IM such as visual exploration differ in quality and quantity from child to child and that these early differences may have an influence on intellectual growth later in childhood.

3.4 Developmental Theory and IM

While the theoretical accounts reviewed thus far focus explicitly on the process of early perceptual and cognitive development, they also overlap considerably with theories of IM. These correspondences can be highlighted by organizing IM into two categories: knowledge-based approaches (including prediction-based and novelty-based IM) and competence-based approaches (e.g., Baldassarre 2011; Berlyne 1954; Kagan 1972; Oudeyer and Kaplan 2007; Schmidhuber 2009; White 1959).

First, evolutionary theory is consistent with both of the knowledge-based approaches. Evolution provides a "drive" or "instinct" to explore, and in particular, the learning mechanism underlying this exploratory process is predictive. For example, Haith's high firing rate principle helps to drive young infants' eye movements in an anticipatory or future-oriented manner: As infants direct their gaze toward nonhomogeneous regions of the visual field, they learn to predict upcoming visual features and events (e.g., Wentworth and Haith 1998). In addition, evolution also provides a motivation for seeking out novel or unfamiliar visual experiences, both in terms of the underlying neural substrate and the maturational constraints that influence early oculomotor control.

Second, Piagetian theory overlaps both categories of IM. The process of generalizing assimilation is inherently predictive: As infants manipulate and interact with new objects, the application of existing sensorimotor schemes to those objects provides an implicit prediction of their properties. For example, by biting an object, the infant implicitly predicts it will be rigid or solid. An unexpected result (e.g., the object makes a sound) triggers accommodation, which enables the infant to modify existing schemes and potentially generate new ones. Similarly, Piaget's moderate novelty principle offers an explicit role during exploration for the trade-off between familiarity and novelty, and more importantly, it suggests that infants actively seek out experiences that are just beyond their level of understanding. Finally, the same principle—as well as the notion that assimilation and accommodation are modulated through the process of equilibration—is also consistent with the competence-based approach to IM. In particular, equilibration drives the infant toward finding a balance between assimilation and accommodation, which is presumably manifested as a motivation to achieve mastery (i.e., fully developed schemes).

Third, like evolutionary theory, information-processing theory is also consistent with knowledge-based IM. For example, template-matching theory integrates the roles of prediction and novelty by proposing that infants compare their ongoing experiences to stored long-term representations. Like Piaget's sensorimotor schemes, these representations provide an implicit basis for predicting event outcomes, and in particular, template-matching theory proposes that a mismatch between expected and experienced events increases attention and exploration.

4 Visual Exploration and the Development of Visual Selective Attention

As I noted earlier, one of the primary goals of this chapter is to propose that visual exploration is an early manifestation of IM that provides a foundation for the development of several essential cognitive components. In order to support this claim, I present in this section a detailed description of a collaborative research project that investigates the development of oculomotor skill and object perception in young infants (Amso and Johnson 2006; Johnson 2004; Johnson et al. 2004; Schlesinger et al. 2007a,b, 2011). The project incorporates and integrates many of the themes and ideas presented thus far in this chapter, including the following: (1) the role of an underlying neural substrate that constrains the development of visual attention, (2) the systematic changes in oculomotor behavior that reflect the transition from exogenous to endogenous control of vision, and (3) the dynamic interplay between visual salience and visual novelty, which work together to shape visual exploration in real time. It should be noted that our work thus far has focused largely on the first two issues, but as I highlight in the final section, we are also beginning to address the third theme.

Before describing our work, however, it is important to remember that our use of the term IM focuses on how it directs or causes visual exploration rather than as a learning signal that modifies visual-exploratory behavior. From this perspective, both our behavioral and modeling work reveal important developmental changes in visual exploration, which reflect progressive improvements in how infants scan the visual world and collect information about objects and events. In addition, our behavioral findings provide clear evidence that these improvements are closely associated with infants' developing abilities to perceive objects, while our modeling results suggest the underlying neural mechanisms that may explain the developmental pattern.

The specific component of visual exploration that we are investigating is *visual selective attention*, which is defined as the ability to deploy attention in a systematic manner while ignoring irrelevant stimuli. In particular, our work seeks to identify the specific mechanisms—both neural and behavioral—that underlie the development of visual selective attention. How does our work inform the study of IM in young infants? This question can be answered in at least two ways.

First, visual exploration does not become a manifestation of IM until it is *autonomous*, that is, until infants are at least partially capable of determining where they look and to which features of the visual environment they attend. Thus, it is the shift from reflexive orienting to systematic scanning of the visual world that marks the beginning of visual exploration. It is precisely on this early developmental achievement that our behavioral and modeling work focuses.

Nevertheless, and perhaps counterintuitively, we investigate the shift to exogenous control of vision by employing a salience-based model. The use of this modeling approach is not intended to suggest that visual salience (i.e., bottom-up visual input) plays a central role in the developmental process. Instead, as I highlight below, the salience-based model provides a compact and convenient framework for representing the processing pathway through which visual input is systematically transformed and used to guide visual activity. We account for developmental change, meanwhile, by exploring specific changes in neural activity. Therefore, our work informs the study of IM in young infants by providing a comprehensive explanation for the emergence of autonomous visual exploration in early infancy.

Second, a long-term goal of our model is to provide an account for how IM shapes the specific pattern of visual exploration observed in young infants (e.g., as illustrated in Fig. 1). However, our work to date has focused on the modulation of bottom-up visual input through early attentional mechanisms. This leaves neglected the role of top-down influences on visual exploration such as novelty and curiosity.

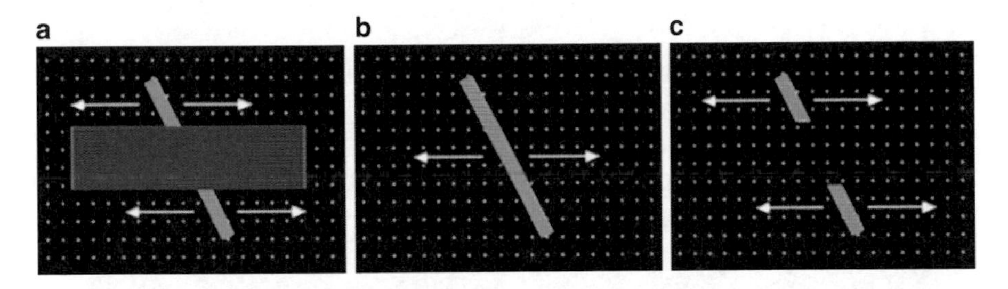

Fig. 2 Illustration of the stimuli used to test the development of perceptual completion in young infants. (**a**) The occluded-rod display, (**b**) the solid-rod display, and (**c**) the broken-rod display

We have made some recent progress on this issue, and as I highlight at the end of this section, there are a number of relatively straightforward ways in which the model we are investigating can be extended and elaborated to explicitly simulate the role of IM on visual exploration.

Our current approach is designed to address a number of questions. First, how do changes in visual selective attention during early infancy give rise to new (and more effective or efficient) patterns of scanning behavior? Second, as new scanning strategies emerge, what effect, if any, do they have on the development of object perception? As a specific case study, consider the developmental problem of learning to perceive partially occluded objects as coherent wholes. To help illustrate the problem, Fig. 2a presents a snapshot from an animation event, in which a green rod moves laterally behind a large, blue screen (the arrows indicate the direction of motion). In the unity perception task, infants are first presented with this occluded-rod display until they habituate (i.e., their looking time decreases by 50 %). After habituating, infants then watch the displays illustrated in Fig. 2b, c on alternating test trials: During the solid-rod display (Fig. 2b), a single rod moves laterally, while two smaller, aligned rod segments move synchronously during the broken-rod display (Fig. 2c).

The tendency to look longer at one of the two test displays is assumed to reflect a novelty preference (e.g., Gilmore and Thomas 2002) and provides a basis for inferring whether infants perceive the occluded rod as a single object or two disjoint segments moving synchronously. Thus, infants who look longer at the broken-rod test display are referred to as perceivers because their looking pattern suggests that they perceive the occluded rod as a single, coherent object. Alternatively, infants who look longer at the solid-rod test display are referred to as non-perceivers because their looking pattern suggests instead that they perceive the occluded rod as two disconnected segments.

How does unity perception develop? Interestingly, between birth and age 2 months, infants look longer at the solid-rod display (e.g., Slater et al. 1996) and therefore appear to lack unity perception. By age 4 months, this preference switches, and infants begin to look longer at the broken-rod display (Johnson 2004). This developmental pattern suggests that unity perception is not present at birth, but instead rapidly develops in the first few months of postnatal life.

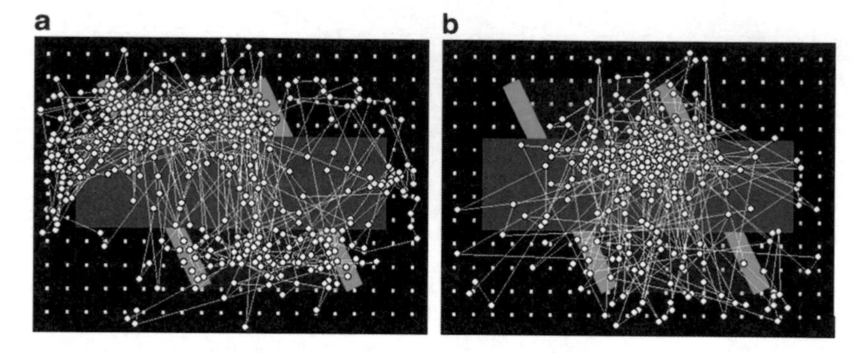

Fig. 3 Gaze patterns produced by two 3-month-old infants while viewing the occluded-rod display. The infant on the *left* (**a**) focused on the movement of the rod, while the infant on the *right* (**b**) distributed attention to other parts of the display, including the occluding box and the background dots

An important question—suggested by Piagetian theory—is whether the development of unity perception depends on improvements in oculomotor skill. For example, do perceivers and non-perceivers scan the occluded-rod (habituation) display in a comparable manner, or are there measurable differences in how they distribute their attention? Johnson et al. (2004) addressed this question by tracking the eye movements of 3-month-olds as they viewed the occluded-rod display. Each infant in the study then viewed the solid-rod and broken-rod test displays and was subsequently assigned to either the perceiver or non-perceiver group, depending on which of the two test displays the infant preferred to view.

Figure 3 presents examples of scan plots from two infants in the study (each dot represents a single fixation). Figure 3a, which was produced by an infant in the perceiver group, includes a large proportion of fixations toward the rod segments and comparatively fewer toward the occluding box. In contrast, Fig. 3b was produced by an infant in the non-perceiver group. Note that this second scan plot illustrates the opposite pattern: Many fixations are generated toward the occluding box, and relatively few are generated toward the moving rod. This qualitative pattern was investigated in a follow-up study by Amso and Johnson (2006), who divided the occluded-rod display into a series of regions of interest (ROI). Figure 4 illustrates the 6 ROIs, including the top and bottom portions of the occluded rod (ROIs 1 and 2) and the four quadrants of the background and occluding box (ROIs 3–6). They defined *rod scans* as gaze shifts within or between the rod segments and *vertical scans* as gaze shifts from the upper to lower quadrants, or vice versa (e.g., from 6 to 3).

Based on the findings from Johnson et al. (2004), Amso and Johnson (2006) predicted that 3-month-old perceivers would produce significantly more rod scans than 3-month-old non-perceivers. Since vertical scans do not provide information about the occluded rod, they also predicted that perceivers and non-perceivers would not differ in the percent of vertical scans produced. Figure 5a presents the proportion

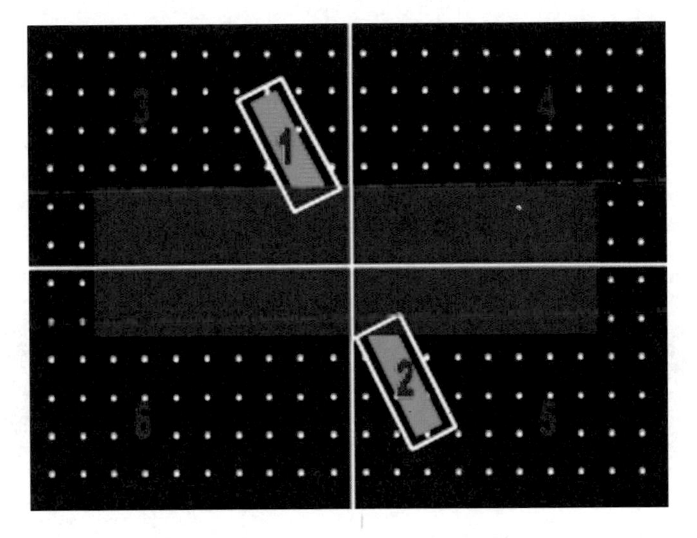

Fig. 4 The six regions of interest (ROIs) used by Amso and Johnson (2006) to measure which aspects of the occluded-rod display were fixated by 3-month-old infants

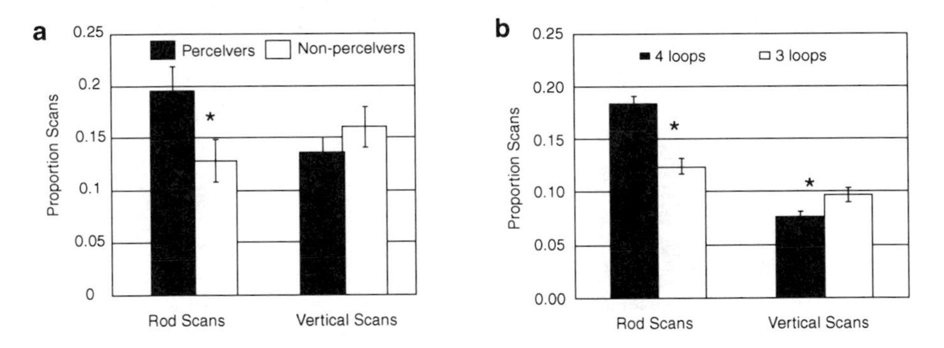

Fig. 5 Proportion of rod scans and vertical scans produced during the occluded-rod display. (**a**) Behavioral data acquired from 3-month-old infants and (**b**) simulation data generated by an eye-movement model

of rod scans and vertical scans produced by the two groups of infants. As predicted, 3-month-old perceivers generated significantly more fixations to the rod segments than non-perceivers, while there was no significant difference in the percent of fixations between the upper and lower halves of the occluded-rod display.

Taken together, the findings from these two studies not only show that perceivers are more effective at scanning the occluded-rod display, but they also provide support for the idea that effective scanning is a necessary prerequisite for unity perception. However, the data do not provide a direct explanation for why infants make the transition from non-perceivers to perceivers between ages 2 and 4 months. What underlying developmental mechanism drives this process? In particular,

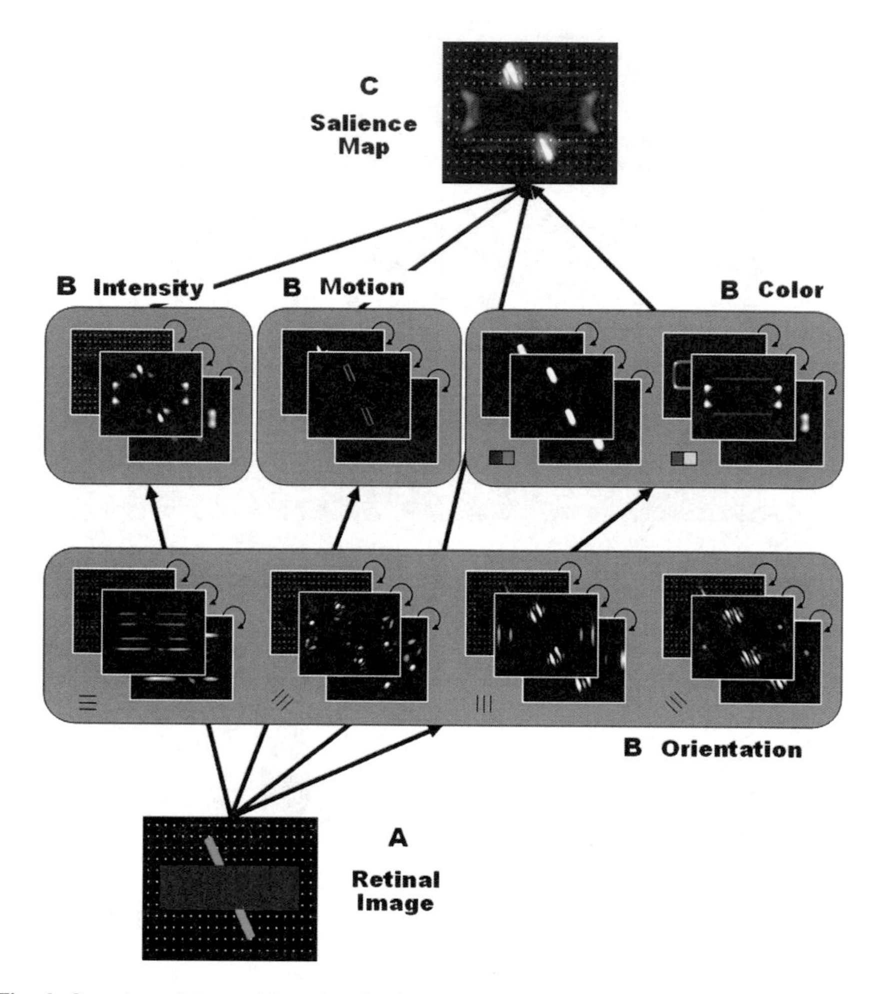

Fig. 6 Overview of the model used to simulate infants' visual exploration. (**a**) The retinal image, (**b**) feature abstraction and spatial competition, and (**c**) summation of the feature maps into a salience map

what enables young infants to scan the occluded-rod display more systematically so that they subsequently detect and attend to the key features of the display?

In order to explore these questions, we adapted a computational model of early visual processing (originally designed by Itti and Koch 2000; see also Itti and Koch 2001) to simulate the development of early visual processing in young infants (Schlesinger et al. 2007a,b). The model represents visual processing through a series of optical transformations that occur over four stages. (In the details presented below, note that all of the modeling work was hand-coded within the MATLAB environment, based on the architecture and algorithms presented by Itti et al. 1998.) Figure 6 illustrates the first three of these stages:

1. During the first stage, a 480×360 still-frame image is taken from the rod-and-box animation event and projected onto the simulated retina (Fig. 6a). Note that the model employs a monocular vision system and that the simulated visual receptors are uniform in size and evenly distributed on the retina (i.e., the retina is not divided into a fovea and periphery). In addition, the number, size, and arrangement of the receptors are assumed to be in 1-to-1 correspondence with the input image (i.e., 480×360 pixels).
2. In the second stage, the retinal image is used to produce 24 feature maps, which are distributed over four feature channels: one intensity or luminance channel, one motion channel, two color channels (i.e., blue–yellow and red–green opponent pairs), and four oriented-edge channels (i.e., 0°, 45°, 90°, and 135°). During this stage, the feature maps are created through a three-step process. First, each feature is extracted from the input image at three spatial scales (i.e., fine, medium, and coarse), resulting in a total of 24 feature maps (see Fig. 6b). Second, a center-surround receptive-field contrast filter is then applied to each feature map, which mimics the inhibitory–excitatory organization found in early visual processing (i.e., retinal ganglion cells and LGN). This filter also enhances feature contrast within each of the feature maps.

   During the third and final step of the feature-map process, each map passes through a spatial-competition filter. Note that application of the spatial-competition filter is a recurrent, iterative process (see below) and is indicated in Fig. 6b by the circular arrows at the corner of each of the feature maps. The spatial-competition process is implemented by convolving each feature map with a difference of Gaussian kernel: a narrowly tuned 3D Gaussian combined with a weak, broadly tuned 3D Gaussian, which corresponds to short-range excitatory and longer-range inhibitory interactions, respectively, in early visual processing.
3. The salience map is produced during the third processing stage by summing the 24 feature maps (Fig. 6c). In the current implementation, the feature maps are weighted equally; note that an alternative strategy, which represents the role of top-down modulation of the salience map, would be to assign unique weights to each of the feature maps before summing.
4. During the final processing stage (not illustrated), a stochastic selection procedure is used to select a target on the salience map, which enables the model to shift its virtual fixation point from one location on the map to another. First, the 100 most-active locations on the salience map are identified. Second, a fixation probability is assigned to each of these locations, proportional to the activation level at the corresponding location. This weighting strategy biases selection toward highly salient locations while also allowing other less-salient locations to occasionally be fixated. Finally, a location is randomly selected as a target for the next fixation from this weighted distribution.

   In order to simulate a sequence of eye movements over the entire event, the model is then presented with the animation display, one frame at a time. Activity on the salience map accumulates after each frame of the animation is presented, and roughly five times per second, a highly active (i.e., perceptually salient) location on the salience map is selected as a target for fixation. Concurrent with activity buildup on the salience map, activity at the current gaze point decays at the rate of 0.6 on each time step; this decay process allows salience to decrease at the current gaze point and enables the model to disengage fixation and produce a gaze shift to a new location (i.e., it implements an inhibition-of-return mechanism).

A critical parameter in the model is used during the second processing stage (see Fig. 6b). The value of this parameter, which varies from 0 to 10, controls the duration (i.e., the number of iterations or repetitions) of a spatial-competition process, in which features at different locations within the same channel or dimension (e.g., color) compete for activation. To help demonstrate this process, Fig. 7 presents an input image, followed by the corresponding salience map that is produced after running the spatial-competition process for 0, 2, 5, 8, and 10 iterations. As Fig. 7 illustrates, low values of the spatial-competition parameter (e.g., 0 or 2) are associated with shallow salience maps and multiple activation peaks. In contrast, high values (e.g., 8 or 10) are associated with steeper maps and fewer, more pronounced activation peaks.

The spatial-competition parameter has direct relevance for understanding how IM and visual selective attention are related during the development of visual exploration. In particular, this parameter plays a fundamental role not only at the computational level but also at the level of neurophysiology. First, note that because parameter values near 0 produce salience maps with numerous peaks, the resulting gaze patterns include frequent fixations to information-poor areas of the display, such as the center of the occluding box and the background texture dots. Conversely, parameter values near 10 result in fixations to highly informative areas of the display, such as the rod segments and the edges of the occluding box. Therefore, at a computational level, changes in the value of the spatial-competition parameter are clearly related to adaptive changes in the scanning behavior of the model.

Second, the computational process of spatial competition can also be interpreted as an analog for neural processing in the posterior parietal cortex (PPC), an area of the brain that is associated with the encoding of visual salience and the modulation of visual attention (e.g., Gottlieb et al. 1998; Shafritz et al. 2002). In particular, the feature maps produced during the second processing stage (Fig. 6b) correspond to the retinotopic maps found in PPC, which represent salient locations, objects, and prospective targets for action (e.g., an eye movement and reach). Given this correspondence, the spatial-competition parameter can be interpreted as controlling the temporal duration of recurrent processing in the PPC: Low values correspond to rapid processing, with brief pauses between synchronous bursts or "pulses" of activity, while high values correspond to slower processing and longer pauses between neural pulses.

It then makes sense to ask: Does the duration of recurrent parietal processing develop systematically in early infancy, thereby modulating the quality of visual exploration? In order to investigate this question, we systematically hand-tuned the value of the spatial-competition parameter from 0 to 10 iterations and then measured the proportion of rod scans and vertical scans produced by the model during the

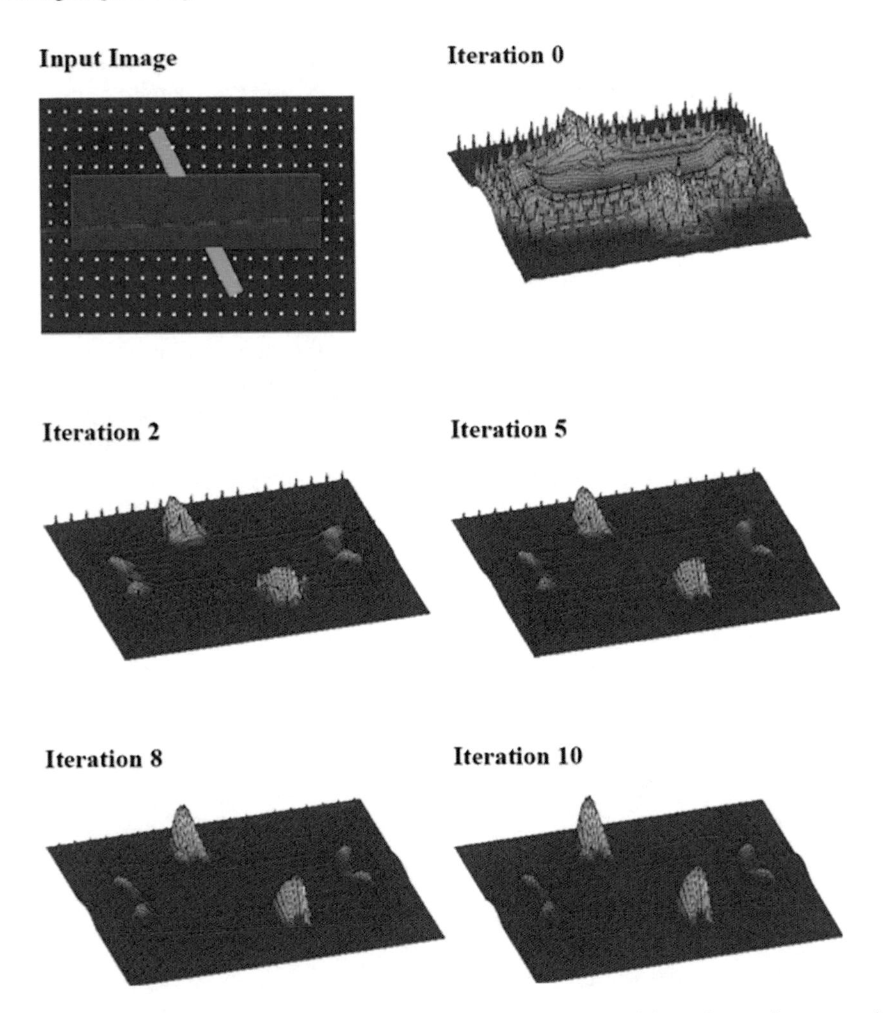

Fig. 7 Illustration of the spatial-competition algorithm. The original input image is presented, followed by the corresponding salience map that is created after 0, 2, 5, 8, and then 10 iterations of the spatial-competition algorithm

occluded-rod display for each value of the parameter. As Fig. 5b illustrates, a key finding from this simulation study was that the model replicated the scan patterns produced by non-perceivers when the parameter was set at three iterations, while the scan patterns produced by perceivers were reproduced when the parameter was set at four iterations (Schlesinger et al. 2007b).

Thus, the model not only succeeds in capturing the real-time behavior of both perceivers and non-perceivers, but it also suggests that maturational growth or development in the posterior parietal cortex may play a central role in the shift from exogenous to endogenous control of vision during early infancy. However, there are some important limitations in the current implementation of our model that should be noted. First, the developmental pattern produced by the model depends on hand tuning of the spatial-competition parameter (i.e., the number of spatial-competition iterations). While this modeling strategy provides valuable data, a better alternative is for the model to adaptively self-tune the parameter instead.

Consequently, we are currently pursuing the use of a prediction-learning system. In particular, we are implementing a forward model that learns to anticipate a series of visual inputs, based on the eye movements produced by the salience-based system. Our long-term goal is to link these systems together so that an error signal in the prediction-learning system can be used to adaptively tune the spatial-competition parameter in the salience-based system. While this work is underway, our preliminary findings demonstrate that increasing the duration of spatial competition results in faster learning in the prediction-learning system (Schlesinger et al. 2011). This result provides a strong indication that improvements in the prediction-learning system are positively correlated with longer durations of spatial competition. Second, a related limitation of the model is that it employs monocular visual input, and in addition, interaction with the physical world is limited to visual scanning (i.e., the model lacks the ability to grasp and manipulate objects). This approach is suitable for very young infants (i.e., 0–3 months), as the current model was specifically designed to simulate infants' performance on visual tasks such as the perceptual-completion task and visual search. However, it does not yet scale developmentally to older infants and more complex skills. In contrast, related models of visual attention and visual–motor coordination may provide greater versatility and flexibility (e.g., Ognibene et al. 2010). One of the ways that we are addressing this limitation is by porting our model to the iCub platform, which provides not only binocular visual input and a humanoid body but also a realistic 3D environment.

5 Summary and Open Questions

I began this chapter with two questions: What engages young infants' visual-exploratory activity, and how does this activity develop in the first few months of life? In this section, I begin by summarizing the main ideas and research findings that I raised. I then conclude by highlighting four open questions that serve as key challenges to the study of IM in young infants and suggesting potential strategies for addressing these questions.

First, the development of visual exploration is strongly influenced by the growth of the neural systems that support oculomotor control. For the first 2–4 months, infants are learning to focus their eyes, to trace complex contours and follow moving objects, and to shift their gaze rapidly and accurately toward targets of interest. These skills are made possible in part by neural growth that includes structural changes not only at the retinal level but also within and between cortical areas (e.g., PFC, V1, and PPC). Second, and in parallel with changes in the underlying neural substrate, infants are also establishing control over their eye movements at the behavioral level. In particular, their gaze patterns are becoming predictive or anticipatory, and they are also more efficient at scanning visual stimuli. These changes suggest that the mechanism responsible for driving visual exploration in young infants undergoes a major qualitative shift in early infancy. Thus, while newborn infants look at things in a somewhat reflexive or stimulus-driven manner, by age 3 months infants look at things in a more purposeful or deliberate manner. In other words, the newborn looks because it has to, while the older infant looks because it wants to.

Although it is clear that both physiological and behavioral factors play an important role in the development of oculomotor skill, neither of these levels provides a complete answer to the question of what motivates visual exploration. In other words, what is the function or purpose of visual-exploratory activity? I approached this question from three theoretical perspectives. First, according to evolutionary theory, visual exploration is a behavior pattern that has evolved in the human species to promote brain development. By this view, visual exploration is analogous to an instinct or innate behavior. Second, while Piaget agrees that visual activity is initially a reflex-like behavior, he suggests that with practice and repetition, it becomes an elaborate sensorimotor skill. In particular, he proposes that infants are constantly searching for new objects to assimilate and that this search process is biased toward objects that are moderately novel. Finally, information-processing theory complements Piaget's approach but also extends it by suggesting specific internal mechanisms (e.g., template-matching theory) through which novelty motivates visual exploration.

After reviewing the theoretical approaches to IM and visual exploration, I then provided a detailed overview of recent work on the development of visual selective attention in young infants. Three major findings were described. First, at age 3 months, some infants have developed the ability to perceive a partially occluded object as a coherent whole (i.e., perceptual completion), while others have not yet reached this milestone. Second, systematic comparisons of how infants scan occluded objects suggest that perceptual completion is the result of efficient, systematic visual exploration. Finally, a series of simulation studies provide additional support for the role of skilled oculomotor behavior in the development of perceptual completion and, more importantly, also suggest that growth in an area of the brain associated with spatial processing and visual attention (i.e., PPC) may underlie changes in visual exploration during early infancy.

The ideas and work discussed thus far provide an important foundation, not only for the study of visual exploration but also more broadly for the study of IM. Nevertheless, there are a number of issues that remain unaddressed. I highlight here four key questions:

1. Is visual exploration in early infancy the earliest form of IM? To answer this question, it is important to remember that the focus in this chapter has been on IM as a mechanism that directs or causes behavior, rather than as a learning signal that modifies behavior. Thus, the question can be broken into two problems: (a) What are the earliest forms of exploratory behavior, and (b) how are these

behaviors integrated within or influenced by a more general IM mechanism (e.g., novelty seeking, prediction learning, and skill development)?

As a preliminary step toward answering these questions, it may be useful to note that there are a number of similarities between how young infants explore the world visually, and how older infants, children, and adults explore through more elaborate forms of action. Indeed, Piaget proposed that the same underlying mechanism can be used to explain infants' exploratory activities, both in early infancy and then again at later stages. Thus, he noted that between 12 and 18 months, infants engage in a pattern of behavior he called a tertiary circular reaction: At this stage, infants systematically manipulate objects, in order to discover novel properties or functions. For example, a child might discover that dropping an object from a high chair makes an interesting sound and then attempt to drop different objects, one after another, in order to figure out which ones make the loudest sounds.

Other later-developing behaviors might also be included within the spectrum of IM, such as the emergence of pretend or symbolic play in early childhood and the development of academic skill and mastery motivation in middle childhood. The possibility that IM begins to take root in early infancy is an important question for developmental psychologists. If in fact these different forms of IM are related, then it should be possible to predict the quality of later forms on the basis of how prior ones emerge and develop. For example, recall that individual differences in visual-processing speed and efficiency during infancy are associated with comparable differences in IQ during later childhood. These findings provide support for the idea that curiosity and novelty-seeking behavior in infants have a measurable impact on learning and cognitive skill in older children.

2. What role does salience play in the development of visual exploration? As I noted earlier, our use of a salience-based model is not intended to suggest that visual exploration in young infants is entirely driven by bottom-up perceptual salience. Rather, our simulation findings provide clear evidence that internal modulation of salience, through maturational or developmental changes in attentional mechanisms, may play a fundamental role in shaping the development of visual exploration and, in particular, in the shift from endogenous to exogenous control of vision.

   Nevertheless, salience is an important dimension of IM, insofar as salient objects and events not only drive attention but are also associated with brain areas that involve dopaminergic activity (e.g., Barto et al. 2004; Bromberg-Martin et al. 2010; Redgrave and Gurney 2006; Redgrave et al. 2012). An important open question, therefore, is not only what role perceptual salience plays in IM during early infancy but also how it interacts with or is related to top-down forms of salience that involve prediction or appraisal (e.g., motivational salience and incentive salience; see Bromberg-Martin et al. 2010).

A related and equally important issue concerns the fact that perceptual and cognitive development in young infants is often assessed with a preferential-looking method, such as *habituation-dishabituation*, which relies on the tendency for infants to look longer at things that are novel or unfamiliar. This raises several questions: What are the neural bases of novelty detection in young infants (for related discussions, see Merrick 2012; Nehmzow et al. 2012)? How and when does this substrate develop? Is the underlying mechanism predictive? An intriguing, though admittedly speculative hypothesis is that, at least for very young infants (e.g., 2–3 months), it is the comparatively fast visual pathway from the retina to the superior colliculus that may play a key role in the detection of unexpected events and perceptual-motor learning (e.g., Isoda and Hikosaka 2008; Redgrave and Gurney 2006).

3. Is IM a general attribute, or is it skill and domain specific? A third question concerns the knowledge structures that are formed in the process of exploratory behavior. One possibility is that IM is a general attribute. According to this view, a particular child can be characterized as preferring a certain level of novelty or familiarity. For example, an infant may show a strong preference for familiar objects, situations, and actions. The idea that there is a single, unified drive or mechanism for IM, which spans a diverse range of knowledge domains, has been proposed by Schmidhuber (2009). Alternatively, IM may be highly domain specific. In this case, an infant may show a preference for familiarity in one domain or skill context (e.g., when interacting with people) while showing a preference for novelty in other domains (e.g., food, toys, books).
4. Where is the "best place" to explore? The final question is relevant not only to developmental psychologists but also to researchers in machine learning as well. In particular, Piaget's moderate novelty principle suggests a strategy for guiding the exploratory process: Exploration, and as a result, learning is best achieved at the "edges" of the state space. In other words—rather than randomly probing the environment, or alternatively, exhaustively sweeping through all possible states—Piaget's theory advocates for a relatively conservative approach to exploration, in which new experiences are sought that modestly extend known regions of the environment (i.e., hierarchical, cumulative learning). Interestingly, it should be noted that this approach complements Vygotsky's notion of the *zone of proximal development* (Vygotsky 1978), which is the gap or space between what a child can do alone and what they can do with the assistance of others.

References

Albright, T., Stoner, G.: Contextual influences on visual processing. Annu. Rev. Neurosci. **25**, 339–379 (2002)

Amso, D., Johnson, S.P.: Learning by selection: Visual search and object perception in young infants. Dev. Psychol. **42**, 1236–1245 (2006)

Antinucci, F.: Cognitive Structure and Development in Nonhuman Primates. Erlbaum, Hillsdale (1989)

Baldassarre, G.: What are intrinsic motivations? A biological perspective. In: Cangelosi, A., Triesch, J., Fasel, I., Rohlfing, K., Nori, F., Oudeyer, P.-Y., Schlesinger, M., Nagai, Y. (eds.) Proceedings of the International Conference on Development and Learning and Epigenetic Robotics (ICDL-EpiRob-2011). IEEE, New York, Frankfurt, Germany (2011)
Banks, M., Bennett, P.: Optical and photoreceptor immaturities limit the spatial and chromatic vision of human neonates. J. Opt. Soc. Am. **5**, 2059–2079 (1988)
Barborica, A., Ferrera, V.: Modification of saccades evoked by stimulation of frontal eye field during invisible target tracking. J. Neurosci. **24**, 3260–3267 (2004)
Barto, A., Singh, S., Chentanez, N.: Intrinsically motivated learning of hierarchical collections of skills. In: UCSD Institute for Neural Computation I. (ed.) Proceedings of the 3rd International Conference on Development and Learning, San Diego (2004)
Berlyne, D.: A theory of human curiosity. Br. J. Psychol. **45**, 180–191 (1954)
Bjorklund, D.: The role of immaturity in human development. Psychol. Bull. **122**, 153–169 (1997)
Bornstein, M., Sigman, M.: Continuity in mental development from infancy. Child Dev. **57**, 251–274 (1986)
Bowlby, J.: Attachment. Basic Books Inc, New York (1969)
Bromberg-Martin, E., Matsumoto, M., Hikosaka, O.: Dopamine in motivational control: Rewarding, aversive, and alerting. Neuron **68**, 815–834 (2010)
Bronson, G.: Infant differences in rate of visual encoding. Child Dev. **62**, 44–54 (1991)
Canfield, R., Kirkham, N.: Infant cortical development and the prospective control of saccadic eye movements. Infancy **2**, 197–211 (2001)
Case, R.: Intellectual Development: Birth to Adulthood. Academic, New York (1985)
Charlesworth, W.: The role of surprise in development. In: Studies in Cognitive Development: Essays in Honor of Jean Piaget, pp. 257–314. Oxford University Press, Oxford (1969)
Dannemiller, J.: Competition in early exogenous orienting between 7 and 21 weeks. J. Exp. Child Psychol. **76**, 253–274 (2000)
Edelman, G.: Neural Darwinism. Basic Books Inc., New York (1987)
Ferrera, V., Barborica, A.: Internally generated error signals in monkey frontal eye field during an inferred motion task. J. Neurosci. **30**, 11612–11623 (2010)
Fox, N., Kagan, J., Weiskopf, S.: The growth of memory during infancy. Genet. Psychol. Monogr. **99**, 91–130 (1979)
Gilmore, R.O., Thomas, H.: Examining individual differences in infants' habituation patterns using objective quantitative techniques. Infant Behav. Dev. **25**, 399–412 (2002)
Ginsburg, H., Opper, S.: Piaget's Theory of Intellectual Development. Prentice Hall, Englewood Cliffs (1988)
Gottlieb, J.P., Kusunoki, M., Goldberg, M.E.: The representation of visual salience in monkey parietal cortex. Nature **391**, 481–484 (1998)
Greenough, W., Black, J.: Experience, neural plasticity, and psychological development. In: Experience, Neural Plasticity, and Psychological Development, pp. 29–40. Johnson and Johnson Pediatric Institute, New York (1999)
Haith, M.M., Hazan, C., Goodman, G.: Expectations and anticipation of dynamic visual events by 3.5-month-old babies. Child Dev. **59**, 467–479 (1988)
Haith, M.: Rules that babies look by: The organization of newborn visual activity. Erlbaum, Hillsdale (1980)
Haith, M., Wentworth, N., Canfield, R.: The formation of expectations in early infancy. Adv. Infancy Res. **8**, 251–297 (1993)
Hess, R., Field, D.: Integration of contours: New insights. Trends Cogn. Sci. **3**, 480–486 (1999)
Isoda, M., Hikosaka, O.: A neural correlate of motivational conflict in the superior colliculus of the macaque. J. Neurophysiol. **100**, 1332–1342 (2008)
Itti, L., Koch, C.: A saliency-based search mechanism for overt and covert shifts of visual attention. Vis. Res. **40**, 1489–1506 (2000)
Itti, L., Koch, C.: Computational modelling of visual attention. Nat. Rev. Neurosci. **2**, 194–203 (2001)

Itti, L., Koch, C., Niebur, E.: A model of saliency-based visual attention for rapid scene analysis. IEEE Trans. Pattern Anal. Mach. Intell. **20**, 1254–1259 (1998)

Johnson, M.: Cortical maturation and the development of visual attention in early infancy. J. Cogn. Neurosci. **2**, 81–95 (1990)

Johnson, S.: Development of perceptual completion in infancy. Psychol. Sci. **15**, 769–775 (2004)

Johnson, S., Slemmer, J., Amso, D.: Where infants look determines how they see: Eye movements and object perception performance in 3-month olds. Infancy **6**, 185–201 (2004)

Kagan, J.: Motives and development. J. Pers. Soc. Psychol. **22**, 51–66 (1972)

Klahr, D., MacWhinney, B.: Information processing. In: Cognitive, Language, and Perceptual Development, vol. 2, pp. 631–678. Wiley, New York (1998)

Maurer, D., Salapatek, P.: Developmental changes in the scanning of faces by young infants. Child Dev. **47**, 523–527 (1976)

McCall, R., Carriger, M.: A meta-analysis of infant habituation and recognition memory as predictors of later iq. Child Dev. **64**, 57–79 (1993)

Merrick, K.E.: Novelty and beyond: Towards combined motivation models and integrated learning architectures. In: Baldassarre, G., Mirolli, M. (eds.) Intrinsically Motivated Learning in Natural and Artificial Systems, pp. 209–233. Springer, Berlin (2012)

Nehmzow, U., Gatsoulis, Y., Kerr, E., Condell, J., Siddique, N.H., McGinnity, M.T.: Novelty detection as an intrinsic motivation for cumulative learning robots. In: Baldassarre, G., Mirolli, M. (eds.) Intrinsically Motivated Learning in Natural and Artificial Systems, pp. 185–207. Springer, Berlin (2012)

Ognibene, D., Pezzulo, G., Baldassare, G.: Learning to look in different environments: An active-vision model which learns and readapts visual routines. In: From Animals to Animats, vol. 11, pp. 199–210. Springer, Berlin (2010)

Oudeyer, P.-Y. Kaplan, F.: What is intrinsic motivation? A typology of computational approaches. Front. Neurorobot. **1**, 1–14 (2007)

Piaget, J.: The Origins of Intelligence in Children. International Universities Press, New York (1952)

Redgrave, P., Gurney, K.: The short-latency dopamine signal: A role in discovering novel actions? Nat. Rev. Neurosci. **7**, 967–975 (2006)

Redgrave, P., Gurney, K., Stafford, T., Thirkettle, M., Lewis, J.: The role of the basal ganglia in discovering novel actions. In: Baldassarre, G., Mirolli, M. (eds.) Intrinsically Motivated Learning in Natural and Artificial Systems, pp. 129–149. Springer, Berlin (2012)

Ruthazer, E., Stryker, M.: The role of activity in the development of long-range horizontal connections in area 17 of the ferret. J. Neurosci. **16**, 7253–7269 (1996)

Schlesinger, M., Amso, D., Johnson, S.: The neural basis for visual selective attention in young infants: A computational account. Adap. Behav. **15**, 135–148 (2007a)

Schlesinger, M., Amso, D., Johnson, S.: Simulating infants' gaze patterns during the development of perceptual completion. In: Berthouze, L., Prince, C.G.and Littman, M., Kozima, H., Balkenius, C. (eds.) Proceedings of the Seventh International Workshop on Epigenetic Robotics: Modeling Cognitive Development in Robotic Systems, pp. 157–164. Lund University Cognitive Studies, Lund, New Brunswick, New Jersey (2007b)

Schlesinger, M., Amso, D., Johnson, S.: Increasing spatial competition enhances visual prediction learning. In: Cangelosi, A., Triesch, J., Fasel, I., Rohlfing, K., Nori, F., Oudeyer, P.-Y., Schlesinger, M., Nagai, Y. (eds.) Proceedings of the International Conference on Development and Learning and Epigenetic Robotics (ICDL-EpiRob-2011). IEEE, New York, Frankfurt, Germany (2011)

Schmidhuber, J.: Simple algorithmic theory of subjective beauty, novelty, surprise, interestingness, attention, curiosity, creativity, art, science, music, jokes. J. SICE **48**, 21–32 (2009)

Shafritz, K.M., Gore, J.C., Marois, R.: The role of the parietal cortex in visual feature binding. Proc. Natl. Acad. Sci. U. S. A. **99**, 10917–10922 (2002)

Siegler, R., Jenkins, E.: How Children Discover Strategies. Erlbaum, Hillsdale (1989)

Slater, A., Johnson, S., Brown, E., Badenoch, M.: Newborn infants' perception of partly occluded objects. Infant Behav. Dev. **19**, 145–148 (1996)

Sokolov, E.: Perception and the Conditioned Reflex. Pergamon, New York (1963)
Sporns, O., Edelman, G.: Solving bernstein's problem: A proposal for the development of coordinated movement by selection. Child Dev. **64**, 960–981 (1993)
Vygotsky, L.: The Mind in Society: The Development of Higher Psychological Processes. Harvard University Press, Cambridge (1978)
Wentworth, N., Haith, M.: Infants' acquisition of spatiotemporal expectations. Dev. Psychol. **34**, 247–257 (1998)
White, R.: Motivation reconsidered: The concept of competence. Psychol. Rev. **66**, 297–333 (1959)

Part VI
Tools for Research on Intrinsic Motivations

A Novel Behavioural Task for Researching Intrinsic Motivations

Tom Stafford, Tom Walton, Len Hetherington, Martin Thirkettle, Kevin Gurney, and Peter Redgrave

Abstract We present a novel behavioural task for the investigation of how actions are added to an agent's repertoire. In the task, free exploration of the range of possible movements with a manipulandum, such as a joystick, is recorded. A subset of these movements trigger a reinforcing signal. Our interest is in how those elements of total behaviour which cause an unexpected outcome are identified and stored. This process is necessarily prior to the attachment of value to different actions [Redgrave, P., Gurney, K.: The short-latency dopamine signal: A role in discovering novel actions? Nat. Rev. Neurosci. **7**(12), 967–975 (2006)]. The task allows for critical tests of reinforcement prediction error theories [e.g. Schultz, W., Dayan, P., Montague, P.: A neural substrate of prediction and reward. Science 275, 1593–1599 (1997)], as well as providing a window on a number of other issues in action learning. The task provides a paradigm where the exploratory motive drives learning, and as such we view it as in the tradition of Thorndike [Animal intelligence (1911)]. Our task is easily scalable in difficulty, is adaptable across species and provides a rich set of behavioural measures throughout the action-learning process. Targets can be defined in spatial, temporal or kinematic/gestural terms, and the task also allows the concatenation of actions to be investigated. Action learning requires integration across spatial, kinematic and temporal dimensions. The task affords insight into these (and into the process of integration).

T. Stafford (✉) · T. Walton · L. Hetherington · M. Thirkettle · K. Gurney · P. Redgrave
Adaptive Behavior Research Group, Department of Psychology, University of Sheffield, Sheffield, UK
e-mail: t.stafford@sheffield.ac.uk; t.walton@sheffield.ac.uk; l.hetherington@sheffield.ac.uk; m.thirkettle@sheffield.ac.uk; k.gurney@sheffield.ac.uk; p.redgrave@sheffield.ac.uk

G. Baldassarre and M. Mirolli (eds.), *Intrinsically Motivated Learning in Natural and Artificial Systems*, DOI 10.1007/978-3-642-32375-1_15,

1 Introduction

We present here, for the first time, a novel behavioural task for the investigation of intrinsically motivated action learning. We are not concerned to define precisely "intrinsically motivated" (for a treatment of this issue, see Barto 2012; Mirolli and Baldassarre 2012), rather we wish to establish a novel method which allows us to inspect those components of action learning which involve exploration and making of movements which are not predefined by the task or previous learning. Core to our approach is the idea that we can assess a component of action learning which is prior to the processes of long-term value attribution.

In the task, free exploration of the range of possible movements with a manipulandum, such as a joystick, is recorded. A subset of these movements trigger a reinforcing signal. Our interest is in how those elements of total behaviour which cause an unexpected outcome are identified and stored. Because we record all movement in the exploratory phase of the task, we are able to closely inspect the processes involved in action discovery. We define an action as a stereotyped movement, or parameter-defined family of movements, made by an agent, whether habitual or goal-directed. During exploration an agent will make many movements, usually of multiple effectors simultaneously. The process of action discovery is the identification of the subset of movements which are causally related to outcomes. It is in identifying these computations and mechanisms fundamental to action discovery in biological architectures that we believe this task has a role to play. Once identified, the computations and/or mechanisms can be embedded in an artificial agent which performs action discovery.

The motivation for the development of the task came from our critique (Redgrave and Gurney 2006; Redgrave et al. 2008) of the dominant computational theory of action learning, reinforcement learning (Sutton and Barto 1998) and the association of the short-latency dopamine (DA) signal in the basal ganglia with reward prediction errors (Schultz et al. 1997). Although we have reservations about the ability of DA neurones to signal reward, we think DA might play a critical role in the intrinsically motivated discovery of agency and the development of novel actions. This task, we believe, can play a role in the investigation of this. As well as allowing critical tests of our theory (Redgrave and Gurney 2006; Redgrave et al. 2008), we believe the task will allow productive new insights into processes which support intrinsically motivated action learning, as well as clues to their mechanistic underpinnings in the brain.

In this chapter we first discuss the ambitions and limitations of experimental tasks in relation to computational theories and use this discussion to guide an abstract description of what a good task for use in experiments on intrinsically motivated action discovery would look like. We then describe the task in more detail and show pilot data from current implementations of the task for use with humans and rats. We show how the task matches the desired features of a task for use in experiments on intrinsically motivated action discovery. We compare and contrast the focus of this task with other tasks used by major alternative approaches to action learning, highlighting the as-yet-unaddressed need for an account of action discovery and the unique contribution our task can make. Finally we provide an overview of experiments which we have underway using the task and of the prospects for future possible contributions of the task.

1.1 The Role of Behavioural Testing

In the context of a book with contributions dominated by roboticists and computational theorists, it may be worth giving a short overview of our ambitions as experimentalists.

At its most fundamental, an experiment can give a systematic demonstration of some phenomenon, for example, Kish (1955) showed the existence of non-rewarded, that is, "intrinsically motivated", operant conditioning. This was an important early indication that although primary rewards, such as food, could strongly influence an animal's rate of responding, responding could also be affected by "mere" sensory consequences of an action, such as "microswitch clicks, relay noises, and stimuli produced by a moving platform" (Kish 1955 citing work by Kish and Antonitis 1956).

An experimental procedure can also provide a forum for the careful characterisation of the features of a behavioural phenomenon. In this sense, it is a kind of structured observation. This observation is particularly useful when a phenomenon has not been studied before or where the phenomenon is to be studied in two very different circumstances (e.g. as manifested in different species).

However, for many of the phenomenon of behaviour, including learning, we are all familiar with the appearance of the phenomenon, and even sophisticated theories can be compared immediately to our atheoretical impression of the phenomenon for superficial validity. In order to distinguish theories from each other, or in order to yield new data which can be used to advance theories, experiments must be carefully designed according to theoretical motivations. It is not enough to "see what happens".

We wish to relate our measurements directly to theoretical constructs that are important to the theories we are testing. For example, if an animal tends to choose brighter objects to explore first, this observation cannot advance any reasonable theory of intrinsic motivation. By measuring how bright an object must be in order to be selected first, and how this quality trades-off against other features - which we might understand under the heading of "salience", we can then begin to ask questions about the mechanism that computes salience and thus impacts on intrinsically motivated exploration.

Computational theory can play a number of roles with respect to experimental investigation. Theory is required to outline the scope of possibilities, to make predictions and to provide a benchmark against which data can be compared. All these purposes of modelling make use of the assumption of optimality that if there is a "best" way to compute something, then the brain will have found a way to do this computation. As far as this assumption is true, we can discover facts about the brain and make predictions by theoretical effort alone. By developing theories of how various functions can or should be computed, we are discovering facts which will also be true of the optimal brain. The limitation of this approach is that it is only useful as far as the brain is optimal, or—more precisely—to the extent that the brain is optimising the same thing that we suppose in our theories of it. If, for example, the brain optimises metabolic efficiency or robustness across the vagaries of evolutionary time, an informationally optimal computation may be shunned in favour of a suboptimal one (e.g. Stafford and Gurney 2007). This divergence from our model of optimality is often the most interesting thing to the experimentalist. As experimentalists, we strive to construct situations in which contingent truths about the brain and behaviour are shown, rather than necessary truths. The heuristics and biases programme in cognitive psychology is an example of the successful prosecution of this approach (Kahneman et al. 1982; Kahneman and Tversky 1979; Tversky and Kahneman 1981).

Even when behaviour does conform exactly to some computationally optimal or elegant theory, the experimental neuroscientist is still compelled to ask questions of mechanism. That is, how is some function implemented? What is the biological basis which comprises the mechanistic underpinning of the function? Marr (1982) provides the canonical discussion of computational, algorithmic and mechanistic levels of investigation of brain function.

Ideally an experimental procedure will allow for precise measurement in a situation that is highly replicable. Too much freedom on the part of the participant in the experiment will prevent meaningful comparison between different participants or conditions of the task. This issue of variability arising from different subjects is particularly relevant to studies of intrinsic motivation, since any study of intrinsic motivation must allow, by definition, a degree of freedom of choice in the experimental participant's actions. Conversely, it was in order to reduce variability that the early and successful approach of skinner was adopted (one action—pressing the lever, one dependent variable—rate of response). As will become clear later in this chapter, we believe that the experimental analysis of behaviour has now progressed to a point where important gains can be made by allowing a slight increase in the freedom allowed to participants in action-learning tasks.

1.2 Requirements of a Task for Investigating Intrinsically Motivated Action Learning

With these considerations in mind, let us characterise those features that a task for investigating intrinsically motivated action learning would ideally have. In contrast to famous procedures established by Skinner for the investigation of action learning (Ferster and Skinner 1957), we do not seek to minimise extraneous movements of the biological or artificial subject. Since we are interested in the role of intrinsic motivation, we seek a task where some spontaneously emitted behaviour is the focus, not a regrettable side effect. Since we believe that reward-based learning is an important but not complete element of action learning, we would ideally have a task where primary rewards (e.g. economic, metabolic or reproductive utility) can be added but are not integral (see White 1989 for a discussion of the distinction between "reward" and 'reinforcement". Briefly, "reinforcement" is the wider class, referring to all mnemonic effects, while "reward" is the narrower class, referring to stimuli which immediately elicit overt approach behaviour). We desire a task where exploratory movements can be recorded and their conversion into definite actions observed. Perhaps also, it is desirable, in order to gain some leverage on the nature of intrinsic motivation, that the elements of our task which do turn out to be reinforcing can be analysed as to why they are reinforcing, be it, for example, novelty and surprise or, for example, compression gain (Schmidhuber 2009).

No behavioural task, on its own, can provide insights into the neurobiological mechanisms required for its performance. For this, cross validation with *in vivo* imaging, invasive neurobiological procedures (e.g. lesions, pharmacological manipulations, electrophysiological and haemodynamic recording) or post-mortem investigation is required. These are all facilitated if the task can be carried out by non-human animals. Some insight into mechanism is also afforded by the use of stimuli or response domains for which the neurobiological mechanisms have also been uncovered. It would therefore be advantageous if the stimuli or responses involved in the task were flexible, so that they could be tailored to the requirements of particular studies which require highly specified stimuli or responses.

Empirical investigation is also constrained by practical requirements such as the expense of the equipment needed and the time taken to run a procedure. So ideally our task would be cheap and quick to run. Unlike computational models, human and non-human animal participants in an experiment learn and adjust according to their experiences and cannot be "reset" to a position of naivety. Normally psychologists take steps to ensure or confirm that their experiments are not confounded by significant learning effects. When the topic under investigation *is* learning effects, this becomes more difficult. One approach might be to only use naive participants. This is the situation with many action-learning paradigms—once the rat has learnt to press the lever, you need a new rat. This approach introduces delay and expense to the procedure. An ideal task would find some way of avoiding these inconveniences.

2 The Task

Here we describe the essentials of the task and its variants. The essence of the task is that the subject's free movements are recorded, either via a manipulandum, such as a joystick, or directly via a touch screen. Certain movements, henceforth "targets", result in a sign or signal, henceforth the "reinforcement signal". The aim of the

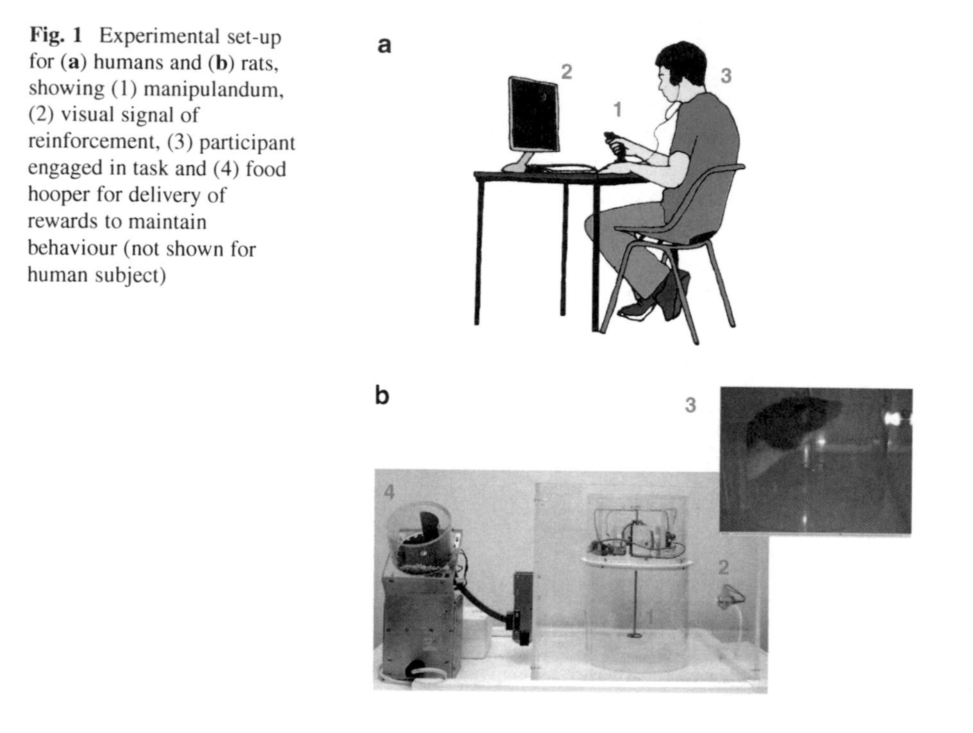

Fig. 1 Experimental set-up for (**a**) humans and (**b**) rats, showing (1) manipulandum, (2) visual signal of reinforcement, (3) participant engaged in task and (4) food hooper for delivery of rewards to maintain behaviour (not shown for human subject)

task is to discover what characteristics of movement of the manipulandum evoke a phasic stimulus (which may or may not be a reward). The target may be defined in terms of absolute spatial position, in which case it is a "hotspot", or in terms of a relative motion anywhere in absolute space, in which case it is a "gesture". The target can even be related to the timing of the movement, for example, onset or speed, regardless of its spatial characteristics. The success of most real-life actions will depend on all of these components, which refer to as the "where", "when" and "what" of action. For different experiments with the task, the target can be defined in terms of one or more of these dimensions, so it is possible to investigate the discovery of different components of an action independently of the others. When one target has been learnt, the criteria for reinforcement are simply changed and a new action has to be discovered. This therefore affords the requirements of repeated measures.

2.1 Examples of Data from the Task

Figure 1 shows the apparatus for running the experiment with both human and rat participants. Note that in the human set-up, the computer display is used only to deliver signals that the target motion has been made; it provides no visual feedback on the recorded position of the joystick. For the rat version, a long-handled

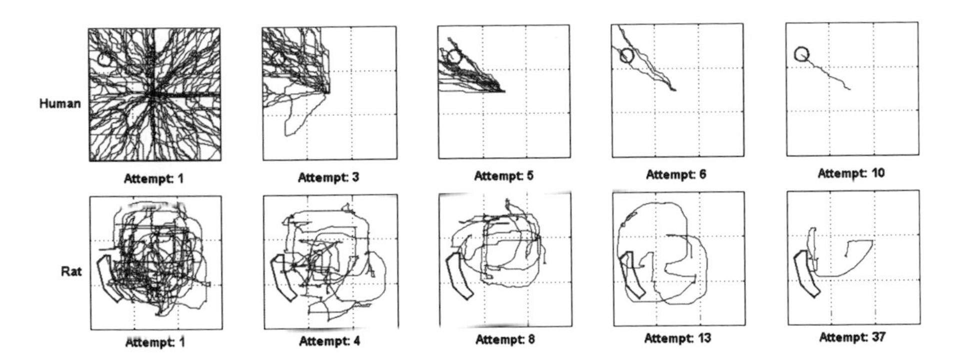

Fig. 2 Movement traces (*blue*) for a spatial target (outlined in *red*) for typical (**a**) human and (**b**) rat participants

manipulandum hangs from the ceiling of the rat's enclosure, to give it sufficient mechanical advantage. It can be moved with precision by the animal using a mouth or forepaw grip or less precisely using a full body or tail swipe. Once moved, the rat joystick is engineered so that it maintains position rather than returning to the centre point. While a typical computer-literate human participant can be simply instructed to make exploratory motions with the joystick, rat participants require more direction. For the rat versions of the task, so far, we have shaped the animal's behaviour by initially reinforcing any movement of the joystick and subsequently refining the required target. A full description of the mechanics and procedures involved in running this task with rats is in preparation. Similarly, we are also preparing a full description of the procedures involved in the human version of the task.

As alluded to, the task affords a complete record of the movements of the manipulandum. Figure 2 shows typical continuous traces from both human and rat subjects as they initially explore and then refine their movements so as to home in on a spatially defined target (a "hotspot"). Note the similarity in the plots. Although rats take longer to refine movements into a stereotyped action, the similarity in the progression of behaviour in this "where" version of the task suggests that we are tapping the same process that relies on similar underlying machinery of action discovery.

From the raw, total, data of participant movements, various statistics can be computed which reveal the progress of action learning. Figure 3 shows a sample statistic—total time to find hotspot—which reveals the progress of action learning during a trial with a typical human participant, where "trial" refers to all attempts at finding a particular target. Note that it is also possible to calculate other statistics, such as the total distance traversed by the manipulandum.

Figure 4 shows typical learning statistics from a rat. Note that within-trial learning is evidenced, but not significant across-trial learning.

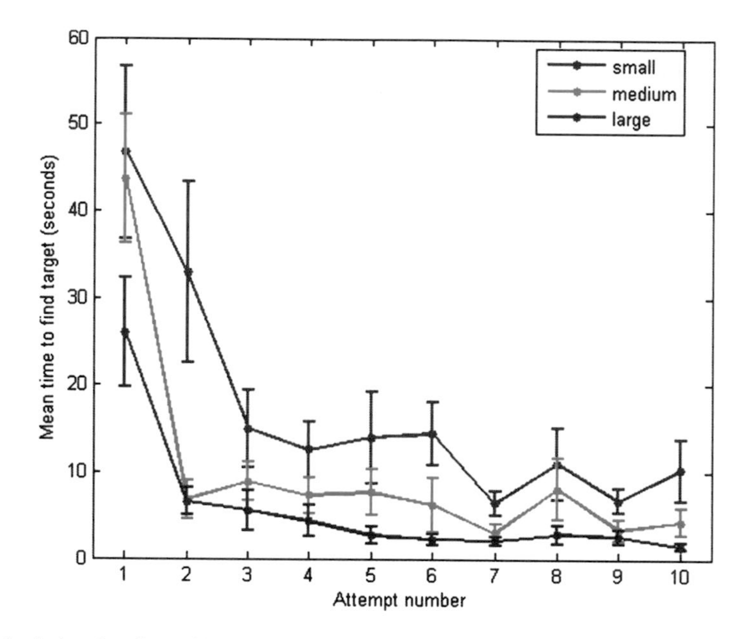

Fig. 3 Statistics showing within-trial learning for typical human participants ($n = 29$, standard error bars shown)

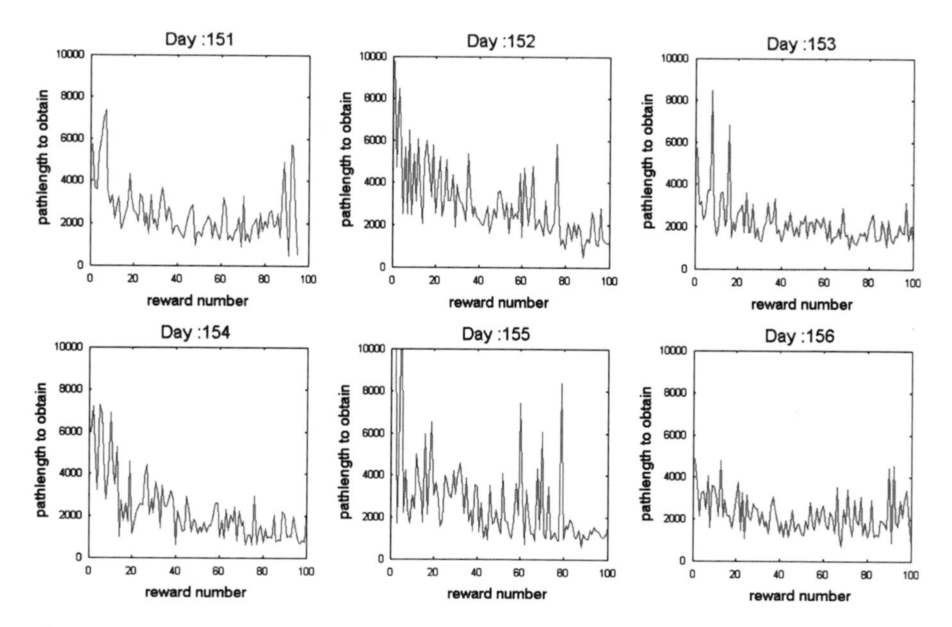

Fig. 4 Average within-trial learning on six consecutive days on the rat version of the task ($n = 6$)

2.2 *Benefits of the Task*

A prime benefit of the task is that it does not take long to perform, and once a particular target has been learnt, the target can be switched so that the same non-human animal or human participant can repeat the process of action learning. This allows experiments with repeated-measures designs (which allow analyses of greater statistical power) as well as greatly reducing the expense and time-cost of experimentation in comparison with those tasks that require fresh subjects for each trial.

The task enjoys a number of other practical benefits. It is scalable in difficulty, simply altering the required precision of the target. For example, in the spatial version of the task, this corresponds to the size of the hotspot. This means that task performance can be equated across different populations (e.g. patients versus controls, lesioned and non-lesioned animals).

The task provides a rich set of behavioural measures. The moment-by-moment recording of the discovery of actions can give insight into the micro-features of action learning. For example, one issue we have considered is the extent to which accidental or coincidental movement features that are present during a first successful movement will be preserved and reinforced. We have supposed that unexpected events provoke inspection of a limited record of motor output, the equivalent to the eligibility trace in reinforcement learning. Identification of the time window relative to an outcome for which non-causal movement features are not eliminated from an action as it is refined may be revealing of the temporal extent of this record of motor output. The manipulation of delay between target movements and reinforcement signal may also be revealing of these internal processes.

The rich set of behavioural measures can also be converted into robust statistics which show the progression of learning throughout a trial. Candidate statistics include total length of movement in between reinforcement signals, time taken to complete movement and various measures of movement complexity and efficiency.

The task affords a number of benefits to the investigator of intrinsically motivated action learning. It is a simple paradigm where the exploratory motive drives learning. There are different qualifications to this claim for the case of human and non-human participants. Human participants cannot be said to be solely intrinsically motivated, since they are induced or instructed to participate in the task by a high-level set of priorities (cash payment, course credit, amicable obligation or even charitable idealism). Once participating, however, the aspect of their behaviour which we record is driven by intrinsic exploratory motives (indeed the before-cited priorities are not posed at the right descriptive level to play an explanatory role in our understanding of moment-by-moment behaviour in the task). For non-human animals, any high-level priorities are less obvious and are certainly not given to the animal by the experimenter. Animals are simply placed in the apparatus and their behaviour recorded. In pilot studies with rats, we have, however, used food rewards to maintain behaviour. These are presented at a fixed time after the signal is delivered indicating that a target motion has been made. This was done because although action discovery can be motivated by neutral as well as traditional rewarding stimuli, the neutral stimuli are often not as effective at maintaining behaviour once the causal relation between action and outcome has been discovered (Reed et al. 1996). In both cases, we are happy to say that the moment-by-moment behaviour of the participants in our task is intrinsically motivated, and this is obviously the focus of our investigation.

Aside from the appropriateness of the task for assessing, what we argue is a key aspect of, action learning, it is also distinct from other tasks (see Sect. 3). Staddon and Niv (2008) note that it is a "historical curiosity that almost all operant-conditioning research has been focused on the strengthening effect of reinforcement and almost none on the question of origins, where the behavior comes from in the first place". We believe that this task can play a role in addressing this neglect.

It is important for the usefulness of the task that it shows convincing within-trial learning while being relatively robust to across-task learning. We must be able to see participants' learning of individual targets without too much interference from their learning (or not) of the task as a whole. We have in preparation details of the experimental support we have gathered for this requirement (see Fig. 4 which shows that for a rat doing the task performance, improvements (learning) found during a given trial are also found in subsequent trails, showing that carry-over of performance improvements between trials has been minimised).

The target domain can be altered in the task, so that it is defined with respect to what movement a participant makes, or where, when or even how fast. Contrasting different domain versions of the task may also help to reveal the common functional and anatomical core of action discovery. Elsewhere we have suggested that the basal ganglia are ideally anatomically situated to play the role of this core, communicating via looped feedback circuits with disparate brain regions which may contain information relevant to different target domains (Alexander et al. 1986).

Once learnt in the context of the task, actions can then be paired with rewards or paired with different value outcomes in different contexts. It should also be possible to demonstrate the concatenation of actions in sequences or routines and the subsumption of actions in hierarchies. This is obviously a core interest of this book as a whole and a topic of considerable theoretical interest (Botvinick et al. 2009).

3 Extant Approaches to Action Learning

The task is distinct from existing tasks used to investigate action learning. Here we describe existing tasks used to investigate action learning and the theoretical frameworks associated with them, emphasising the distinct contribution which can be made by our new task.

3.1 *Distinct from Operant Conditioning and Reinforcement Learning*

Our task has a different focus from those that look at the attachment of value to actions. The way outcome value (and aspects of outcome delivery) determines the distribution of effort once eliciting actions have been discovered is the focus of operant conditioning experiments and reinforcement learning theory. We instead focus on the process of action discovery. This is a problem which necessarily must be solved before the problem of how to value actions can be solved. This is, namely, that of identifying which movements in the entire space of possible movements create distinct outcomes in the world and so are worth storing and repeating as actions. Reinforcement learning (Sutton and Barto 1998) gives a principled computational account of the credit assignment problem in operant conditioning, but assumes a given set of states, or actions, to which credit can be optimally assigned. Our task aims to address a prior requirement of action learning, that of identifying what movements should be stored as actions.

It is worth noting that the primary technology of operant conditioning research, the Skinner box, makes automatic the recording of response rate at the cost of making invisible the processes leading up to the selection of the response. Skinner's procedure involves familiarising the animal with the box, so that other behaviours have already diminished, and thus the "attentional problem" is solved for the animal. Only the lever, the novel element, is the subject of exploration, and so this exploratory element is minimised and controlled for, to allow the experimental focus on response rates alone [this is discussed by Skinner himself (Skinner 1969)]. Thorndike's procedure required a "stamping out" of all behaviours which did not allow the cat out of the box, and so is closer to the aspects of action learning upon which we want to focus. Skinner showed that the relation between effects and actions could be systematically studied, but Thorndike's demonstration that, from many movements, the critical components for causing a particular outcome could be identified and refined into a stereotyped action has been relatively ignored (Staddon and Niv 2008).

3.2 *Distinct from Motor Learning*

There is a considerable literature which deals with the topic of motor learning and the computational theory of optimal control, in the engineering sense (Wolpert et al. 2001). It is worth noting that the problems upon which motor control theories tend to be based involve a single action, or small set of actions, which are "declared" by the experimenter. By providing continuous feedback on motor performance, the motor learning studied in these tasks may be understood computationally as a form of supervised learning (Wolpert et al. 2001). The Thorndikian process of action discovery is thus avoided. The tasks used for such studies of motor learning, in our view, focus on the "how" of motor control, rather than the "what" which is the subject of our interest. In biological terms, this relates to the parameterisation of an action so that it may be efficiently and correctly performed (i.e. timing and force of muscle contractions). Studies of motor learning tasks have found a heavy involvement of the cerebellum in this process (Diedrichsen et al. 2005; Jueptner and Weiller 1998).

3.3 Distinct from Action-Outcome Learning

Tony Dickinson has provided a compelling and thorough account of what he has called "action-outcome" learning (Adams and Dickinson 1981; Dickinson 2001). This action-outcome learning is contrasted with habit learning, and it is part of a goal-directed learning system in which the outcome associated with an action is integral to its representation. We would view action learning of the sort studied in our task as necessary but not sufficient for this kind of action-outcome learning. Dickinson and colleagues have shown convincingly that rats can select actions according to the outcome associated with them, an important cognitive capacity which is beyond the reach of mere operant conditioning of actions (the habit system). Both these systems, we claim, are predicated upon the discovery of novel actions. Once discovered, actions can both be reinforced by their consequences and associated with outcomes.

One test of the distinctiveness of action-outcome learning in the Dickinsonian sense from action discovery as present in our task may be the sensitivity of performance to delays in the reinforcement signals. It has been shown that delays of more than 2 s dramatically interfere with action-outcome learning (Dickinson 2001; Elsner and Hommel 2004). This sensitivity provides a signature which we can compare with the timing sensitivity of action discovery in our new task.

4 Prospects

4.1 A Prior Requirement of Action Learning

As discussed, we view intrinsically motivated action learning as prior to the above kinds of learning. In Staddon and Niv's (Staddon and Niv 2008) terms, we are focussing on the "origins and refinement of behavioural variety". We see this as in the tradition of Thorndike (Thorndike 1911), in that the emphasis is on exploration as a route to action discovery. Variation between movements is required to identify which components of previous behaviour were truly causal in provoking an outcome and which were merely coincidentally associated. In Thorndike's task, the question of value ("how much was that action worth?") is deprioritised (escaping the box is unambiguously very high value). Rather the question of the moment is "what was it I just did?".

As discussed, reinforcement learning does have an account of how credit is assigned to previous actions, but this framework assumes that the space of possibly relevant actions is given. Our concern is how the brain builds representations for actions, rather than accords them value. One caveat to this claim about reinforcement learning is that it applies to conventional non-hierarchical interpretations of reinforcement learning. As this task concerns the learning of collections of movements in what we have termed an action, so it could be an analogue for hierarchical reinforcement learning algorithms where higher level representations or "options" are built from smaller actions.

4.2 *Intrinsic Motivation, Rewards and Latent Learning*

It is not our claim that this task avoids all involvement of extrinsic motivation. Indeed, in the animal version of the task, food rewards are provided. The delivery of these rewards is separated in time from the reinforcement signal, since we wish to isolate the neurological effects of these two events, but it is not the case that behaviour in this task is guided only by intrinsic motivations. We view the task as capturing for our scientific inspection an effect—action learning—that is a purported reason for the existence of intrinsically motivated behaviour. Elements of behaviour in the task—namely, the exploration—are not constrained directly by extrinsic rewards, and therefore, the task reveals the basic processes of action acquisition which we suppose are a key mechanism in intrinsically motivated learning. We do not wish to claim that this a purely intrinsically motivated task, but that it will reflect important aspects of intrinsically motivated behaviour in general.

An instructive historical comparison may be to studies of "latent learning" (Thistlethwaite 1951). Tolman (Tolman 1948; Tolman and Honzik 1930) famously described how rats, allowed to familiarise themselves with a maze, showed dramatic improvements in their time to run the maze once a food was introduced at the end of the maze. The conventional reading of this finding is that non-rewarded behaviour—the intrinsically motivated exploration of the maze—can still induce learning, which can be recruited in the service of goal-orientated behaviour at a later point. For our present purposes, it is worth noting that a long debate among behavioural psychologists failed to establish that the learning which occurred in these experiments was truly without reinforcement (Jensen 2006). In other words, the learning still involved the strengthening of stimulus response links due to experience, albeit in the absence of directly extrinsic rewards such as food. Similarly, we believe, it would be impracticable to construct a practical experimental task which can be proved to contain no elements of extrinsic rewards, so we do not attempt it.

Although we do not wish to establish that our task has no elements of extrinsic motivated behaviour, we do believe that action acquisition in this task is an important example of the mechanisms and processes which support intrinsically motivated cumulative learning. Our task allows us to focus on the behavioural variation which is shaped into novel actions.

4.3 Planned Tests of Theories of Intrinsically Motivated Action Learning Using the New Task

Since it makes the processes of intrinsically motivated action acquisition conveniently observable for the first time, there are a plethora of uses of this task. However, in the first instance, we envisage two major uses in the context of intrinsically motivated and cumulative learning.

Firstly, the task allows us to carry out a series of tests of our theoretical proposals about the biological basis of action discovery in the mammalian brain (Redgrave and Gurney 2006; Redgrave et al. 2008). One of these tests involves running the task with Parkinsonian patients. Our theory predicts that patients with Parkinson's disease will have a specific learning deficit concerning action discovery. The easy calibration of the task for difficulty means that we should be able to show that the movements required in the task can be performed by the patients, but that the patients have a deficit with respect to action discovery compared to age-matched healthy controls. Another specific test of our theory involves running the task with reinforcing signals which are specialised for cortical and subcortical visual routes (see Smith et al. 2004; Sumner et al. 2002). This will allow us to discern the importance of the signals carried by these routes in allowing action discovery.

Secondly we will use the task to collect data on biological action-discovery systems (i.e. rats, monkeys and humans). This will demonstrate the utility of the task for investigating action discovery and provide a normative data set that artificial models of action discovery must try and match. Specifically, the task allows us to ask questions of the nature of the representations formed during intrinsically motivated action discovery. The paths formed by animal in the course of learning an action are a rich data set, which should allow us to ask what elements of behaviour are reinforced—are the speed, final position and/or trajectory of successful movements retained?

Acknowledgements Our thanks to Michael Port for building the rat joystick and thanks to Lisa Walton for drawing TW performing the human version of the joystick task and Ashvin Shah for useful discussions of reinforcement learning. This chapter is written while the authors were in receipt of research funding from the Wellcome Trust, BBSRC and EPSRC. This research has also received funds from the European Commission 7th Framework Programme (FP7/2007–2013), "Challenge 2—Cognitive Systems, Interaction, Robotics", Grant Agreement No. ICT-IP-231722 and Project "IM-CLeVeR—Intrinsically Motivated Cumulative Learning Versatile Robots".

References

Adams, C., Dickinson, A.: Instrumental responding following reinforcer devaluation. Quart. J. Exp. Psychol. Sect. B **33**(2), 109–121 (1981)

Alexander, G., DeLong, M., Strick, P.: Parallel organization of functionally segregated circuits linking basal ganglia and cortex. Annu. Rev. Neurosci. **9**(1), 357–381 (1986)

Barto, A.G.: Intrinsic motivation and reinforcement learning. In: Baldassarre, G., Mirolli, M. (eds.) Intrinsically Motivated Learning in Natural and Artificial Systems, pp. 17–47. Springer, Berlin (2012)

Botvinick, M., Niv, Y., Barto, A.: Hierarchically organized behavior and its neural foundations: A reinforcement learning perspective. Cognition **113**(3), 262–280 (2009)

Dickinson, A.: The 28th Bartlett memorial lecture. Causal learning: An associative analysis. Quart. J. Exp. Psychol. B Comp. Physiol. Psychol. **54**(1), 3–25 (2001)

Diedrichsen, J., Verstynen, T., Lehman, S., Ivry, R.: Cerebellar involvement in anticipating the consequences of self-produced actions during bimanual movements. J Neurophysiol. **93**(2), 801 (2005)

Elsner, B., Hommel, B.: Contiguity and contingency in action-effect learning. Psychol. Res. **68**(2–3), 138–154 (2004)

Ferster, C., Skinner, B.: Schedules of Reinforcement. Prentice-Hall, Englewood Cliffs (1957)

Jensen, R.: Behaviorism, latent learning, and cognitive maps: Needed revisions in introductory psychology textbooks. Behav. Anal. **29**(2), 187–120 (2006). undefinedPMCID: 2223150

Jueptner, M., Weiller, C.: A review of differences between basal ganglia and cerebellar control of movements as revealed by functional imaging studies. Brain **121**(8), 1437 (1998)

Kahneman, D., Slovic, P., Tversky, A.: Judgment Under Uncertainty: Heuristics and Biases. Cambridge University Press, Cambridge (1982)

Kahneman, D., Tversky, A.: Prospect theory: An analysis of decision under risk. Econ. J. Econ. Soc. **47**(2), 263–291 (1979)

Kish, G.: Learning when the onset of illumination is used as the reinforcing stimulus. J. Comp. Physiol. Psycho. **48**(4), 261–264 (1955)

Kish, G., Antonitis, J.: Unconditioned operant behavior in two homozygous strains of mice. J. Genet. Psychol. **88**, 121–129 (1956)

Marr, D.: Vision: A Computational Investigation into the Human Representation and Processing of Visual Information. Henry Holt and Co., New York (1982)

Mirolli, M., Baldassarre, G.: Functions and mechanisms of intrinsic motivations: The knowledge versus competence distinction. In: Baldassarre, G., Mirolli, M. (eds.) Intrinsically Motivated Learning in Natural and Artificial Systems, pp. 49–72. Springer, Berlin (2012)

Redgrave, P., Gurney, K.: The short-latency dopamine signal: A role in discovering novel actions ? Nat. Rev. Neurosci. **7**(12), 967–975 (2006)

Redgrave, P., Gurney, K., Reynolds, J.: What is reinforced by phasic dopamine signals? Brain Res. Rev. **58**(2), 322–339 (2008)

Reed, P., Mitchell, C., Nokes, T.: Intrinsic reinforcing properties of putatively neutral stimuli in an instrumental two-lever discrimination task. Learn. Behav. **24**(1), 38–45 (1996)

Schmidhuber, J.: Driven by compression progress: A simple principle explains essential aspects of subjective beauty, novelty, surprise, interestingness, attention, curiosity, creativity, art, science, music, jokes. In: Anticipatory Behavior in Adaptive Learning Systems, From Psychological Theories to Artificial Cognitive Systems, Pezzulo, G., Butz, M.V., Sigaud, O., and Baldassarre, G. (Eds). Lect. Notes in Compt. Sci. Springer-Verlag, Berlin, Germany **5499** pp. 48–76 (2009)

Schultz, W., Dayan, P., Montague, P.: A neural substrate of prediction and reward. Science **275**, 1593–1599 (1997)

Skinner, B.: Contingencies of Reinforcement: A Theoretical Analysis. Appleton-Century-Crofts, New York (1969)

Smith, P., Ratcliff, R., Wolfgang, B.: Attention orienting and the time course of perceptual decisions: Response time distributions with masked and unmasked displays. Vis. Res. **44**(12), 1297–1320 (2004)

Staddon, J., Niv, Y.: Operant conditioning. Scholarpedia **3**(9), 2318 (2008)

Stafford, T., Gurney, K.: Biologically constrained action selection improves cognitive control in a model of the stroop task. Phil. Trans. R. Soc. B Biol. Sci. **362**(1485), 1671 (2007)

Sumner, P., Adamjee, T., Mollon, J.: Signals invisible to the collicular and magnocellular pathways can capture visual attention. Curr. Biol. **12**(15), 1312–1316 (2002)

Sutton, R., Barto, A.: Reinforcement Learning—An Introduction. MIT, Cambridge (1998)

Thistlethwaite, D.: A critical review of latent learning and related experiments. Psychol. Bull. **48**(2), 97 (1951)

Thorndike, E: Animal intelligence. Macmillan Co., New York (1911)

Tolman, E.: Cognitive maps in rats and men. Psychol. Rev. **55**(4), 189–208 (1948)

Tolman, E., Honzik, C.: Introduction and removal of reward, and maze performance in rats. Univ. Calif. Publ. Psychol. **4**, 257–275 (1930)

Tversky, A., Kahneman, D.: The framing of decisions and the psychology of choice. Science **211**(4481), 453 (1981)

White, N.: Reward or reinforcement: What's the difference? Neurosci. Biobehav. Rev. **13**(2–3), 181–186 (1989)

Wolpert, D., Ghahramani, Z., Flanagan, J.: Perspectives and problems in motor learning. Trends Cogn. Sci. **5**(11), 487–494 (2001)

The "Mechatronic Board": A Tool to Study Intrinsic Motivations in Humans, Monkeys, and Humanoid Robots

Fabrizio Taffoni, Domenico Formica, Giuseppina Schiavone, Maria Scorcia, Alessandra Tomassetti, Eugenia Polizzi di Sorrentino, Gloria Sabbatini, Valentina Truppa, Francesco Mannella, Vincenzo Fiore, Marco Mirolli, Gianluca Baldassarre, Elisabetta Visalberghi, Flavio Keller, and Eugenio Guglielmelli

Abstract In this chapter the design and fabrication of a new mechatronic platform (called "mechatronic board") for behavioural analysis of children, non-human primates, and robots are presented and discussed. The platform is the result of a multidisciplinary design approach which merges indications coming from neuroscientists, psychologists, primatologists, roboticists, and bioengineers, with the main goal of studying learning mechanisms driven by intrinsic motivations and curiosity. This chapter firstly introduces the main requirements of the platform, coming from the different needs of the experiments involving the different types of participants. Then, it provides a detailed analysis of the main features of the mechatronic board, focusing on its key aspects which allow the study of intrinsically motivated learning in children and non-human primates. Finally, it shows some preliminary results on curiosity-driven learning coming from pilot

---

F. Taffoni (✉) · D. Formica · G. Schiavone · M. Scorcia · E. Guglielmelli
Laboratory of Biomedical Robotics and Biomicrosystems, Università Campus Biomedico, Rome, Italy
e-mail: f.taffoni@unicampus.it; d.formica@unicampus.it; g.schiavone@unicampus.it; m.scorcia@unicampus.it; e.guglielmelli@unicampus.it

A. Tomassetti · F. Keller
Laboratory of Developmental Neuroscience, Università Campus Biomedico, Rome, Italy
e-mail: a.tomassetti@unicampus.it; f.keller@unicampus.it

E.P. di Sorrentino · G. Sabbatini · V. Truppa · E. Visalberghi
Unit of Cognitive Primatology, Institute of Cognitive Sciences and Technologies, CNR, Rome, Italy
e-mail: eugenia.polizzi@istc.cnr.it; gloria@istc.cnr.it,sabbatini@istc.cnr.it; valentina.truppa@istc.cnr.it; elisabetta.visalberghi@istc.cnr.it

F. Mannella · V. Fiore · M. Mirolli · G. Baldassarre
Laboratory of Computational Embodied Neuroscience, Institute of Cognitive Sciences and Technologies, CNR, Rome, Italy
e-mail: francesco.mannella@istc.cnr.it; vincenzo.fiore@istc.cnr.it; marco.mirolli@istc.cnr.it; gianluca.baldassarre@istc.cnr.it

G. Baldassarre and M. Mirolli (eds.), *Intrinsically Motivated Learning in Natural and Artificial Systems*, DOI 10.1007/978-3-642-32375-1_16,

experiments involving children, capuchin monkeys, and a computational model of the behaviour of these organisms tested with a humanoid robot (the iCub robot). These experiments investigate the capacity of children, capuchin monkeys, and a computational model implemented on the iCub robot to learn action-outcome contingencies on the basis of intrinsic motivations.

1 Introduction

Behavioural sciences encompass all the disciplines that explore the activities and the interactions among organisms in the natural world. They involve a systematic rigorous analysis of human and animal behaviour through controlled experiments and naturalistic observations (Klemke 1980). Behaviour is anything that a person or an animal does. In behavioural studies, several approaches to observe and measure human and animal behaviours are used (Martin and Bateson 1998). Especially in the past, while psychologists focused on the proximate causation of behaviour and on general processes of learning in few animal species (namely, those that better adapted to laboratory conditions), ethologists were typically interested in studying the ultimate causation of behaviour, especially in nature where spontaneous behaviours and the role played by the environment could be better appreciated. These two fields are now increasingly integrating (Wasserman and Zentall 2006), also thanks to neuroscience that contributes to clarify the neural mechanisms underlying observable behaviours.

The autonomous acquisition of new skills and knowledge is one of the most astonishing capacities that can be observed in humans and animal models. The driving force that shapes this process is unknown. Children seem to acquire new skills and know-how in a continuous and open-ended manner (Kaplan and Oudeyer 2007). Before developing tool-use ability, for example, children show typical exploratory behaviours based on trial and error which could be considered as a self-generated opportunity for perceptual learning (Lockmann 2000). Most importantly, this process is not directly related to biologically relevant goals but seems to serve the acquisition of skills and knowledge themselves. According to Thelen and Smith (1994), this process follows a well-defined path strictly linked to the development of cognitive and morphological structures, which are related to the new acquired skills (e.g. tool use). How children learn to use these skills in a different context to reach a specific goal is unknown. Also non-human primates show the capability of learning new skills through exploratory behaviours (see White 1959). Even if distinguishing food-seeking exploration from generic exploration is problematic, several studies have shown that non-human primates learn to efficiently manipulate mechanical puzzle whose solution is not rewarded with food or water (Harlow 1950; Harlow et al. 1950). Exploration in chimpanzees has been studied by Welker 1956: in this work, several pairs of objects were put in front of the chimpanzees to understand their preferences for one or the other. In this way, size, brightness, and heterogeneousness were shown to be important features for eliciting interest towards the stimuli. Chimpanzees also spent a greater time exploring objects that could be moved and changed or could emit sound and light. Apart from the perceptual features of objects, it has also been suggested that interest and interaction can be strengthened by the opportunity to exert control over the environment (Glow et al. 1972; Glow and Winefield 1978).

In order to study which is the driving force that shapes exploratory behaviours underlying learning processes in humans and non-human primates, we designed a new mechatronic tool for behavioural analysis called "mechatronic board" (or "board" for ease of reference). In the construction of the board, we focused our attention on the experimental needs related to tests involving children, the New World tufted capuchin monkeys (*Cebus apella*), and humanoid robots. To show an example of the use of the board, we illustrate here some pilot experiments involving these three types of participants and directed to test if the free exploration of the board driven by intrinsic motivations allows the participants to acquire actions and action-outcome associations that improve their capacity to solve subsequent biologically relevant tasks (Baldassarre 2011). The pilot experiments run with the board and involving children and monkeys are being modelled with biologically constrained computational models tested in the humanoid robot iCub (Natale et al. 2012) engaged with the same board used to test children. The aim of these models is to understand the computational and biological mechanisms underlying the behaviours and the learning processes observed in the real participants.

2 The Mechatronic Board

The mechatronic board is an innovative device specifically designed for inter-species comparative research on intrinsically motivated cumulative learning in children and non-human primates. The board can be also used to test computational models with humanoid robots. This platform has been designed to be modular and easily reconfigurable, allowing to customise the experimental setup according to different protocols devised for children and monkeys (Taffoni et al. 2012). The mechatronic board is the result of a multidisciplinary design process, which has involved bioengineers, developmental neuroscientists, primatologists, and roboticists to identify the main requirements and specifications of the platform. The main requirements, which guided the design and fabrication of the board, are as follows:

- To allow the accomplishment of experiments involving intrinsic and/or extrinsic motivations, that is, respectively, curiosity-driven and rewarded actions, and, moreover, to allow the learning of actions in a cumulative learning fashion.
- To embed non-intrusive technologies and to be formed by elements that are ecological and small/light enough to be suitably manipulated by capuchin monkeys and children.

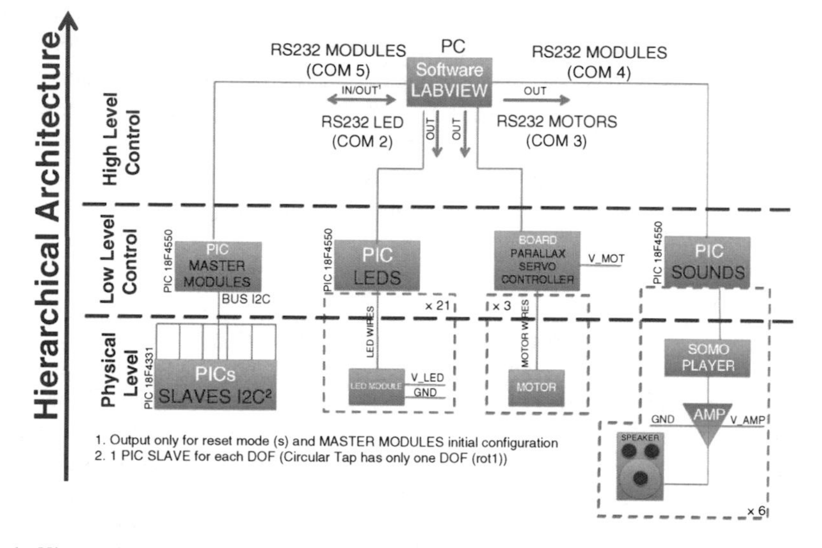

Fig. 1 Hierarchical architecture of the board: physical level made by the interfaces with participants, local low-level control based on microcontrollers, and high-level control running on a remote laptop

- To be equipped with instrumented interchangeable objects stimulating different kinds of manipulative behaviours so as to allow recording several kinds of actions (e.g. rotations, pushing, pulling, repetitive hand movements, and button pressing).
- To record synchronised multimodal information for behavioural analysis and to allow the generation of several different stimuli: visual, acoustic, and tactile.
- To allow the performance of a set of reprogrammable actions and to allow rewarding them (e.g. food for monkeys, small toys or stickers for children) and to allow the participants to see such rewards and at the same time to prevent their retrieval if necessary (done with automatically closing/opening boxes with transparent covers).
- To be made of materials, mechanisms, and electronic components robust enough to resist actions of monkeys and children.
- To prevent any manipulation or interaction which could be potentially dangerous for the participants or detrimental for the board.

To easily reconfigure the experimental setup responding to the requirements detailed above, a hierarchical *three-level control architecture* was chosen (see Fig. 1). The *physical level* is made by the interfaces that participants can directly interact with: modules and rewarding mechanisms. This level is mechanically and electronically decoupled by the other higher levels allowing, on the one hand, an easy change of mechatronic modules and, on the other, an improvement in the robustness of the apparatus. The microcontroller-based *middleware-level control* manages low-level communication with mechatronic modules, reward mechanisms, and audiovisual stimuli. The *high-level control* is a control programme running on

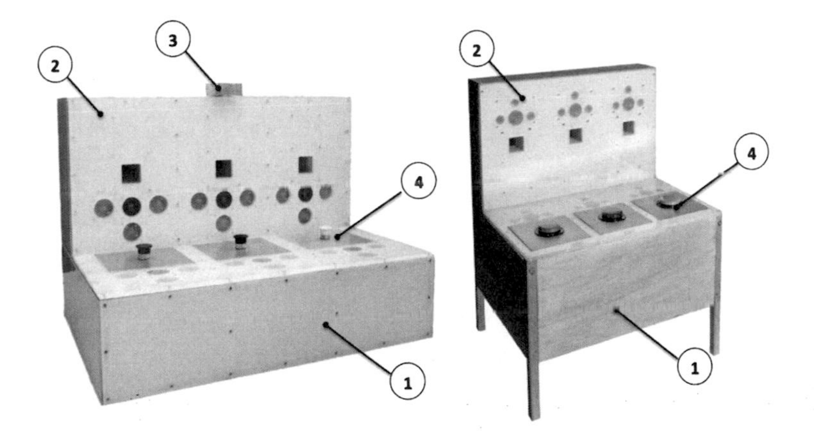

Fig. 2 The mechatronic board for monkeys (*left*) an children (*right*): (1) planar base, (2) reward-releasing unit (the squares are boxes that can open to deliver the reward, the nine grey circles are coloured lights, the three dark grey circles are loudspeakers), (3) local wide-angle camera (only in the monkey board), and (4) mechatronic modules—in this setting simple push buttons. The stimuli/reward system is not visible by the participants, and it controls the aperture and closure of the reward boxes as well as the visual and acoustic stimuli

a remote laptop which allows supervising the acquisition of data and programming the *arbitrary association between actions and outcomes*.

The mechatronic board has been designed and built in two versions for experiments with capuchin monkeys and children. The two versions of the board are slightly different to take into account the differences between the two groups of participants. The monkey version of the board is heavier, bigger, waterproof (as monkeys could urinate on it), made of non-varnished materials (as monkeys like to remove the paint with their teeth and nails), and robust enough to resist to actions such as hitting, rubbing, and biting. The children version of the board is similar to the monkey version, but is scaled in dimension and mainly made of wood (see Fig. 2).

Both versions of the board are formed by the following components (Fig. 2):

1. One planar base (800 × 600 × 200 mm for the monkey board, 650 × 500 × 450 mm for the children board): it is provided of three slots (200 × 200 mm, 180 × 180 mm) where the buttons or the different mechatronic modules can be easily plugged in.
2. The reward-releasing unit (800 × 200 mm, 650 × 120 × 400 mm): it is mounted on the back area of the planar base and contains the reward boxes where rewards are placed by the experimenter. The boxes are made by transparent material so that the participants can always see inside them. The rear side of the board is provided of suitable openings that allow the experimenter to easily insert the reward in the boxes.
3. A local video camera: embedded on the top of the reward-releasing unit in the monkey version and external for children. This camera allows recording videos of the work space during the experiments.

4. Pushable buttons and mechatronic modules: each of them is provided with a specific set of sensors and a local microcontroller unit that sends data to the microcontroller-based middleware level through a communication bus (I2C bus). Each module is identified by a hardware address, which guarantees the modularity and the reconfigurability of the system allowing to easily collect data from the different peripherals. For the mechatronic modules, only optical sensors were used in order to physically separate electronics and physical interfaces in order to avoid any direct interaction between participants (monkeys or children) and the electronics of the board. The current architecture allows reconfiguring the platform by substituting the modules (a total of three modules can be plugged at the same time); newly designed modules can also be plugged in as long as they have a unique I2C address.

   The board is currently equipped with a set of button modules and three complex mechatronic modules. The button modules allow the detection of a simple pressing action, or they can be programmed to respond to more complex interactions such as multiple consecutive presses or a hold press (the time interval can be arbitrarily set by the high-level control system). There are also other modules that support the execution of more sophisticated actions. The first mechatronic module, called circular tap, measures rotations and vertical translation of about 30 mm. The second one, called fixed prism, allows to assess horizontal rotation and translation. The third one, called three-degree-of-freedom cylinder (3 DOF cylinder), records the movements during the interaction with three different affordances. In the 3 DOF cylinder, the effect of interaction can be direct, if the participant rotates the central cylinder or translates it using the horizontal handle, or mediated by an inner mechanism, which translates the rotation of the lateral wheel in an horizontal translation of the cylinder along its main axis. Figure 3 shows the affordances and the degrees of freedom of the three mechatronic modules.
5. Stimuli and reward system: the whole platform is provided with a set of different stimuli (acoustic and visual) to provide various sensory feedbacks associated to the manipulation of the mechatronic objects. The stimuli come both from the mechatronic objects (object stimuli) and from the reward-releasing boxes (box stimuli). The acoustic stimuli are managed by a low-level sound module (Somo-14D manufactured by 4D Systems) that can playback a set of pre-stored audio files; the files that can be used during the experiments can be chosen among a bigger database of natural and artificial sounds. The visual stimuli consist of a set of 21 independent multicoloured lights. The actions on the mechatronic objects produce the activation of the audiovisual stimuli and/or the opening of the reward boxes, as defined by the experimental protocol. The reward system is conceived so that the participant can retrieve the reward only if he/she performs the correct action on the mechatronic modules. The reward-releasing mechanism was designed to be not backdriveable (so that the participant cannot force the opening: see Fig. 4).

   A Parallax Continuous Rotation Servo motor (maximal torque: 0.33 Nm) has been used to drive the box opening mechanism. The motor is coupled to

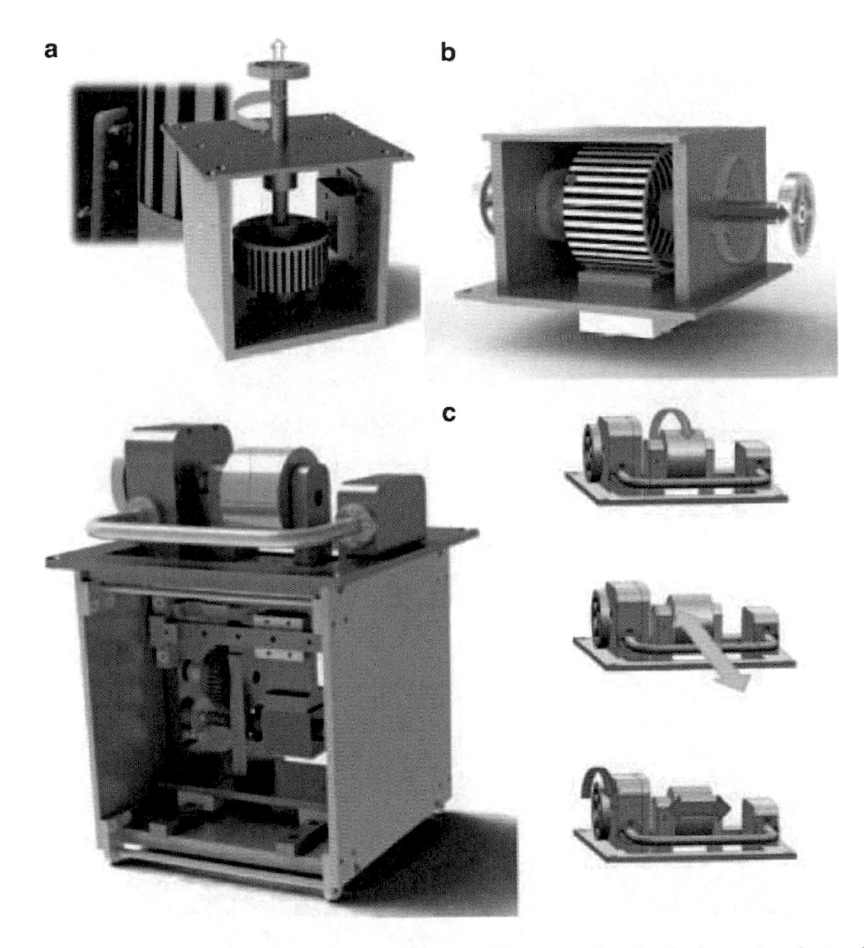

Fig. 3 Mechatronic modules. (**a**) Circular tap: overall layout and a detail of encoder electronics for rotation measurement. (**b**) Fixed prism: the frontal wall has been removed allowing to see inner mechanism. (**c**) Three DOF cylinder: the overall layout is shown on the *left*, whereas the degrees of freedom on the *right* (adapted from Taffoni et al. 2012)

the sliding door by a worm-wheel low-efficiency mechanism ($\eta_{\text{tot}} = 0.3$). The low torque of the motor and the low efficiency of the transmission make the mechanism not harmful if the participants' hand is caught in the sliding door; furthermore, since the mechanism is not backdriveable, it does not allow the participant to force the opening of the sliding door. The action-outcome associations are managed by the high-level control system and are fully programmable according to the experiment requirements.

All the electronics of the microcontroller-based middleware level have been integrated in a single motherboard that could be embedded into the planar base. The motherboard was connected to the audio/video stimuli boards and to the mechatronic modules using ten-way flat cables (see Fig. 5).

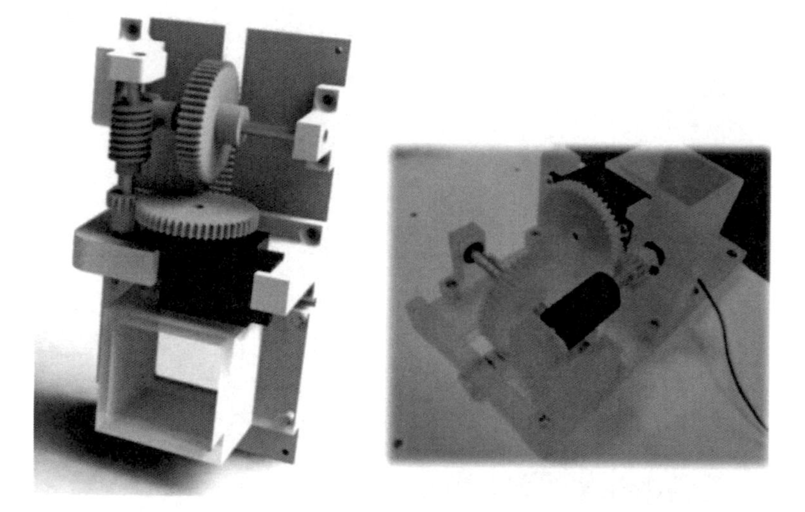

Fig. 4 Reward-releasing mechanism. *Left*: rendering of the mechanism. *Right*: the developed mechanism

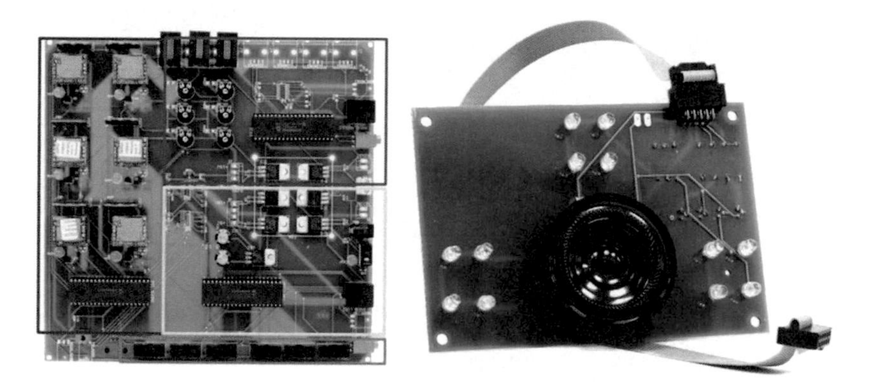

Fig. 5 *Left*: motherboard with the electronics of the microcontroller-based middleware system: PIC master for mechatronic modules (within the *top-right blue rectangle*), PIC for LED control (*centre-right yellow rectangle*), PIC for sounds control (*left green rectangle*), and connectors for audio/video stimuli board (*bottom orange rectangle*). *Right*: audiovisual stimuli board

3 Experiments with Children, Monkeys, and the iCub Robot

Here, we provide an example of experimental use of the mechatronic board equipped with push buttons. Pilot experiments were carried out at the day-care centre "La Primavera del Campus" (Universita Campus Bio-Medico, Rome, Italy) with children aged between 24 and 51 months; at the "Primate Centre" (Institute of Cognitive Sciences and Technologies, CNR, Rome) with a New World primate species, the tufted capuchin monkey (*Cebus apella*); and at the Laboratory of Computational

Embodied Neuroscience (Institute of Cognitive Sciences and Technologies, CNR) with the iCub humanoid robot. The goal of the experiments was to verify if intrinsic motivations can drive monkeys, children, and a computational model tested on a humanoid robot to spontaneously explore the board and so acquire knowledge on the possible action-outcome associations that characterise it (e.g. the pressure of certain buttons opens certain boxes). The acquisition of this knowledge is tested in a second experimental phase where the achievement of a certain outcome, for example, the opening of a box, is made desirable by associating with it a reward (e.g. a food or sticker is inserted into a particular box that can be opened by pressing a certain button). The ease with which a certain outcome is accomplished is a measure of the knowledge acquired on the basis of intrinsic motivations in the previous exploration phase.

3.1 Experimental Protocols

3.1.1 Children

The experiments are performed by placing the board in an empty room where the child is introduced by his/her teacher. The teacher invites the child to explore the board by saying, "*Look at this new toy. What is this? What can it do?*", without saying anything about what the board actually does. As mentioned, the experimental protocol is divided in two phases, a training phase and a test phase, and involves two groups of participants, an experimental group and a control group.

During the training phase, which lasts 10 min, the children of the experimental group can discover by spontaneous exploration that they can open each box (empty in this phase) by pressing a certain button for more than one second. When a box is opened, a light inside the box turns on, and a sound of an animal cry is produced (a different one for each button: a rooster, a frog, and a cat). For both groups, the simple press of a button makes the lights close to the button to turn on and produces a single xylophone note (three different notes are set for the three buttons). For both groups, the blue button (Bb) opens the left box (LB), the red button (Rb) the right box (RB), and the green button (Gb) the central box (CB) (see Fig. 6).

In the test phase, equal for the two groups, the reward (a sticker) is pseudo-randomly placed in one of the three closed boxes where it is clearly visible to the participants. The child is invited to retrieve the sticker without receiving any indication on which action to perform to open the box. As in the training phase, the box can be opened by pushing and holding the particular button associated to the box for more than one second. Pressing a button also causes the other stimuli as in the training phase.

Once the participant opens the box and reaches the sticker, this is given to the child as a reward. If the participant does not retrieve the sticker after 2 min, the sticker is moved to the next box. The test phase ends after nine successful openings of the boxes (three for each box) or after 18 min.

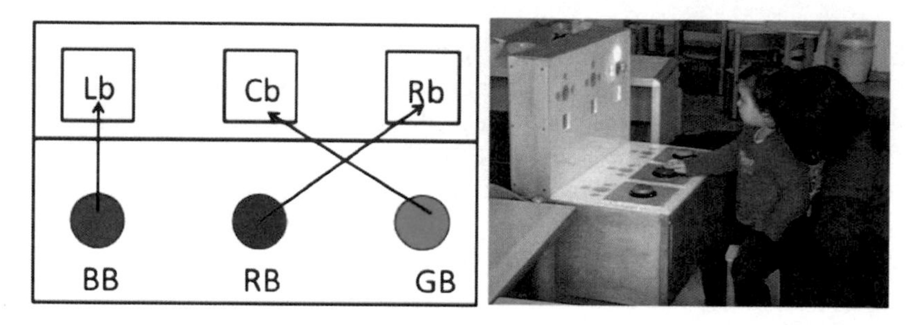

Fig. 6 *Left*: schematic representation of the arrangement of buttons and their association with boxes from the perspective of the user. *Right*: a snapshot of the experiment during the training phase

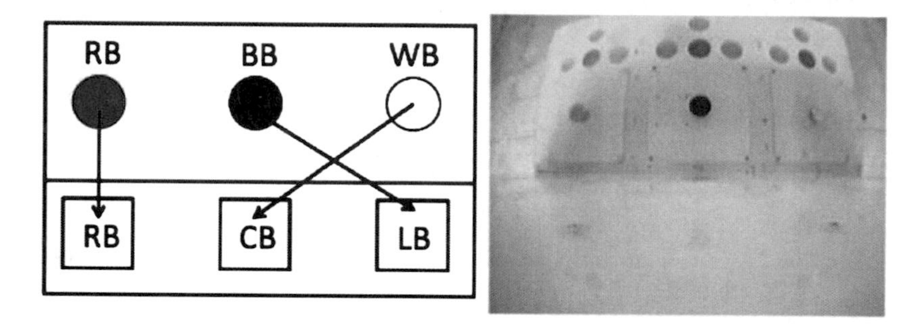

Fig. 7 Configuration of buttons and their association with boxes from the monkey's perspective (adapted from Taffoni et al. 2012)

3.1.2 Monkeys

In the experiment with monkeys, the board has three buttons of different colours (white, black, and red) placed about 25 cm apart from one another along the same line (see Fig. 7). The buttons can be discriminated by trichromatic and dichromatic subjects (male capuchin monkeys are all dichromats, whereas females can be either dichromats or trichromats, Jacobs 1998). The pressure of each button produces a specific combination of audio and visual stimuli along with the opening of one of the three boxes. Each subject is separated from the social group it belongs to just before the experimental session. Subjects are not food deprived and water is freely available at all times. The pilot experiment includes two phases as for the children protocol. During the training phase, the correct action performed by the subject (i.e. pressing a button at least once) produces a specific combination of audio and visual effects together with the opening of one box. The box does not contain any reward. The training phase lasts 20 min.

In the test phase, the reward (one peanut kernel) is located in one of the three boxes in clear view of the subject. The reward can be obtained by pressing the associated button. Each subject receives nine trials. The reward position was balanced across boxes. The test phase ends after nine trials or when 40 min elapses. For all subjects, the white button (WB) opens the central box (CB), the black button (BB) the left box (LB), and the red button (RB) the right box (RB) (see Fig. 7). Thus, the spatial relation between button and associated box is crossed for WB and BB and frontal for RB. The pilot experiment is videotaped by a camera (Sony Handycam, DCR-SR35) and by the camera embedded in the board. The ELAN software was used to synchronise the videos obtained by the two cameras.

3.1.3 Robot

The iCub robot was used to test a computational model of the board experiment run with monkeys and children (see Fig. 8). The model was built in order to formulate an operational hypothesis on the neural and computational mechanisms that might underlie the behaviours observed in the experiments with real participants.

The test with the robot is divided in two phases as the experiments involving the real participants. In the learning phase, the robot can press any button of the board. The pressure of a button causes the opening of a box. For simplicity, the buttons and boxes spatially correspond, and no sound nor light is caused by the button pressure. The opening of a box causes a surprising, unexpected event that leads the robot to learn the action-outcome association between the action executed and its effect (box opening). In the test phase, one particular outcome (e.g. box 1 opening) is given a high value (to this purpose, for now the neural representation of the outcome is manually activated). As a consequence, if the robot has suitably learned the action-outcome associations related to that outcome during the learning phase, it is expected to be able to immediately recall the correct action to obtain the reward.

We now explain the model architecture (see Fig. 9) and functioning (see Baldassarre et al. 2012 for further details on the model and its results). The empirical experiments show that when monkeys and children face the board experiment for the first time, they are already endowed with a suitable action repertoire that allows them to explore the board by performing quite sophisticated actions: for example, they focus their attention on various parts of the board quite efficiently and execute various actions such as "reach", "touch", "press", and "scratch". For this reason, the computational model is formed by two main components: a sensorimotor component (SMc), which learns and executes the movements needed to implement arm and eye actions, and a decision-making component (DMc), which learns to select and trigger the execution of such actions in the correct context.

Sensorimotor Component. As mentioned above, this component is responsible for executing the movements that implement the actions (such as reach and press) when they are selected by the DMc. This component might correspond to cortico-cortical sensorimotor pathways of dorsal neural pathways of the brain (Caligiore et al. 2010; Goodale and Milner 1992). The actions are acquired with suitable learning

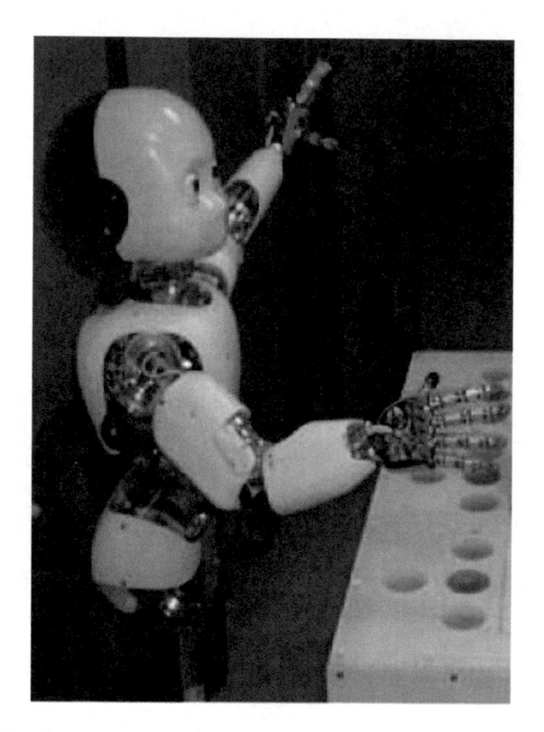

Fig. 8 The iCub robot that interacts with the board

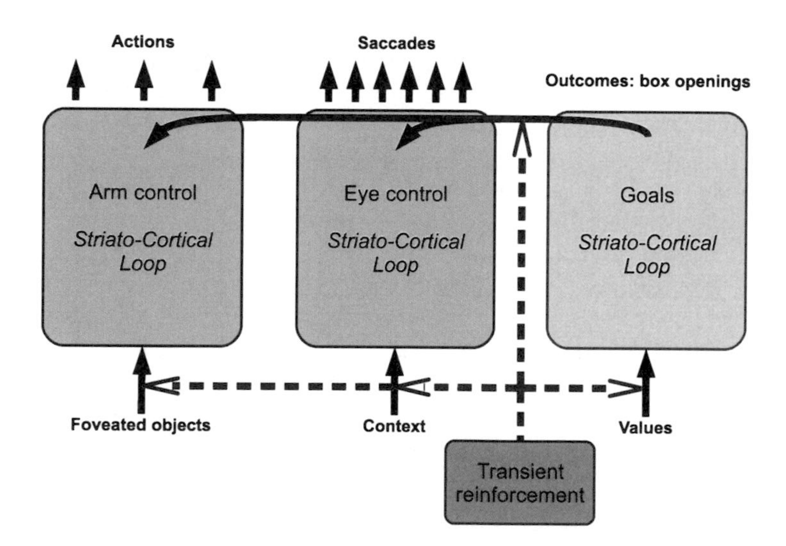

Fig. 9 The architecture of the computational model controlling the robot. *Blue boxes*: striato-cortical loops involving premotor and parietal cortex and controlling the arm and eye movements. *Yellow box*: loop selecting desired outcomes (goals). *Red box*: dopamine centres

processes before the system tackles the two phases of the experiment, so mimicking the acquisition of skills by monkeys and children before the experiment with the board. The actions used by the model were six actions for the eye ("look at button x" and "look at box y", where x and y were respectively the three buttons and the three boxes) and three arm actions ("press the looked object" and other two dummy actions introduced to test the learning capabilities of the system). Each action was learned on the basis of a sensorimotor mapping where the sensory and motor spaces were represented with maps of receptive or motor fields (cf. Lee et al. 2007). Given the focus of this chapter on the high-level cognitive aspects of the experiments with children and monkeys, the SMc of the system is not further discussed here.

Decision-Making Component. This component is responsible for deciding the actions to perform based on mechanisms putatively implemented by three *striato-cortical loops* of brain (Yin and Knowlton 2006). Striato-cortical loops are formed by basal ganglia, subcortical nuclei responsible for learning to select actions in the correct context, and various frontal cortical regions responsible for performing different actions such as reach, press, and look at a particular place in the environment and for encoding action outcomes. In the model, two loops involving the premotor and parietal cortex are responsible for selecting respectively eye actions (e.g. "look at a particular button or box") and arm actions (e.g. "press" the object you are looking). The third loop, involving the prefrontal cortex, is responsible for encoding action outcomes (e.g. "box 1 is opening"; cf. Miller and Cohen 2001).

During the learning phase, the model initially selects and performs random actions by looking various parts of the board and by executing arm action on them. Based on this exploration, the model learns to associate particular experienced outcomes with particular actions, for example, the fact that when button 1 is pressed box 1 opens. This learning process involves the formation of connections between the loop encoding outcomes and the other two loops selecting actions based on a Hebbian rule. This learning process is driven by learning signals putatively corresponding to the production of dopamine, a neuromodulator playing an important role in trial-and-error learning processes taking place in striato-cortical loops and in frontal cortex (Houk et al. 1995). Following Redgrave and Gurney (2006), in the model these learning signals are produced by the perception of the sudden opening of boxes: this surprising event activates another component of the system, putatively corresponding to the superior colliculus, that in turn causes the dopamine signal. The dopamine signal also drives a second learning process involving the striato-cortical loops, and this causes the model to repeat the last performed actions several times. This facilitates the learning process that forms the action-outcome association mentioned above (this mechanism is called "repetition bias"; Redgrave et al. 2012).

An important aspect of the model is the fact that the dopamine learning signal is *transient*: it progressively fades away if the surprising event (e.g. opening of box 1) is experienced several times (Mirolli et al. 2012). In turn, the decrease of the leaning signal causes an unlearning process within the striato-cortical loops, and this causes a decrease of the tendency to produce the actions that lead to the outcome. In this way the system can focus its activity on other action outcomes to be learned.

Table 1 Children involved in the pilot experiment

Subject	Group	Age (months)
CBM08	EXP	24
CBM06	CTRL	24
CBM11	EXP	33
CBM09	CTRL	32
CBM17	EXP	48
CBM19	CTRL	51

Table 2 Number of interactions of each participant with the board during the training phase

Participant	Presses	Correct actions[a]	Activation box 1 (%)	Activation box 2 (%)	Activation box 3 (%)
CBM08	142	57	14.03	42.11	44.86
CBM06	292	27	18.51	33.33	48.16
CBM11	92	19	21.05	36.84	42.11
CBM09	102	59	25.42	30.51	44.07
CBM17	239	49	12.24	48.98	38.78
CBM19	365	36	36.11	30.56	33.33

"a" refers to the percentage of button pushes lasting longer than 2 s

3.2 *Preliminary Results*

3.2.1 Children

Six children aged between 24 and 51 months were involved in the experiment. All children were identified as right-handed by their teachers (in future experiments, we plan to assess manual preference using the Oldfield inventory). Children were age-matched according to three age groups and assigned to the experimental group (EXP) or the control group (CTRL) (see Table 1):

- *Age group 1*, two children, mean age 24 months
- *Age group 2*, two children, mean age 31.5 months
- *Age group 3*, two children, mean age 49.5 months

During the training phase, both CTRL and EXP groups were exposed to the board for 10 min. As illustrated in Sect. 3), the box openings were disabled for the CTRL group. Table 2 summarises the interaction of each participant with the board during this phase.

Younger participants (age groups I and II) seem to prefer middle and right presses (respectively Rb and Gb) possibly because participants are right-handed. Such preference is not observed in children of group age III. Interestingly, there is a progressive increase of the number of pushes of the Lb from the younger to older age. No significant differences in terms of number of correct actions were observed between the experimental and control groups.

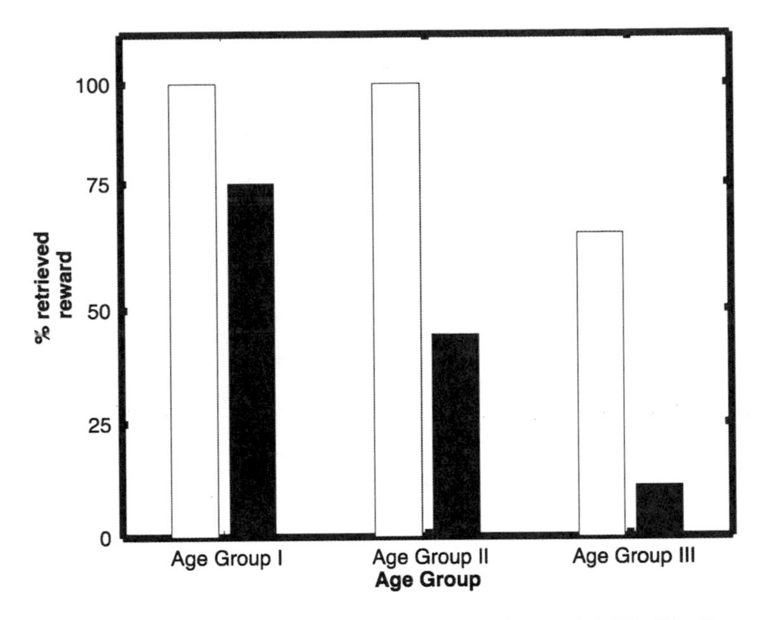

Fig. 10 Retrieved rewards (%): comparison between EXP (*white*) and CTRL (*black*) groups

Table 3 Differences in the SRI between EXP and CTRL group

Subject	SRI simple (mean ± SD)	SRI crossed (mean ± SD)
CBM08	0.39 ± 0.24	0.24 ± 0.10
CBM06	0.20 ± 0.22	0.14 ± 0.17
CBM11	0.95 ± 0.1	0.62 ± 0.23*
CBM09	1	0.08 ± 0.12*
CBM17	0.34 ± 0.01	0.45 ± 0.28
CBM19	0.32 ± 0.01	0.33 ± 0.01

$^{*}p < 0.05$

To assess the transfer of motor skills into the new context, during the test phase, participants were asked to retrieve a sticker inserted into one of the three boxes. Nine stickers were used (three for each box), and the insertion order was random (see Sect. 3). Participants in the experimental group were found to retrieve a higher number of rewards. The training effect increases dramatically with age (Fig. 10).

To assess if participants have learned the spatial relationship between buttons and boxes, we defined a *spatial relationship index* (SRI) as

$$\text{SRI} = \frac{\text{Number of correct pushes}}{\text{number of total pushes per trial}} \qquad (1)$$

According to this index, if a participant presses only the button which controls the opening of the box where the reward is placed, such index will tend to one; if a

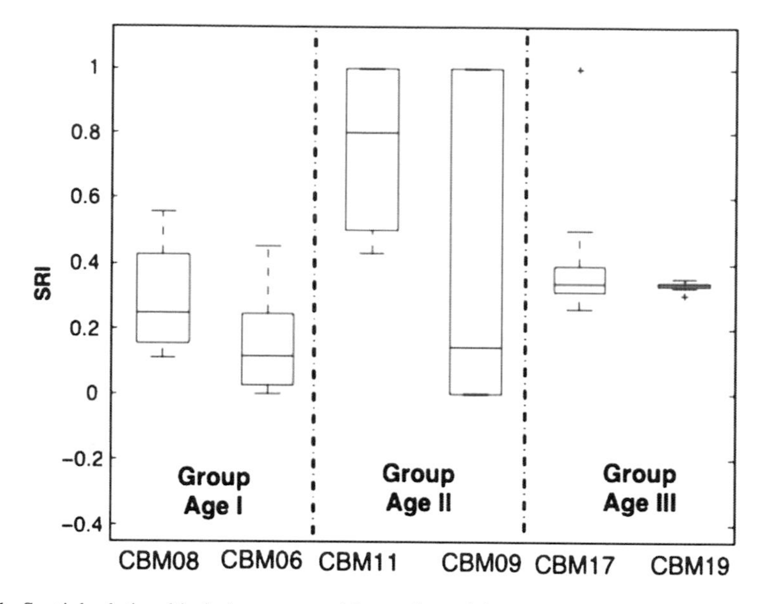

Fig. 11 Spatial relationship index measured for each participant

participant presses randomly all the buttons, such index will tend to 0.33; and if a participant learns a wrong relationship, such index will tend to zero.

Figure 11 presents the box plot of the SRI values for the six participants involved in the experiment. Red lines represent the median value of the index. Younger participants (age group I) do not seem to have learned the spatial relationship between buttons and boxes; in age group II, the two medians seem to suggest that there could be a difference between the CTRL and the EXP group: in particular the CTRL group seems to behave in a random way. Children of age group III do not show any difference and seem to act in a random way. This suggests that the children in the EXP group have learned that pressing a button for a longer period opens the boxes and are able to exploit this knowledge to retrieve the reward. However, they did not discover the spatial relationship between the buttons and the boxes. Considering separately the trials where reward was placed in boxes CB and RB cross related to buttons opening them, children of age group II seem to show a statistically significant difference ($*F(1, 10) = 25.72$, $p = 0.0007$) in SRI between CTRL and EXP.

3.2.2 Monkeys

The subjects of the pilot experiments were three adult capuchin monkeys (Pedro, Robiola, and Robin Hood). During the training phase, two subjects contacted the board within a few sec (Robiola, 6 s, and Robin Hood, 37 s) whereas Pedro took much longer (6 min and 27 s). Robiola performed her first push directed towards a button 1 min and 15 s after the beginning of the trial, whereas the other subjects

Table 4 Association between boxes and buttons

	Left box Black button	Central box White button	Right box Red button
Mean number of pushes per subject per trial ± SE	1.9 ±0.8	0.8 ±0.3	1 ±0.25
Mean number of incorrect responses per subject per trial ± SE	1.2 ±0.2	3.7 ±0.7	1.2 ±0.3
Mean holding time per subject per trial ± SE	0.2 ±0.05	0.25 ±0.03	0.3 0.11

never did it. Robiola pressed all the buttons at least twice, for a total of 14 pushes. The average time during which she held the button pressed was 0.17 s (SE: ±0.008). The average time of contact of the subjects with the board was 5 min and 5 s (Robiola, 10 min and 38 s; Pedro, 3 min and 55 s; Robin Hood, 3 min and 11 s). Each button was manipulated for a mean of 15.55 s (SE: ±2.02) during Phase 1. The overall mean scratching rate (used as a behavioural measure of stress) occurred at 0.4 events/min (SE: ±0.02).

During the test phase seeing a reward in one of the boxes prompted subjects attention towards it and increased his/her motivation to manipulate the board. Capuchins readily visually explored the baited box; this behaviour was much more frequent than in the previous phase (Pedro, 170 times; Robin Hood, 132; Robiola, 20). Indeed, subjects spent much more time on the board (mean ± SE, 19 min and 10 s ± 2.76) and manipulated each button much longer (mean ± SE, 40 s ± 8.03). Scratching occurred at a higher rate than in Phase 1 (mean ± SE, 0.6 events/min ± 0.05).

Table 4 shows for the three box-button associations the mean number of incorrect responses before pushing the correct button, the number of times each button is pressed, and the mean holding time of each button. Overall, the frontal association (right box red button) had a mean number of errors similar to the left box black button crossed association, whereas the other crossed association (central box-white button) scored a higher level of errors (see also Fig. 2). The black button located in the central position (operating the left box) was pressed almost twice the other two buttons, therefore increasing the probability to open the left box. Consequently, the comparison between frontal and crossed associations should be carried out by comparing the performances in the right and in the central box. Since the mean number of errors per trial per subject was 1.2 (right box) and 3.7 (central box), we suggest that spatial proximity plays a primary role in learning an association between action and outcome. The SRI for the three subjects involved in the experiment highlights an easier understanding of direct spatial relation (SRI = 0.76) with respect to the crossed ones (SRI = 0.51 for the black button left box and SRI = 0.34 for white button central box).

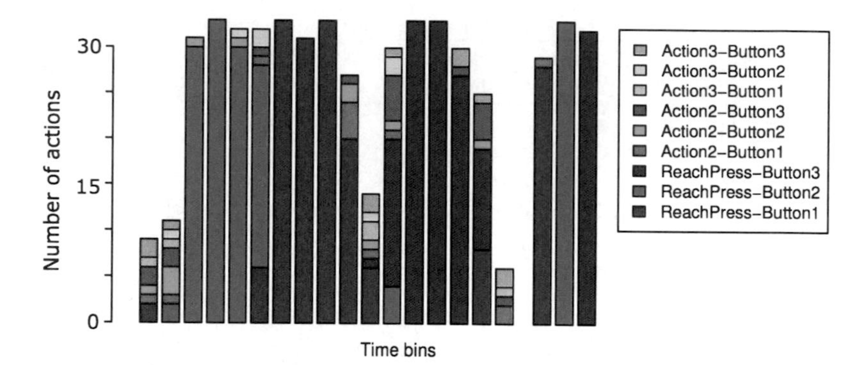

Fig. 12 Behaviour of the model during the training phase and the test phase. The y-axis shows the actions performed during time bins (x-axis) of 5 % of the total time of the experiment (120 min). The y-axis represents the number of selections and executions of the three arm actions on the three buttons when these are looked by the eye (nine combinations in total). The actions directed to the boxes are omitted for simplicity. The first 17 bins refer to the learning phase. The last three bins refer to the test phase: for each bin, one of the three goals was manually activated. Notice how the model initially performs actions randomly, then focuses on pressing one button (from bin 2 to bin 6), then on pressing a second button (from bin 7 to bin 10), then on pressing the last button (from bin 12 to bin 15), and finally on exploring again (last bin). Also notice how the system executes the correct actions during the last three bins of the test, thus demonstrating goal-directed behaviour

3.2.3 Robot

Figure 12 shows the behaviour of the computational model tested with the iCub robot during the training phase and during the test phase. Each histogram bar shows the percent of times the system performs the three action compounds involving an action of the eye and one of the arm: "look at button x and press button x" indicated with different colours for the three buttons. The graph also reports the other six action compounds of the type "look at button x and arm performs dummy action y on button x" (recall that there are two dummy actions). Notice how during training the system initially performs actions randomly, then focuses on performing the correct arm action (press) on button 2, then focuses on performing the correct action on button 1, then focuses on performing the correct action on button 3, and finally performs again random actions as at the beginning. This result shows that the repetition bias allows the model to focus its attention on a particular button for a certain period of time and then to repeat the press action several times. This leads the model to quickly learn to associate the outcome (box opening), represented in the prefrontal cortex loop, to the eye action of looking at the pressed button, represented in the eye loop, and to the arm action of pressing that button, represented in the arm loop.

The last three histogram bars of Fig. 12 indicate the behaviour of the model when, during the testing phase, each of the three goals is manually activated in prefrontal cortex for a certain period of time (the three bars refer to the three different goals). The graph shows that when an outcome is activated, the system is capable of recalling the suitable action compound that allows the system to achieve that outcome. For example, when the outcome "opening of box 1" is activated, the system looks at button 1 and presses it.

4 Discussion

The tendency of young children to explore more frequently central and right push buttons could affect the way in which they learn new skills. Preliminary results seem to suggest that children who were given the chance of discovering a new skill based on intrinsic motivations had a higher chance of employing that skill to later obtain valuable outcomes. However, neither the experimental nor the control groups did learn more complex spatial relationships. These results suggest to focus on an age range between 36 and 48 months in order to avoid problems related to motor control development.

Regarding monkeys, the results suggest that capuchin monkeys were not very interested in the buttons during the learning phase, whereas their interest towards the board significantly increased during the test phase due to the view of the reward. In this phase the board triggered a variety of behaviours, such as visual exploration, prolonged contact with the apparatus, and pressing the buttons. These behaviours may eventually lead capuchins to learn specific action-outcome associations. The association between boxes and buttons in the crossed condition was perceived by monkeys as more challenging than the frontal association, while there was a strong bias towards the central black button that decreased the number of errors when opening its associated box (the crossed left box). Although we did not collect specific data on subjects' positions on the board, this effect was probably due to the fact that monkeys spent more time at the centre of the board, where the black button was placed, than at the left and right sides. Overall, the results highlight the role of extrinsic rewards and spatial proximity as critical factors affecting capuchins' learning processes and point out the importance of choosing suitable objects that promote interest and manipulation. Very likely, buttons were too simple and afford only the action of pressing. We may thus suggest that the use of the mechatronic board equipped with modules rather than buttons would likely elicit an increase in capuchins' interest towards the apparatus.

The results obtained with the computational model and the robot have shown that the model is able to focus on performing actions that produce interesting events on the board. This focusing is transient, and when the system has acquired experience on one aspect of the board, it gets bored and starts to explore other aspects. Moreover, the model is capable of recalling the execution of suitable actions when a goal representation is activated by some internal event based on the experience acquired with intrinsic motivations. For now the mechanism that activates the goals is hardwired, but in the future it will be substituted by extrinsic motivation mechanisms based on the amygdala (a set of brain nuclei that play a key role in motivations and the assignment of subjective value to stimuli). The added value of the model resides in the fact that it explains the target phenomena by furnishing detailed computational mechanisms that might underlie the target behaviours. Moreover, the overall architecture of the model and the functions ascribed to its components has been constrained on the basis of neuroscientific knowledge on the relevant parts of the brain that are known to play important functions for the production of such behaviours. In this respect the model, although preliminary in many aspects, represents an important base for the future development of further models and a sound understanding of how intrinsic motivations drive learning and exploitation of actions in real organisms. Aside its scientific value, this knowledge can also contribute to guide the design of fully autonomous learning robots.

5 Conclusions

In this work we presented a new mechatronic platform, called the *mechatronic board*, for studying intrinsically motivated learning in children, monkeys, and robots. This chapter has presented a thorough discussion of the main design principles and implementation features of the platform and has illustrated three examples of how it can be exploited to investigate intrinsic motivations based on three pilot experiments run with children, monkeys, and the humanoid robot iCub. The preliminary data so obtained clearly indicate that the platform can be effectively used for the behavioural analysis of humans, non-human primates, and robots engaged in acquiring skills based on intrinsic motivations. Despite the fact that these preliminary experiments were carried out using the platform equipped only with buttons, more challenging mechatronic objects allowing different possibilities of interaction have been designed and will be used in future comparative studies. An important issue for future research is to develop an experimental paradigm involving the board with which to investigate the different kinds of intrinsic motivations that different subjects (e.g. monkeys and children) have. In particular, we are interested in developing a paradigm with which to experimentally assess the presence, in animals and humans, of the competence-based intrinsic motivations (Mirolli and Baldassarre 2012) that have been suggested by recent computational models (Baldassarre and Mirolli 2012; Schembri et al. 2007a,b,c; Stout and Barto 2010).

Acknowledgements This research was supported by the European Community 7th Framework Programme (FP7/2007–2013), "Challenge 2: Cognitive Systems, Interaction, Robotics", Grant Agreement No. ICT-IP-231722, and Project "IM-CLeVeR: Intrinsically Motivated Cumulative Learning Versatile Robots". It was also supported by the Italian Ministry of Educationg Universities and Research, FIRB Research Program 2006, no. RBAP06SPK5.

References

Baldassarre, G.: What are intrinsic motivations? A biological perspective. In: Cangelosi, A., Triesch, J., Fasel, I., Rohlfing, K., Nori, F., Oudeyer, P.-Y., Schlesinger, M., Nagai, Y. (eds.) Proceedings of the International Conference on Development and Learning and Epigenetic Robotics (ICDL-EpiRob-2011), pp. E1–8. IEEE, Piscataway (2011)

Baldassarre, G., Mannella, F., Fiore, V., Redgrave, P., Gurney, K., Mirolli, M.: Intrinsically motivated action-outcome learning and goal-based action recall: A system-level bio-constrained computational model. Neural Netw. (2012, in press)

Baldassarre, G., Mirolli, M.: Deciding which skill to learn when: Temporal-difference competence-based intrinsic motivation (TD-CB-IM): In: Baldassarre, G., Mirolli, M. (eds.) Intrinsically Motivated Learning in Natural and Artificial Systems, pp. 255–276. Springer, Berlin (2012)

Caligiore, D., Borghi, A., Parisi, D., Baldassarre, G.: Tropicals: A computational embodied neuroscience model of compatibility effects. Psychol. Rev. **117**(4), 1188–1228 (2010)

Glow, P., Roberts, J.S., Russell, A.: Sound and light preference behaviour in naïve adult rats. Aust. J. Psychol. **24**, 173–178 (1972)

Glow, P., Winefield, A.H.: Response-contingent sensory change in a causally structured environment. Anim. Learn. Behav. **6**, 1–18 (1978)

Goodale, M.A., Milner, A.D.: Separate visual pathways for perception and action. Trends Neurosci. **15**(1), 20–25 (1992)

Harlow, H.F.: Learning and satiation of response in intrinsically motivated complex puzzle performance by monkeys. J. Comp. Physiol. Psychol. **43**(4), 289–294 (1950)

Harlow, H.F., Harlow, M.K., Meyer, D.R.: Learning motivated by a manipulation drive. J. Exp. Psychol. **40**, 228–234 (1950)

Houk, J.C., Adams, J.L., Barto, A.G.: A model of how the basal ganglia generate and use neural signals ghat predict reinforcement. In: Houk, J.C., Davids, J.L., Beiser, D.G. (eds.) Models of Information Processing in the Basal Ganglia, pp. 249–270. MIT, Cambridge (1995)

Jacobs, G.: A perspective on colour vision in platyrrhine monkeys. Vis. Res. **38**, 3307–3313 (1998)

Kaplan, F., Oudeyer, P.: In: search of the neural circuits of intrinsic motivation. Front. Neuorosci. **1**, 225–236 (2007)

Klemke, E.D. (ed.): Introductory Readings in the Philosophy of Science. Prometheus Books, New York (1980)

Lee, M.H., Meng, Q., Chao, F.: Staged competence learning in developmental robotics. Adap. Behav, **15**(3), 241–255 (2007)

Lockmann, J.J.: A perception-action perspective on tool use development. Child Dev. **71**(1), 137–144 (2000)

Martin, P., Bateson, P. (eds.): Measuring Behaviour: An introductory guide, Cambridge University Press, Cambridge (1998)

Miller, E.K., Cohen, J.D.: An integrative theory of prefrontal cortex function. Annu. Rev. Neurosci. **24**, 167–202 (2001)

Mirolli, M., Baldassarre, G.: Functions and mechanisms of intrinsic motivations: The knowledge versus competence distinction. In: Baldassarre, G., Mirolli, M. (eds.) Intrinsically Motivated Learning in Natural and Artificial Systems, pp. 47–72. Springer, Berlin (2012)

Mirolli, M., Santucci, V.G., Baldassarre, G.: Phasic dopamine as a prediction error of intrinsic and extrinsic reinforcements driving both action acquisition and reward maximization: A simulated robotic study. Neural Netw. (2012, submitted)

Natale, L., Nori, F., Metta, G., Fumagalli, M., Ivaldi, S., Pattacini, U., Randazzo, M., Schmitz, A., Sandini, G.: The icub platform: A tool for studying intrinsically motivated learning. In: Baldassarre, G., Mirolli, M. (eds.) Intrinsically Motivated Learning in Natural and Artificial Systems, pp. 433–458. Springer, Berlin (2012)

Redgrave, P., Gurney, K.: The short-latency dopamine signal: A role in discovering novel actions? Nat. Rev. Neurosci. **7**(12), 967–975 (2006)

Redgrave, P., Gurney, K., Stafford, T., Thirkettle, M., Lewis, J.: The role of the basal ganglia in discovering novel actions. In: Baldassarre, G., Mirolli, M. (eds.) Intrinsically Motivated Learning in Natural and Artificial Systems, pp. 129–149. Springer, Berlin (2012)

Schembri, M., Mirolli, M., Baldassarre, G.: Evolution and learning in an intrinsically motivated reinforcement learning robot. In: Almeida e Costa Fernando, Rocha, L.M., Costa, E., Harvey, I., Coutinho, A. (eds.) Advances in Artificial Life. Proceedings of the 9th European Conference on Artificial Life (ECAL2007). Lecture Notes in Artificial Intelligence, vol. 4648, pp. 294–333, Lisbon, Portugal, September 2007. Springer, Berlin (2007a)

Schembri, M., Mirolli, M., Baldassarre, G.: Evolving childhood's length and learning parameters in an intrinsically motivated reinforcement learning robot. In: Berthouze, L., Dhristiopher, P.G., Littman, M., Kozima, H., Balkenius, C. (eds.) Proceedings of the Seventh International Conference on Epigenetic Robotics, vol. 134, pp. 141–148. Lund University, Lund (2007b)

Schembri, M., Mirolli, M., Baldassarre, G.: Evolving internal reinforcers for an intrinsically motivated reinforcement-learning robot. In: Demiris, Y., Mareschal, D., Scassellati, B., Weng, J. (eds.) Proceedings of the 6th International Conference on Development and Learning, pp. E1–6. Braga, Portugal, July 2007. Imperial College, London (2007c)

Stout, A., Barto, A.G.: Competence progress intrinsic motivation. In: Kuipers, B., Shultz, T., Stoytchev, A., Yu, C. (eds.) IEEE International Conference on Development and Learning (ICDL2010). IEEE, Piscataway (2010)

Taffoni, F., Vespignani, M., Formica, D., Cavallo, G., Polizzi di Sorrentino, E., Sabbatini, G., Truppa, V., Mirolli, M., Baldassarre, G., Visalberghi, E., Keller, F., Guglielmelli, E.: A mechatronic platform for behavioral analysis on nonhuman primates. J. Integr. Neurosci. **11**(1), 87–101 (2012)

Thelen, E., Smith, L.: A Dynamic Systems Approach to the Development of Cognition and Action. MIT, Boston (1994)

Wasserman, E., Zentall, T.: Comparative Cognition: Experimental Explorations of Animal Intelligence. Oxford University Press, New York (2006)

Welker, W.L.: Some determinants of play and exploration in chimpanzees. J. Comp. Physiol. Psychol. **49**, 84–89 (1956)

White, R.W.: Motivation reconsidered: The concept of competence. Psychol. Rev. **66**, 297–333 (1959)

Yin, H.H., Knowlton, B.J.: The role of the basal ganglia in habit formation. Nat. Rev. Neurosci. **7**(6), 464–476 (2006)

The iCub Platform: A Tool for Studying Intrinsically Motivated Learning

Lorenzo Natale, Francesco Nori, Giorgio Metta, Matteo Fumagalli, Serena Ivaldi, Ugo Pattacini, Marco Randazzo, Alexander Schmitz, and Giulio Sandini

Abstract Intrinsically motivated robots are machines designed to operate for long periods of time, performing tasks for which they have not been programmed. These robots make extensive use of explorative, often unstructured actions in search of opportunities to learn and extract information from the environment. Research in this field faces challenges that need advances not only on the algorithms but also on the experimental platforms. The iCub is a humanoid platform that was designed to support research in cognitive systems. We review in this chapter the chief characteristics of the iCub robot, devoting particular attention to those aspects that make the platform particularly suitable to the study of intrinsically motivated learning. We provide details on the software architecture, the mechanical design, and the sensory system. We report examples of experiments and software modules to show how the robot can be programmed to obtain complex behaviors involving interaction with the environment. The goal of this chapter is to illustrate the potential impact of the iCub on the scientific community at large and, in particular, on the field of intrinsically motivated learning.

1 Introduction

Developmental robotics is a young field of research that attempts to build artificial systems with cognitive abilities (see Lungarella et al. 2003 for a review). In contrast to other, more traditional, approaches, researchers in this field subscribe

L. Natale (✉) · F. Nori · G. Metta · M. Fumagalli · S. Ivaldi · U. Pattacini · M. Randazzo · A. Schmitz · G. Sandini
Department of Robotics, Brain and Cognitive Sciences, Istituto Italiano di Tecnologia, Genova, Italy
e-mail: lorenzo.natale@iit.it; francesco.nori@iit.it; giorgio.metta@iit.it; M.Fumagalli@ewi.utwente.nl; serena.ivaldi@isir.upmc.fr; ugo.pattacini@iit.it; marco.randazzo@iit.it; schmitz@sugano.mech.waseda.ac.jp; giulio.sandini@iit.it

G. Baldassarre and M. Mirolli (eds.), *Intrinsically Motivated Learning in Natural and Artificial Systems*, DOI 10.1007/978-3-642-32375-1_17,

to the hypothesis that cognition is not hard coded but that, on the contrary, it emerges autonomously from the physical interaction between the agent and the environment (Weng et al. 2000; Zlatev and Balkenius 2001). Developmental robotics is a strongly interdisciplinary field that brings together researchers from behavior and brain sciences (psychology, neuroscience), engineering (robotics, computer science), and artificial intelligence, motivated by the conviction that each field has a lot to learn from the others. Roboticists in particular have realized that the real world is too complex to be modeled and too dynamic to hope that static models are of any use. For this reason, they have started to seek inspiration from biological systems and how they deal with the complexity of the world in which they live.

The study of humans and biological systems confirms that nature solved this problem by designing systems that undergo a constant physical and behavioral adaptation. As humans we are probably the most convincing example in this respect, since learning and adaptation are so evident in the first period of our lives. For these reasons, developmental approaches to robotics assume that intelligent behavior and cognition emerge autonomously through development.

Experimental evidence in the field of developmental psychology shows that motor and perceptual development happen as a result of the constant physical interaction between the body and the world (Bushnell and Boudreau 1993; Needham et al. 2002; von Hofsten 2004). Newborns spend a considerable amount of time exploring the world. They do so by experimenting with their own actions and by exploring correlations between what they do and what is measured by their sensory streams.

Unfortunately, today's machines demonstrate learning abilities that are not comparable to the ones that we observe in animals or in infants. Learning in artificial systems is often applied to specific, predefined tasks, and it requires a certain degree of human supervision for parameter tuning or data preparation. Finally, exploration, acquisition of new data, learning, and exploitation are distinct processes. On the other hand, learning in humans is something that happens continuously. Children seem to be always actively searching for learning opportunities; they show what has been defined an intrinsic motivation to engage in activities that involve exploring the environment in search for novel things to learn. Intrinsic motivations and curiosity are clearly required ingredients to design machines that are able to autonomously discover not only how to solve certain tasks (like object manipulation or perception) but also how to learn or develop new abilities based on current knowledge (see Mirolli and Baldassarre 2012 and Barto et al. 2004; Kaplan and Oudeyer 2008; Oudeyer and Kaplan 2007).

Progress in developmental robotics and intrinsically motivated learning has been somewhat slow. In our opinion, this is in part due to the fact that research in these fields requires experimental platforms whose design and construction are difficult. We list here some of the aspects that characterize human development that have deep implications in the design of the hardware and software architecture of such platforms:

- Motion during development is at times dominated by exploratory unstructured behaviors (sometimes referred to as "motor babbling").
- Failure in performing a task is the norm rather than the exception.
- Learning is not cheap, the acquisition of new competences on the contrary require lots of trials and considerable efforts.
- The development of perceptual abilities requires sophisticated interaction with the world.
- Perception is intrinsically multimodal, and multisensory integration is critical for learning.
- Learning is open ended, that is, it is an incremental process in which new abilities provide support and opportunities for gathering newer ones.

This implies that developing robots need to be robust and able to operate for several hours (maybe days) in frequent and unpredictable physical interaction with the environment. They need to have articulated mechanical structure that allows interacting with the world in a sophisticated way. For example, they should be able to locomote, manipulate objects, and use tools. Their sensory system should include diverse and redundant modalities ranging from vision and sound to touch and force. Finally, their software architecture should be flexible enough to allow development of interconnected modules that receive sensory streams, perform control, and exchange information. The software should be modular to support reusability of components so that existing capabilities can work as building blocks to construct newer, more complex ones.

One of the goals of the RobotCub project[1] was the design and construction of a platform that satisfies the aforementioned constraints. The resulting platform is the iCub, a humanoid robot with 53 degrees of freedom and a rich sensory system. The iCub is an open system: researchers have full access to the details of the platform and can customize it depending on their particular needs.[2]

In this chapter, we provide an overview of the platform, focusing on the functionalities that we consider more interesting for researchers in the field of developmental robotics and intrinsically motivated learning. Section 2 provides an overview of the hardware platform, the mechanical structure, the actuation system, and the sensors. Section 3 describes the software architecture and the motivations that have driven its design. Section 4 describes three examples of software modules in which actuators and sensors are used for controlling the interaction with the environment, namely, force control, detection of grasp using the sensors on the hand, and reaching. Section 5 demonstrates a complete behavior in which the robot grasps objects on the table. Finally, Sect. 6 draws the conclusions.

---

[1]The RobotCub project was funded by the European Commission, Project IST-004370, under Strategic Objective 2.3.2.4: Cognitive Systems.

[2]The iCub software and hardware are licensed under the GNU General Public License (GPL) and GNU Free Documentation License (FDL), respectively.

2 The Hardware Platform

The iCub (Metta et al. 2008; Tsagarakis et al. 2007) was designed specifically for manipulation and locomotion (Fig. 1). This is reflected on how the degrees of freedom (DOF) are allocated on the robot. Each arm has 16 motors, 3 of which control the orientation of the hand (roll–pitch–yaw) and 4 the shoulder and the elbow. Each hand has five fingers and is actuated by nine motors. Thumb, index, and middle fingers are independently actuated, while the fourth and fifth fingers are connected to a single motor. The joints that are not driven by dedicated motors are mechanically coupled. As usual in these cases, the coupling is elastic to allow better adaptations to the objects. A motor on the palm is responsible for controlling the fingers' abduction. This DOF is critical to better adapt the hand to objects with various shapes and size. A detailed description of the fingers and their actuation is reported in Fig. 2.

The initial design criteria of the legs aimed to allow the robot to locomote by crawling on the floor (see Fig. 1). From an early analysis, it was determined that five DOF were sufficient. To allow standing and walking, it was later decided to add an additional motor at the ankle. Overall in the current design, the legs of the iCub have six DOF each.

Three motors control the orientation of the robot at the level of the torso. This turns out to be an important feature because it significantly extends the workspace of the arms. The iCub can bend forward to reach for a far object or turn the attention to different areas while maintaining the arms within their optimal workspace. The head comprises a three-DOF neck (tilt, pan, and roll) and cameras that can rotate around a common tilt and independently around pan axes to control the gaze direction and the angle of vergence.

Another design choice was to shape the robot as a three-and-a-half-year-old child (approximately 100 cm high). The overall weight of the robot is 22 kg. The mechanics and electronics had to be optimized to fit in the available space. The actuation solution adopted was a combination of a harmonic drive reduction system (100:1 ratio for all the major joints) and a brushless, frameless motor. The harmonic driver gears provide zero backlash and high reduction ratios in small space with low weight, while the brushless motors guarantee appropriate performance in terms of speed, torque, and robustness. An important decision in this respect was to use frameless motors. These motors are provided without housing and bearings in separate components that can be integrated directly inside the structure of the robot thus minimizing size, weight, and dimensions. In the majority of the cases, torque is transmitted from the motors to the joints using steel tendons routed in complex ways via idle pulleys. Most of the motors are thus placed closer to the body and away from distal links. The motors of the shoulder (placed in the torso) and the hand (placed in the forearm) are examples of this. One of the advantages of this solution is that the robot has lower inertia and as a consequence turns out to be easier to control and safer during interaction with humans.

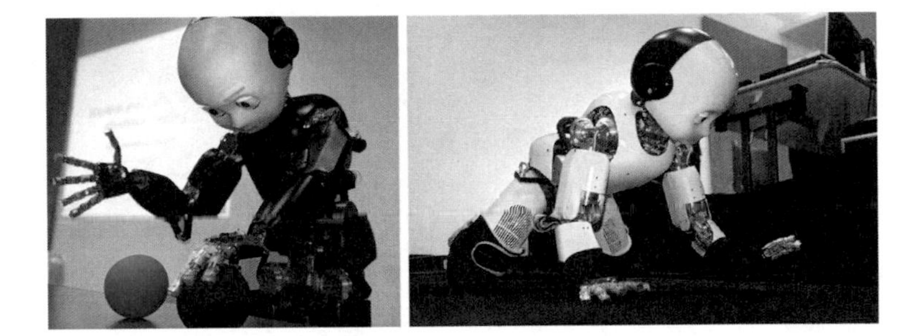

Fig. 1 The iCub

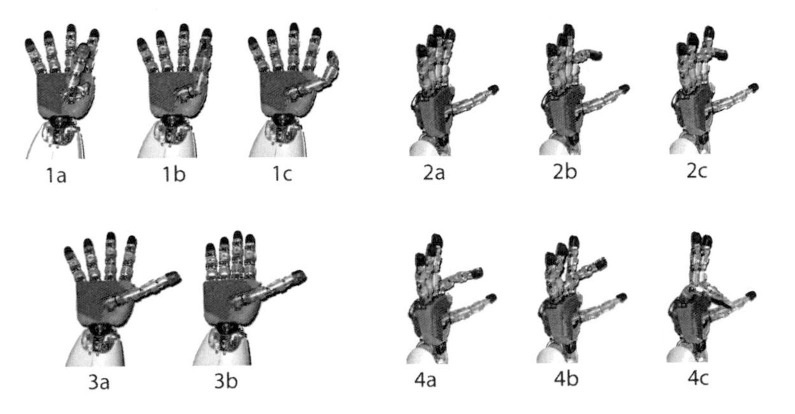

Fig. 2 Hand details. All fingers have three moving phalanges. The middle and distal phalanges are mechanically coupled to bend in a natural way. The coupling is elastic to allow better adaptation to the objects. The thumb has an additional joint that allows it to rotate at the base to oppose different fingers. Pictures 1a–c demonstrate the degrees of freedom of the thumb; in particular, picture 1c shows the coupled motion of the middle and distal phalanges. Pictures 2b and c show the coupled motion of the proximal phalanges of the index and middle finger, respectively (compare with 2a). Index and middle fingers can rotate at the level of the proximal phalanges (4a and 4b). All the phalanges of the fourth and fifth fingers are coupled together and are actuated by a single motor (4c). Finally, 3a and 3b demonstrate the abduction of the fingers

Clearly the decision to use electric motors was dictated by practical considerations, considered that at the beginning of the project (and still now, at the time of writing), it was the only solution that met the specifications in terms of speed, torque, and size. The choice of the reduction system originated from similar considerations. Electrical motors, especially when equipped with large reductions, are difficult to backdrive and in general are easier to be controlled in position mode. This is a clear limitation for the targeted research and applications,[3] so we equipped the robot with

---

[3]In position control, potentially large forces are produced to achieve a desired position. This is dangerous when unexpected interaction with the environment occurs because the robot is learning,

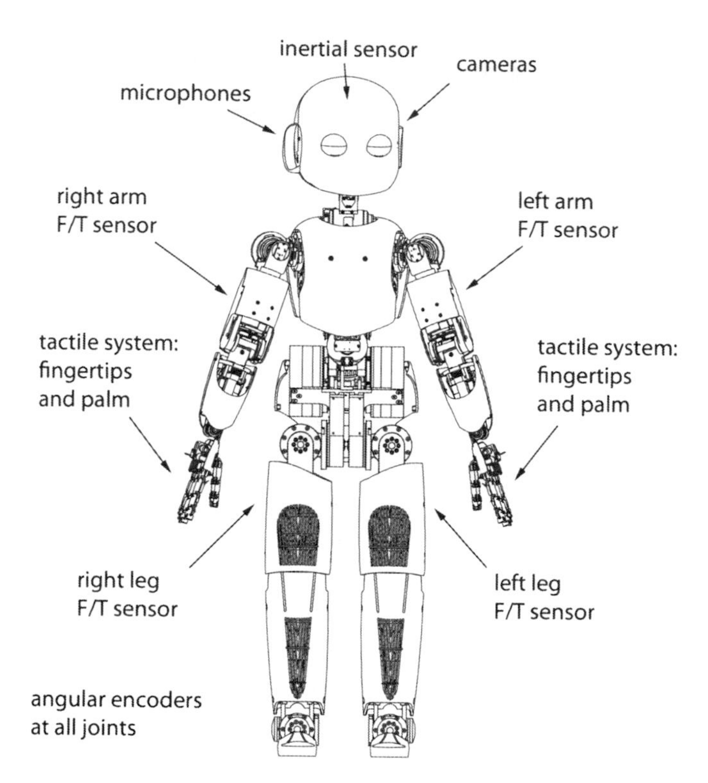

Fig. 3 The iCub sensory system

various sensors that allow measuring contact forces (torque and tactile sensors) and we implemented torque and impedance control. Section 4 in this chapter shows some results on these topics.

The robot is endowed with a complete sensory system, which includes (Fig. 3):

- Vision: two color cameras attached to the eyes. We employ commercial Dragonfly cameras from Point Grey.[4] Images are acquired by the PC104 computer mounted on the head and streamed to the network at the maximum rate of 60 Hz and resolution of 640×480 pixels.
- Sound: two microphones are mounted on the head (condenser electrets microphones). A mechanical structure similar to the human pinnae produces spatial filtering that can be used for sound localization (Hörnstein et al. 2006).

---

exploring, or interacting with humans. In this scenario, as explained in Sect. 4.1, force control is a preferable approach.

[4] Point Grey Research, Inc.: http://www.ptgray.com.

- Inertial sensor: the Xsens MTx sensor from Xsens Technology[5] contains three gyroscopes, three linear accelerometers, and a compass. This sensor is mounted inside the head and provides absolute orientation and angular acceleration (the signal from the compass is quite noisy and in practice of scarce utility, probably because of the interference with the mechanical structure of the robot).
- Forces and torques: we mounted custom 6-axis force/torque sensors in the arms and legs. These sensors are mechanically similar to commercial sensors usually used in robotics (in particular the ATI Mini-45 sensor[6]). Our sensor embeds the electronics that perform signal conditioning and A/D conversion. Signals are transmitted to a CAN bus at the maximum frequency of 1 kHz. In addition, we have been working to embed joint-level torque measurement in the shoulder (Parmiggiani et al. 2009).
- Proprioception: all motors and joints are equipped with angular encoders. It is therefore possible to recover the position of all joints, including those that are elastically coupled to the actuation.
- Touch: recent versions of the iCub mount tactile sensors on the hands. These sensors are based on capacitive technology and provide contact and pressure information. Overall each hand has 108 sensors, 12 in each fingertip and 48 on the palm (Schmitz et al. 2010).

The sensory system is one of the key features of the iCub. The availability of a rich sensory system makes it possible to use the robot to study algorithms that exploit and integrate different sensory modalities (e.g., sensory fusion, multimodal calibration, and multimodal perception to mention a few). The force and tactile sensors on the limbs enable the implementation of control strategies to monitor and regulate the interaction forces between the robot and the world. This is crucial for applications that involve autonomous exploration and learning or the interaction with humans.

3 Software Architecture

Very often academic research laboratories need robotic platforms as tools for testing and experimenting new ideas or algorithms. The robotic platforms that are built within these laboratories are not the main goal of the research, but are considered as useful tools whose development is just a preliminary effort before the real work. When the research focuses on the robot itself (e.g., when it involves the study of mechanical solutions, actuators, or sensors), it only produces results that rarely go beyond the status of prototypes. In fact the research community gives reward

[5] Xsens 3D Motion Tracking: http://www.xsens.com.

[6] ATI Industrial Automation: http://www.ati-ia.com.

mainly to publication of new ideas or principles. This happens for good reasons, and in this chapter, we do not want to criticize this approach. It is true, on the other hand, that this trend has several drawbacks that make research in robotics suffer in different aspects. The first we discuss here is the *lack of off-the-shelf solutions for common problems*: with some notable exceptions (OpenCV,[7] OROCOS,[8] and more recently ROS[9]), it is difficult to find good implementations of existing algorithms, especially that work on a given platform and for applications in humanoid robotics. Often a researcher working on a specific topic has to start from scratch the development of even the most basic functionalities (like control of attention or reaching). This clearly slows down research that involves the implementation of complex behaviors (like grasping or human–robot cooperation) and contributes to a second fundamental problem: the *lack of a scientific methodology* that, by comparing different techniques, allows the identification and promotion of better algorithms.

The iCub software architecture intends to mitigate these problems. We review here the key design choices that drove its development: ease of use, modularity, and scalability.

3.1 Ease of Use

One of the design choices of the software platform was to reduce as much as possible the learning curve for new users. We tried to minimize the time a new user would have to spend in order to get accustomed not only with the software itself but also with the developmental environment. Particular attention was taken to avoid forcing people to a particular development environment, be it the operating system, compiler, or IDE. The iCub software is fully working on Windows and Linux (and with minimal effort on MacOS), and more importantly, a mix of the two. Users can take advantage of the platform that best suits their needs and skills. For example, psychologists find it more natural to use Windows, and it is not unusual to have to interface the robot software with off-the-shelf devices that are supported only in the Windows operating system (i.e., an eye tracker). Linux, on the other hand, appears the natural choice of people that have a more technical background. Similar considerations apply to the development environment. In addition, and to a more limited extent, the software provides interoperability with other languages like

[7]Open Computer Vision Library: http://sourceforge.net/projects/opencvlibrary.

[8]Open Robot Control Software: http://www.orocos.org.

[9]Robot Operating System: http://www.ros.org.

Python, Java, and MATLAB. Winning choices in this respect have been the use of open-source tools like CMake,[10] SWIG,[11] and ACE.[12]

3.2 Modularity

The iCub software architecture was built on top of YARP (Fitzpatrick et al. 2008). YARP is an open-source software middleware that supports code reuse and development in robotics. In YARP, software is organized as *modules* (usually executables) that communicate using objects called *ports*. Ports are entities that receive or transmit data with each other. Modules are executed on a set of computers (*nodes*) and cooperate through ports. On top of this, YARP allows creating devices that have a standard C++ interface and support remotization of these devices across the network. Code development is intrinsically modular; functionalities are added to the system as modules that have a specific interface. With time modules that become obsolete can be easily replaced with new ones that offer the same interface. Clearly the advantage of a distributed architecture is that it is easily scalable; as long as resources are available, new modules can be added to the system. Connections between modules can be created and destroyed dynamically, so the system does not need to be stopped when new modules are added or, for any reason, moved across machines. The other advantage of YARP is that the system can be made of heterogeneous nodes (i.e., nodes running different operating systems).

The robot offers a YARP interface to communicate with its motors and sensory system. All that the users need to know is how to use the interface to send commands to the robot and access the sensory information. The complexity of the networking, low-level hardware and device drivers is completely hidden to users. This is beneficial because it allows nonexperts to use the robot and it avoids that changes to the low-level hardware have catastrophic impacts on the user code.

A good example of modularity is the iCub simulator (Tikhanoff et al. 2008). This software component is implemented using the ODE dynamics engine,[13] and it simulates all the sensors, actuators, and degrees of freedom of the iCub to provide the same software interface of the real robot (i.e., the simulator and the real robot provide compatible YARP ports). Software modules can be developed using the simulator and later plugged to the real robot without effort. It is important to point out that the simulator was not designed to simulate the dynamics of the robot with accuracy. Nonetheless, it can be a fundamental tool for fast prototyping and testing,

---

[10] Kitware, Cross Platform Make: http://www.cmake.org.

[11] Simplified Wrapper and Interface Generator: http://www.swig.org.

[12] The ADAPTIVE Communication Environment: http://www.cs.wustl.edu/~schmidt/ACE.htm.

[13] Open Dynamics Engine: http://www.ode.org.

in particular of learning algorithms that are time consuming and require that large number of experiments are performed.

We mentioned modularity as a requirement for long-term development. In the iCub, architecture modules are loosely coupled and are easily developed by different people with minimal interference. At the time of writing, the iCub community is made of roughly 40 active developers and a larger number of users scattered in different parts of the world. Modularity makes it possible for all these developers to coexist and cooperate within the same project.

3.3 Scalability: From Modules to Applications

The iCub software architecture defines the concept of *application* as a collection of modules that achieve a particular functionality. Examples of applications are the attention system (Ruesch et al. 2008), the reaching behavior (Pattacini et al. 2010), or the exploration of object affordances (Montesano et al. 2008) (other applications are reported in Table 1 in Sect. 6). Applications are obtained by instantiating a set of modules. Since modules can be configured depending on the context, an application should also store the information about how these modules are configured. In other words, applications are somewhat abstract entities that consist of a list of modules and instructions for running them.

Unfortunately, the execution of an application that is fragmented in many modules can be complicated and time consuming, especially for people who have not participated in its development. Good documentation can partially mitigate this problem, but the effort required to run a certain application has a strong influence on the probability that the application will be reused. The risk is that developers do not perceive the advantages of a modular approach and start developing monolithic applications. Modularity can prevent scaling from simple experiments involving a few modules to complex behaviors obtained by instantiating many modules (and maybe other applications).

The iCub software contains a *manager* that simplifies running applications. Each application is associated to an *application descriptor* (i.e., an xml file) that contains all the information required to instantiate it, including the modules to run, the set of parameters, the name of the machines on which modules will be executed, and how modules should be connected. From this information, the manager is able to execute all modules on the desired machines, configure them appropriately, and establish connections between the ports involved. In other words, the manager automates common tasks like starting and stopping an application or monitoring its status. Like modules, applications can be uploaded in the repository, documented, and shared across developers. The idea is that the users do not instantiate modules individually, but rather from the application descriptors available in the repository (this process is exemplified in Fig. 4).

Another limit to the growth of the system is imposed by the delay introduced by the communication between modules. Latencies are heavily dependent on the

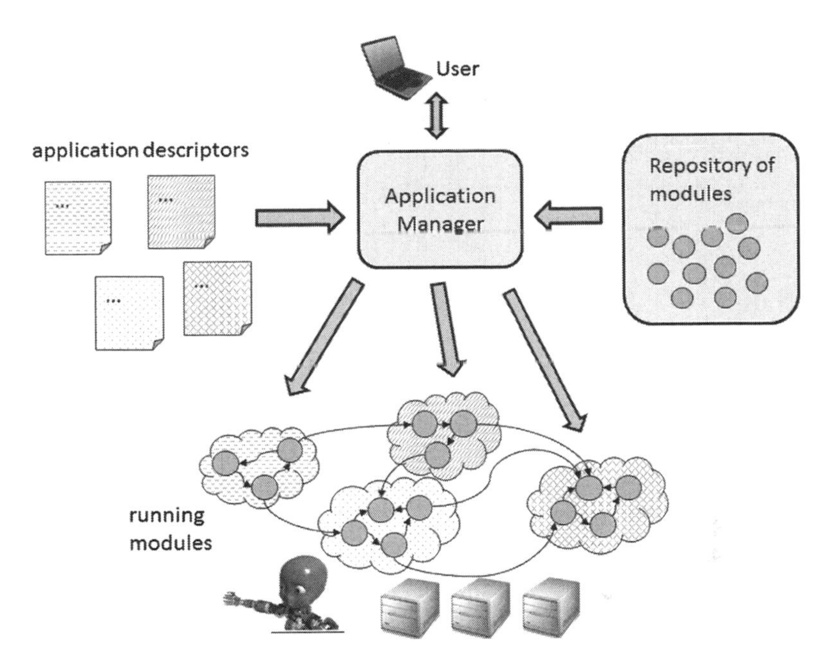

Fig. 4 Managing applications and modules

computing infrastructure and for this reason are difficult to estimate. YARP was implemented and designed to be efficient and minimize overheads, and so far it has demonstrated to behave well in this respect (we have measured that the delay introduced by a port is below 300 μs for small packets, see Natale 2009). An important design principle driving software development in iCub is to avoid introducing coupling between the timing of the modules. The reason for this is that we want to avoid that the performance of slow modules have a negative impact on the others. Among the different communication paradigm available in YARP, we favor "streaming" communication in which no synchronization between sender and receiver is required or enforced. When large packets are sent to multiple receivers (i.e., packets containing images), we use the *multicast* protocol to minimize the associated overhead.

Finally, a clear limitation to the scalability of the system is dictated by the available resources: computing power and network bandwidth. In developing modules and applications, it is important to monitor the available resources and avoid saturating them. Our experience has shown that with some attention it is possible to create applications made of a large number of modules (our largest applications involve running at least 20 interconnected modules, e.g., "imitation, learning object affordances," or "objects and actions learning" in Table 1). In addition, since technology has been progressing at a steady pace in these aspects, we believe this is unlikely to be a problem in the near future.

Table 1 A list of the functionalities that have been implemented on the iCub. The table reports the name of the functionality and a description. When available references to the scientific papers that present the work are reported in the *right column*

Overview of high-level functionalities on the iCub		
Functionality	Description	References
Attention system	Control of attention using visual and auditory cues	Ruesch et al. (2008)
Log-polar attention system	Control the attention using visual cues in log-polar space	The iCub "contrib" software repository
Reaching	Control the arm to reach for a point in space with the hand	Pattacini et al. (2010)
Force control	Control the amount of force exchanged between the arm, legs, and the environment	Fumagalli et al. (2010)
Skin spatial calibration	Automatic calibration of the tactile system, compute the spatial location of each taxel	Del Prete et al. (2011)
Head calibration	Perform automatic calibration of the head using vision and inertial information	Santos et al. (2010)
Crawling	Locomotion on the legs and arms	Dégallier et al. (2011)
Cognitive architecture	A cognitive architecture for the iCub robot implementing gaze control	Vernon et al. (2011)
Imitation learning and grasping	The robot learns a grasp model from a first demonstration of a hand posture which is then physically corrected by a human teacher pressing on the fingertips	Sauser et al. (2012)
Kinesthetic teaching	An action acquisition model based on multiple time-scales recurrent neural network and self-organizing maps; the robot learns multiple behaviors through demonstration	Peniak et al. (2011a)
Imitation, learning object affordances	The robot learns a representation of object affordances and uses it to imitation actions	Montesano et al. (2008)
Objects and actions learning	Learning under human supervision, includes visual object recognition and actions	The iCub "main" software repository
Object learning	Replication of the "modi experiment" from developmental psychology literature	Peniak et al. (2011b)
Reaching with force fields and obstacle avoidance	Plan a trajectory in space while avoiding obstacles; obstacles are represented as force fields	The iCub "main" software repository
Body schema: hand detection and localization	The robot learns autonomously to visually identify its own hand and arm	Ciliberto et al. (2011); Saegusa et al. (2011)
Online learning machine	An incremental learning algorithm for regression	Gijsberts and Metta (2011)

4 Examples of Software Modules

In the previous sections, we have described the iCub hardware and software platforms. In this section, we describe some software modules that exploit the available sensors and actuators to control the interaction with the environment. These and other modules are available open source and documented in the iCub software repository.[14] We report data from experiments with the goal of demonstrating some of the current capabilities of the robot that appear more relevant with respect to the topic of this chapter.

4.1 Force Control

Force control is a well-known technique that is commonly used to better control the interaction between the robot and the environment, especially in the presence of uncertainties (Sciavicco and Siciliano 2005). Recently force control has obtained renewed importance since researchers and industries have started to propose applications that see robots working in close interaction with humans. Safety and uncertainty handling have pushed the need for robots that can control or limit the amount of force they exert on the external world (De Santis et al. 2008; Schiavi et al. 2009). Among the possible solutions that allow achieving safety (light-weight designs, intrinsically compliant actuations, see Haddadin et al. 2009; Zinn et al. 2004), force control has the advantage that it does not require an increase in the complexity of the system.

We employ 6-axis force and torque (F/T) sensors, integrated within the two arms and legs. The F/T sensors of the arms are placed in the upper arm, between the shoulder and the elbow, while those employed for the legs are placed between the hip joints and the knee (see Fig. 3). These F/T sensors employ semiconductor strain gages (SSG) for measuring the deformation of the sensing elements.

Commonly force sensors are placed at the end effector. The adopted solution however has some advantages; in particular it allows to:

- Estimate forces and torques due to the internal dynamic of the links
- Measure external forces exerted on the whole arm
- Derive the torques at each joint

The drawback is that, if not compensated for, dynamic forces due to the links are detected as external forces (something that does not happen when the F/T sensor is placed at the end effector). To properly compensate forces acting on the whole arm, we need to know their point of application. Since the latter information is not available without tactile feedback in this work, we assumed that all forces are applied at the end effector (to remove this hypothesis, we have recently installed a

[14] iCub software documentation: http://www.icub.org

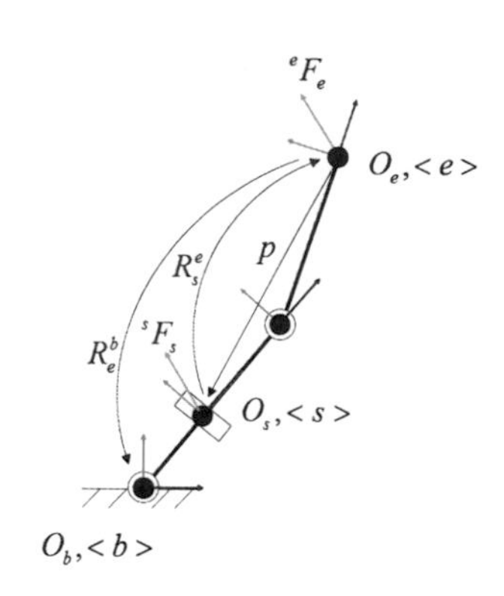

Fig. 5 Schematic representation of the reference frames and coordinate transformations involved in the computation of the joint torques from the measures of the F/T sensor. See text for details

distributed tactile sensing system on the arms, see Del Prete et al. 2011; Schmitz et al. 2011). In addition, we suppose also that the contribution of the internal dynamics of the manipulator is known and compensated for (e.g., see Murray et al. 1994). Under these hypotheses, the actual external wrench and the measured F/T vector are related with pure kinematic relations, and it is possible to estimate the corresponding joint-level torques.

With reference to Fig. 5, the output of the F/T is a wrench ${}^{s}F_{s} \in \mathbb{R}^{6}$ represented in the sensor reference frame $\langle s \rangle$. We can compute an equivalent wrench that, applied to the end effector, produces the same effect. This clearly depends on the vector $p_{s}^{e} \in \mathbb{R}^{3}$–the relative distance of the center of the sensor reference frame $O_{s} \in \mathbb{R}^{3}$ with respect to the position of the end effector–and on the rotation matrix relating $\langle s \rangle$ with $\langle e \rangle$. Formally:

$$ {}^{b}F_{e} = T_{e}^{b} H_{s}^{e}\, {}^{s}F_{s} \tag{1} $$

in which ${}^{b}F_{e} \in \mathbb{R}^{6}$ is the external force (represented in the reference frame $\langle b \rangle$) and H_{s}^{e} and $T_{e}^{b} \in \mathbb{R}^{6\times 6}$ are defined as:

$$ H_{s}^{e} = \begin{bmatrix} R_{s}^{e} & 0 \\ -S(p)R_{s}^{e} & R_{s}^{e} \end{bmatrix}, \tag{2} $$

$$ T_{e}^{b} = \begin{bmatrix} R_{e}^{b} & 0 \\ 0 & R_{e}^{b} \end{bmatrix}. \tag{3} $$

Here $R_{a}^{b} \in \mathbb{R}^{3\times 3}$ represents the rotation matrix from $\langle a \rangle$ to $\langle b \rangle$, and $S(.) \in \mathbb{R}^{3\times 3}$ is the matrix operator of $p\times$.

From ${}^{b}F_{e}$, it is straightforward to compute the joint-level torques:

$$ \hat{\tau} = J^{T}(q)\, {}^{b}F_{e}, \tag{4} $$

where $J(q) \in \mathbb{R}^{6\times n}$ is the Jacobian of the n-joints manipulator, and q is the vector of joint positions. Given the value of $\hat{\tau}$ corresponding to the current reading ${}^{b}F_{e}$, the following control strategy:

$$ u = \mathrm{PID}(\hat{\tau} - \tau_{\mathrm{d}}), \tag{5} $$

employs a proportional–integral–derivative controller (PID) to compute the motor command $u \in \mathbb{R}^n$ that achieves a desired value of joint torques τ_d (which, in turn, produce a corresponding net force exerted by the arm at the end effector).

A simple way to demonstrate force control is to implement an impedance controller.[15] At the joint level, this is easily achieved by computing τ_d as in:

$$\tau_d = -K(q - q^\star), \tag{6}$$

being $K \in \mathbb{R}^n$ the vector of virtual joint stiffnesses. This controller simulates virtual springs attached to each joint i, with stiffness K and equilibrium point at $q_i^\star$.

When the value of the stiffness K is low, the arm exhibits a "compliant" behavior, as demonstrated in the following experiment. The controller maintains $q^\star$ or, equivalently, a certain position of the arm. We apply disturbances by means of variable forces applied at the end effector. Forces produce a displacement of the end effector; depending on the stiffness K, the controller tries to oppose the external disturbances with a restoring force proportional to the displacement (Fig. 6). This situation is similar to what happens when the arm interacts with the environment. In theory if K is large enough, $q \to q^\star$ and we can use this controller to achieve any desired configuration of the arm. In practice, however, we would like to use small values of the stiffness K so to reduce the effects of unwanted collisions. To better validate the control system, in Fig. 7, we report the plot of torque versus displacement with constant and variable values of the parameter K (respectively, left and right).

4.2 *The Sensors on the Hand: Grasp Detection*

The sensory system of the iCub allows us to determine when the fingers get in touch with an object. To this purpose, we can exploit the encoders in the joints of the fingers and the tactile sensors on the fingertips and palm. Let us first focus on the former approach.

We have implemented a mechanism to perform contact detection using the springs mounted on the phalanges of the hand. Due to the elastic coupling between the phalanges (see Sect. 2 and, in particular, Fig. 2), the fingers passively adapt when they encounter an obstacle (i.e., when they touch the surface of an object). The amount of adaptation can be indirectly estimated from the encoders on the joints of the fingers. In other words, the idea is to measure the discrepancy between the finger motion in presence of external obstacles (e.g., objects or the other fingers) and the one that would result in normal operation (in absence of obstacles/free movement).

[15] An impedance controller drives the arm by simulating virtual springs attached between the arm and a desired equilibrium point.

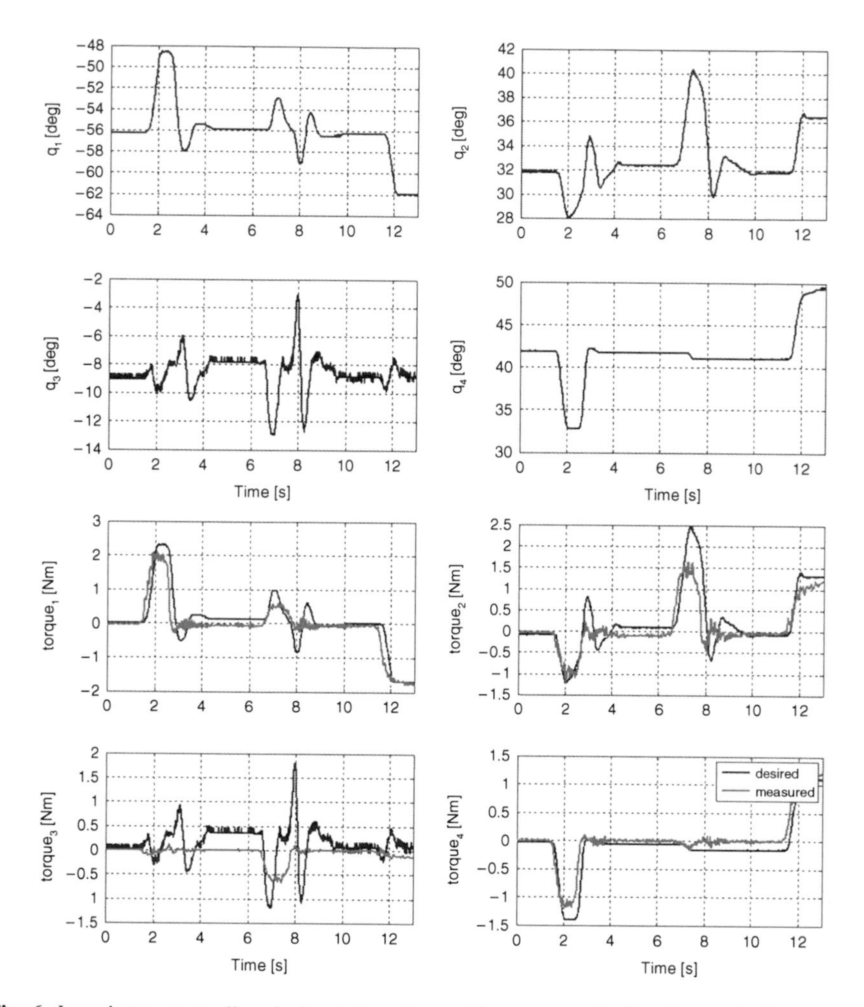

Fig. 6 Impedance controller during interaction with an external disturbance (only the four shoulder joints are considered). The external disturbance is applied to the arm at roughly $t_1 \approx 2$ s, $t_2 \approx 4.5$ s, and $t_3 \approx 12$ s. *Top plots*: displacement of each joint during interaction (q_1, q_2, q_3, and q_4). The *solid line* shows the encoder value. During the whole experiment, the reference value requested to each joint is maintained stationary. The compliant behavior of the arm is demonstrated by the fact that during the interaction with the disturbance, the joints are allowed to move away from the reference position. *Bottom plots*: requested (*black line*) versus actual (*gray line*) torques at the joints (torque$_1$, torque$_2$, torque$_3$, and torque$_4$). The requested torques increase when the joints move away from the desired position and attempt to restore the desired position of the arm (forces are proportional to the displacement)

In a calibration phase, we estimate the (linear) relationship between the joints of the fingers in absence of contact. In normal operation, we detect contact by comparing how much this model fits the current encoder readings.

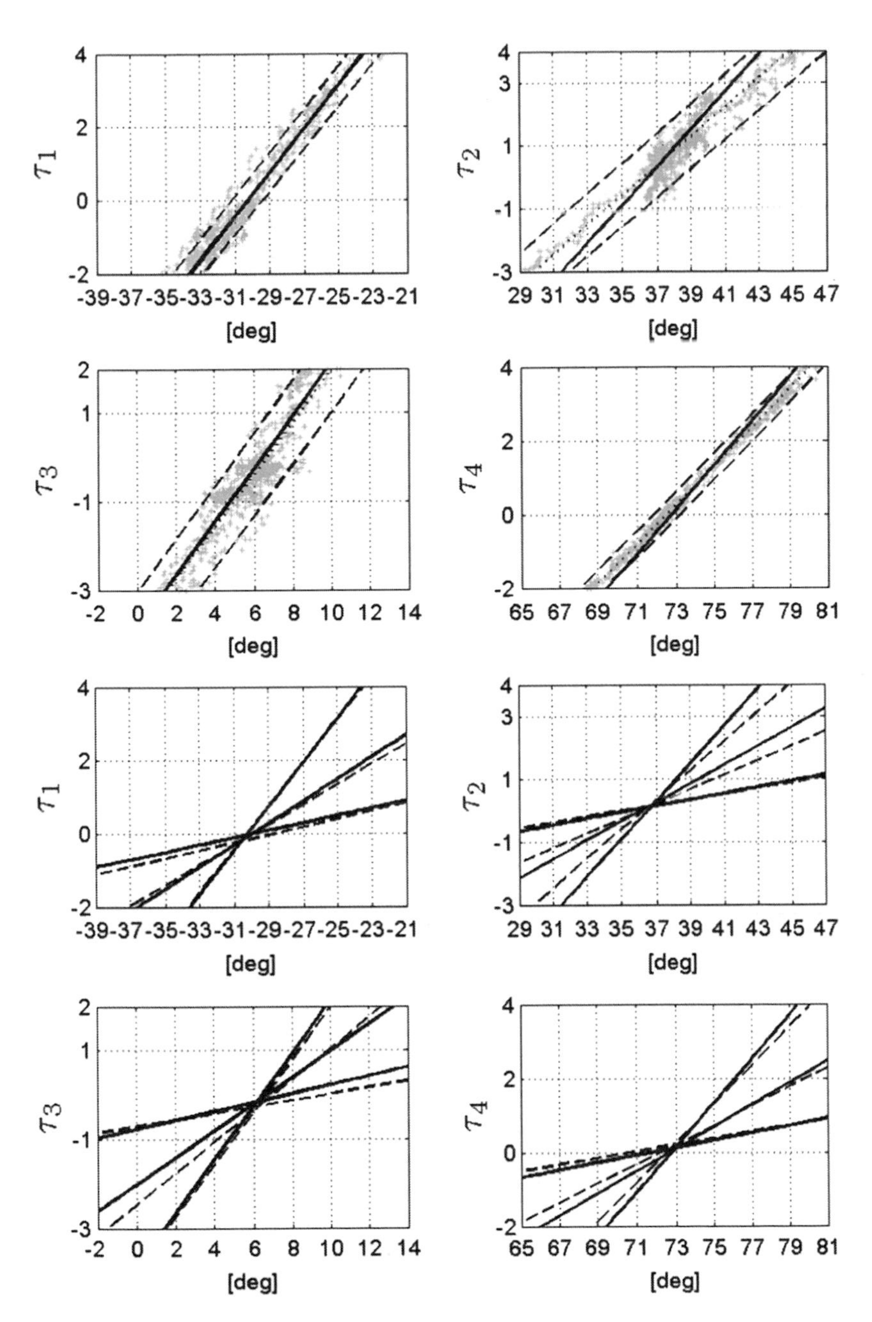

Fig. 7 Measuring the stiffness of each joint (only the four shoulder joints are considered). In these experiments, the virtual springs have a constant equilibrium point at $q = (-30, 37, 6, 73)^{\circ}$. *Top rows*: all joints maintain a certain stiffness; the plots show the values of torques versus position. *Crosses* represent measured values, *dashed lines* 95 % confidence interval for the measured stiffness, and least square linear fit. *Solid line* is the value of K used in the controller. *Bottom plots*: in this case, we tested three different values of K. We plot the ideal response that would be obtained using the desired value of K (*solid lines*) versus least squares fit (*dashed lines*)

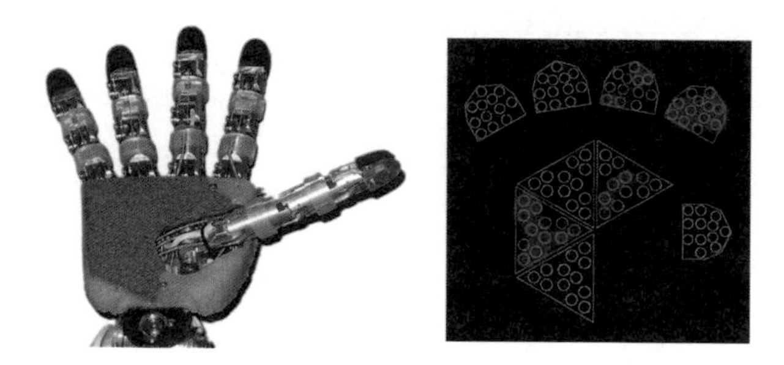

Fig. 8 The skin system on the hands consists of units of 12 capacitive sensors each: 5 units are installed in the fingertips and 4 cover the palm. Overall 108 sensors are available on each hand. *Left*: a picture of the hand. *Right*: schematic representation of how the units and sensors are distributed on the fingers and palm

Let us group together those joints of the fingers that are actuated by the same motors and that are coupled with elastic elements. For each of these groups, we define generic n-dimensional vectors $q \in \mathbb{R}^n$, each collecting the values of all the n joints that are actuated by the same motor (e.g., for the thumb, index, and middle distal phalanges $n = 2$ each, while for the ring and small fingers $n = 6$, as explained in Fig. 2). For each motor, the following parametric equation, r, models the mechanical coupling:

$$r : q = k_0 + k_1 \times s, s \in [s_{\min}, s_{\max}] \quad (7)$$

where s is the free parameter to be chosen in $[s_{\min}, s_{\max}]$. In a calibration phase, we can fit this model to a set of joint positions recorded in absence of external forces. Once we have determined the values of the parameters k_0 and k_1, we can determine if a given value of encoders q fits the mode in Eq. (7). The idea is that the higher the effect of the external perturbation to the fingers, the larger the error with which the model in Eq. (7) predicts the value q. This algorithm was implemented in a software component that is available in the iCub software repository, along with a more detailed description of the algorithm.[16]

The hand is equipped with a skin system made of interconnected units providing a total of 108 sensing elements distributed as in Fig. 8. The details of the technology are reported elsewhere (Schmitz et al. 2008, 2011).

We now report a series of grasping experiments in which we show that the sensors of the hand (joint encoders and tactile system) can detect when the fingers touch an object. The robot was programmed to perform a series of grasping actions on different objects. The objects were placed on the same position, and grasping was completely preprogrammed. We collected the information from the grasp detector (the output of the module, i.e., the error between the measured data and the model)

[16] *graspDetector*: see iCub Software Documentation, http://www.icub.org

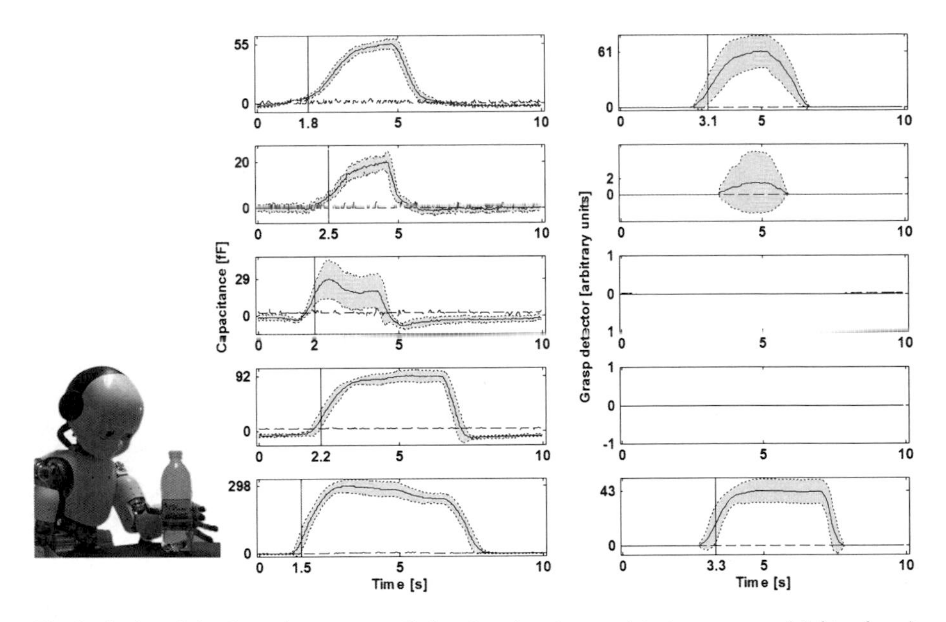

Fig. 9 A plot of the fingertips response (*left column*) and grasp detector response (*right column*) while grasping a plastic bottle. *Rows* correspond to different fingers. From the *top* to the *bottom*: thumb, index, middle, ring, and little finger. The *dashed line* is the response when the grasp action is performed without object. The *solid line* is the average response in 20 trials. The *shaded region* is the standard deviation in 20 trials. The *horizontal axis* reports also the detection time instant (vertical segment): this instant has been obtained on the basis of a threshold chosen on a 95 % confidence interval. Data from other objects is reported in Schmitz et al. (2010)

and the output of one of the taxel of the fingertips (i.e., the taxel whose activation was strongest). As a reference, we also collected data when the hand performed the same movement but in absence of an object. Figure 9 reports the data we collected averaged across 20 consecutive trials. The plots clearly show that both signals allow detecting when the finger gets in touch with the object. More details on this experiment are reported by Schmitz et al. (2010).

4.3 Reaching

We here describe a software component that controls the position and orientation of the hand.[17] Given a target position and orientation of the hand in the Cartesian space, a first stage of processing employs a nonlinear optimization technique to determine the arm joints configuration q_d that achieves the desired posture. The second stage of processing consists in a biologically inspired controller that computes the velocity

[17] *iKinArmCtrlF*: see iCub software documentation: http://www.icub.org

$\dot{q}$ of the motors to produce a humanlike quasi-straight trajectory of the end effector. The details of this algorithm are reported by Pattacini et al. (2010) so we report here a brief description of its functionalities.

The solver module computes the value of the joint encoders $q^\star \in \mathbb{R}^n$ that achieves a given position $x_d \in \mathbb{R}^3$ and orientation $\alpha_d \in \mathbb{R}^3$ of the end effector while, at the same time, satisfies a set of given constraints expressed as inequalities. Formally, this can be expressed as:

$$q^\star = \arg\min_{q \in \mathbb{R}^n} \left(\|\alpha_\mathrm{d} - K_\alpha(q)\|^2 + \lambda \cdot (q_\mathrm{rest} - q)^T W (q_\mathrm{rest} - q) \right)$$
$$\text{s.t.:} \begin{cases} \|X_\mathrm{d} - K_x(q)\|^2 < \epsilon \\ q_L < q < q_U \end{cases}, \qquad (8)$$

where K_x and K_α are the forward kinematic functions that respectively compute position and orientation of the end effector from the joint angles q, q_rest is a preferred joint configuration, W is a diagonal matrix of weighting factors, λ is a positive scalar (< 1), and ϵ is a small number. The cost function in Eq. (8) requires that the final orientation of the end effector matches the desired value α_d and that the arm joints are as close as possible to a preferred "resting value" q_rest. The weights W determine which joints receive more importance during the minimization, whereas the scalar λ determines the overall importance given to this part of the cost.

In addition, the solution to the problem has to comply with a set of constraints. We here enforce that the position of the end effector is arbitrarily close to the desired value X_d.[18] Other constraints can be imposed as well; here, for example, we require the solution to lie between lower and upper bounds of physically admissible values. To solve the minimization problem, we employ an interior-point optimization technique; in particular, we use the *Ipopt* library, a public domain software package designed for large-scale nonlinear optimization (Wächter and Biegler 2006). As demonstrated in Pattacini et al. (2010), this technique has several advantages, such as speed, automatic handling of the singularities, and possibility to incorporate complex constraints as inequalities in the problem.

The controller module is responsible for computing a series of joint-space velocities $\dot{q}$ that drive the arm from the current configuration q to the desired final state $q^\star$ computed by the solver in the previous step. The approach we follow in this case is similar to the multi-referential dynamical systems approach (Hersch and Billard 2008). Two dynamical systems operate in joint and task space with the same target position and generate desired commands for the arm. The coherence constraint between the two tasks is enforced with the Lagrangian multipliers method. This can be used to modulate the relative influence of each controller.

[18] In doing so, we ensure that this constraint receives higher priority in the minimization (Pattacini et al. 2010). This part of the task is fulfilled with a precision up to the value of the constant ϵ that is selected to be practically negligible (in our case 10^{-6} m).

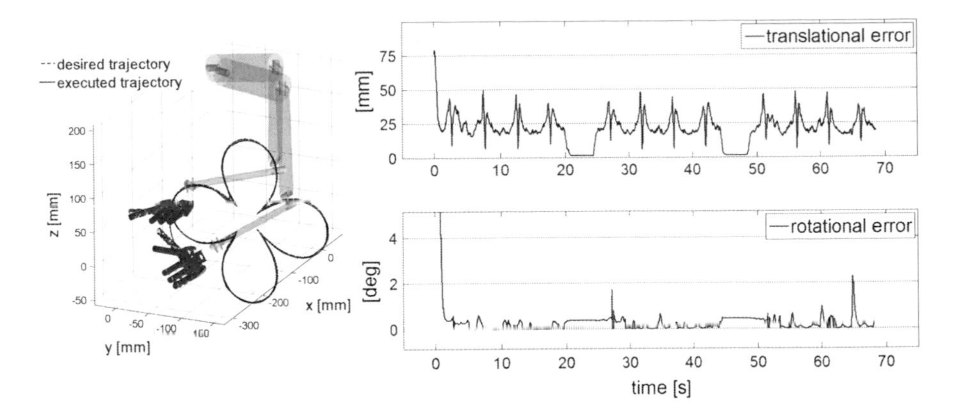

Fig. 10 Tracking a desired trajectory with a lemniscate shape in the operational space. *Left*: trajectory in Cartesian space. For better understanding, the figure shows two configurations of the arm: the *lower one* depicts the starting pose, while the *upper one* shows the commanded hand orientation during the task. *Right*: tracking error during the same experiment

The joint-level controller produces straight trajectories in joint space, while the task-level controller produces straight trajectories in the task space. Both controllers have their own advantages, the former allows to avoid joint limits, while the latter make sure the arm follows rectilinear bell-shaped trajectories in the task space. Instead of the second-order dynamical systems proposed by Hersch and Billard (2008), we use a third-order system whose coefficients are tuned to better approximate a minimum jerk profile (Flash and Hogan 1985) . This allows production of smoother trajectories of the arm, both in the joint and task space (Pattacini et al. 2010).

To simplify the use of the *reaching controller*, YARP defines an interface that specifies methods for task-space control of a robotic structure. The purpose is twofold: (1) it achieves better modularity and (2) hides the implementation details of the controller behind a set of immutable interfaces. Examples of these methods are *go_to_pose(), get_pose(), and set_trajectory_time()*.[19] The functionalities of this module are also available through the *iKin* library; this is a general-purpose kinematics library that can be configured to represent the forward kinematics of any serial link.

Figure 10 shows the Cartesian position of the end effector while tracking a desired pose in the operational space; in this particular example, 10 degrees of freedom are controlled (7 for the arm along with the pitch, the roll, and the yaw joints of the torso): one cycle of the lemniscate-shaped desired trajectory in front

[19] A complete list of available methods is available on the documentation page of the *ICartesianControl* interface in the YARP software documentation: http://www.yarp.it

of the robot frontal plane was executed in 20 s, whereas the time control gain T for point-to-point movements was set to 0.5 s. Our experiments show that the controller can easily run in real time and has good response in terms of accuracy and smoothness.

5 An Integrated Behavior

We present an example of a grasping behavior that was implemented on the robot using modules in the repository as building blocks. The earliest stage of the visual processing is the attention system (e.g., see Ruesch et al. 2008), which consists in detecting regions in the (visual) space toward which directing gaze. A commonly adopted solution is to employ a set of filters (each tuned to features like colors, orientations, and motion) and combine their output to obtain a saliency map. This saliency map is then searched for local maxima which correspond to "interesting" regions in the visual scene. The gaze of the robot is finally directed toward these saliency regions using a certain criteria (in this case, using a "winner-take-all" approach, but other strategies like random walk could be thought). Each feature can be given more importance: in this case, it was decided to give more priority to motion so that moving objects are more likely to attract the attention of the robot. The gaze control module controls the motor of the head to bring salient regions at the center of the cameras. A low-level segmentation algorithm groups together areas in the images that have uniform color and extract the center of the area that is closer to the center of the image. The process described above exploits visual information from one camera and extracts only the location of the target in image coordinates. Since the extraction of 3D information is difficult and easily imprecise, we decided to take a pragmatic approach and compute the missing information from the assumption that all relevant objects lay on a table whose height is determined by touch. With this assumption, the visual processing module computes the Cartesian position of the target with respect to a known reference frame.

The reaching subsystem receives the Cartesian position of the target object and computes the trajectories of the joints to achieve the desired posture. Once the hand is above the object, the finger closes, with a predefined movement, until the robot detects the contact with the object. If grasping is successful, the robot lifts the object; otherwise, it opens the hand and brings the arm back to the initial position. The whole sequence is exemplified in Fig. 11.

This behavior, although already sophisticated, makes several simplifying assumptions about the locations of the objects and, to a certain extent, their shape. In the context of this chapter, this experiment shows an example of how basic modules can be integrated to perform a meaningful behavior that involves the interaction between the sensory system and the controllers of different body parts. Finally, this behavior could be, itself, a building block for an even more complicated behavior involving the interaction with the environment (e.g., learning of affordances or human–robot cooperation to mention a few).

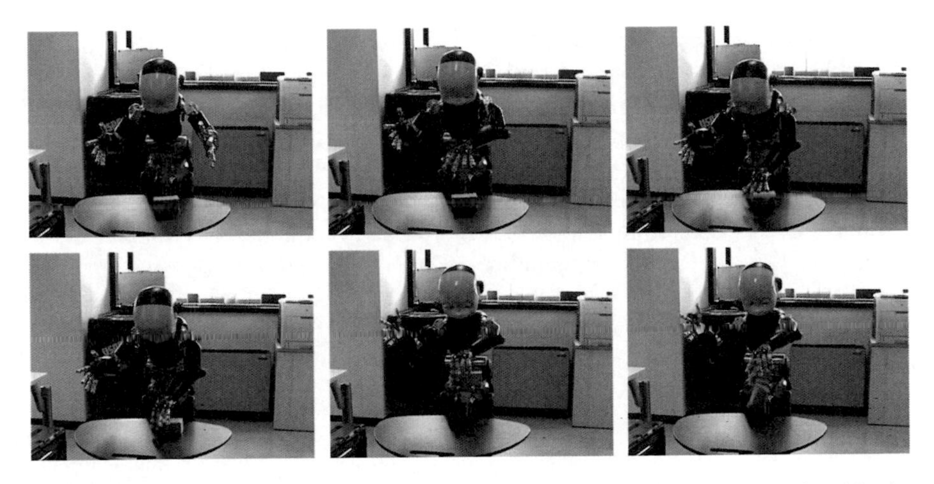

Fig. 11 A grasping sequence. From *top left* to *bottom right*, an object is placed on the table; the robot moves the hand above the object and closes the hand. When a successful grasp is detected, the robot lifts the object and eventually drops it

6 Conclusions

The design of the robot started with difficult constraints. The targeted research area required the robot to have a certain degree of complexity to allow sophisticated interaction with the environment. Fitting 53 degrees of freedom and all the sensors in a small, integrated platform was one of the most difficult design challenges. The iCub had to be built in multiple copies, to be used by people who did not participate in its development and likely to have a mixed background ranging from engineering and computer science to biology and psychology. For these reasons, the robot had to go beyond the level of a simple prototype but rather be a mature, documented, and robust platform. The software had to minimize the learning curve and be usable by nonexpert users. Finally, one of the goals of the project was to create a community of people working on the same robots, sharing results and algorithms.

In recent years, the community of iCub users has been rapidly growing around the 20 robots that have been distributed, the mailing list, the summer schools, and the use of the software simulator. As a whole, the community is contributing to the iCub at various levels: from basic functionalities like routines for calibration, control of attention, or grasping to more sophisticated ones like learning of object affordances and learning by demonstration (a representative list of these functionalities is reported in Table 1).

In this chapter, we have provided an overview of the iCub platform. We have covered aspects of the software and hardware architecture that make the platform suitable for research in the fields of developmental robotics and cognitive systems in general. We have also provided a description of the available functionalities, with particular focus on those that are more relevant for controlling the manual interaction with the environment, namely, force control and touch-based control of the arms and hands (references to other functionalities implemented on the iCub are in Table 1). These features support the implementation of exploratory behaviors in that they allow safe and prolonged interaction with the environment. The iCub sensory system also provides a wealth of information opportunities for learning. The software architecture is intrinsically modular; it allows experimenting with learning architectures in which complex abilities are formed on the basis of simpler ones. Overall we believe these functionalities make the iCub particularly interesting to the community of researchers studying intrinsically motivated learning. As we have demonstrated, the iCub is a unique integrated platform that embeds most of what is needed to tackle the problems that are challenging the research community in this field.

Acknowledgements The research leading to these results has received funding from the European Union Seventh Framework Programme FP7/2007-2013 under grant agreements 231500 (ROBOSKIN), 214668 (ITALK), and 215805 (CHRIS).

References

Barto, A., Singh, S., Chentanez, N.: Intrinsically Motivated Learning of Hierarchical Collections of Skills. In: International Conference on Developmental and Learning, La Jolla, California, October 20–22 (2004)

Bushnell, E.W., Boudreau, J.P.: Motor development and the mind: The potential role of motor abilities as a determinant of aspects of perceptual development. Child Dev. **64**(4), 1005–1021 (1993)

Ciliberto, C., Smeraldi, F., Natale, L., Metta, G.: Online multiple instance learning applied to hand detection in a humanoid robot. In: IEEE/RSJ International Conference on Intelligent Robots and Systems, San Francisco, California, USA (2011)

De Santis, A., Siciliano, B., De Luca, A., Bicchi, A.: An atlas of physical human–robot interaction. Mech. Mach. Theory **43**(3), 253–270 (2008)

Dégallier, S., Righetti, L., Gay, S., Ijspeert, A.: Towards simple control for complex, autonomous robotic applications: Combining discrete and rhythmic motor primitives. Auton. Robots **31**(2), 155–181 (2011)

Del Prete, A., Denei, S., Natale, L., F., M., Nori, F., Cannata, G., Metta, G.: Skin spatial calibration using force/torque measurements. In: IEEE/RSJ International Conference on Intelligent Robots and Systems, San Francisco, California, USA (2011)

Fitzpatrick, P., Metta, G., Natale, L.: Towards long-lived robot genes. Robot. Auton. Syst. **56**(1), 29–45 (2008)

Flash, T., Hogan, N.: The coordination of arm movements: An experimentally confirmed mathematical model. J. Neurosci. **5**(3), 1688–1703 (1985)

Fumagalli, M., Nori, F., Randazzo, M., Natale, L., Giorgio, M., Giulio, S.: Exploiting proximal F/T measurements for the iCub torque control. In: IEEE/RSJ International Conference on Intelligent Robots and Systems, Taipei, Taiwan (2010)

Gijsberts, A., Metta, G.: Incremental learning of robot dynamics using random features. In: IEEE International Conference on Robotics and Automation, Shanghai, China (2011)

Haddadin, S., Albu-Schaffer, A., Hirzinger, G.: Requirements for safe robots: Measurements, analysis and new insights. Int. J. Robot. Res. **28**(11–12), 1507–1527 (2009)

Hersch, M., Billard, A.: Reaching with multi-referential dynamical systems. Auton. Robots **25** (1–2), 71–83 (2008)
Hörnstein, J., Lopes, M., Santos-Victor, J.: Sound localization for humanoid robots—building audio-motor maps based on the HRTF. In: IEEE/RSJ International Conference on Intelligent Robots and Systems, pp. 1170–1176, Beijing, China (2006)
Kaplan, F., Oudeyer, P.-Y.: Intrinsically motivated machines. In: Lungarella, M., Iida, F., Bongard, J., Pfeifer, R. (eds.) 50 Years of AI, pp. 303–314. Lecture Notes in Computer Science, vol. 4850. Springer, Berlin (2007)
Lungarella, M., Metta, G., Pfeifer, R., Sandini, G.: Developmental robotics: A survey. Connect. Sci. **15**(4), 151–190 (2003)
Metta, G., Sandini, G., Vernon, D., Natale, L., Nori, F.: The iCub humanoid robot: An open platform for research in embodied cognition. In: PerMIS: Performance Metrics for Intelligent Systems Workshop, Washington DC, USA, August 19–21 (2008)
Mirolli, M., Baldassarre, G.: Functions and mechanisms of intrinsic motivations. In: Baldassarre, G., Mirolli, M. (eds.) Intrinsically Motivated Learning in Natural and Artificial Systems. Springer, Berlin (2012, this volume)
Montesano, L., Lopes, M., Bernardino, A., Santos-Victor, J.: Learning object affordances: From sensory–motor coordination to imitation. IEEE Trans. Robot. **24**(1), 15–26 (2008) (Special Issue on Biorobotics)
Murray, R.M., Sastry, S.S., Zexiang, L.: A Mathematical Introduction to Robotic Manipulation. CRC, Boca Raton (1994)
Natale, L.: A study on YARP performance. Technical report, Department of Robotics, Brain and Cognitive Sciences, Istituto Italiano di Tecnologia (2009)
Needham, A., Barret, T., Peterman, K.: A pick-me-up for infants exploratory skills: Early simulated experiences reaching for objects using sticky mittens enhances young infants object exploration skills. Infant Behav. Dev. **25**(3), 279–295 (2002)
Oudeyer, P.-Y. Kaplan, F.: What is intrinsic motivation? A typology of computational approaches. Front. Neurorobot. **1**(6), doi:10.3389/neuro.12.006.2007 (2007)
Parmiggiani, A., Randazzo, M., Natale, L., Metta, G., Sandini, G.: Joint torque sensing for the upper-body of the iCub humanoid robot. In: IEEE-RAS International Conference on Humanoid Robots, Paris, France (2009)
Pattacini, U., Nori, F., Natale, L., Metta, G., Sandini, G.: An experimental evaluation of a novel minimum-jerk Cartesian controller for humanoid robots. In: IEEE/RSJ International Conference on Intelligent Robots and Systems, Taipei, Taiwan (2010)
Peniak, M., Marocco, D., Tani, J., Yamashita, Y., Fischer, K., Cangelosi, A.: Multiple time scales recurrent neural network for complex action acquisition. In: International Joint Conference on Development and Learning and Epigenetic Robotics (ICDL-EPIROB), Frankfurt am Main, Germany (2011a)
Peniak, M., Morse, A., Larcombe, C., Ramirez-Contla, S., Cangelosi A.: Aquila: An open-source gpu-accelerated toolkit for cognitive and neuro-robotics research. In: International Joint Conference on Neural Networks (IJCNN), San Jose, California (2011b)
Ruesch, J., Lopes, M., Bernardino, A., Hörnstein, J., Santos-Victor, J., Pfeifer, R.: Multimodal saliency-based bottom-up attention a framework for the humanoid robot iCub. In: IEEE—International Conference on Robotics and Automation, Pasadena, California (2008)
Saegusa, R., Natale, L., Metta, G., Sandini, G.: Cognitive robotics—active perception of the self and others. In: 4th International Conference on Human System Interaction, Yokohama, Japan (2011)
Santos, J., Bernardino, A., Santos-Victor, J.: Sensor-based self-calibration of the iCub's head. In: IEEE/RSJ International Conference on Intelligent Robots and Systems, Taipei, Taiwan (2010)
Sauser, E., Argall, B.D., Metta, G., Billard, A.: Iterative learning of grasp adaptation through human corrections. In: Eric L. Sauser, Brenna D. Argall, Giorgio Metta, Aude G. Billard (eds.), Robotics and Autonomous Systems, Elsevier **60**(1), 55–71 (2012)

Schiavi, R., Flacco, F., Bicchi, A.: Integration of active and passive compliance control for safe human–robot coexistence. In: IEEE International Conference on Robotics and Automation, Kobe, Japan (2009)

Schmitz, A., Maggiali, M., Natale, L., Bonino, B., Metta, G.: A tactile sensor for the fingertips of the humanoid robot iCub. In: IEEE/RSJ International Conference on Intelligent Robots and Systems, Taipei, Taiwan (2010)

Schmitz, A., Maggiali, M., Randazzo, M., Natale, L., Metta, G.: A prototype fingertip with high spatial resolution pressure sensing for the robot iCub. In: IEEE-RAS International Conference on Humanoid Robots, Daejeon, Republic of Korea (2008)

Schmitz, A., Maiolino, P., Maggiali, M., Natale, L., Cannata, G., Metta, G.: Methods and technologies for the implementation of large scale robot tactile sensors. IEEE Trans. Robot. **23**(3), 389–400 (2011) (Special Issue on Robot Sense of Touch)

Sciavicco, L., Siciliano, B.: Modelling and control of robot manipulators. In: Advanced Textbooks in Control and Signal Processing, 2nd edn. Springer-Verlag London Limited 2000, printed in Great Britain (2005)

Tikhanoff, V., Fitzpatrick, P., Metta, G., Natale, L., Nori, F., Cangelosi, A.: An open source simulator for cognitive robotics research: The prototype of the iCub humanoid robot simulator. In: Workshop on Performance Metrics for Intelligent Systems, Washington, D.C (2008)

Tsagarakis, N., Becchi, F., Righetti, L., Ijspeert, A., Caldwell, D.: Lower body realization of the baby humanoid—iCub. In: IEEE/RSJ International Conference on Intelligent Robots and Systems, San Diego, California (2007)

Vernon, D., von Hofsten, C., Fadiga, L.: A roadmap for cognitive development in humanoid robots. In: Cognitive Systems Monographs (COSMOS), vol. 11. Springer, Berlin (2011)

von Hofsten, C.: An action perspective on motor development. Trends Cogn. Sci. **8**(6), 266–272 (2004)

Wächter, A., Biegler, L.T.: On the implementation of an interior-point filter line-search algorithm for large-scale nonlinear programming. Math. Program. **106**(1), 25–57 (2006)

Weng, J., McClelland, J., Pentland, A., Sporns, O., Stockman, I., Sur, M., Thelen, E.: Autonomous mental development by robots and animals. Science **291**(5504), 599–600 (2000)

Zinn, M., Roth, B., Khatib, O., Salisbury, J.K.: A new actuation approach for human friendly robot design. Int. J. Robot. Res. **23**(4–5), 379–398 (2004)

Zlatev, J., Balkenius, C.: Why "epigenetic robotics"? In: Balkenius, C., Zlatev, J., Kozima, H., Dautenhahn, K., Breazeal, C. (eds.) International Workshop of Epigenetic Robotics, vol. 85, pp. 1–4. Lund University Cognitive Studies, Lund (2001)

Printed by Publishers' Graphics LLC
MO20130412.15.36.105